ORAL MEDICINE

THIS BOOK IS DEDICATED TO A PIONEER IN
FURTHERING BETTER RELATIONS BETWEEN
MEDICINE AND DENTISTRY

MILTON CHARLES WINTERNITZ
FRIEND, TEACHER, AND SCIENTIST

Introduction

The strongest motives, leading most patients to seek the services of a dentist, are probably relief or avoidance of pain and the improvement or maintenance of facial appearance. Before and during the War, however, and from now on probably more than ever, increasing numbers of the laity have wider horizons. They know better what health means in terms of personal satisfaction and achievement, and they will be more insistent on getting what they want; and the more far-seeing dentist will be prepared, and will keep prepared, to meet these growing demands.

"For as the body is one, and hath many members, and all the members of that one body, being many, are one body: . . ." In these words Paul expressed the relationship between the individual and the Church. They are no less appropriate if applied in the fields of national and international affairs, of politics, or of economics. The idea owes its forcefulness and appositeness to what everyone can see and no one can deny. The physical body of man is composed of parts, but functions as a whole. Its parts are interrelated, one with another, and with the body as a whole.

The oral cavity, first segment of the digestive tract by virtue of its position, is also in close relation with the respiratory system. Inheritable and constitutional factors influence its development and reactivity. Blood vessels, lymphatics, and nerves insure rapid intercommunication between it and the rest of the body. It is affected by nutrition, metabolism, and endocrine balance or imbalance. It benefits by the general basic defense mechanisms of the body. In many ways it reflects, as a mirror, the state of systemic health and, unfortunately, it is one of the areas in the body most vulnerable to endogenous and exogenous insults and irritants.

To practice rationally, the dentist takes the history of the patient, examines him, makes a diagnosis, prepares a plan of treatment or management, and carries out that plan. If the history and examination are limited only to the local oral condition, the diagnosis will often represent only a part-truth, and part-truths are sometimes most misleading. The dentist in his periodic check-up of the patient has a unique opportunity to recognize the earliest signs of a disease while still curable or controllable, where neglect would bring tragedy. Case-planning without due regard to extra-oral conditions may do, and has done, much more harm than good.

The viewpoints and objectives expressed above are not new but relatively few dentists carry them out to their logical conclusions in daily practice. Dentistry has not yet reached the position and recognition among the health services which the importance of its field and its potentialities deserve: nor will it until the general practitioner has prepared himself to take advantage of his opportunities—opportunities which are also obligations.

I have had the privilege of reading Doctor Burket's book in manuscript and am delighted with this addition to our literature: comprehensive, well-organized, authoritative, and thoroughly practical.

The practitioner of medicine, physician and internist, would do well to read at least the Table of Contents. If he does that, I believe he'll delve deeper. It should convince him that the mouth contains much more than that doubly unruly member, the tongue. There are many situations and ways in which he can help the neighboring dentist, and the dentist can in turn help him, to speed recovery. Both physician and dentist will benefit, but the patient will benefit most.

Between the covers of this book, the dentist will find much which he should know in order to do his clinical job, the job that is his for the asking. Here is a "must" for those who are eager to accept a larger share of responsibility for their patients' health, and to meet that responsibility competently and with inner satisfaction.

J. L. T. APPLETON
Dean, School of Dentistry
University of Pennsylvania

Preface

Oral Medicine discusses the many important relationships between oral and systemic disease, and it suggests opportunities for a more universal and intimate co-operation between the medical and dental practitioners in giving the best possible health service to our common patient.

When an author plans a book, his first problems are the selection of the subjects with which he will deal, their relative importance for the purpose in mind, and their arrangement. A further obligation is that what he writes truly represents the best current knowledge available; and, finally, he should realize how much his reader will appreciate clarity and brevity.

The attention given to the various diseases in this book is believed to be commensurate with their importance to the dentist and to the physician or intern interested in the dental aspects of various systemic diseases. The author well realizes that he has emphasized certain diseases which as pure medical problems are relatively of minor importance, while on the other hand he has devoted little space to certain diseases; e.g., hypertension, whose wide distribution makes them important medically but for which no close oral relationship has yet been established.

In a special Color Atlas, the author has presented a selected group of sixty subjects illustrating oral lesions most commonly encountered by the dentist and physician in daily practice. Arranged in ten plates to be used in conjunction with the Diagnostic Index which immediately follows it, this color section is the distillation of a large collection of color studies gathered by the author over many years of clinical investigation. Because they are judged the best and most representative from this collection, it is felt that the student and practitioner will find in these color illustrations a much needed synopsis and guide to diagnosis and treatment. The Diagnostic Index is similarly arranged, with the principal diseases classified and grouped in logical order for study and reference as this book is used both in the classroom and in practice. Likewise, the many illustrations in black and white throughout the text are shown life-size, to be of greatest value.

No attempt is made to cover the entire scope of Medicine, but rather to give to the dental practitioner a sufficient knowledge of Medicine that he may adequately fulfill his professional responsibilities to his patient and co-operate intelligently with the physician. By demonstrating the close link that actually exists in the patient between his dental and general health, it is hoped that this book will itself serve as an agent in furthering this co-operation.

Since the ambulatory patient rather than the acutely ill individual is the chief concern of the dentist, he is primarily interested in a knowledge of symptomatic diagnosis on the basis of a dental-medical history, an examination of the oral cavity and exposed body parts, aided by some of the simpler laboratory tests; in brief, "dental-chair medicine."

The author wishes to thank all of his colleagues, friends and family for their many helpful suggestions and valuable criticism. Their interest and sympathetic understanding have been most encouraging and appreciated.

L. W. B.

Contents

SECTION ONE

GENERAL CONSIDERATIONS

SECTION TWO

FUSOSPIROCHETAL INFECTIONS, METAL
INTOXICATION AND INTOLERANCE

SECTION THREE

DISEASES OF THE TONGUE AND DERMATOLOGIC DISEASES OF DENTAL INTEREST, MINOR STOMATITIDES

SECTION FOUR

DISEASES OF THE ORGAN SYSTEMS

SECTION FIVE

NUTRITIONAL DEFICIENCIES AND DISEASES OF METABOLISM

SECTION SIX

DISEASES OF THE BLOOD AND BLOOD-FORMING ORGANS

SECTION SEVEN

THE SPECIFIC INFECTIOUS GRANULOMATA

SECTION EIGHT

FOCAL INFECTION, DENTAL PEDIATRICS AND GERODONTICS, HAZARDS OF DENTAL PRACTICE, DENTAL DISEASES OF OCCUPATIONAL ORIGIN

SECTION TEN

COLOR ATLAS

SECTION ELEVEN

REGIONAL DIAGNOSTIC INDEX

SECTION ONE
GENERAL CONSIDERATIONS

1
Medical-Dental Relations

SCOPE OF DENTISTRY   HEALTH INDICATORS
THE DENTIST AND THE PHYSICIAN

SCOPE OF DENTISTRY

In recent decades the scope and accomplishments of Dentistry have increased. Today the dentist is not only concerned with restorative and prosthetic dentistry but also with the supporting tissues of the teeth and the oral mucosa in both health and disease. Since diseases of these latter structures may have a profound effect on the organism as a whole, or systemic diseases may be first manifested in these tissues, it is evident that the dentist must have an understanding of disease processes elsewhere in the body. In this respect he is no different from any other medical specialist and like any other medical specialist his interest in systemic disease will be modified by the frequency and the extent to which they affect his specialty.

Oral Medicine is assuming greater importance in the practice of Dentistry in America, but few seriously consider Dentistry as a true specialty of Medicine and dentists as being more than mechanics. Dentistry is a true health service profession which requires the same broad biologic background, specialized training, good judgment and technical ability as any other medical specialty. Full or partial denture construction or the filling of a tooth is no more a mechanical operation than an appendectomy or the nailing of a fractured femur. All require an understanding of the underlying anatomic structures and physiologic functions of the affected parts and a high degree of technical skill for their treatment.

HEALTH INDICATORS

The teeth and the oral tissues must be regarded as an intimate part of the human organism and they must be considered in states of health and disease in terms of their effect on the organism as a whole. The oral cavity is analogous to other body cavities with their associated organs. They all are governed by the same physico-chemical laws and physiologic principles and they have a common source of nutrition. The oral cavity and its contained structures however are in intimate relation with the external environment and are subjected to mechanical, chemical and bacterial insults that are rarely if ever experienced by other body cavities which make them unusually vulnerable to disease. For this reason the oral tissues are sensitive indicators of the general health status of the individual and changes in these structures are frequently the first indication of subclinical disease processes in other organ systems. This is particularly true in the nutritional deficiencies, endocrine and gastro-intestinal disturbances, and in certain of the anemias and blood dyscrasias.

The importance of the oral tissues as an indicator of the general health of the individual has not been sufficiently appreciated. The average physician has traditionally neglected not only his own mouth, but also the mouths of his patients. Dentists are too often guilty of the former but rarely of the latter. Sir Wm. Osler recognized and stressed the significance of the oral cavity as a "mirror" of the rest of the body, yet even now the oral cavity is scarcely mentioned in many medical curricula and in only a few is it given the consideration it can justify clinically.

THE DENTIST AND THE PHYSICIAN

It is obvious that the modern dental practitioner must consider the teeth and the oral structures in terms of their cause and effect on the organism as a whole. This requires a broad biologic understanding of the human body and a basic knowledge of disease in other organ systems. The dental practitioner need not know, fortunately, the entire field of Medicine, nor all about any particular disease entity. Neither is the dental practitioner concerned about medical treatment except as this might be dependent on, or be modified by, dental care. Under no circumstances should he assume the role of the family physician in any other respect than that of co-operating in guarding the health and well-being of his patient.

The dentist and the physician are both concerned primarily with the diagnosis, treatment or prevention of the various diseases of the human body. The correct diagnosis and the best treatment at times will require the closest co-operation between the dentist and the physician. The many interrelationships between medical and dental practice are not sufficiently appreciated. As a result, the patient does not always benefit from the co-operative administration of these two professions. It is unfortunate that the fraternal medical-dental relations which are evidenced in written articles and combined medical-dental meetings, are not found more universally in practice.

Much of the antipathy and the lack of understanding between the members of these two professions can be overcome with a little effort on the part of the dentist and the physician. Dentistry, chronologically, is an adolescent compared to Medicine, but this does not imply that as a profession it is inferior in purpose, achievements or service to humanity. Just because Dentistry was practiced in the beginning by barber surgeons does not lessen our right to be considered as a member of the healing arts. Dentistry is regarded by many as a "mechanical" profession. Actually it is no more a mechanical profession than surgery; both specialties require a biologic understanding of anatomy, physiology and pathology in addition to their individual and special technics and training.

It is generally agreed that Dentistry can contribute materially to human comfort, appearance and health. It is time that we evaluate how Dentistry and Medicine can better assist each other in the care of our patients.

Dental consultations and assistance have been infrequently requested in the past as they usually necessitated an explanation of the medical aspects of the case and in many instances the terminology used as well. On occasions when consultations were sought, the dentist at times lacked the necessary biologic background for an understanding of the problems and a scientific justification for the recommended treatment.

Today the prospective dentist receives a biologic training equivalent to that of the prospective physician. He is also given lectures and clinics in internal medicine which further familiarize him with medical terminology and which give him a basic understanding of the common disease entities, their oral symptoms and relations, the associated laboratory findings and the possible complications that might ensue. The recent dental graduate can speak and understand the language of the physician and he can co-operate with him intelligently in the treatment of his patients.

The physician, however, is still prone to consider the oral cavity as the corridor to the tonsils and his knowledge of Dentistry is limited all too frequently by personal experiences which many times are unpleasant. Too many physicians consider Dentistry as the triad composed of decayed teeth, "trench mouth" and "pyorrhea." Medical teaching devotes little if any time to Dentistry and the importance of a proper functioning dental apparatus to the general health of the patient or to the interrelationships of dental and medical practice.

It is not uncommon to find a well-presented course on oral hygiene and Dentistry given to the student nurses in hospitals associated with medical schools and nothing given to the medical students. This is a serious medical curricular defect which is preventing better understanding and more fruitful co-operation between these professions. The physician must have a general knowledge of our problems, our abilities and limitations as dentists as well as a basic knowledge of oral diseases of medical importance before we can best serve him. Considering the importance of oral health in general medical practice and in most of the specialties the young physician should receive adequate undergraduate instruction which includes clinical demonstrations of oral disease.

The dentist can do much, however, to improve medical dental relations by the intelligent and diplomatic handling of patients referred to him by the medical profession. A dental consultation carries a definite responsibility which should be discharged in a manner that will impress both the patient and the referring doctor of your ability, thoroughness, honesty and assistance in the particular case.

2

The Dental Consultation

| IMPORTANCE OF CASE HISTORY | THE QUESTION OF TREATMENT |
| X-RAYS | FEE |

The dental consultation should always be arranged by the physician or dentist treating the case. Patients will frequently be encountered who seek the advice of another dentist concerning the correctness of the proposed treatment or the quality of the work being done. These cases should not be seen unless they are referred by the original dentist.

IMPORTANCE OF CASE HISTORY

The dental consultant should be given a brief summary of the case. The nature of the medical complaint should be given in sufficient detail to permit the dentist to fulfill his duties to the best of his abilty. It is not enough for the physician to say that the patient has arthritis. He should specify the type of arthritis which is present and furnish any pertinent clinical or laboratory findings that are available. The patient seen in consultation will require the same history and clinical examination as outlined in Chapter 3. A complete roentgenologic examination of the mouth is essential even in the clinically edentulous patient. Careful examination of certain teeth by means of the electric pulp tester or their reaction to heat or cold may be indicated. In some instances, tissue must be removed for biopsy studies.

The results of the consultation should not be discussed with the patient unless they are fully aware of its specific purpose. In most cases, the findings should be given only to the physician or referring dentist. The complete clinical and laboratory findings should be transmitted in writing so that they may form an integral part of the patient's history. The physician or dental practitioner does not have the time to listen to your verbal report and, if his assistant takes down your findings, there are opportunities for errors and mistakes. The manner in which the dental consultant presents his findings will do much to encourage or discourage additional consultations.

X-RAYS

It is not necessary that the dental roentgenograms be sent to the physician. The dentist is better trained in their interpretation than the physician. When the films are requested by the physician for examination it is desirable to arrange to read them with him. In this way large bone trabeculae or normal anatomic landmarks will not be mistaken by the physician for pathologic changes and the confidence of the patient and the physician lost.

THE QUESTION OF TREATMENT

At the conclusion of the presentation of his findings, the dental consultant should make his recommendations for the particular case. The fact that you have been selected as consultant does not give you the privilege of treating the patient. It may be that the physician, knowing the physical status of the patient, does not feel this treatment is indicated or safe at the present time, and, in other cases, the actual treatment of the patient may be justifiably performed by another dentist. The dentist should always thank the referring physician or dentist and express an interest in the future outcome of the case. In this way he can frequently follow the results of his recommendations for treatment.

FEE

The consultation fee should be a just compensation for the consultant's time and experience, but it should be within the financial ability of the patient. The fee is collected by the consultant from the patient. The recognition of any man as a consultant in his field is an honor and a responsibility that carries with it the confidence and respect of his professional colleagues.

3

The Patient's History

VALUE TO DENTIST	PSYCHOLOGY OF THE INTERVIEW

VALUE TO DENTIST

A detailed and informative history is one of the most important steps in making a diagnosis of unusual oral lesions and it should be a routine procedure for every new patient. It should always precede the examination of the patient except in cases of emergency. A complete history and its critical analysis accounts in no small part for the success of the so-called "diagnostician." Every dentist can and should be his own diagnostician. The ability to take and write a history, omitting the irrelevant facts and arranging the significant ones according to their relative importance, is an accomplishment of which the dental intern, consultant or practitioner may well be proud.

The history should include a certain amount of routine information, such as the patient's name, address, telephone number, racial stock, occupation, age, sex, marital status, date and the name and address of the referring dentist or physician. A properly printed record form will assure that this essential information is not omitted.

SCHOOL OF DENTISTRY, UNIVERSITY OF PENNSYLVANIA
ORAL MEDICINE DEPARTMENT

Name Pt. ....
Last name First name

Age......... Sex......... Race......... Master No. ....

Address .... Phone No. ....

Referred by:..................... Address.........................

FIG. 1. History-taking form in use at the School of Dentistry, University of Pennsylvania.

The history should be written and it should include negative findings since they may be of significance in later years, but the order of the various parts of the history is largely a matter of choice. The historian should make notes while the patient is talking so that he can later organize the essential material in the proper chronologic sequence and with the proper emphasis on the various symptoms.

PSYCHOLOGY OF THE INTERVIEW

A good practical and psychologic beginning is to ask the patient to express in his own words his Chief Complaint (C.C.), i.e., "a painful sore on the tongue." The history should then include a running narrative of the date of onset, the mode of development, the symptomatology and the treatment, if any, of the C.C. This portion of the history is frequently known as the present illness (P.I.) as distinguished from the Past Medical History (P.M.H.). It may be necessary to inquire judiciously as to certain features of the P.I. but the historian should never assume the role of an inquisitor, as significant points may be missed. Leading questions should be avoided, and it is unwise at this time to point out any errors in the patient's use of technical terms or their misinterpretation of symptoms. The patient should be encouraged to mention all related phenomena or symptoms which were experienced during the P.I., although they may be considered to be unrelated. While it is admitted that the intelligence of the individual patient and his powers of observation are important in obtaining a good history, the end result will depend largely on the ability, the patience and the experience of the historian.

Following the P.I. the patient should be questioned concerning his Past Medical History (P.M.H.). Patients are likely to forget past illnesses and to minimize their significance. It is helpful to ask the patient if he has been confined to bed for more than three or four days for the past 5 years. A history of past operations may also furnish pertinent information. This part of the history may or may not contribute to the actual diagnosis of the C.C., but it furnishes the clinician with some background as to the physical makeup of the patient and his susceptibility to infection. A brief review of the Family History (F.H.), social and occupational history, and personal habits may be important in special cases.

A review of the different organ systems is next in order. In the usual case presenting oral lesions this does not require detailed questioning. It is practical and, in fact, desirable to have a tabulation of the various organ systems printed on one portion of the history form so that omissions will not be made.

The author finds that an attempt to formulate some diagnostic possibilities at this time enables him to examine the patient more intelligently. A brief review of the history will usually furnish one or more diagnostic possibilities which should be kept in mind during the examination of the patient.

THE EXAMINATION OF THE PATIENT

The examination should not be confined to the oral cavity, as much information can be obtained from a careful visual examination of the exposed body parts. The general appearance of the individual is important. The texture of the skin, the presence of petechiae or eruptions, as well as the tex-

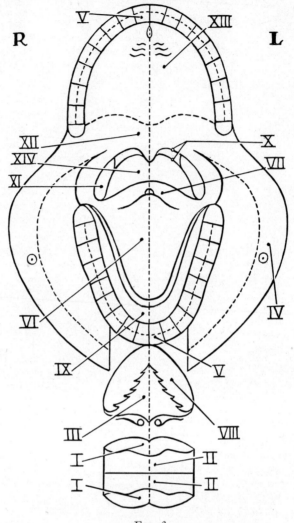

R   L

FIG. 3

I. External labial mucosa. II. Vestibular labial mucosa. III. Frenulum. IV. Buccal mucosa with papilla and orifice of Stenson's duct. V. Gingiva—The dotted line separates the labial (buccal) gum. The lines at right angles to the dotted line permit one to indicate the region involved, in relation to the neighboring teeth. VI. Tongue (dorsal). VII. Tongue (base) with lingual tonsil and foramen cecum. VIII. Tongue (ventral), plica fimbriata, plica sublingualis, and orifice of submaxillary duct. IX. Floor of mouth. X. Faucial arches (anterior and posterior). XI. Faucial tonsils. XII. Soft palate with uvula. XIII. Hard palate with incisal pad, rugae and foveae palatinae. XIV. Pharynx with pharyngeal tonsil.

(The chart was designed by Herman R. Churchill, D.D.S., Dr. med. dent., Professor of Dental Histology and Histo-Pathology, School of Dentistry, University of Pennsylvania. It is based largely upon the experience gained in a nutritional study of patients with periodontal diseases, conducted by H. T. Kelley, M.D., J. H. Gunter, D.D.S., M.D., and Dr. Churchill.)

ture and quality of the hair, should be noted. The conjunctivae should be examined for early evidences of jaundice, petechiae or other abnormalities. The reaction of the pupils to light and to accommodation can be easily determined by the dentist, as well as evidence of exophthalmos.

The examination of the lips, oral mucosa, the tongue, pharynx and teeth are then next in order. A definite routine should be developed by the practitioner so that these structures will be examined efficiently and thoroughly. A semidiagrammatic anatomic representation of these parts is used frequently to insure a complete examination and to furnish a convenient form for recording significant findings. The lips, the gingiva, the oral mucosa, the palate, tongue, tonsillar and pharyngeal regions and the teeth are usually examined in that order. Good light is essential and the small low voltage diagnostic lights are frequently helpful.

Special attention should be given to the location, appearance, symptomatology and distribution of all lesions in the mouth. Rubber gloves or finger cots should be used when the lesions are palpated and frequently additional information can be secured when bidigital or bimanual palpation is used. This is especially true when examining lesions on the cheeks, tongue and floor of the mouth. A careful examination of the tonsillar fossae and oropharynx should be made. Lastly, the dental structures should be examined for possible cavities, occlusal trauma, faulty restorations or contact points, fistulae, evidences of periodontal disease, etc.

It is advisable to examine the neck for lymphadenopathy after the intraoral examination has been made, as in this manner special attention can be given to the regional lymph nodes that drain the area of the lesion. The superficial and deep lymph nodes of the neck are best examined from behind with the patient's head inclined forward sufficiently to relax the tissues overlying the lymph nodes. Distension of the superficial veins of the neck as well as evidences of thyroid enlargement should be recorded.

The author feels that examination of the thoracic and abdominal regions should be left to our medical colleagues, except in special circumstances. The rate and the physical characteristics of the pulse should be determined, as this affords some estimation of the condition of the cardiovascular system. There is no reason why the dentist cannot take blood pressure readings, but he should be cautious about mentioning any findings suggestive of hypertension, especially if they are based on a single determination. The observation of the respiratory rate, depth and audibility of breathing offer valuable information if general anesthesia is contemplated. Lastly, the extremities can be observed for evidence of edema or swelling.

After the detailed examination of the oral structures and the visual appraisal of the patient's exposed body parts, with the background furnished by the history, a definite diagnosis may have been made or at least one or more possibilities have been suggested. Laboratory aids such as roentgenograms, hematologic or bacteriologic studies, blood chemical or serologic findings or biopsy studies may be required, but they should be requested only when necessary. In most instances, they only confirm the clinical impression and seldom are they the sole clue to the diagnosis. The patient should be asked to return after the laboratory studies have been completed. In painful cases symptomatic treatment should be given, as the patient will have little respect for the most capable clinician if he does not attempt to alleviate the pain. It is best to withhold the diagnosis until the laboratory reports have been received. The diagnosis will require occasional revision and such change does not inspire confidence in the patient or the referring doctor.

Even after a careful review of the history and repeated examination of the patient, including laboratory studies, a definite diagnosis cannot always be made. The dentist should realize that an "Undetermined Diagnosis" may be a tribute to his honesty, rather than a reflection on his ability.

4

Laboratory Procedures

INTRODUCTION

Laboratory procedures may be required to establish or to confirm the diagnosis of oral lesions. They should not be relied upon to the exclusion of a careful history and clinical examination. The experienced clinician uses laboratory studies more for confirming the diagnosis than establishing it. Laboratory studies concerned with nutritional adequacy, such as vitamin levels in the body, gastric analysis, gallbladder studies and absorptive function tests of the small intestine, are becoming more important in the diagnosis of certain disturbances of the oral tissues which are associated with nutritional deficiencies.

The laboratory procedures used in dental practice are for the most part those widely used in medicine. They are necessary for the diagnosis of oral lesions which are secondary to such diseases as diabetes, leukemia, pernicious anemia, hyperthyroidism, syphilis and tuberculosis. A few laboratory procedures have been devised solely for dental use, such as the tests for caries susceptibility (Fosdick, Bunting-Jay, Gore, Hill) and Gutzeit's short wave provocative radiation and sedimentation test for detecting oral foci of infection of systemic significance.

The procedures used most frequently in dental practice are comparatively simple and they can be mastered readily by the dental practitioner or his assistant. Included in this category are the complete blood count or hemogram, the determination of the bleeding time and clotting time, the examination of stained bacterial smears, the taking of bacterial cultures, routine urine analyses and the simple "patch tests." Gastric analyses, the various blood chemical analyses, animal inoculations, the erythrocyte sedimentation rate and biopsy examinations, the preparation of autogenous vaccines and the various serologic tests for syphilis require special training and facilities. These studies can best be performed by a reputable hospital or commercial laboratory.

The result of a single laboratory examination is of less significance, and consequently of less assistance in diagnosis, than the study of a series of examinations made at appropriate intervals. If abnormal findings are obtained, a series of reports will permit an evaluation of the rapidity and the direction of the departure from normal values. The result of a single laboratory examination, especially if it is at variance with the clinical history and physical findings, should be accepted with caution. Additional laboratory examinations should be requested.

COMPLETE BLOOD COUNT (HEMOGRAM—C.B.C.)

The complete blood count is of considerable value in determining the systemic response to oral infections, and in ruling out certain systemic diseases as the cause of oral lesions. The complete blood count does not require elaborate or expensive equipment and the technic can be easily mastered by the dentist or his assistant, or the patient can be referred to his own physician or to a reputable laboratory. The dentist should know the normal values and pathologic variations of the hemogram in the common diseases.

The routine blood count includes: (1) an enumeration of the total number of erythrocytes (RBC) and leukocytes (WBC) per cu. mm. blood; (2) a differential leukocyte count; (3) a hemoglobin estimation (Hgb.) and (4) an objective report of the stained blood smear.

Equipment

(1) Red blood cell diluting pipette
(2) White blood cell diluting pipette
(3) Hematocytometer (counting chamber)
(4) Hemoglobin pipette
(5) Hemoglobinometer
(6) Diluting solutions for (1), (2) and (4)
(7) Wright's stain
(8) Lancet
(9) Glass slide 1" x 3"
(10) Microscope

Hemoglobin Determination

The hemoglobin is determined by filling the hemoglobin pipette to the proper mark and mixing this blood with a suitable diluent. The color of the resulting solution is compared with a standard and the hemoglobin in Gm./100 cc. blood is determined. Technics for Hgb. determination vary in their accuracy and complexity. The Sahli method is simple and reasonably accurate.

Hemoglobin determinations reported only in per cent are of little value as 100% may represent any value from 13.6 to 18 Gm./100 cc. of blood. Fourteen and one-half Gm./100 cc. blood can be considered as an average value for 100% Hgb.

Erythrocyte and White Blood Cell Counts

The red blood cell count is made by drawing blood into the red cell diluting pipette to the first mark, and then filling the pipette to the second mark

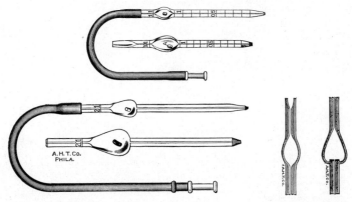

FIG. 4. Various diluting pipettes for counting blood cells. Above, the Thoma pipettes, left, Trenner automatic pipettes and right, cross sections of the Thoma and Trenner pipettes. (Kracke and Parker, Textbook of Clinical Pathology, Williams & Wilkins.)

with Hayem's or some other diluting fluid. After a thorough shaking, several drops of the diluted blood are discharged and a single drop of the diluted blood is placed beneath the cover glass of the hemocytometer and the red cells are counted in five of the small ruled central squares. The numerical result, multiplied by 100,000, gives the red blood cells/cu. mm. blood.

The white blood cell count is obtained in a similar fashion by diluting an accurately measured quantity of blood with a 2% acetic acid solution (to lake the erythrocytes) in a white blood cell diluting pipette. After shaking and discharging a few drops of this diluted blood, a drop of the solution is placed under the cover glass of the hemocytometer and the cells are counted in four of the large corner squares. This numerical result multiplied by 50 gives the white blood cells/cu. mm. of blood.

Differential Leukocyte Count (Stained Blood Smear)

The blood smear for the differential count may be made in several ways. Smears made with regular 1 x 3 microscopic slides produce satisfactory results for routine studies. A clean, grease-free slide is just touched to the bleeding point of the finger or ear, care being taken not to touch the skin. The end of a second or "pusher slide" is placed at an angle of 45° to the

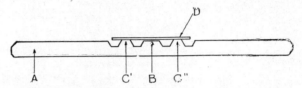

FIG. 5. Counting chamber. Side view. (A) Longitudinal section of chamber. (B) Ruled area. (C', C") Supports for coverslip. (D) Coverslip. Note space between (B) and (D). (Kracke and Parker, Textbook of Clinical Pathology, Williams & Wilkins.)

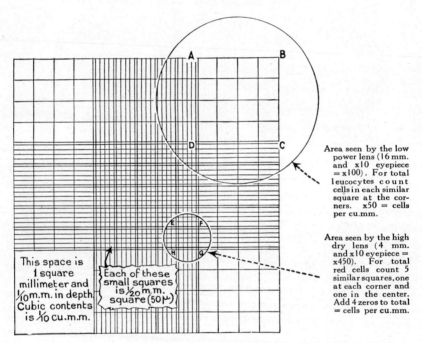

Area seen by the low power lens (16 mm. and x10 eyepiece = x100). For total leucocytes count cells in each similar square at the corners. x50 = cells per cu.mm.

Area seen by the high dry lens (4 mm. and x10 eyepiece = x450). For total red cells count 5 similar squares, one at each corner and one in the center. Add 4 zeros to total = cells per cu.mm.

This space is 1 square millimeter and $\frac{1}{10}$ m.m. in depth. Cubic contents is $\frac{1}{10}$ cu.m.m.

Each of these small squares is $\frac{1}{20}$ m.m. square (50μ)

FIG. 6. Improved Neubauer ruling on a hemocytometer. (After Nicholson, Laboratory Medicine, Lea & Febiger.)

first and gradually drawn towards the drop of blood until contact is made. The tilted slide is then pushed smoothly away from the drop of blood, producing an even thin film of blood. When dried, the blood film is stained with Giemsa's or Wright's stain.

Wright's Staining Technic for Blood Films.*

(1) The slide is placed on a flat surface and Wright's stain is added drop-by-drop (counting the drops) until the slide is completely covered. Avoid adding so much stain that it runs off the slide.

(2) In 1 to 3 minutes add to the stain an equal number of drops of distilled water or buffer solution (pH 6.4 to 6.7).

(3) In 3 or 4 minutes the stain is rapidly washed off. Unless considerable water is used, a precipitate may be formed.

(4) After drying, the smear is examined under the oil immersion lens.

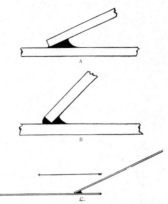

The differential leukocyte count is obtained by determining the number of the various cell types in at least 100, better 200, and, in some cases, 500 leukocytes. The results are usually given in percentages, but more information is obtained by also reporting the absolute numbers of each cell type. This is done by multiplying the total leukocyte count by the percentage values. The absolute count affords a clearer picture of the actual hematologic findings, particularly in such diseases as malignant neutropenia.

FIG. 7. (A) Showing how the blood collects behind the edge of the spreader when the angle between the two slides is small. (B) Showing how blood collects in front of the edge of the spreader slide when the angle is too great. (C) Showing the direction in which the slide is moved to make the blood film. (Kracke and Parker, Textbook of Clinical Pathology, Williams & Wilkins.)

When the differential count shows a percentage increase of any one cell type, without an increase in the absolute number of cells, it is referred to as a "relative" increase of the particular cell type. When there is an actual increase in the absolute number of any cell type, it is spoken of as an "absolute" increase of the particular cell type.

The normal percentage and absolute cell values for the leukocyte count are given in Table I.

TABLE I
AVERAGE PERCENTAGE AND ABSOLUTE VALUES FOR THE DIFFERENTIAL LEUKOCYTE COUNT

Types of Cells	Percent	Absolute Numbers
Neutrophils	60–70	3,000 to 7,000
Basophils	0.1–1	0 to 100
Eosinophils	1–3	50 to 300
Lymphocytes	20–35	1,000 to 3,500
Monocytes	2–6	100 to 600

The blood smear is also noted for variations in size (anisocytosis); shape (poikilocytosis); degree of hemoglobin content, stippling and other unusual findings. The blood platelets are noted as "numerous" or "few."

* Wright's stain can be purchased prepared from a laboratory or biologic supply house.

TABLE II

Conditions Associated with Leukocytosis and Leukopenia

LEUKOCYTOSIS	LEUKOPENIA
Physiologic leukocytosis— exercise—digestion—fear and pain	Typhoid—paratyphoid fevers
Acute and chronic infections	Influenza—measles
Polycythemia	Undulant fever
Leukemia	Kala-azar
	Malignant neutropenia
	Catarrhal jaundice
	Reaction to certain drugs— amidopyrine, barbiturates, sulfonamides
	Banti's and Gaucher's disease

TABLE III

Diseases Commonly Associated with Numerical Variations of the Different Leukocytes

POLYMORPHONUCLEARS	LYMPHOCYTES
INCREASE	INCREASE
Myelogenous leukemia	Lymphocytic leukemia
Acute infectious disease	Mumps—German measles
Erythroblastosis fetalis	Whooping cough
Intoxications by drugs and poisons	Chronic infections
	Convalescence from acute infections
DECREASE	DECREASE
Malignant neutropenia	Aplastic anemia
Aplastic anemia	Myelogenous leukemia
Lymphocytic leukemia	

MONOCYTES	EOSINOPHILS
INCREASE	INCREASE
Monocytic leukemia	Eosinophilic leukemia
Infectious mononucleosis	Allergic diseases
Hodgkin's disease	Scarlet fever
Gaucher's disease	Hodgkin's disease
Malaria—kala-azar	Some skin diseases
Tuberculosis	Protozoan diseases— trichinosis
Subacute bacterial endocarditis	DECREASE
DECREASE	Typhoid fever
Aplastic anemia	Aplastic anemia

TABLE IV

Platelet Changes Associated with Some Common Diseases of Dental Interest
(Normal values 250,000-500,000 cu. mm. of blood)

ESSENTIALLY NORMAL	DECREASE IN PLATELETS (Thrombocytopenia)
Malignant neutropenia	Thrombocytopenic purpura (Werlhoff's disease)
Scurvy	Symptomatic purpura hemorrhagica due to:
Infectious mononucleosis	Chemical or physical agents
Hemophilia	Acute and chronic leukemias
Simple purpura	Aplastic anemia
INCREASE IN PLATELETS (Thrombocytosis)	Pernicious anemia
Polycythemia vera	Hemolytic jaundice
Hemolytic anemias	Banti's disease
Chronic myelocytic anemia	Gaucher's disease
Acute rheumatic fever	Bacterial endocarditis

A more detailed study of the polymorphonuclear neutrophils such as that suggested by Schilling and others, permits the clinician to follow slight changes in the host's response to a particular infectious process. The neutrophils are placed in one of four groups according to their degree of maturation as judged by the configuration and arrangement of the nucleus. The nucleus is small and round in Group I, slightly indented in Group II, band-formed (nonsegmented) in Group III and it presents the typical lobulated form in Group IV. When there is an increased percentage of the younger forms (Groups I, II and III), it is spoken of as a "shift to the left." This terminology is derived from the fact that the percentage of neutrophils in each group is usually written on a horizontal line beginning with Group I. (See Table V.)

TABLE V

NORMAL FINDINGS IN SCHILLING COUNT AND TYPICAL VARIATIONS

	Groups			
	I	II	III	IV
Percentage of normal distribution....................		2	3	63
"Shift to the left" without increase in percentage of polymorphonuclear neutrophiles..		4	12	47
"Shift to the left" with an increase in the percentage of polymorphonuclear neutrophiles.....................	1	6	20	55

Color Index (C.I.)

The color index is a measure of the amount of hemoglobin carried by the individual erythrocyte. It is a valuable aid in classifying and diagnosing various anemias.

The color index is derived by the following formula.

$$\frac{\% \text{ Hb. compared to normal (15.5 Gm./100 cc. blood)}}{\% \text{ R.B.C. compared to normal (5,000,000 per c. mm.)}} = \text{C.I.}$$

The normal values of the C.I. are 0.9-1.2. Values less than one are generally associated with secondary anemias, and a C.I. greater than one is associated with macrocytic anemias (i.e. pernicious anemia, sprue, and certain parasitic infections).

BLEEDING TIME (DUKE'S METHOD)

Equipment

Lancet
Filter paper

This method furnishes skin bleeding time which is not necessarily an indication of the bleeding time of the deeper tissues or infected, ulcerated mucous surfaces.

The lobe of the ear or the tip of a finger is cleaned with 70% alcohol and allowed to dry and a puncture wound 2-3 mm. deep is made. The first drop of blood is wiped away. If sufficient blood is not obtained from the initial puncture, rather than producing bleeding by pressure, a second puncture should be made.

A piece of filter paper or white blotting paper is touched to the bleeding point at 30 second intervals until a blot is no longer obtained. The bleeding

---

The Thomas W. Evans Museum and Dental Institute, School of Dentistry University of Pennsylvania
Form 133-E   **ORAL MEDICINE LABORATORY REPORT**

Patient_ David, Alan _____Date_ 7/23/43 _____Master No._45679
Instructor_ Dr. Jones _____Dept._ O.M._Student_____
R.B.C._ 4700000 _cu.mm.   HB._Klett 152.8_gms./100 cc. blood___ 97 _%
W.B.C._ 7500 _____cu.mm.   Bl. Time_____Cl. Time_____C.I._ 1.0 _
   DIFFERENTIAL (100) cells counted   Time_____

	Absolute No.	%	
NEUTROPHILES	4875	65	Sediment. Rate
Seg.	4425	59	Wassermann React.
Non-seg.	450	6	URINE
EOSINOPHILES	150	2	ALBUMIN
BASOPHILES	75	1	SUGAR
LYMPHOCYTES	1950	26	SPEC. GRAV.
MONOCYTES	375	5	REACTION
TRANSITIONAL	75	1	SEDIMENT.

Remarks_____ Signed_ E.J. Smith _Date_7/23/

FIG. 8. Form used in Oral Medicine Laboratory, School of Dentistry, University of Pennsylvania, for recording the result of a complete blood count. The W.B.C. and differential leukocyte count are essentially normal. There is a slight anemia present.

time in minutes is determined by dividing the number of blots by 2. A bleeding time of over 6 minutes is considered to be abnormal.

COAGULATION TIME

Capillary Tube Method

Equipment

Lancet
Capillary glass tubing

This test can be performed simultaneously with the bleeding time.

Capillary glass tubes 1-2 mm. in diameter are filled with blood from a lancet wound. At 30 second intervals a short length of the filled capillary tubing is carefully broken off until a fibrin strand is observed connecting the 2 pieces of capillary tubing.

The interval of time between the filling of the capillary tube and the formation of fibrin is the coagulation time. Normal coagulation time with this method varies from 1 to 5 minutes.

This method is useful for routine examination prior to dental extractions since it does not require venipuncture. It is less accurate than the test tube method which should be performed in cases giving higher-than-normal values.

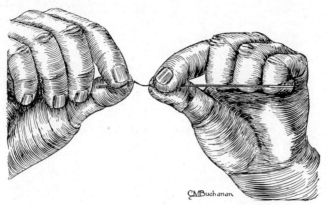

Fig. 9. The determination of coagulation time by capillary tube method. The capillary tube is broken between the fingers and the strand of fibrin is suspended between the broken edges. (Kracke and Parker, Textbook of Clinical Pathology, Williams & Wilkins.)

Test Tube Method

Equipment

Dry glass syringe
Dry test tube
Tourniquet

Approximately 5.0 cc. of venous blood are withdrawn in a dry syringe and placed in a dry test tube. The test tube is tilted at 30-second intervals until the blood no longer flows. Normal coagulation time by this method varies from 5 to 20 minutes.

Clot Retraction

When normal blood clots, there is a retraction of the clot with a separation of the serum. This can be readily observed if several cc. of blood are allowed to clot in a small test tube. Delay or failure of clot retraction is characteristic of diseases associated with a low platelet count.

THE TOURNIQUET TEST—CAPILLARY FRAGILITY FINDINGS (RUMPELL-LEED PHENOMENON)

Equipment

Sphygmomanometer cuff, or rubber tourniquet
or
Negative pressure apparatus
Hand lens

The tourniquet test is a measure of capillary resistance and is not specifically diagnostic for any disease. A sphygmomanometer cuff (or rubber tubing tourniquet) is placed about the upper arm and inflated to the mean value between systolic and diastolic pressure and held there for 5 minutes. The pressure is then released and the skin of the forearm is examined for petechial hemorrhages. Numerous petechiae are seen in scarlet fever, thrombocytopenic purpura, scurvy, and perhaps in vitamin-P deficiency states.

A rough quantitative estimate of the vitamin-C nutritional status of the individual is believed to be obtained by slight modifications of the tourniquet test in which the number of petechiae are counted in a 2.5 cm. diameter circle which is situated a fixed distance below the elbow crease. This method, while more time consuming, is a more accurate measure of capillary resistance than the so-called negative pressure or "suction pump methods."

TABLE VI

COAGULATION TIME, BLEEDING TIME, CLOT RETRACTION TIME, AND CAPILLARY
FRAGILITY FINDINGS IN SOME COMMON DISEASES OF DENTAL INTEREST

Diseases	Coagulation Time	Bleeding Time	Clot Retraction Time	Capillary Fragility
Pernicious anemia..........	Normal	Prolonged	Poor	Negative
Aplastic anemia............	Normal	Prolonged	Poor	Variable
Malignant neutropenia.....	Normal	Normal	Normal	Negative
Acute leukemia............	Normal	Prolonged	Poor	Variable
Infectious mononucleosis....	Normal	Prolonged	Normal	Negative
Hemophilia................	Prolonged	Normal	Normal but delayed	Negative
Purpura hemorrhagica......	Normal	Prolonged	Poor	Positive
Hereditary hemorrhagic telangiectasia..............	Normal	Normal	Normal	Negative

BLOOD PRESSURE DETERMINATION

Equipment

Sphygmomanometer
Stethoscope

A blood pressure determination is within the capabilities of every dentist. It will afford some information as to the cardiovascular system of the patient. The patient should be seated and the left arm (preferably) placed on a table or desk at approximately the same level as the heart. The pressure cuff is wrapped smoothly about the upper arm with its lower border approximately 2 inches above the elbow. The cuff is then connected to the sphygmomanometer.

The bell of the stethoscope is placed in the antecubital fossa to determine the proper time to take the readings of the systolic and diastolic pressure. The pressure cuff is inflated until the sphygmomanometer reads around 200 mm. Hg. The pressure is decreased gradually by manipulating the control valve until the pulse beat is heard in the stethoscope. This sound is usually definite, clear and sharp. It is heard over a relatively narrow range on the manometer. The point at which this sound is first heard clearly represents the systolic pressure.

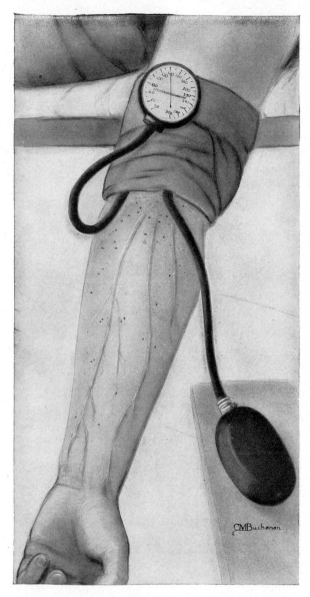

FIG. 10. Showing petechial spots on forearm in a positive capillary resistance test after the diastolic pressure has been maintained for five minutes. Some workers prefer to maintain the pressure midway between the diastolic and systolic for three minutes. There is no reason to do this test on a patient who shows spontaneous purpuric spots. (Kracke, Diseases of the Blood, J. B. Lippincott Company.)

As the pressure in the cuff is allowed to decrease a second pulse sound is gradually heard which reaches a maximum and then disappears gradually. This second sound is softer, deeper and it is heard over a relatively wider range on the manometer. The manometer reading at the point of maximum intensity represents the diastolic pressure. This sequence of inflation and deflation of the cuff may be repeated over the range of the sounds to verify the initial readings.

The blood pressure is recorded as the systolic pressure/diastolic pressure, i.e., 120/95. A casual blood pressure reading made on a nervous or an excitable patient may give abnormally high figures. A systolic pressure of over 150 mm. Hg and a diastolic pressure of over 100 mm. Hg may indicate cardiovascular disease. In general, it is undesirable to inform the patient of his blood pressure.

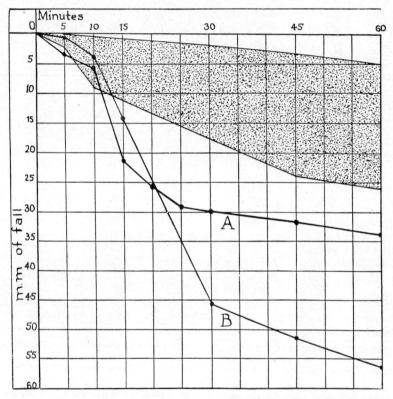

Fig. 11. A graph showing curves of sedimentation of red cells. Any curve within the shaded area is considered normal. Curve A represents a moderately increased rate, and curve B an extremely fast rate. (Kracke and Parker, Textbook of Clinical Pathology, Williams & Wilkins.)

ERYTHROCYTE SEDIMENTATION RATE (SEDIMENTATION RATE—S.R.)

The rate at which red blood cells, suspended in blood serum, settles varies in different disease states although it is not specific for any one disease. It is used for indicating the presence, the relative severity, or the progress of such conditions as rheumatic fever, tuberculosis and suspected infection (focal infection).

Equipment

Dry syringe
Glass vials containing dried anticoagulant
Sedimentation tubes

Venous blood is collected in a dry syringe and placed in vials containing an anticoagulant, usually ammonium oxalate. A graduated sedimentation tube is then filled with the oxalated blood and placed in an absolutely vertical position. The erythrocyte level is read at ten-minute intervals and at the end of the hour. A time-sedimentation curve may be drawn, or only the reading at the end of the hour reported.

The generally accepted normal sedimentation rates are:

Males 0 to 10 mm. in 60 minutes
Females 0 to 20 mm. in 60 minutes

There is considerable difference of opinion relative to the significance of the erythrocyte sedimentation rate in relation to chronic oral (periapical) infections.

URINE ANALYSIS

Equipment

Test tubes
Benedict's solution
Glacial acetic acid
Urinometer
Litmus or nitrazine paper
Bunsen or alcohol flame
Microscope
Glass slides

A routine urine examination consists of a report of (1) the macroscopic appearance of the specimen, (2) the reaction (pH), (3) specific gravity, (4) qualitative test for sugar and albumin and (5) microscopic examination of the sediment for casts, cells or organisms.

The examination should be made on the first urine voided in the morning. A few drops of toluol will avoid glycolysis and the deterioration of casts and cells.

The color and clarity of the specimen are noted, and its reaction is determined by means of litmus or nitrazine paper. Unless the urine is freshly voided the reaction is of little significance. The specific gravity is read with an urinometer. When the volume is insufficient to make this determination a report of Q.N.S. (quantity not sufficient) is made.

Test for Albumin (Heat and Acetic Acid Test). A test tube is filled ⅔ full of clear urine—filter if necessary. The top portion of the urine in the tube is carefully boiled. A few drops of 5% acetic acid are then added, after which the tube is again heated a few minutes. If albumin is present, a white cloud forms which is reported as follows:

+ A barely visible cloud
++ A faint cloud
+++ A definite cloud
++++ A heavy cloud

The use of a dark background will facilitate the readings.

Test for Sugar (Benedict's Qualitative). About 8 drops of urine are added to 5 cc. of Benedict's qualitative reagent. The solutions are mixed and heated for 5 minutes, preferably in a boiling water bath. A turbid green to red color develops if sugar (reducing substances) are present. The results are reported as follows:

+ No reduction on boiling, but a
    green color appears on cooling
++ Green-yellow color
+++ Orange-yellow color
++++ Orange-red color

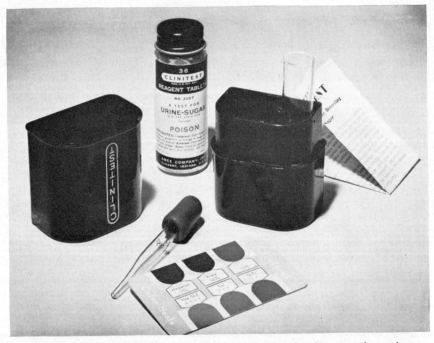

Fig. 12. Compact unit for making copper reduction test for urine-sugar. Place five drops of specimen in the test tube. Rinse dropper and add ten drops of water. Drop in tablet containing chemicals and heat producing agent. Wait fifteen seconds after boiling has ceased and then compare with the color scale. ("Clinitest" set manufactured by Ames Co., Inc., Elkhart, Indiana.)

If sugar is demonstrated in the first specimen of urine voided in the morning it indicates definite disturbance of carbohydrate metabolism. In early diabetes sugar may be demonstrated only in the specimen voided in the evening. The failure to demonstrate sugar in a single urine specimen does not rule out diabetes.

A simple kit comprising a test tube, tablets containing the reacting and heat-producing substances, and a color guide are available at moderate cost.

THE THOMAS W. EVANS MUSEUM AND DENTAL INSTITUTE
SCHOOL OF DENTISTRY UNIVERSITY OF PENNSYLVANIA
ORAL MEDICINE LABORATORY REPORT

Patient James Smith   Date 8 Jan 1945   Master No. 6152

Instructor A. Jones   Dept. O.M.   Student A. Barnes

R.B.C. ____cu.mm.   HB. ( ) ____gms./100 cc. blood____%

W.B.C.____cu.mm.   Bl. Time____Cl. Time____C.I.____

DIFFERENTIAL (00) cells counted   Time____

	Absolute No.	%	
NEUTROPHILES	cu. mm.	____	Sediment. Rate ____
Seg.			Wassermann React. ____
Non-seg.			URINE
EOSINOPHILES			ALBUMIN neg.
BASOPHILES			SUGAR neg.
LYMPHOCYTES			SPEC. GRAV. 1016
MONOCYTES			REACTION acid
TRANSITIONAL			SEDIMENT. none

Remarks____   No casts or bacteria

Signed M.A.S.   Date 9 Jan. 1945   seen

Form 133-E

Fig. 13. Form used in Oral Medicine Laboratory, School of Dentistry, University of Pennsylvania, for recording results of a routine urine analysis. The findings given are normal.

This kit affords the dentist a rapid, accurate and convenient means of testing the urine for sugar.

Urinary Sediment. Microscopic examination of the urinary sediment will reveal the presence of urinary casts, red and white blood cells and bacteria. Cells and casts are usually reported in numbers per high power field (H.P.F.) or numbers per low power field (L.P.F.). If the urine is obtained under sterile conditions, the sediment may be stained and examined for bacteria. A typical urine report with essentially normal findings is shown in the illustration.

STAINED BACTERIAL SMEARS

A smear will indicate in a few minutes the probable type of infection and the relative proportion of the various organisms that are present. The technic is simple and the information obtained is considerable in proportion to the time consumed. While stained bacterial smears are most useful in the examination of sites that are normally sterile they nevertheless furnish valuable information, if interpreted intelligently, when taken from nonsterile fields such as the oral cavity.

Bacterial smears may aid in the diagnosis of fusospirochetal, streptococcal, pneumococcal and Neisserian stomatitides, oral moniliasis and oral tuberculous ulcerations. The technic for making and fixing the smear is essentially similar for all diseases even though different staining procedures may be used in certain cases.

Making and Fixing the Bacterial Smear

Equipment

Clean 1″ x 3″ glass slide
Glass marking pencil
Toothpick or explorer
Bunsen or alcohol flame
Stains
Microscope

The 1″ x 3″ glass slides should be chemically and physically cleansed and kept in 70% alcohol for ready use. When material is studied from several sites, the respective areas should be indicated on the slide by means of a glass marking pencil or the slides can be readily ruled into 6 or more areas by means of a carborundum disk. The patient's name and date can be written in pencil on a small ground area in the center of the slide. Slides so prepared can be used repeatedly.

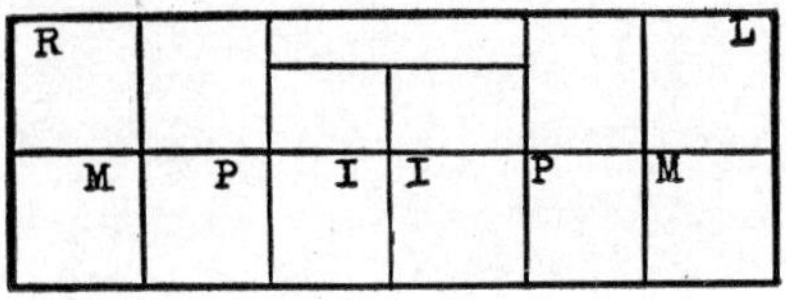

FIG. 14. Slide ruled with carborundum stone in preparation to making bacterial smears from different areas of the mouth. (From Appleton's Bacterial Infection, Lea & Febiger.)

Material for the smear should be obtained, in most instances, from the deeper portions of the lesions. A flat toothpick or a pointed applicator stick is satisfactory for transferring the material to the slide. It may be necessary to dilute the material with a drop of water to permit satisfactory microscopic examination when stained. The smears are allowed to dry naturally after which they are fixed by passing the slide through an alcohol or Bunsen flame three times. Overheating the smear destroys the morphologic characteristics of the organisms and cells.

If the practitioner does not have access to a microscope, the fixed smear can be sent to a laboratory for staining and interpretation. The laboratory selected should be familiar with the criteria for a positive smear for an oral fusospirochetal infection. Laboratories should report the numbers of the various organisms in a number of fields rather than attempt a diagnosis; e.g., "In 10 fields examined, there was an average of countless numbers of spirochetal forms, 30 fusiform bacilli, 3 leukocytes, 5 cocci and 3 bacilli."

Staining the Smear

(Staining technics will vary, depending on the disease suspected.)

Gram's Stain for Routine Morphologic Study

(1) The fixed bacterial smear is stained with Hucker's crystal violet for 2 minutes when it is washed with water.

(2) Gram's iodine solution is then applied for 1 or 2 minutes.

(3) The slide is then washed with 95% ethyl alcohol for a few seconds until the smear has a slate gray appearance. The slide is then washed with water.

(4) The decolorized slide is counterstained with 2% safranin for 1 minute and washed again.

(5) The slide is allowed to dry and is then examined under the oil immersion objective.

Staining of Smears from Suspected Fusospirochetal Infections

Single Staining Method. Immediately after fixing the slide *and while it is still warm,* apply half-saturated crystal violet stain. Wash off immediately under running tap water and allow to dry in air or blot gently.* Examine under the oil immersion objective.

Double Staining Method. Flood the slide with carbolfuchsin and immediately wash off under running tap water. Apply methylene blue for about 30 seconds and again wash in running tap water.* Allow the slide to dry in air or blot gently. Examine under an oil immersion objective. Both methods are of equal diagnostic value but the Double Staining Method will show more cellular detail.

A positive smear for oral fusospirochetal infection consists of overwhelming numbers of the fusospirochetal organisms as compared with the usual oral flora. Daley has classified smears for oral fusospirochetal infection as "negative," "potentially positive" and "positive."

The "potentially positive" smears refer to those cases in which the fusospirochetal organisms are present without obvious clinical symptoms of the disease. There may be some merit to this classification since it seems desirable in the "potentially positive" cases to take steps to eliminate these organisms and to establish satisfactory oral hygiene.

Staining of Smears from Suspected Tuberculous Lesions

A drop of carbolfuchsin is placed on the fixed smear. On this drop put a strip of filter paper large enough to cover the film. Drop more carbolfuchsin on this paper, but not enough to float it away. This will keep the film covered with the dye and greatly lessen the chances of staining the fingers or of "cooking" the preparation.

Steam, by passing the slide through the flame rather slowly once or twice, when thin clouds of steam will be seen rising from the surface of stain. Set aside until the clouds subside. The dye on the paper should be replenished

---

* I am indebted to Miss Newman for suggesting the following method of washing the stain off a slide, which practically eliminates the objectionable splashing of the stain. The stained slide is dipped gently several times into a paper cup which is two-thirds full of water. This removes the concentrated stain from the slide and dilutes it. The contents of the cup can be conveniently emptied into the cuspidor, wash basin or sink without much danger of splashing or staining.

several times during the staining process, to prevent drying. The stain under no circumstances should be brought to the boiling point.

When this step is finished, the paper and the dye can be washed off in running tap water. Decolorize with 5% sulfuric acid until the red color has been removed from the film and this has regained its original dull gray tone even after washing in tap water. Wash the acid off in tap water and apply methylene blue for 5 seconds. Wash off in tap water and blot dry. Put a drop of immersion oil on the film and examine with an oil immersion lens.

It may be impossible to demonstrate the acid-fast organisms in repeated direct smears. Before a clinically suspicious lesion is considered to be non-tuberculous, guinea pig inoculations and biopsy study of material obtained from the lesion should be performed in addition to clinical roentgenologic studies.

Examination of Smears from Suspected Actinomycotic Lesions

The pus or discharge from the lesion should be spread out in a thin layer, as in a petri dish. This will help one to find the macroscopic "sulfur granules." One of these granules is then placed on a slide which contains a drop of 20% NaOH. A cover glass is added and the material is crushed and examined with subdued light under the low-power objective. The typical actinomycotic granule appears as a mass of radiating mycelia with clubs at their extremities. The radiating configuration of the colonies accounts for the term "ray fungus."

If the clinical history and findings are suggestive of actinomycosis, cultural examination should follow negative microscopic results. Anaerobic cultural methods should be employed using serum or blood agar.

Examination of Smears from Suspected Monilial Infections

Scrapings from suspected monilial lesions can be placed on a slide containing a drop of 20% NaOH. A cover slip is added and the preparation is observed under the low-power objective for mycelial structures or budding forms. A drop of gentian violet stain will aid in recognizing the mycelial structures.

BACTERIAL CULTURES OF TOOTH APICES

Bacterial cultures of tooth apices are frequently requested by the physician for verification of a suspected periapical infection or for the purpose of making autogenous vaccines. Cultures made from the apical region of extracted teeth by any of various technics must be interpreted with caution because of the technical difficulties involved in removing teeth without contamination with the oral flora.

From the standpoint of the bacteriologic technic an external approach or root amputation method of culturing is preferable. Because of the additional surgical procedures required in this culturing technic it is seldom agreed to by the patient. Furthermore, this method is best applied to anterior teeth and single rooted teeth, preferably those in the maxilla. A modification of this method, devised by Coriell, utilizes a small dental trocar for obtaining material for culture before the removal of the tooth. While this device overcomes some of the objections of the root amputation technic it is not generally applicable for the examination of all teeth.

The difficulty in obtaining bacteriologically significant cultures arises not because of the inability to maintain an aseptic operating technic but because of the difficulty in rendering the operative field, particularly the gingival crevice, sterile. The repeated application of the usual topical medicaments is ineffective in sterilizing this area. Actual cauterization of the gingival crevice by heat just prior to the extraction is the most effective method of sterilizing the gingival crevice.

A bacteriologic check can be made of the effectiveness of the method employed for sterilization. This consists of painting a suspension of *Serratia marcesens* in the gingival crevice prior to sterilization. If these organisms are recovered in the cultures made from the apical region of the extracted tooth, it indicates that the sterilization of the gingival crevice was ineffective and that the tooth apex has been contaminated during extraction with organisms from the gingival crevice. Under these circumstances, the cultural findings could not be considered as representing the true bacteriologic status of the tooth apex.

BLOOD CULTURES

Blood cultures are used to demonstrate the presence of a bacteremia. They are particularly useful in cases of severe sepsis, typhoid fever and subacute bacterial endocarditis, etc. They will seldom be necessary in dental practice. The demonstration of a bacteremia is dependent on the number of organisms which are present in the circulating blood and the time when the cultures are taken. Like many other laboratory studies, negative results do not rule out the possibility of a bacteremia.

The technic for taking a blood culture is identical to that for a venipuncture with special attention being paid to asepsis. Media should be used which will permit the growth of both aerobic and anaerobic organisms. Sufficient medium should be used (50 cc.) so that any bacteriostatic substances in the blood stream will be sufficiently diluted. Certain substances, such as saponin, may be added to the culture medium to increase the frequency of positive cultures when few organisms are present in the circulating blood. If sulfonamides are being administered, the culture media should contain paraaminobenzoic acid to inhibit the bacteriostatic effect of the sulfonamides.

PATCH TESTING FOR CONTACT STOMATITIS

Patch testing may be required to establish a diagnosis of stomatitis venenata. Best results are obtained when the test is performed on the same tissues which presented the lesions. Goldman & Goldman devised a simple and practical method for contact testing of the buccal mucosa and gingivae. They found that a soft rubber suction cup, such as is used to fasten display advertisements by suction, was an effective carrier for the test substances. For use under the lips the rubber suction cups should be cut down to a diameter of 1.2 to 1.4 cm. Suction cups 1.0 cm. high, 2.5 cm. in diameter across the top and approximately 0.7 cm. in diameter at the bottom of the bowl should be used for the application of the test substance to the palate.

Collodion is placed in the central depression of the cup and a small piece of cotton is partly imbedded in it. The liquid, cream or paste to be tested is then applied to the cotton. Small pieces, or scrapings of denture material, can be fastened to the cotton by means of collodion. Care should be taken

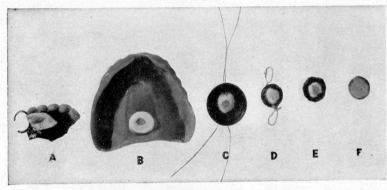

Fig. 15. The different materials which may be used for contact testing of the buccal mucous membrane. (A) Partial denture with cotton pad fixed to denture with collodion. (B) Complete denture with cotton pad fixed to it with collodion. (C) Large suction cup with dental floss attached. (D) Small suction cup with dental floss ties. (E) Small suction cup without dental floss. (F) Cotton pad. (Goldman, L., and Goldman, B., Arch. Dermat. & Syph., 50:79-84, 1944.)

to see that the material to be tested is not completely imbedded in the collodion. The suction cup is fixed in position for testing the sensitivity of the palatal, gingival, cheek or lip mucosa to the test substance by dental floss. If the suction cup is fastened to the maxillary anteriors with the base of the cup next to the teeth, the inner surface of the lip can be examined from time to time by simply turning up the lip.

A less accurate but somewhat easier method for testing the sensitivity of suspected substances consists of their application to the skin surface. A small gauze square or piece of filter paper, moistened with the material to be tested, is applied to the skin of the upper arm and held in place with adhesive tape. In suspected cases of allergy to vulcanite or acrylic denture bases, scrapings of the denture material may be employed instead of the entire denture. The use of denture scrapings does not entail the discomfort and hazard of "wearing" the denture on the arm for several days. Suitable control substances should be tested and it is also advisable to have the test performed on a second individual.

The patch test should be allowed to remain for 24 to 48 hours and in the case of denture scrapings it is often necessary to allow them to remain in contact with the tissues for 3 days. The patient should be told to remove the test material as soon as itching or a mild burning sensation is experi-

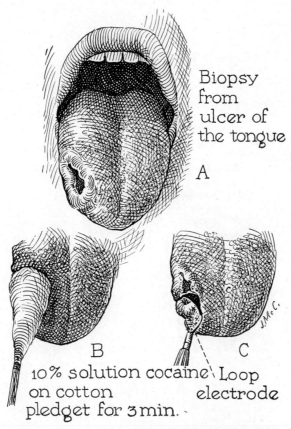

Biopsy
from
ulcer of
the tongue

A

B
10% solution cocaine
on cotton
pledget for 3 min.

C
Loop
electrode

FIG. 16. Biopsy of an ulcer of the tongue follow-ing local application of 10 per cent cocaine solu-tion. The cutting current with a loop electrode is an excellent method of removing such biopsies. (Ferguson, Surgery of the Ambulatory Patient, J. B. Lippincott Company.)

enced. A positive reaction is indicated by local irritation which may be ac-companied by vesiculation and pigmentation.

The patch test is of no value in the diagnosis of stomatitis medicamentosa. A small "test dose" of the suspected drug should be administered to see whether there is an exacerbation of symptoms.

In suspected cases of allergic stomatitis or angioneurotic edema associated with food or other protein sensitization, skin testing by the scratch, intradermal or multiple pressure method should be performed by an allergist. Skin testing of bacterial vaccines is used infrequently.

BIOPSY EXAMINATION

Histologic study of the tissue from an oral lesion may be required to make a definite diagnosis. If the lesion is shown to be neoplastic, information concerning the relative malignancy and radiosensitivity is also obtained. Tissue removed for diagnostic purposes is known as a biopsy.

The oral surgeon is better equipped to perform a biopsy because of his familiarity with surgical technic and his knowledge of the type of specimen desired by the pathologist. The general practitioner can however remove tissue for diagnosis if a few general rules are observed.

(1) The date of the biopsy, the name, age, sex of the patient, the area of the biopsy specimen and a brief description of the clinical appearance of the lesion and associated symptoms along with the tentative clinical diagnosis should accompany the specimen.

(2) Iodine-containing surface antiseptics should be avoided as they have a tendency to stain certain tissue cells permanently. The type of anesthetic used and a statement whether the tissue was removed with the scalpel (generally preferred) or with the electrocautery should be noted. In suspected malignant lesions, the electrocautery is the method of choice of some surgeons, particularly when the entire growth cannot be removed.

(3) The biopsy specimen should include not only the lesion but some clinically normal adjacent tissue. Small lesions should be removed completely when the biopsy is done. In all instances sufficient tissue should be obtained. In certain suspected lesions, i.e., tuberculous, it may be desirable to use a part of the biopsy for animal inoculations, injections or other bacteriologic procedures.

(4) The portion of the biopsy to be used for histologic study should be placed at once in a suitable fixing solution—usually 4 to 10% formalin—and sent to the hospital or pathologic laboratory.

The pathologist's report will require 5 days to a week. If the specimen contains calcified tissue a longer time is required. Even after biopsy study it is not always possible to make a diagnosis but many times the pathologist can suggest certain diagnostic possibilities as a result of a study of the pathologic processes observed in the tissues.

SEROLOGIC TESTS FOR SYPHILIS (S.T.S.)

The serologic tests for syphilis are not specific in the sense that the antigens used are obtained from luetic animals or individuals. These reactions are of two general types: (1) the complement fixation tests which require a hemolytic system for reading the results, and (2) flocculation reactions. The Wassermann reaction is a complement fixation test while the Eagle, Hinton, Kahn, Kline and Mazzini tests are flocculation reactions. In general the complement fixation tests are more "specific" and the flocculation tests are more "sensitive."

Rein has described a microscopic test that can be performed by the dental practitioner but the time required for its performance and the possibility of inaccurate findings when performed by inexperienced individuals limit its usefulness.

Most of these serologic tests, with the exception of the Kline and Eagle, require a quantity of blood that must be obtained by venipuncture. The Wassermann reaction is frequently reported as "negative" or + to + + + + and some of the flocculation tests are simply reported as "negative" or "positive" and many laboratories report all tests as "negative," "doubtful" or "positive." Because of differences in sensitivity and methods used, the results of all the tests are not always in agreement. Leprosy, yaws, malaria and occasionally infectious mononucleosis are associated with positive Wassermann reactions in the absence of syphilis.

Since these tests are somewhat complicated and accurate results can be achieved only by the experienced, it is impractical for the dentist to perform the test himself. If a serologic test for syphilis is required for the diagnosis of an oral lesion, the patient should be referred to a physician for this procedure and a physical examination.

GASTRIC ANALYSIS

Analysis for hydrochloric acid will furnish information as to the secretive function of the stomach. A deficient secretion of HCl has a marked effect on the absorption of many foods and accessory food factors. To obtain a measure of the secretive function of the stomach, a test meal consisting of crackers and a couple of glasses of water, alcohol ingestion or histamine injection is used to stimulate gastric secretion.

Gastric acidity is expressed in degrees (°), which indicate the number of cc. of 0.1 normal NaOH that is required to neutralize 100 cc. of the gastric secretion. Normal values for gastric acidity (free acid) using the test meal described (modified Ewald) vary between 20° and 60°. Values above 60° indicate hyperacidity, and those below 20°, hypoacidity. Values for the combined gastric hydrochloric acid are usually ½ those of the free acid.

Achlorhydria is found in pernicious anemia, gastric carcinoma, pellagra, sprue and in many subclinical nutritional deficiencies. Hyperchlorhydria is common in individuals with duodenal ulcer, gastric ulcer, gastric hypermotility and certain neurotic disturbances.

SHORT WAVE PROVOCATIVE RADIATION AND SEDIMENTATION RATE TO DETERMINE FOCI OF INFECTION OF SYSTEMIC SIGNIFICANCE

Gutzeit and Kuchlin claimed that after short wave currents are applied to the area of the dental infection the erythrocyte sedimentation rate becomes noticeably accelerated for from 2 to 4 hours after the treatment if the dental focus is responsible for the systemic manifestations. The diagnostic value of this test has not been established.

THE PELS-MACHT TEST

The Pels-Macht test is a phytopharmacologic test which is used by some clinicians as an aid in making a clinical diagnosis particularly in pemphigus. The toxic effect of the vesicle fluid or blood serum of such patients on the growing roots of lupine seedlings is compared with the root growth of similar seedlings grown under standard conditions. From these values, a phytopharmacologic index is derived that is said to be diagnostic.

BASAL METABOLIC RATE (B.M.R.)

The B.M.R. is an estimate of the rate of metabolic processes in the body. It is used chiefly in the diagnosis of thyroid disease. The B.M.R. should be determined preferably on hospitalized patients although tests made on ambulatory patients are of value when properly obtained and interpreted. The normal B.M.R. range varies from at least -10% to $+10\%$, with even greater variation in an occasional, clinically normal individual. It is determined by measuring the amount of oxygen consumed during a unit of time while the individual is under certain prescribed conditions.

An approximation of the B.M.R. may be obtained from the pulse rate and the blood pressure findings by the use of a simple formula suggested by Read.

$$\tfrac{3}{4} \, (\tfrac{3}{4} \; P.R. + P.P.) - 72 = B.M.R.$$

where P.R. is the pulse rate and P.P. is the pulse pressure. If the B.M.R. calculated by this formula is beyond a range of -20% to $+20\%$ it should be determined by more accurate methods.

TABLE VII

SYSTEMIC CONDITIONS COMMONLY ASSOCIATED WITH VARIATIONS IN THE BASAL METABOLIC RATE (B.M.R.)

Increased + 15	*Decreased* − 15
Hyperthyroidism	Hypothyroidism
Leukemia	Hypoadrenalism
All fevers	Hypopituitarism
Acromegaly at times	Starvation
Pituitary basophilism	
Certain drugs—caffeine	
Exercise—digestion	
Pregnancy	
Emotional disturbances	

BLOOD PHOSPHATASE

Phosphatase is an enzyme which is directly related to the functional activity of tissue cells. Its action liberates inorganic phosphorus from the phosphoric esters in the tissues.

Normal plasma phosphatase values in adults range from 1.5 to 4 Bodansky units and from 4 to 15 Bodansky units in children. Elevated plasma phosphatase values are found in certain bone diseases such as osteitis fibrosa cystica, Paget's disease and osteogenic sarcoma. More recently, elevation of the "acid" phosphatase has been shown to be associated with the development of certain neoplasms, particularly those of the prostate gland.

Elevated plasma phosphatase values were obtained from the gingival blood of patients with periodontal disease. The phosphatase elevation coincided roughly with the clinical rapidity of the disease.

PREGNANCY TESTS

Aschheim-Zondek and Friedman Tests

The Aschheim-Zondek and Friedman Tests are biologic tests for pregnancy.

TABLE VIII

AVERAGE VALUES FOR THE COMMON BLOOD CHEMISTRY DETERMINATIONS

Average Values in Mg. per 100 cc.
Unless Otherwise Stated

Glucose	80-110
CO_2 combining power	55-65 vols., %
Total nonprotein nitrogen (N.P.N.)	25-40
Blood urea nitrogen (B.U.N.)	8-18
Uric acid	2-4
Free cholesterol	40-50 (average 47)
Cholesterol ester	190-200 (average 192)
Prothrombin time (plasma)	10-20 sec. (Quick's method)
Chlorides (as Cl)	352-383
Sodium	315-340 (average 330)
Potassium	16-22 (average 19)
Calcium	9-11
Phosphorus (as inorganic phosphate)	2-5 Adults / 4-7 Children
Phosphatase	1.5-4.0 Adults / 4-14 Children } Bodansky units

REFERENCES

LABORATORY PROCEDURES

Bernier, J. L.: Indications and technique for the biopsy, Army Dent. Bull., 8:4, 1942.

Cahn, L. R.: Pitfalls in histologic diagnosis: A clinico-pathologic study, Am. J. Orthodontics & Oral Surg., 28:504, 1942.

Gettinger, Raymond: Biopsy in oral surgery, J. A. D. A., 25:451, 1938.

Goldman, L., & B. Goldman: Contact testing of the buccal mucous membrane for stomatitis venenata, Arch. Dermat. & Syph., 50:79-84, 1944.

Hume, E. E.: Contributions of the Medical Corps of the Army to the Public Health Laboratory, Science, 97:293-9, 1943.

Macht, D. I., & M. B. Macht: Phytotoxic reactions of some blood sera, J. Lab. & Clin. Med., 26:597, 1941.

Mallory, T. B.: The interpretation and reliability of reports of serologic tests for syphilis, New England J. Med., 223:441, 1940.

McCulloch, A. J.: The presentation of case records, Illinois Dent. J., 12:450, 1943.

Rault, C. V.: The value of routine blood sedimentation tests in dental patients, Mil. Surgeon, 83:132, 1938.

Rein, C. R., & M. H. Feldman: A simple method for detecting syphilis in routine dental practice, J. A. D. A., 18:1203, 1935.

Shuttleworth, C. W. T.: Bacteriology in diagnosis, Brit. Dent. J., 75:150, 1943.

FUSOSPIROCHETAL INFECTIONS, METAL INTOXICATION AND INTOLERANCE

5

Fusospirochetal Infections

Fusospirochetal infections occur throughout the body. They can be divided into (1) extra-oral and (2) intra-oral.

EXTRA-ORAL

Fusospirochetal infections of the nares, conjunctivae and middle ear are rare. They result usually from self-inoculation or extension of oral infections. The dentist should take precautions during the treatment of oral fusospirochetal disease to minimize the possibility of conjunctival infections, especially if pressure sprays are used.

Upper Respiratory and Pulmonary

Tracheal, pharyngeal or bronchial involvement are also usually secondary to oral lesions. Oral fusospirochetal infections in patients with bronchiectasis or lung abscess should receive energetic local treatment in order to minimize the possibility of the spread of these organisms to the tracheobronchial tree or abscess cavity. General anesthesia should not be given to patients with oral fusospirochetal disease. Secondary fusospirochetal infections of lung abscesses or tuberculous cavities produce a particularly foul odor. Such complications are more easily prevented than cured.

Genitalia

Lesions of the external genitalia associated with the fusospirochetal symbiosis are usually auto-inoculated or the result of perverted sexual practices although some authorities claim that smegma normally contains spirochetes. In the male, the prepuce or foreskin is a common site of the lesion—fusospirochetal balanitis. Phagadenic ulcerations of the penis, seen by von Ham in the tropics, are an example of fusospirochetal infection. The clinical appearance of these lesions and the subjective symptoms are similar to the oral lesions. These are best treated with non-caustic topical medicaments. Vulval lesions associated with oral fusospirochetal infections have been reported by Cleveland & Hanestein and McDonagh. These vulval lesions must not be confused with the periodic vulval ulcerations which occur at times during the menses.

Intestinal and blood stream infections with these organisms are rare. Larson & Barron reported a case of Vincent's stomatitis and osteomyelitis with a positive blood culture for the *Fusiformis fusiformis*. Williams reported 2 cases of arthritis in which the *F. fusiformis* and *Borrelia vincentii* were both recovered from the blood stream as many as 11 times. One patient was edentulous and did not exhibit the typical oral lesions. Fusospirochetal organisms were not found in the urine, stools or urethral discharge by culture or by dark-field examination. The source of the infection was considered to be the tonsils in one instance and a rat bite in the other. Fusospirochetal infections of the brain, heart and viscera have been reported.

Human Bite Wounds (*Morsus humanus*)

All wounds produced by human teeth are potentially dangerous and result frequently in serious infections in which the *Bor. vincentii* and *F. fusiformis* are believed to play an important role. The incidence of infection following human bites is roughly related to the cleanliness of the teeth producing the wound.

Human bites may be inflicted intentionally but more frequently they occur accidentally. During fights it is not uncommon for the clenched fist to be lacerated by the adversary's teeth. These wounds are especially dangerous, as following the injury, the parts relax and the infection is carried deep into the tissue and the tendon spaces where conditions are favorable for the growth of anaerobes.

The dentist may receive wounds caused by human teeth during the administration of general anesthesia or when an instrument slips. The mental or epileptic patient and the incorrigible child are other sources of tooth-inflicted wounds in dental practice. No one method of treatment has given uniformly good results. Sulfanilamide locally and by mouth has been used. Zinc peroxide should be effective if access can be gained to the wound and intravenous arsphenamine should be tried. Radical surgical treatment may be necessary.

INTRA-ORAL: ACUTE FUSOSPIROCHETAL STOMATITIS

Oral fusospirochetal infections may present a variety of clinical forms varying from the acute, in which ulcerations or membranous lesions may predominate to the chronic forms where actual hypertrophic changes are often seen. The infection may be generalized or localized to certain areas of the mouth.

Terminology

The terms oral fusospirochetosis, Vincent's infection, Plaut-Vincent's disease, trench mouth, phagedenic stomatitis, necrotic stomatitis (gingivitis) or ulceromembranous stomatitis, have been employed to designate this disease entity. The term fusospirochetal stomatitis (or gingivitis) is preferable, as it indicates the supposed etiology and the inflammatory nature of the disease. It is more specific than necrotic or ulceromembranous gingivitis which might be used correctly in describing a wide variety of oral lesions. Oral fusospirochetosis, while acceptable, does not convey an accurate impression of the pathosis which is characterized by a local inflammatory reaction with ulceration. The terms Vincent's infection and trench mouth should be avoided as patients frequently consider these "diseases" a reflection on their social and personal habits.

Incidence

Fusospirochetal infections of the mouth occur in epidemic but more often endemic or sporadic forms. In the San Luis Valley (Colorado) epidemic in 1932 approximately 40% of the 9,404 individuals examined had positive clinical and laboratory findings. Endemic outbreaks are common in jails, asylums, orphanages, army encampments, on board ship, among hospital staffs and student groups. The incidence of oral fusospirochetal infections is related to social customs, nutritional factors, general physical status and oral hygiene of the individual. The disease is most common in adolescents and young adults. The element of fatigue and emotional stress must also play a causative role. It is likely to be high during and after school vacation periods. This may be related to insufficient rest, inadequate nutrition, the increased consumption of alcoholic beverages or indiscriminate kissing.

Oral fusospirochetal diseases may develop, however, in individuals who have excellent oral hygiene as well as in those who do not smoke. Clinical and bacteriologic studies of above-average young women were made to determine the prevalence of the infection. Numerous spirochetes and fusiform bacilli were found in 139 of the 462 mouths studied. Mild but definite clinical symptoms were observed in 113 of the positive smear group and two had typical acute fusospirochetal stomatitis.

Oral fusospirochetal infections are believed to be transmitted by direct contact, through salivary droplets, by means of contaminated eating, cooking, or drinking utensils, by kissing, by toilet articles, or through infected dishwater.

Etiology

The etiologic agents responsible for oral fusospirochetal infections are outlined below. The predisposing factors in most cases appear to be of major importance in determining the clinical onset of the disease.

(1) Exciting.
  (a) *Borrelia vincentii* (Vincent's spirochete).
  (b) *Fusiformis dentium* (Fusiform bacillus).
  (c) Other oral flora.
(2) Predisposing causes.
  (a) Local.
    (1) Erupting or malposed teeth—associated gum flaps.
    (2) Poor dentistry in the form of overhanging gingival margins of fillings, ill-fitting crowns or prosthetic appliances. Poor or inadequate contact points due to caries or faulty restorations.
    (3) Areas of traumatic occlusion, local areas of poor oral hygiene, food impaction.
    (4) Local interference with the nutrition of the marginal and interseptal gingiva due to calculus, orthodontic appliances or metallic deposits (Bi) in the tissues.
  (b) Systemic.
    (1) Vitamin deficiencies C and B complex.
    (2) Gastro-intestinal disturbances—intestinal hyperirritability, chronic gallbladder disease.
    (3) Chronic malnutrition.
    (4) Certain blood dyscrasias, leukemia, aplastic anemia.

The etiologic importance of the fusospirochetal organisms is questioned by some since these organisms are frequently found in small numbers in "normal" mouths. Pneumococci are frequently recovered from the throat without clinical evidence of pneumonia and yet we recognize their etiologic role in certain types of pneumonia. Many ulcerative lesions of the mouth such as the decubital ulcerations secondary to ill-fitting dentures, severe allergic reactions, oral aphthae and many times the ulcerations associated with malignant neutropenia contain few oral spirochetal forms. The fusospirillary organisms are present in such overwhelming numbers in fusospirochetal infections of the mouth and ears, lungs and the external genitalia that it is difficult to explain their preponderance on any other basis.

The *F. fusiformis* is a non-motile, cigar-shaped, straight or slightly curved organism about the same length as the diameter of a red blood cell. It stains readily with carbolfuchsin and when a double staining technic with methylene blue is used a barred or beaded appearance is frequently observed.

The *Bor. vincentii* is longer than the *F. fusiformis,* being 12-15 μ in length, or about twice the diameter of the red blood cell. They have from 4 to 8 coils in contrast to the 10 to 20 turns exhibited by the *Tr. pallidum.* In dark field preparations, the *S. vincenti* moves with a snake-like lashing motion in contrast to the corkscrew undulation of the *Tr. pallidum.* The *Bor. vincentii* stains with ordinary aniline dyes. Vibrios, the other oral spirochetes and bacterial flora are probably of importance in the production of this disease.

Experimental Production of Fusospirochetal Infections

Many attempts have been made to produce this disease experimentally in the hope of obtaining more definite knowledge concerning its etiology, pathosis and treatment. Vincent and Tunnicliffe were unable to produce the disease in animals. Lichtenburg found that healthy guinea pigs had no spirochetal organisms in their mouths but if these animals were anesthetized and the gums were lacerated, 14 days later typical Vincent's organisms could be demonstrated by means of smears. Kline produced gangrene in guinea pigs following the injection of material from patients with Vincent's infection. Rosenthal has found that the saliva from a healthy mammal (except man) stops the motility of the spirochetes. Rosebury demonstrated conclusively that the oral fusospirochetal organisms were the causative agents of pulmonary gangrene. He also found that if tissue injury was produced when the inoculations were made in the groins of animals, typical abscesses and gangrene resulted. Experimental oral lesions were produced when there was tissue injury in addition to the inoculum. Goldman presented experimental evidence (monkey) that Vincent's infection may not be a contagious disease but a manifestation of a dietary disease with the fusospirochetal flora superimposed.

Contagious Nature of the Disease

Under experimental conditions the disease is not particularly contagious. Diseased dogs have been permitted to run in the same room with healthy animals and to eat from the same pan. The healthy animals did not develop the infection. Swabs from the gingival pockets of infected animals were inserted beneath the gingival margins of healthy dogs also with negative results. Grossman and Schwartzman could not transmit experimentally the disease in children and they concluded that it was not contagious. The British and American navies have observed that when facilities are not available for the sterilization of the mess utensils the incidence of "Vincent's" is high. This was also noted in World War I. It is believed that the disease is transmitted by contaminated water which is used for dishwashing. The public health authorities of 20 states require the reporting of cases.

Endemics in fraternity and boarding houses, private and public schools furnish abundant clinical evidence of its contagiousness. The author has seen numerous instances where one and then other members of a family have contracted the disease.

Pathogenesis

While some authorities state that the presence of teeth is a requisite for the development of the oral lesion, this view does not seem logical. Vincent's angina has been noted in infants before the eruption of any teeth and on 2 occasions the disease has been described in the edentulous adult. Gootzeit and Rosenthal have demonstrated these organisms in the edentulous mouths of adults. A break in any mucous membrane, or skin, where favorable growth conditions exist can serve as an initial site for the development of the disease.

A local irritation alone or in combination with some systemic predisposing factor may lower the resistance of the marginal gingiva or interdental papilla sufficiently for a slight erosion to develop. In these areas of damaged tissue the fusospirochetal organisms become implanted. The small ulcer which develops rapidly is surrounded by a zone of coccal and fusiform organisms. Polymorphonuclear leukocytes are few in number in the region of the lesions. Deeper within the tissues are observed the spirochetal forms which are considered by many the aggressive organism.

Subjective Symptoms

In an acute infection, local pain is an outstanding and universal symptom. It may prevent the maintenance of the usual oral hygiene, the chewing of food and normal rest. Even speaking, the passage of cold air or food over the affected tissues is painful. The slightest pressure on the ulcerated areas is exquisitely painful—an important diagnostic sign. The patient complains of an intense burning of the oral tissues. Sialorrhea is an early and constant symptom and when marked it may cause the patient much discomfort. The saliva is frequently bloody from the bleeding ulcerations. Spontaneous hemorrhages are observed frequently in children, often during sleep as is evidenced by blood on the pillow. Regional adenopathy may be present.

A metallic taste and a foul odor are also characteristic symptoms of acute infections. The taste is described as similar to that resulting from the action of weak acids on copper or brass. The odor, while difficult to describe, is readily recognized after it is once experienced. There is a loss of taste sensation. The teeth are frequently elongated, sensitive to pressure and slightly mobile. The patient at times complains of a "woody" sensation of the teeth resulting from periodontal membrane involvement.

The general subjective symptoms are variable. The patient complains sometimes of weakness. This is due partly to the infection and to the lowered food intake due to the inflamed oral tissues. It may be impossible to eat solid foods, and citrus fruits or their juices are irritating and painful because of their acidity. The patient observes that the usual pleasure is not derived from smoking.

Constitutional symptoms are usually insignificant in adults, but they are more common and more severe in children; occasionally, however, adults are markedly prostrated and require hospitalization. In severe conditions where there is pharyngeal involvement there may be difficulty in swallowing. Headache, mild back and joint pains and general malaise are common. In children, temperatures of 103° F. are not unusual and temperatures of even 104° F. have been reported in adults, but since most of these cases terminated fatally the hyperpyrexia may have been due to secondary factors. The elevation of the pulse rate out of proportion to the temperature is said to indicate the toxic nature of the disease.

Objective Symptoms

The ulcerative and membranous lesions are the characteristic objective findings. The typical fusospirochetal ulcerations appear as small punched-out lesions that develop first on the interdental papilla or the marginal gingiva. At times all that remains of the interdental papilla is a small triangular-shaped mass of necrotic tissue. Acute pain and bleeding result from the slightest pressure on these areas.

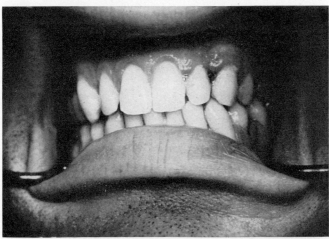

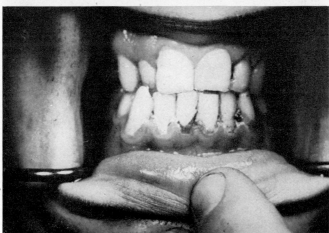

FIG. 17 (*Top*). Early fusospirochetal lesions of the interdental papillae between the maxillary left second incisor and canine and the mandibular left premolars. Note the good oral hygiene in this patient.

FIG. 18 (*Bottom*). Acute fusospirochetal gingivitis with necrosis of the interdental papillae between the mandibular left second incisor and canine teeth with ulceration and pseudomembrane formation on the labial marginal gingivae.

In severe cases, the ulcerations are found on the palate, on the inner surfaces of the cheeks and lips. The palatal ulcerations develop by direct extension of the gingival lesions while buccal and labial lesions result from contact of these tissues with the gingival ulcerations.

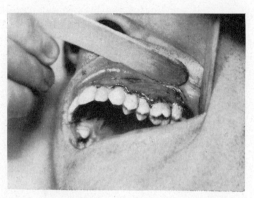

FIG. 19. Gingival lesions in acute fuso-spirochetal gingivostomatitis.

In acute cases, a yellowish or grayish white pseudomembrane is present. It is removed with comparative ease, leaving a cup-shaped bright red ulceration which bleeds readily. This punched-out appearance of the ulceration is particularly noticeable on the interdental papillae and the palate. If the

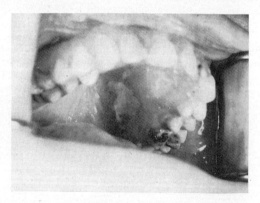

FIG. 20. Palatal extension of the gingival lesions in a patient with fusospirochetal gingivitis.

ulcerative process continues, as it may in untreated cases, the alveolar process becomes exposed and the teeth and bone are sequestrated.

When hemorrhage is a prominent symptom, the mucous membrane and the teeth are stained a deep brown from the decomposing blood. The tongue is usually coated due to neglected oral hygiene or therapy with oxidizing agents. The contact ulcers which develop occasionally on the tongue are exquisitely painful. The saliva is thick, viscid and increased in amount. The salivary glands are often sore and painful. Fusospirochetal infections limited

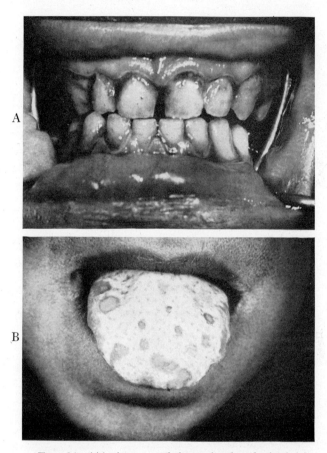

Fig. 21. (A) Acute oral fusospirochetal gingivitis in a 12-year-old girl. Note the loss of the interdental papillae and the pseudomembrane on the marginal gingivae. The tooth discoloration is due to the gingival hemorrhage. (B) Fusospirochetal ulcerations of the tongue in the same patient. The tongue lesions, which were very painful, responded rapidly to the topical application of 10% sodium carbonate.

to the salivary glands have also been reported. A heavy, foul odor is associated with all fusospirochetal infection or cultures of these organisms. It is so characteristic that, once experienced, it is rarely mistaken. Prinz believes that it is the outstanding symptom of the acute oral fusospirochetosis.

In all cases of oral fusospirochetal infection the tonsils should be carefully examined for lesions which may serve as a primary incubation zone. If present, both sites of the disease must be treated simultaneously. The regional lymph nodes are usually enlarged, if not visibly so, at least palpably. The lymphadenopathy is variable, depending on the individual, the severity

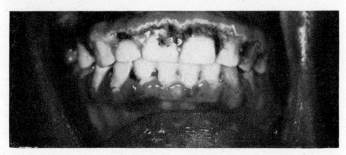

FIG. 22. Acute necrotizing fusospirochetal gingivitis of approximately eight hours' duration.

of the disease and amount of secondary infection. Adenopathy is common in children and in cases of circumcoronal infections about erupting third molars.

Laboratory Diagnostic Aids

Bacteriologic Smear. The diagnosis of fusospirochetal infection should not be made on the basis of the smear alone. It is a confirmatory finding for the experienced clinician and a valuable diagnostic aid to the less experienced. It is most useful in the diagnosis of the subacute and chronic forms

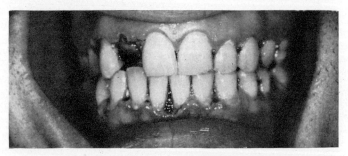

FIG. 23. Acute fusospirochetal gingivitis about the maxillary teeth following fracture of the right maxillary second incisor. The destruction of the interdental papillae in the mandibular incisor region is a typical finding in chronic fusospirochetal infections.

of the disease and it furnishes important information as to the effectiveness of treatment. Fine has shown that the accuracy of diagnosis based on smears alone may be as high as 88%. The material for the smear must be taken from the interdental ulcerated areas, the gum tissue adjacent to erupting teeth or other primary incubation zones. The technic for taking and staining the smear is given in the chapter on Laboratory Procedures.

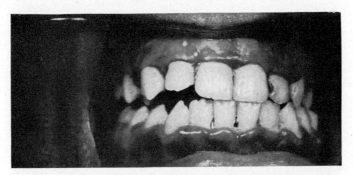

FIG. 24. Chronic fusospirochetal gingivitis with destruction of the interdental papillae and hypertrophy of the marginal gingivae. This form of fusospirochetal gingivitis is too frequently unrecognized.

If the dentist does not interpret the smear, he should be certain that the laboratory performing this service knows the criteria of a positive smear for this disease. The finding of an occasional fusospirochetal organism is of little significance; they must be present in overwhelming numbers.

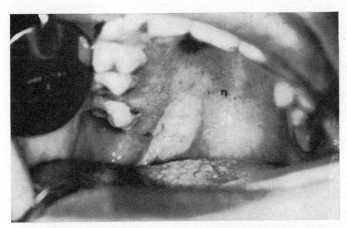

FIG. 25. Palatal ulceration in a patient with fusospirochetal gingivitis. This ulcer started originally as an extension of a lesion of the palatal marginal gingiva about the upper right second molar.

The blood count is of little positive value in the diagnosis of fusospirochetal infections. It will aid in eliminating those diseases whose oral lesions might be confused with fusospirochetal ulcerations, i.e., malignant neutropenia, the leukemias and aplastic anemia.

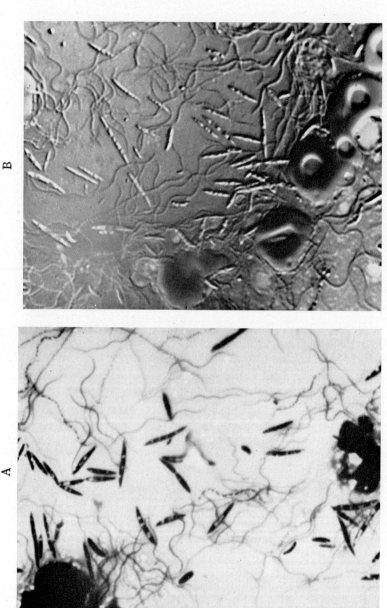

FIG. 26 (A) Typical smear findings in acute fusospirochetal stomatitis. Note the predominance of the oral spirochetes and fusiform bacilli. (B) Smear findings in acute fusospirochetal infection. Photomicrograph taken with dimensional lighting. (Photomicrographs by Wardlaw M. Hammond, Research Associate in Micrography, School of Dentistry, University of Pennsylvania.)

The hemogram in acute fusospirochetal infections fails to show an alteration in keeping with the clinical nature of the lesions and the subjective symptoms. Tarnow observed a leukocytosis of from 8,000 to 14,000 cells cu. mm., with a relative increase in the percentage of lymphocytes and mononuclears. Bryant reported that the total and absolute count findings in 22 cases were essentially within normal values. Stine believed that the blood picture is of no help in making a diagnosis of Vincent's infection, and, in fact, may be confusing in that it suggests the possibility of other conditions which might produce ulcerative lesions. In one of his cases the blood count was 40,000 leukocytes cu. mm. with 81.5% lymphocytes and in another it was 3,744 leukocytes cu. mm. with 27% neutrophiles.

A complete blood count should be done in all cases of acute ulcerative lesions of the mouth if (1) there is any doubt that the condition is a fusospirochetal infection or (2) if the lesions fail to respond promptly to local treatment. Any case of ulcerative stomatitis that fails to respond to the usual treatment within 3 to 4 days should have a hemogram and other laboratory studies that may be indicated.

The hemograms of 110 patients being treated for fusospirochetal infections in the Oral Medicine Clinic were studied. The total leukocyte counts varied from 2,900 to 16,000 cells cu. mm. with 78% of the counts falling within the normal range of 5,000 to 10,000 cells cu. mm. The absolute neutrophile and lymphocyte cell counts of this group of patients and 110 patients with periodontal disease were studied. Thirty of the absolute lymphocyte counts as compared to 25 in the periodontal group, were not in the generally accepted range of values. Twenty-two of the 30 absolute lymphocyte counts in the periodontal patients and 21 of the absolute lymphocyte counts in the periodontal groups were above the generally accepted range of values.

These findings do not indicate that a relative lymphocytosis is a common feature of fusospirochetal disease; however, when abnormal absolute lymphocyte counts are obtained, they are usually above the normal range of values.

THE WASSERMANN REACTION. The Wassermann reaction or other serologic tests for syphilis are negative in oral fusospirochetal infections in the absence of syphilis or other conditions which might give a positive reaction.

URINALYSIS. In severe cases a slight albuminuria may be observed. This is the renal manifestation of the toxemia.

BLOOD CULTURE. The blood culture may be of value when the deeper tissues are involved. The difficulty of growing these organisms minimizes its importance.

Diagnosis

The sudden development of punched-out ulcerations on the marginal gingiva or the interdental papilla, the symptoms of acute pain and hemorrhage from slight pressure on these lesions, sialorrhea, and a metallic taste and the characteristic foul odor of the breath in a patient with comparatively mild systemic symptoms should suggest a clinical diagnosis of oral fusospirochetal disease. The clinical impressions should be corroborated by a bacteriologic smear. In chronic infections, where clinical symptoms are less striking, the disease is often unrecognized unless smears are routine.

Differential Diagnosis

The conditions most likely to be confused with fusospirochetal infections are herpetic and streptococcal stomatitis, the oral lesions of malignant neutropenia (agranulocytosis) leukemia, diphtheria, syphilis and tuberculosis.

Malignant Neutropenia. The sudden onset and the similar clinical appearance of the lesions of malignant neutropenia and fusospirochetal infections may present problems in diagnosis. In malignant neutropenia the ulcerations do not elicit an acute inflammatory response and they are usually less painful. They have frequently a greenish black base which is not found in fusospirochetal ulcerations.

Herpetic Stomatitis. Oral herpetic lesions involve primarily the smooth mucosal surfaces and rarely the gingival tissues. The vesicle stage is extremely transitory and the lesion has a slightly dull yellowish appearance which can be readily differentiated from the punched-out painful ulcerations of fusospirochetal disease.

Streptococcal stomatitis and staphylococcal stomatitis are rare. The diffuse involvement of the marginal and alveolar gingivae in these diseases with the absence of ulcerative lesions at the marginal gingivae and interdental papillae will enable a clinical differentiation.

Acute Syphilis. The mucous patches of acute syphilis may be confused with fusospirochetal stomatitis; however, the former occur rarely on the marginal gingivae and the interdental papillae. The mucous patches have a translucent raised appearance and are less painful. A Wassermann reaction will assist in the diagnosis.

Diphtheritic lesions of the pharyngeal and tonsillar region may be confused with fusospirochetal ulcerations. The patient with diphtheria presents more severe toxic constitutional symptoms. The diphtheritic membrane is tougher and harder to remove, having a tendency to tear rather than lift away. Suggestive evidence of a diphtheritic infection can be obtained on the basis of bacterial smears and verified by culture on Loeffler's medium.

It must be emphasized that uncommon oral lesions, many times secondary to serious general disease, are frequently first diagnosed as oral fusospirochetal infections. The dentist and the physician both should be critical of their diagnosis of oral fusospirochetal infections.

Treatment

The treatment of oral fusospirochetal infections is directed towards eliminating the painful subjective symptoms and the predisposing causes of the disease. Surgical procedures are definitely contraindicated in the acute bacterial phase of the infection. Since dental operations are required in most cases to eliminate some of the predisposing causes of the disease, the treatment of this infection falls naturally and correctly to the dentist. The use of arsenicals alone only ameliorates the subjective symptoms without eliminating the predisposing causes. This results in frequent recurrences or the persistence of a chronic infection which often results in considerable tissue destruction and which may lead to more serious periodontal diseases. When the deeper structures are affected, intravenous therapy may be desirable and beneficial. It should be administered only by the physician.

Objectives. The general objectives in the treatment of oral fusospirochetal infections are (1) the reduction of the numbers and possibly the virulence of the oral bacteria through mechanical means such as mouth washes, douches and topical medication, (2) the elimination or correction of as many of the local and general predisposing factors as is possible and (3) measures taken to increase local and general tissue resistance. The procedures discussed under (1) relieve the acute subjective symptoms, while those discussed in (2) and (3) are more important for the actual control and successful elimination of the infection.

General Recommendations. In acute infections, several general measures are recommended. Rest, preferably in bed, is desirable and beneficial. A mild saline cathartic can be administered. The diet should be semi-solid, bland, nutritious and contain an abundance of "protective" foods and citrus fruits. If the citrus fruits cause undue pain, the synthetic vitamin C may be administered (300-500 mg. per day). While a high vitamin C diet has no specific curative effect, it seems to augment the usual treatment, probably by its beneficial effect on wound healing.

Nicotinic acid has been reported as being almost specific for the treatment of fusospirochetal infections. The most favorable results have been noted by King. Nicotinic acid in large doses, 1,000 mg. per day, have been ineffective in our experience in controlling or treating effectively the fusospirochetal infections which are not secondary to a nutritional deficiency. Miller *et al.* reported unsatisfactory results when this disease was treated only with nicotinic acid. Goldberg & Thorp's nicotinic acid excretion studies, made on patients with acute fusospirochetal disease, revealed no evidence of a nicotinic acid deficiency or an increased requirement of this component of the vitamin B complex. Administration of the entire vitamin B complex during the acute phases of the infection is a desirable form of systemic therapy, but as a specific curative measure it is ineffective.

If the fusospirochetal infection is secondary to heavy metal therapy, such as bismuth injections, the injections should be stopped during the early stages of treatment. Smoking and alcoholic beverages are strictly prohibited. If the patient refuses to co-operate in this respect, treatment will rarely be more than moderately satisfactory. Highly spiced and seasoned foods should be avoided.

The general recommendations which are given routinely to the patients in the Oral Medicine Clinic follow:

Fusospirochetal stomatitis (Vincent's infection) is a serious disease. Its successful and rapid cure requires your strict co-operation. Failure to cure the acute disease may result in permanent destruction of the gum tissue and even the jaw bones.

INSTRUCTIONS FOR PERSONAL CARE

(1) Body rest is important in controlling the disease. Rest as much as possible, preferably in bed.
(2) Take a saline cathartic such as citrate of magnesium or Epsom Salts. Repeat if necessary to keep your bowels open.
(3) *Smoking and alcohol* in any form *are strictly prohibited*. Do not brush your teeth until advised.
(4) *Fusospirochetal gingivitis is contagious*. You should use separate eating utensils, glasses, toilet articles and handkerchiefs during the acute stage. Avoid kissing.
(5) Do not eat coarse rough foods, hot or highly spiced food. Eat a soft diet containing an abundance of milk, eggs, fruits (especially citrus fruits), fresh green vegetables, meat soups or chopped meats.
(6) Use the mouth wash as directed, forcing the liquid between the teeth. Use the entire glass, and mix freshly each time.
(7) The disappearance of the acute symptoms such as pain and bleeding does not mean you are cured. Failure to receive complete treatment will result in recurrence of the disease and other complications.

ORAL MEDICINE DEPARTMENT
PERIODONTIC SECTION
DENTAL SCHOOL
UNIVERSITY OF PENNSYLVANIA

Local Treatment. All surgical procedures and subgingival curettage are contraindicated in acute infections, although obvious sources of irritation such as supragingival calculus should be eliminated, provided this can be accomplished without trauma to the inflamed tissues. The accumulated necrotic material and debris should be removed by means of large cotton swabs moistened with hydrogen peroxide or normal saline solution. Small cotton applicators similarly moistened are required to remove the necrotic tissue from the interdental spaces. Avoid tissue trauma.

The importance of thorough mouth irrigation cannot be overemphasized for office, hospital or home care. The heat and mechanical action of the irrigating solution are more important than its composition. Normal saline is effective, inexpensive and can be easily prepared. Half-strength hydrogen peroxide is also efficacious. The irrigations can be accomplished by using a pressure spray, or a fountain syringe with a glass medicine dropper at the end of the rubber tubing. The syringe is fastened about two feet above the level of the head as it is inclined over a basin. Two quarts of hot solution (120° F.) are used for each irrigation and special attention is given to flushing the interdental areas and beneath the flaps of erupting teeth. If mouth irrigation is impossible or impractical, satisfactory results can be obtained by means of effective mouth washing.

TOPICAL MEDICATION. Hundreds of drugs have been advocated for the treatment of oral fusospirochetal infections with no critical means of evaluating their effectiveness. Rosenthal devised a novel method of determining the antibacterial efficiency of the various medicaments, which closely simulates the conditions under which they are used in the mouth.

The effectiveness of the medicaments was determined by their ability to cause cessation of motility of the oral spirochetes, vibrios and bacilli and by their ability to produce negative subcultures of the treated salivary specimen at the end of fifteen minutes' contact. The results obtained with the commonly used medicaments are shown in Table IX.

TABLE IX

EFFECT OF MEDICAMENTS ON ORAL FLORA
(Method and Results Reported by Rosenthal)

	Spirochetes	Vibrios	Bacilli	Rosenow Brain Broth	Blood Agar	Blood Agar Anaerobic
				Subcultures		
Chromic acid............	5	2	2	+	+	+
Sod. perborate sat.	15	15	15	+	+	+
H₂O₂ 3%..............	15	15	15	+	+	+
Lugol's solution........	contact	contact	contact	0	0	0
Acriviolet 1%..........	4½	10	10	+	+	+
Mercurochrome 2%......	15	15	15	+	+	+
Tr. metaphen untinted...	contact	contact	contact	0	0	0
Mercuric cyanide 1%....	3½	9	15	+	+	+
Arsphenamine 10%......	contact	contact	contact	0	few	few
Arsphenamine in glycerine	5-15	8-15	15	+	+	+
Sulfathiazole 15%.......	15	15	15	+	+	+
Zephirin..............	contact	contact	contact	0	0	0
Sodium carbonate 10%...	contact	contact	contact	0	0	0
Eugenol..............	contact	contact	contact	0	0	0
Surgical pack..........	....	....	....	reduction	reduction	reduction
Penicillin..............	Variable results. This antibiotic cannot be accurately tested by this method.					

H_2O_2 3%

Figures represent the time required for loss of motility in minutes. Contact—instant loss of motility. Organisms still motile at the end of 15 minutes are marked 15. All solutions are aqueous unless otherwise noted.

$$0 = \text{no growth} \brace + = \text{growth} \Big\} \text{non-motile organisms.}$$

These results should indicate more accurately the therapeutic effectiveness of these drugs in clinical use where saliva, mucin and cellular debris are present than the more widely used phenol or Rideal-Walker coefficient.

The various medicaments can be conveniently grouped as follows: (Those starred (*) are preferred by the author.)

OXYGEN LIBERATING AGENTS
** Zinc peroxide
 * Hydrogen peroxide
   Sodium perborate
   Potassium chlorate
   Potassium permanganate

MERCURIAL DERIVATIVES
** Tinct. Metaphen 1:200 (untinted)
 * Mercuric cyanide 1%
   Merthiolate 1:1,000
   Mercuric chloride 1:2,000

SPIROCHETOCIDES (ORAL)
** Sodium carbonate 10% aqueous
 * Arsphenamine 10% aqueous
 * Marpharsen
   Neoarsphenamine
   Fuadin

ESCHAROTICS (CAUSTICS)
 * Copper sulfate and zinc chloride
 * Chromic acid 8% *caution!*
 * Negatan
   ZnCl₂ 8%
   Phenol 95%
   Trichloracetic acid 50%
   Iodine 16.5% and silver nitrate 35%

ANILINE DYES
** Viogen (Berwick's solution)
 * Acriviolet 1%
   Gentian violet 1%
   Acriflavine 1%
   Methylene blue 1%

OTHER AGENTS
 * Surgical pack (zinc oxide —resin, eugenol)
 * Copper sulfate, phenol, glycerine and water
   Sulfonamides in paraffin —especially sulfadiazine
   Vitamins—B and C
** Penicillin—topically

Oxygen Liberating Agents. Oxygen liberating agents are used on the theory that the nascent oxygen liberated will prevent the growth of anaerobic organisms. The fusospirochetal organisms are facultative microaerobes and they will maintain their motility after 15 minutes' contact with a concentrated sodium perborate solution. The favorable clinical response following the use of oxygen liberating agents may be due to the minute mechanical cleansing action of the liberated oxygen on the ulcerated areas.

Zinc peroxide was introduced by Meleney in 1936 for the treatment of gangrenous lesions of the oral cavity and the neck region. This substance in an activated or inactivated form will relieve the pain of fusospirochetal ulcerations. Its action is believed due to the slow liberation of nascent oxygen over a period of 24 to 36 hours. A zinc peroxide-water paste is an ideal preparation for office treatment and it may be safely prescribed for home use. It is effective for the relief of pain, it reduces the bacterial flora and it practically eliminates the odor. Burns or undesirable reactions have not been experienced or reported. Zinc peroxide should be dispensed only by prescription.

Hydrogen peroxide (3%) is also a good oxygen liberating agent. Half-strength hydrogen peroxide can be safely recommended as a mouth wash or irrigating solution for home use. Only fresh peroxide which has been dispensed in a tightly stoppered colored bottle should be used. Hydrogen peroxide has the disadvantage of being acid with a pH of 3.5 in the 3% solution.

Sodium perborate ($Na_2B_4O_7$) has been extensively exploited for the treatment of this infection. The public has been given the erroneous impression that the infection can be adequately treated at home by mouth washes and gargles. Chemical burns result frequently when strong solutions and pastes of these substances are used. These burns are extremely painful, they are often extensive in nature and they require precedence in treatment. Sodium perborate should not be recommended for home treatment.

Patients using oxygen liberating agents, and sodium perborate in particular, occasionally develop a black hairy tongue due to the irritation, hypertrophy and staining of the filiform papillae. These "hairs" can frequently be parted with a tongue depressor, and in extreme cases they touch the soft palate and cause gagging. This complication usually disappears spontaneously when the oxidizing agent is stopped.

Escharotic Agents (Caustics). Any caustic will cause some necrosis of the surface tissues, which furnishes an excellent site for the growth of the anaerobic bacteria including the fusospirochetal organisms. It is said by some that caustics tend to "fix" the organisms in the tissues and thereby prevent further damage. The careless or indiscriminate use of caustics results frequently in more tissue destruction than the original infection. Eskow and Bernuan have shown that more tissue destruction occurs when 5% chromic acid was used than when non-caustic medicaments were used in the treatment of this infection.

Five per cent chromic acid is a widely used caustic. If used, it should be applied by means of a glass applicator, platinum loop or college pliers on the areas of ulceration. The tissues should then be covered with a layer of cotton or gauze for five to ten minutes, after which the mouth is washed with warm water. Another widely used preparation is a 16.5% aqueous solution of iodine which is followed immediately by a 10% solution of silver nitrate. This produces a yellow precipitate of silver iodide which is allowed to remain in place several minutes and is then washed off.

Chromic acid, or any other caustic, should not be applied more often than once a day and never for more than two or three visits. Negatan, a phenol derivative, is a useful mild caustic which has little action on the uninvolved mucosal tissues. It is effective in relieving the pain in acute infections. Other

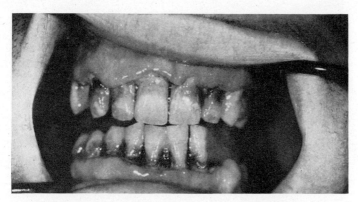

FIG. 27. Extensive loss of the interdental papillae and marginal gum tissue due to long standing fusospirochetal infection. The patient was originally treated with arsenicals (neoarsphenamine) which were administered intravenously. The acute subjective symptoms disappeared, but the disease persisted with tissue destruction.

caustics which have been used are 95% phenol, 35% silver nitrate and 50% trichloracetic acid.

The author is convinced that other medicaments are fully as effective as the caustics and they present none of the dangers associated with their use.

Copper sulfate powder and 8% zinc chloride are properly considered as astringents and fungicides (copper sulfate). A paste of these ingredients is effective when carefully worked into the gingival crevice and interdental spaces. This remedy is not well tolerated in acute infections, but it is particularly effective in the stage of this disease where some gingival edema is present and where, as Francis has shown, a secondary fungus infection may be delaying complete recovery. The emetic action of copper sulfate must be borne in mind.

Mercurial Derivatives. Various mercurial derivatives are effective in the treatment of the acute and chronic stages of this infection. Tincture of Metaphen 1:200 (untinted) is excellent. It has low surface tension, it is practically colorless, and it has been shown by Abel & Clark to have little if any irritant action on the mucosal tissues. Tincture Merthiolate 1:1000 is also effective. Mercuric cyanide 1% has been suggested by Corby and was used with good results in World War I.

Aniline Dyes. While the aniline dyes fail to relieve the pain of the acute infection, they can be utilized advantageously in the treatment of chronic infections when an attempt is made to eliminate the bacteria in the deeper portions of the tissue. They are also good fungicides. One per cent aqueous acriviolet is effective against both Gram (+) and Gram (−) organisms. Berwick recommends the use of the following:

Brilliant green	1.0 Gm.
Crystal violet	1.0 Gm.
Alcohol (ethyl)	50.0 cc.
Water	50.0 cc.

The chief disadvantage of the dyes is their staining property, although with care in application little discoloration of the lips will result. The dyes will readily discolor the usual dental cements and silicates and it is advisable to apply petrolatum or cocoa butter over silicate fillings before application.

Spirochetocides (Oral). The intravenous use of the arsenicals has been discussed previously. The concentration of intravenously administered drugs in the superficial tissues is insufficient to be of value. Since oral fusospirochetal infections develop frequently in individuals who are under intensive treatment for syphilis, it would seem unwise to employ arsphenamine or neoarsphenamine for the treatment of oral fusospirochetal disease in such patients.

Ten per cent sodium carbonate is an excellent topical spirochetocide for the treatment of acute fusospirochetal stomatitis and if carelessly applied it causes little if any tissue damage. This medicament is stable, safe, and effective. It has a pH of 9.5. For psychologic reasons the colorless solution should be tinted with q.s. liquid amaranth.

A 10% aqueous solution of arsphenamine is the best arsenical spirochetocide for topical application. Glucose solutions are more stable but slightly less effective, and those using glycerine have little application in the mouth where solvents of low surface tension are desired.

Other Agents. Fish uses zinc-oxide-eugenol packs or Ward's Surgical Pack for the treatment of oral fusospirochetal disease. After the necrotic tissue has been removed, a paste of these materials is packed in the involved interdental spaces or ulcerated areas and changed at intervals of several days. The author has found this type of treatment very effective, and when the infection is limited to a few teeth or one quadrant of the mouth, it is the method of choice. Spread of infection to additional areas has rarely been observed with this treatment. In extensive cases it requires more time than other methods.

The sulfonamides have been used in the treatment of oral fusospirochetal infections both topically and by allowing the tablets to dissolve slowly in the mouth. The few published reports on the use of sulfathiazole have been favorable, but in most instances this form of treatment has been used in cases of pharyngeal rather than gingival involvement and satisfactory controls have been lacking. Paraffin chewing blocks containing sulfathiazole and sulfadiazine have been used in the Oral Medicine Clinic and also by Gunter,

LaDow and Meloy.* In some cases it is felt that favorable clinical response resulted but in others this form of treatment was not superior if as good as the usual topical application of medicaments. This form of treatment at best can only serve to control the bacterial phase of the infection, dental prophylactic care, the elimination of dental predisposing causes of the infection, and the institution of a satisfactory oral hygiene regime still remain the more important phase of treatment for a permanent result.

The disappearance of pain is a reliable guide to improvement, but it should be considered as an indication that the disease is under control rather than cured. It is imperative that the patient still abstain from smoking and the use of alcoholic beverages. This fact cannot be overemphasized. The disappearance of the acute painful symptoms is an indication that the more important phases of treatment can now be undertaken. These include a thorough oral prophylaxis, the institution of a proper tooth brushing technic (gingival massage) and the correction of the local predisposing causes. Deficient contact points and their associated food impaction areas should be eliminated by the insertion of properly contoured fillings, and other examples of inadequate dentistry should be corrected. The occlusion should be equilibrated if

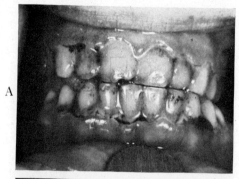
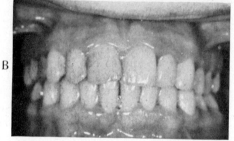

FIG. 28. Case of acute fusospirochetal gingivitis. (A) Before treatment and (B) ten days later. Non-caustic topical medicaments were used.

local areas of overfunction are detected which may serve as causes for repeated recurrences.

The value of home care and co-operation is extremely important. The suggested oral hygiene should be carefully followed by the patient. Interdental stimulation by any of a number of methods is an important aid in restoring the affected interdental papillae to a healthful state.

When Can a Patient with Fusospirochetal Infection Be Considered Cured?

Many recurrences of this disease result from the impression that the disappearance of the acute subjective symptoms means the disease is cured, rather than that the acute bacterial phase is under control. The regular exami-

* Sulfathiazole medicated gum has also been tried.

nation of bacterial smears will reveal a disappearance of the fusospirochetal forms and a return of the usual oral flora. The degree to which the fusospirochetal organisms can be eliminated, as determined by the bacterial smear findings, is dependent on the elimination of (1) all primary incubation zones, (2) the local and general predisposing causes of the infection and (3) the maintenance of a satisfactory oral hygiene regime by the patient.

The patient with a fusospirochetal infection should not be considered cured until (1) the clinical findings are satisfactory, (2) the smear findings on two successive examinations made at a week's interval are negative or contain very few fusospirochetal organisms, (3) the local predisposing factors—such

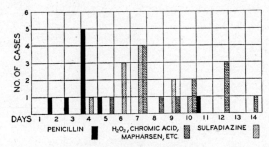

Fig. 29. Comparative therapeutic effect in Vincent's infection of (1) hydrogen peroxide, chromic acid, oxophenarsine hydrochloride and so on, and (2) penicillin. The ordinate indicates the number of cases. The abscissa indicates the days on which smears became negative for Vincent's organisma. (Jour. Amer. Med. Asso., 128:706-710, 1945.)

as unsatisfactory dentistry—have been corrected and (4) the dentist is assured that the patient is following the prescribed oral hygiene regime. The elimination of food impaction areas, local areas of occlusal overfunction, or the institution of interdental stimulation may result in negative smears from areas which had been previously positive. The two negative smear findings should be obtained in the absence of specific therapy and any restriction on the patient's personal habits. The local and general predisposing factors should always be corrected even when satisfactory clinical and smear findings are secured without such dental treatment.

Causes of Failure. Failure to cure the disease satisfactorily or prevent recurrences may be due to ineffective or incomplete professional treatment or the lack of adequate co-operation on the part of the patient. If recurrences occur an undiscovered oral focus of infection should be looked for, such as a periodontal pocket, a third molar gum flap, diseased tonsillar crypt, or an underlying systemic condition such as a subclinical nutritional deficiency or gallbladder disease. The dentist should check carefully whether the patient is following regularly and conscientiously the prescribed home treatment,

Prognosis. The prognosis in oral fusospirochetal infections is good, provided the predisposing causes of the disease can be eliminated and provided the patient co-operates with the proper home treatment. A varying amount of tissue destruction may be unavoidable.

"VINCENT'S" ANGINA

Vincent's (or fusospirochetal) angina should not be confused with fusospirochetal stomatitis. In the former, the ulcerative lesions are confined to the tonsillar or pharyngeal tissues. They tend to involve the deeper structures. Constitutional symptoms are usually more marked. Vincent's angina is a more serious disease than fusospirochetal stomatitis. In recurrent attacks of Vincent's angina the focus for the disease is frequently of oral origin beneath the gum flap of an erupting mandibular molar or a chronic fusospirochetal infection of an interdental papilla. The opposite is often the case, where an infected tonsillar crypt is the focus for a recurrent fusospirochetal stomatitis.

The treatment of Vincent's angina is in the province of the otolaryngologist. Where oral lesions are also present these must be treated simultaneously. Intravenous therapy is frequently beneficial. Shallenberger *et al.* compared the therapeutic results obtained with sodium perborate and hydrogen peroxide, chromic acid and silver nitrate, and oxophenarsine hydrochloride with sulfadiazine as lozenges and local penicillin therapy. The penicillin therapy consisted of swabbing the tissues 4 times daily with a solution containing 250 to 500 units penicillin cu. cm. They found that the penicillin therapy was more rapidly effective than the methods heretofore advocated.

NOMA OR CANCRUM ORIS

Noma connotes a rapidly spreading gangrene of the mucous membranes, or mucocutaneous orifices, such as the lips, the alae of the nose, the external auditory canal, the vulva, the prepuce or the anus. The oral cavity is the most frequent site of involvement and noma of this region is known as cancrum oris.

Cancrum oris is fortunately a rare disease. It occurs usually in children and in the aged. It is more common in the former and in females. Cancrum oris is a frequent and serious complication of kala-azar.

Cancrum oris is considered a malignant form of fusospirochetal infection. The usual oral streptococci and at times diphtheria organisms are recovered from the advanced lesions, but in the areas of beginning necrosis only the fusospirochetal organisms can be demonstrated in large numbers. It is believed by some that the fusospirochetal organisms producing cancrum oris are more virulent than in other forms of fusospirochetal infection. In certain instances, noma appears to be highly contagious. Five cases of noma occurred in a single ward, all beginning in the external auditory canal in which the same syringe had been used for irrigation. As in other fusospirochetal infections, the individual predisposing causes are important factors in the clinical development of the disease.

Since the predisposing causes and the clinical course of cancrum oris in children are different from those in the aged, they will be discussed separately. All forms of the disease have similar histopathologic findings.

In Children. Cancrum oris is uncommon in children who are in good physical condition. It may follow debilitating diseases such as measles, typhoid fever, scarlet fever, pertussis or severe malnutrition, and is frequently

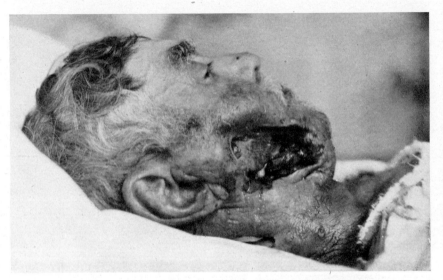

FIG. 30. Noma associated with an infection about the mandibular right second molar. (Case of Dr. Thos. W. Meloy, Philadelphia, Pa.)

found in institutionalized children. Jorge and Garcia reported an epidemic of measles in which 2% of the children developed cancrum oris with a 70% mortality in the affected group.

Cancrum oris may be preceded by a benign-appearing fusospirochetal infection of the oral cavity which is relatively unresponsive to treatment, or by other forms of stomatitis such as oral moniliasis. The pathologic findings in cancrum oris are similar to oral fusospirochetal stomatitis, except that it spreads more rapidly and there is no tendency for the disease to be self-limiting. In most cases, secondary infection supervenes, which hastens the progress of the lesion. In a few cases a line of demarcation develops, the slough separates and healing ensues with marked disfigurement of the parts.

SYMPTOMS. The foul odor of the breath is frequently the first symptom of the disease in young children. When the mouth is examined, a dark purplish red spot is seen on the cheek in the molar region along the interdental line or on the lip. Cancrum oris has also been reported in the edentulous infant. As the lesion progresses, it is accompanied by a marked swelling and brawny edema of the affected parts and the external tissues. The teeth are frequently exfoliated and the alveolar process destroyed. Perforation of the cheeks and lips is common, and since the disease is usually unilateral the extensive tissue slough and necrosis give the patient a horrid and grotesque appearance.

The disease is accompanied by a marked increase in salivary flow. When the lesion becomes secondarily infected, the odor is extremely offensive and it necessitates isolation of the patient. Pain is not severe and it may be entirely absent. The average duration of the disease is 5-10 days. Death is usually due to secondary infection, bronchopneumonia or lung abscess.

DIAGNOSIS. The extremely rapid extension of the necrotic process, the comparatively slight local and systemic reaction before secondary infection develops, when it occurs in a malnourished child or one recovering from a debilitating disease, are highly suggestive of a diagnosis of cancrum oris. The putrid odor is characteristic.

TREATMENT. The treatment of cancrum oris consists of isolation of the patient because of the unpleasant odor and the possible contagious nature of the disease. Treatment is directed towards increasing the general resistance of the patient, maintaining an adequate nutrition and local treatment of the gangrenous lesion. General supportive measures such as hypodermoclyses, transfusions and infusions are essential. Maintaining adequate nutrition is extremely difficult and at times impossible. This undoubtedly accounts in part for the unfavorable prognosis.

Radical surgical interference, such as extensive electrocoagulation of the lesion and the adjacent areas, has been advocated. McMillen has successfully treated 7 cases of cancrum oris with the application of 37% formalin to the gangrenous area. Zinc peroxide should be of particular value in the local treatment of the gangrenous process. Specific chemotherapeutic agents such as the sulfonamides or arsphenamine have not been reported. In view of the recent reports of the therapeutic effectiveness of sulfathiazole and sulfadiazine in the treatment of oral fusospirochetal infections, it should be tried in cases of noma. Penicillin should also be tried.

Cancrum oris in children carries a mortality of 75% to 85%, and those surviving usually have marked facial deformities that require plastic surgery.

In the Aged. Cancrum oris in adults is not uncommon in China where the general lack of oral hygiene, the prevalence of periodontal involvement and dietary deficiencies predispose to the disease. Here it is not so fulminating, the mortality is lower and many times recovery occurs without treatment although marked facial deformity results. It has been mentioned before that cancrum oris is the most frequent, characteristic and serious complication of kala-azar. The early and energetic treatment with potassium antimony tartrate, or similar agents, will largely prevent this complication.

In the United States cancrum oris occurs usually in old individuals who are debilitated by a chronic illness. A history of previous trauma at the site of the lesion, such as the extraction of a tooth, a blow on the face, or biting the cheek, is obtained frequently. In edentulous patients, the gums or the alveolar ridges may be involved first. In most instances these individuals have some chronic disease that affects directly or indirectly the cardiovascular system; i.e., chronic glomerulonephritis. There seems to be a close relation between vascular disease and the oral gangrene, since an ischemic dry gangrenous process usually precedes the more infectious state. The edentulous or near edentulous state of such individuals may affect the clinical course of the disease.

The treatment of cancrum oris in adults is similar to that described previously. It is usually unsatisfactory, due to the poor general resistance of the individual. The mortality is between 70% and 90%.

6

Oral Changes Associated with Intolerance to Metals and Other Elements

GENERAL CONSIDERATIONS	ARSENIC
BISMUTH	AURIC STOMATITIS
LEAD INTOXICATION	STOMATITIS DUE TO COPPER, CHRO-
MERCURIALISM	MIUM AND ZINC
FLUORINE INTOXICATION	RADIOACTIVE AGENTS
ARGYRIA	PHOSPHOROUS POISONING

GENERAL CONSIDERATIONS

Oral mucosal lesions secondary to metallic absorption or intoxication constitute an important group of diseases for the dentist. The first evidence of toxicity is frequently manifested in the mouth and in many of the metals the chief symptoms are confined to these tissues.

The predisposing causes of bismuth, lead and mercurial stomatitis are similar to those of fusospirochetal stomatitis. The absorption of these metals and the deposition of their salts in the gingival tissues interfere with the nutrition of the marginal gingiva and interdental papilla, permitting secondary invasion of the mouth bacteria, including the fusospirochetal organisms. In some instances the metallic salts are themselves irritating.

A discussion of many of the metallic stomatitides would fall logically under fusospirochetal disease, but for convenience the oral manifestations resulting from all forms of metallic absorption are presented as a group.

BISMUTH

Intolerance to bismuth may be manifested by an acute reaction resembling nitrite poisoning or an ulcerative stomatitis with pigmentation. A rarer form of stomatitis which follows occasionally the administration of a bismuth compound represents a drug idiosyncrasy.

Bismuth stomatitis constitutes the most important and frequent manifestation of general intolerance to this metal. It is important to differentiate between a bismuth line and bismuth stomatitis. Bismuth stomatitis can be regarded as a fusospirochetal infection secondary to impaired nutrition of the interdental papillae and marginal gingivae resulting from the bismuth deposits in these tissues. The same local factors which predispose to spirochetal infection predispose to the development of bismuth stomatitis.

Incidence

A bismuth line or stomatitis is common in individuals receiving bismuth preparations for long periods. It is doubtful whether anyone receiving intensive bismuth therapy for syphilis does not at some time manifest a bismuth line or evidence of bismuth intolerance in the mouth. The frequency of the various manifestations is determined largely by the oral hygiene habits of the particular individual.

Vigne observed bismuth intolerance in 202 out of 2,390 patients receiving anti-luetic therapy, with ulcerative stomatitis present in 72% of this group. Pigmentation of the oral mucosa was noted in 80% of 511 patients McCarthy examined. Nine per cent of these patients were edentulous. Goodman and Gilman state that "after two injections most patients show pigmentation of the soft palate and inner surface of the cheeks."

Bismuth stomatitis is more prevalent in males because of their general lack of good oral hygiene but it is not uncommon, even in severe form, in the female. Lueth has found that bismuth deposits rarely appear in children or in women during the second half of pregnancy as the skeletal system of the developing fetus serves as a ready storage depot for the absorbed metal.

Etiology

Bismuth stomatitis develops usually as the result of injection or ingestion of bismuth salts for therapeutic purposes. The cutaneous absorption of this metal has not been demonstrated, hence bismuth pigmentation does not result from inunction; however, the use of bismuth compounds on granulating wound surfaces or in fistulous tracts gives rise frequently to acute stomatitis. Occupational sources are unimportant.

Bismuth came into prominence during World War I, in the form of the famous BIP (bismuth, iodoform and paraffin) bone paste. Bismuth stomatitis and even fatalities from the use of this paste were not uncommon. The efficacy of the spirillicide action of bismuth was experimentally demonstrated by Roberts et al. and it was suggested for human use by Sazerac and Levaditi. Today, insoluble bismuth compounds are used almost universally in alternation with some form of arsphenamine in the treatment of syphilis. Sobisminol mass (capsules) is finding limited use in the peroral treatment of syphilis. Meininger and Barnett found that about 18% of the patients taking sobisminol mass develop a bismuth line or stomatitis.

One should not infer a priori that a bismuth line or bismuth gingivitis results from anti-luetic therapy as bismuth salts are used in dermatology, in internal medicine and in the treatment of arthritis. Intramuscular bismuth injections are used by Grossman for the treatment of psoriasis, lupus erythematosus and lichen planus, and empirically in other skin diseases of obscure etiology. Since bismuth therapy in dermatologic conditions is usually less intensive than in lues, the chances of oral pigmentation or stomatitis are not so great.

The soluble subnitrate and subcarbonate salts are prescribed frequently for non-specific forms of diarrhea, colitis, and dysentery and as a protective antacid in gastric ulcer. The oral administration of the loose powder may occasion rapid development of a bismuth line or stomatitis. This may be due in part to the local action of the salts and to their more rapid and complete absorption from the inflamed gastro-intestinal tract.

Bismuth was a constituent of the old Sippy powders, still used in many dispensaries. Long-continued administration of Sippy Powder No. II may give rise to oral bismuth pigmentation or generalized bismuthia. Other antacids such as the aluminum, magnesium and silicate gels have largely displaced Sippy powders.

Sippy Powder No. I		Sippy Powder No. II	
Magnesium oxide	0.6 Gm.	Bismuth subcarbonate	0.6 Gm.
Sod. bicarb	0.6 Gm.	Sod. bicarb	2-3 Gm.

Pathogenesis

Discoloration due to bismuth therapy may appear as: (1) the common narrow blue-black pigmentation of the interdental papillae and the marginal gingivae with or without stomatitis, (2) a discoloration (and at times extensive slough) due to embolic phenomena following the accidental injection of bismuth preparations into artery or vein, and (3) a general, persistent discoloration of the entire skin.

Steinfeld and Meyer in 1885 described the probable mechanism whereby the bismuth circulating in the blood stream is precipitated by H_2S to form the sulfide which mechanically blocks the smaller blood and lymph vessels. Dalche and Villejean noted the typical bismuth line in experimental animals as early as 1887. Almkvist has since enlarged on this hypothesis. His theory accounts for the relationship between bismuth pigmentation and poor oral hygiene, the presence of salivary calculus and the localization of the pigmentation to those areas most commonly associated with oral fusospirochetal infection.

The absorbed salts are believed to unite with the hemoglobin or an acid radical of the blood, forming unknown compounds, which have been demonstrated histologically as a precipitate. This precipitated material plugs some of the capillaries of the marginal gingivae and interdental papillae resulting in nutritional impairment of these tissues, making them less resistant to secondary infection. If the metallic compound itself is irritating (see Mercury) this plays an additional role in the production of the metallic gingivitis.

The typical bismuth sulfide granules are formed by the action of hydrogen sulfide on this precipitated material. The sulfide granules can be demonstrated within the capillary endothelial cells and the outer layers of the connective tissue just beneath the epithelial surface. The hydrogen sulfide is produced by the action of bacteria on the decaying organic material in areas of poor hygiene. Bartels has demonstrated *in vitro* the production of bismuth sulfide by the action of the oral flora on suitable culture medium containing bismuth salts.

Systemic Aspects

The symptoms of acute intoxication are similar to those seen in nitrite poisoning with cyanosis, dyspnea and methemoglobin formation. More chronic manifestations consist of vague gastro-intestinal disturbances, nausea, vomiting, bloody diarrhea, "bismuth grippe" and jaundice. Bismuth "lines" can be demonstrated roentgenologically in the growing ends of bones. Ulcerative stomatitis is definite evidence of general intolerance to bismuth. Lohe and Rosenfeld have reported nephritis with albuminuria as accompanying the buccal and lingual mucosal lesion.

Oral Aspects

Subjective Symptoms. A bismuth line may be present without other symptoms. Usually however the patient complains of an annoying gingivo-

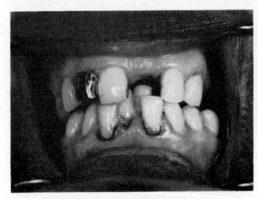

stomatitis with objective findings and symptomatology identical to those described for fusospirochetal gingivitis. The metallic taste is usually marked and the patient complains of a burning sensation of the oral tissues.

Objective Symptoms. In addition, and serving as the predisposing factor, is the blue-black pigmentation which is sharply limited to the marginal gingivae or the contacting tissues. The bismuth line has a well-defined appearance to the naked eye but if it is examined with a hand lens

Fig. 31. Bismuth deposition in the marginal gingiva at the sites of local irritation. Note the localized distribution of the pigmentation in the tissues.

the pigmentation is observed to be diffusely distributed (compare with lead). In mild cases, the interdental papillae may be the only structures affected.

Pigmentation is commonly localized to the gingival tissues about erupting third molars, the lingual gingivae of the lower incisors, especially those with calcareous deposits, malposed teeth and ill-fitting crowns or overhanging filling—the areas susceptible to fusospirochetal infection. The tongue is frequently sore and enlarged. Pigmentation and ulceration may develop where the oral tissues are in contact with calcareous deposits or gingival lesions. These so-called "contact" areas of pigmentation are common on the lips, cheeks and in the third molar area. Regional adenopathy may be present. Brittingham has noted pain in the jaws and in carious teeth soon after bismuth injections. Make described dental "shocks" occurring in teeth of patients receiving bismuth treatments. These latter symptoms are rare.

Diagnosis

An ulcerative stomatitis with a blue-black pigmentation of the interdental papillae or marginal gingivae in a patient receiving intramuscular injections or long-continued oral administration of suspected bismuth compounds is

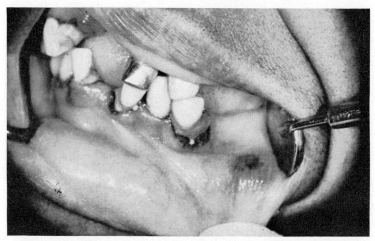

Fig. 32. Bismuth pigmentation localized to areas of poor oral hygiene and irritation. An area of contact pigmentation is present on the lower lip.

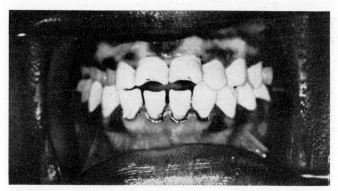

Fig. 33. Bismuth line about marginal gingivae of mandibular incisors of a prenatal luetic patient. Compare the location and intensity of the bismuth and the melanin pigmentation.

sufficient for a diagnosis. The patient is frequently unwilling to admit receiving anti-luetic therapy. The patient's attitude to your questioning constitutes usually a fairly reliable and definite answer.

Bismuth compounds are used for numerous conditions other than syphilis. Always give the patient the benefit of the doubt until you have consulted with his physician. Bismuth pigmentation without symptoms of stomatitis, while definitely objectionable from an esthetic point of view, does not indicate intolerance to the drug. It does not have the serious significance of the

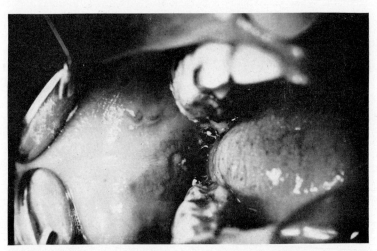

FIG. 34. Painful pigmented ulcer in a patient receiving bismuth injections. These lesions develop usually in the molar region where the cheek mucosa is irritated by calculus, rough crowns or trauma.

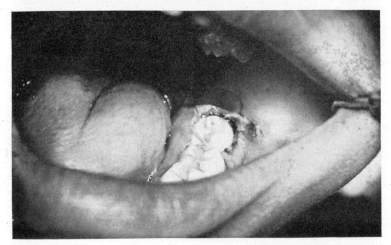

FIG. 35. Acute circumcoronal infection with bismuth pigmentation and traumatic irritation.

lead line. Proper dental treatment will prevent further pigmentation and may reduce that already present.

Laboratory Findings. Laboratory studies are rarely required for the diagnosis of bismuth stomatitis. Biopsy and micro-chemical studies will verify the metal causing the pigmentation.

Differential Diagnosis. In making a diagnosis of bismuth stomatitis it must be determined whether the pigmentation is actually in the gingival

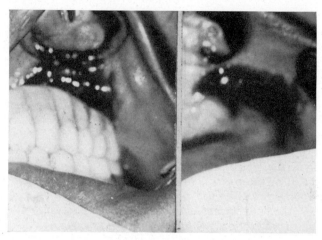

FIG. 36. Bismuth pigmentation persisting in an edentulous patient who had a severe decubital ulcer due to an ill-fitting denture.

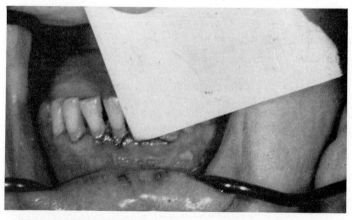

FIG. 37. The "paper test" which is used to differentiate between stain on the root surfaces and pigmentation in the marginal gingival tissues. The dark line on the gums persists after the paper is inserted above the tooth. Case of bismuth stomatitis.

tissue, whether it is bismuth and not some other element or whether it is due to conditions simulating metallic pigmentation.

The "paper test" will demonstrate whether or not the pigmentation is in the gingival tissues. This is performed by inserting the corner of a small piece of paper between the marginal gingiva and the tooth root. If the discoloration is accentuated it is in the marginal gingiva; if it disappears it is due to discoloration of the tooth root. A well-defined blue-black line along the marginal gingivae and the absence of constitutional symptoms usually permit differentiation from lead intoxication. The hemogram will assist in doubtful cases.

The various endogenous and exogenous causes of oral pigmentation, such as that seen in hemochromatosis, Addison's disease, pediculi capitis, and localized areas of melanosis must be considered. Foreign material introduced into the gingival tissue, such as charcoal granules or fragments of pencil lead or amalgam, may be confusing.

Treatment. The ideal and only completely satisfactory treatment of bismuth pigmentation or stomatitis is its prevention. The physician administering bismuth preparations should be aware of, and stress to the patient, the necessity for maintaining scrupulous oral hygiene. In all non-infectious cases the co-operation of the patient's dentist should be obtained before bismuth therapy is commenced. This will prevent the formation of an unsightly bismuth line and the development of a bismuth stomatitis which may necessitate cessation of medication.

The treatment of bismuth stomatitis (not gingival pigmentation) includes immediate cessation of the drug and the local treatment of the oral lesions. Response to treatment is slow. This is due to the circulatory impairment of the marginal gingivae and to the fact that even though the bismuth injections are stopped, there still remain considerable "depot" deposits of bismuth salts which will take weeks and months to deplete. The persistence of these intramuscular depots has been demonstrated by x-rays as long as a year following the last injection. In acute bismuth stomatitis, these deposits of insoluble salts may be evacuated surgically to lessen and shorten the duration of the absorption.

Oral treatment for the ulcerative lesions follows that described for oral fuso-spirochetal disease. Caustics are contraindicated. Special attention should be paid to obtaining and maintaining the best possible oral hygiene. The gingival pigmentation may disappear gradually in the course of months or persist for years even though no additional bismuth is given. The disappearance of the bismuth line is variable and unpredictable. In some cases where the line has developed following bismuth therapy for dermatologic conditions, it has been removed surgically at the request of the patient.

Felsher and Jones suggested the use of a tooth powder composed of 15 parts of sodium hexametaphosphate and 85 parts of talc, to prevent bismuth gingivostomatitis. The patients were instructed to use the powder after each meal and before retiring. There was improvement of the mouth lesions in most of the patients studied and all continued their bismuth and arsenic therapy without interruption. A few of the patients showed previous intolerance to bismuth although proper oral hygiene was maintained. Since the authors presented no controls using talc alone, and since their interpretation of the mechanism of bismuth pigmentation was at variance with that commonly accepted, this form of treatment as a specific for the prevention of bismuth is still being studied. Intravenous injections of sodium thiosulphate have been used to promote the absorption (depigmentation) of bismuth. The results rarely justify this form of treatment.

Prognosis. The prognosis of bismuth stomatitis is good, but response to treatment will not be as rapid as in uncomplicated fusospirochetal infection. The disappearance of the bismuth line is variable and unpredictable.

LEAD INTOXICATION (PLUMBISM-SATURNISM)

Lead produces multiple and varied toxic manifestations. The initial symptoms are usually vague because of the slow absorption of the metal. Lead poisoning is uncommon, although this metal, or its compounds, is used extensively in at least 150 trades. Lead intoxication usually occurs in adult males in association with occupational hazards, but occasionally household or accidental poisonings are found in women and children. Lead is rarely used as a medicine.

Etiology

The respiratory system and the gastro-intestinal tract are the two main channels of absorption. Intoxication develops more rapidly when the lead enters the body through the respiratory tract because a higher concentration of the absorbed metal reaches the general circulation. In absorption from the gastro-intestinal tract a considerable amount of lead is excreted in the bile and never reaches the systemic circulation. Trades in which lead fumes are prevalent such as in lead smelting, storage battery and insecticide manufacturing, brass foundries, and the printing industry are particularly dangerous. Cutaneous absorption does not occur except in the case of fat solvent compounds such as tetra-ethyl lead. There is little danger in using automobile fuel containing tetra-ethyl lead. The real tetra-ethyl hazard is in the manufacture of this substance and in the use of tetra-ethyl gasoline for cleaning purposes.

Domestic intoxication arises from a variety of causes. The making of beer, wine or cider in pottery vessels having a lead-containing glaze has resulted in plumbism. Contamination from lead water pipes was once common. Tooth pastes contained in lead alloy tubes and shot or bullets imbedded in the tissues have given rise to lead intoxication. Lead poisoning in children results from eating from lead-containing dishes, from chewing lead containing paint on toys or cribs, and from the old-fashioned lead nipple shields. Burning old storage battery cases for fuel is another domestic lead hazard.

Symptoms of lead intoxication are largely dependent on its concentration in the general circulation. Lead in the blood soon goes to the bones where it is deposited as the relatively innocuous insoluble tertiary phosphate. A high calcium and phosphorus-containing diet favors the deposition of lead in the skeletal system. Marchoont-Robinson demonstrated that the routine administration of ascorbic acid protects workers exposed to lead dust against chronic lead poisoning. The vague symptoms of chronic lead poisoning may be in reality subclinical scurvy. The pathogenesis of the metallic line and stomatitis has been described under bismuth.

Systemic Aspects

Evidence of lead absorption must be differentiated from symptoms of lead intoxication. Evidences of lead absorption consist of the characteristic "lead line" (Burtonian line) urinary and fecal lead excretion and certain hematologic findings. The lead lines at the epiphyseal ends of growing bones can be demonstrated roentgenographically.

Symptoms of lead intoxication include pallor of the face and lips and frequently emotional instability. Gastro-intestinal symptoms are characteristic. They vary from loss of appetite, nausea and vomiting to the distressing abdominal colic. A peripheral neuritis, affecting primarily the nerve supply of the extensor muscle groups, is responsible for the typical "wrist drop" (radial nerve) and the "foot drop" (peroneal nerve). Lead encephalitis is an infrequent but serious complication.

Oral Aspects

Subjective Symptoms. The "lead line" is pathognomonic of lead absorption and it is only exceeded in importance as an early diagnostic sign by the hematologic findings. It is not necessarily evidence of intoxication. The "lead line" lacks the discreteness of the bismuth line, being more diffusely distributed in the tissues. The gray pigmentation appears a short distance away from the marginal gingivae and when it is studied with a hand lens the "lead line" is seen to be composed of numerous distinct dark granules.

A heavy coating of the tongue is common and when this organ is extended a marked tremor may be observed. Even before the patient becomes aware of the gingival pigmentation they often complain of a peculiar sweetish taste. Salivation is more marked than in bismuth but less so than in mercurialism. The salivary glands are frequently tender.

Objective Symptoms. Any or all of the symptoms of oral fusospirochetal disease may be present. They are secondary to the impaired nutrition resulting from the lead sulfide deposits in the marginal gingivae. This is complicated by the irritating effect of the lead salts in the tissues and in the secreted saliva. While distressing, the oral symptomatology is usually overshadowed by the systemic aspects of the disease.

Diagnosis. The points enumerated under bismuth must be considered in the diagnosis of lead gingivostomatitis. The "peroxide test" described by Prinz may aid in determining the particular metal present if this is not already known from the history. Hydrogen peroxide is applied to the gingival pigmentation; if it is due to lead, the black sulfide is changed to the colorless sulfate in a few minutes. When the lead line is of moderate intensity, the color change is not striking.

LABORATORY STUDIES. One of the earliest and most characteristic findings in lead absorption is a secondary anemia with stippling or punctate basophilia. Stippling may be occasionally found in severe bismuth intoxication, pernicious anemia and leukemia; however, when these cells constitute 1 to 2% of the erythrocytes it is almost pathognomonic of lead intoxication. Workers in trades or occupations exposed to lead have routine hemograms and physical examinations in order to detect abnormal lead absorption. Increased erythrocyte fragility is usually found in lead intoxication. Chemical analysis of the urine, feces and saliva will also show abnormal lead excretion.

Treatment. Treatment of the acute manifestations of lead colic requires the administration of antispasmodics such as atropine or at times morphine. In chronic lead intoxication the treatment is directed toward elimination of further contact and the rapid removal of the lead from the blood and soft tissues by skeletal "fixation." This is accomplished by a high calcium and phosphorus diet which is alkaline in character. Milk is ideal with its optimal calcium-phosphorus ratio, and because it is readily taken even in the presence of a stomatitis.

Deleading, or the gradual elimination of the lead stored in the bones, will occur spontaneously if further contact is eliminated. Kehoes does not recommend deleading by special therapeutic means.

The treatment of lead stomatitis is similar to that described for bismuth. Since more of the lead salts are secreted by the salivary glands, they may contribute to the pain and discomfort in the mouth. Conservative methods with the avoidance of caustics should be used in the treatment of the associated fusospirochetal infection. A decrease in the salivary flow and the contained irritating lead salts can be obtained by the use of atropine $\frac{1}{2}$ mg. or the following preparation.

> Tinct. belladonna   8 cc.
> Camphor water q.s.a.d.   250 cc.
>   Sig. a teaspoonful every hour,
> until the throat becomes dry.
> The dosage should be reduced
> then or given at longer intervals.

Prognosis. The prognosis in lead intoxication is good if permanent nerve damage has not taken place. Aside from the gingival ulceration and the faint pigmentation of the involved tissues, the prognosis is favorable. The oral lesions are usually of secondary importance.

MERCURIALISM (PTYALISM)

Mercurialism is characterized by an ulcerative stomatitis, a marked ptyalism and gastro-intestinal symptoms of varying intensity. Mercurialism was common in the 19th century when patients were "salivated" or given calomel for almost every illness. With the introduction of new drugs for the treatment of syphilis and the reduction of industrial hazards, mercury intoxication has become a rarity.

Mercurialism develops as a result of occupational contact, drug overdosage, suicidal attempts or self-medication with mercurial compounds. Mercury compounds are readily absorbed by inhalation, ingestion, injection and inunction. Mercurial stomatitis has resulted from injecting mercurochrome in sinus tracts and it is even said to have developed from the mercury contained in fillings. The dermatitis and stomatitis often associated with amalgam fillings represent an allergic reaction to this element rather than a true intoxication (see Allergy).

The pathogenesis of the mercury line is similar to that described for bismuth, but the mercuric sulfide is very irritating to the oral tissues. Henrici and Hartzell have produced mercurial stomatitis experimentally in cats.

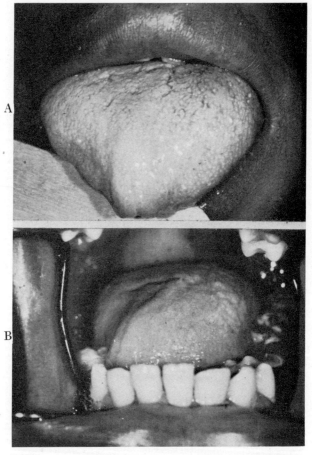

Fig. 38. (A) Acute oral reaction to mercurial "rubs." The marked swelling of the tongue caused it to protrude from the mouth. Also note swelling of upper lip. (B) Same case ten days later following the use of hot physiologic saline irrigations.

Systemic Aspects

The general symptoms of mercurialism include intestinal colic, diarrhea, headache, insomnia, tremor of the fingers and at times the tongue. Renal symptoms indicate severe intoxication and they are usually the cause of death. General manifestations of toxicity are increased by previous renal damage or the use of iodides. When renal damage is present there may be albuminuria.

Oral Aspects

Subjective Symptoms. A marked increase in flow of a ropy, viscid saliva is characteristic of mercurialism. The "hot mouth," itching sensation and metallic taste is due to the mercuric sulfide in the secreted saliva. The lips

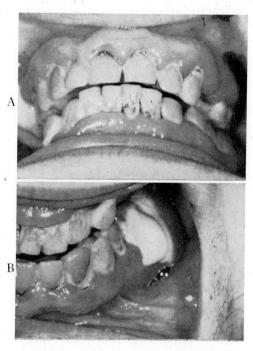

FIG. 39. Acute mercurial stomatitis in a 56-year-old woman resulting from therapy with this metal. (A) Note the marked swelling and hyperemia of the gums with ulceration of the marginal gingivae. (B) The large calcareous mass indicates the poor oral hygiene in this patient.

are dry, cracked and swollen. A faint diffuse grayish pigmentation of the alveolar gingivae is a variable finding. Any or all of the symptoms of oral fusospirochetal infection may be present.

Objective Symptoms. Oral mucosal ulcerations are more prone to occur than in bismuth or lead intoxication and the ulcerations are more likely to spread to the palate, throat and pharynx. A marked periostitis with exfoliation of the teeth or fragments of the jaw occurs in severe cases. The tongue is enlarged and painful and along its borders are indentations produced by the teeth. Ulceration is not uncommon at these areas. The lymph glands and the salivary glands are enlarged and the latter structures are frequently very painful.

Circumoral swelling, a red blotchy eruption on the lips and cheeks, a temperature rise of over 102° F. with swelling of the feet and legs which prevented the wearing of shoes have been reported by Bass due to sensitivity to the mercury contained in amalgam fillings.

Diagnosis

The oral symptoms overshadow usually the systemic complaints. In obscure cases the saliva and urine can be analyzed for this metal. The diagnosis is usually made on the basis of a history of occupational or therapeutic contact with this metal.

Treatment

Systemic treatment includes bed rest and a suitable dietary regime to prevent further renal damage. Intravenous injections of sodium thiosulfate or sodium formaldehyde-sulfoxylate have been advocated. The treatment of the oral lesions follows that described for fusospirochetal stomatitis. Caustics should be avoided. Extractions are contraindicated and if performed may result in extensive tissue necrosis and slough. Atropine or belladonna can be given to lessen the salivary flow and mucosal irritation. Response to treatment is slow.

Prognosis

Death in mercurialism results usually from renal failure. In chronic intoxication the ultimate prognosis is good although extensive destruction of the gingival tissue and even loss of the teeth may occur.

FLUORINE INTOXICATION

Fluorine intoxication may occur as an acute or a chronic process which affects both man and animals. Darmous and gaddar are diseases in animals which are caused by the ingestion of forage contaminated with fluorides.

In man, acute fluoride intoxication occurs chiefly as an occupational disease in cryolite miners, workers in aluminum, fertilizer and insecticide manufacturing plants and those exposed to HFl fumes. Cut-glass workers, brewers, bleachers, dyers and etchers are also prone to develop intoxication. In the conversion of phosphate rock to superphosphate (fertilizer), a large percentage of the fluorine is volatilized causing a definite occupational hazard. Under war conditions phosphates of approved origin are not easily available and those contaminated with fluorine are finding their way into foods prepared for human consumption. Rock phosphate which contains up to 3.5% of fluorine is being imported in increasing amounts from North Africa for use as fertilizers.

Factors other than the absorption of fluorine are important in producing the acute toxic symptoms. Occupational human fluorosis has been observed in a cryolite decomposing factory in Copenhagen, while in Philadelphia a factory handling similar material in the same manner has encountered no cases of acute fluorosis. The toxic effects of fluorine are dependent on both the fluorine intake and the general adequacy of the diet. Individuals with a vitamin C deficiency have a particularly severe form of the disease. In India it has been shown that the consumption of fluorine-containing water coupled with an inadequate diet results in the typical skeletal symptoms.

Systemic Intoxication

The individual with fluorine intoxication complains of gastric symptoms, stiffness and localized or disseminated rheumatic pains. Since fluorine has a particular affinity for bones and teeth, the most characteristic symptoms are seen in these tissues. The thickening of the bony lamina with the disappearance of the normal bony architecture and its replacement by a dense, milky-white opacity is characteristic. The bones become more brittle than normal and there is frequently calcification of the ligamentous attachments. These osteosclerotic changes are particularly noticeable in the vertebrae. An anemia and a susceptibility to severe renal infections are more serious symptoms. The anemia does not respond to any type of antianemic therapy since it is due to the actual crowding of the marrow cellular elements.

Chronic Dental Fluorosis

Chronic fluorine intoxication arises usually from drinking water which contains small amounts of this element. Because of the geographic distribution of the affected individuals, it is frequently called endemic fluorosis. Appreciable quantities of fluorine may also find their way into ingested foods. Products grown on high fluorine-containing soils or those sprayed with fluorine-containing insecticides will add appreciable quantities to that obtained in the drinking water. Soils may contain as much as 6,000 p.p.m. (parts per million), foods from 0.2 to 4.5 p.p.m., and tea, bone products and certain processed foods often higher concentrations. DeEds recently called attention to another possible source of fluorine toxicity in dicalcium phosphate. This salt is used frequently to supplement the diet in pregnancy, for infants and children. Fluorine may be present in dicalcium phosphate due to the sources of the raw material or due to its methods of manufacture. In the samples tested by DeEds, the average daily dose of 1 teaspoonful of dicalcium phosphate containing 0.27% (2,700 p.p.m.) fluorine represents many times the amount of this substance which will result in severe mottling of the enamel.* In random samples fluorine may run from 300 to 1,000 p.p.m. It is desirable to reduce the fluorine content of dicalcium phosphate to a value of 20 to 40 p.p.m.

Mass roentgenologic studies of the skeletal system of individuals residing in areas of endemic fluorosis have failed to reveal the characteristic osteosclerotic skeletal changes associated with fluorine intoxication but an unusually high percentage of spondylitis deformans was discovered. Macheroni

* The sample used in this study was supplied by the Food and Drug Administration.

and Roussi found that in certain localities in Argentina where the fluorine
content of the water was as much as 2 mg. per liter (20 p.p.m.) serious
injury resulted to the bones and teeth.

Linsman and McMurray reported the first case of osteosclerosis due to
fluorine contained in the drinking water. The patient, a 22-year-old male,
had lived his entire life in various communities in Texas, with the exception
of 2 years. The known fluorine content of the drinking water in these communities varied from 4.4 to 12 p.p.m. His teeth showed extensive mottling
of the enamel. The spine, pelvis and thoracic cage all revealed marked osteosclerosis. This patient also had a serious renal infection, which, with the
accompanying anemia, resulted in death. These authors stated that in areas
where chronic fluorosis exists, as manifested by mottled enamel, and where
the fluorine content of the drinking water is over 3 p.p.m., the public should
be systematically studied by the public health authorities to determine the
existence of osteosclerosis. They further advise that all patients with dental
fluorosis who show symptoms of anemia and renal impairment should have
x-ray examinations of the skeletal system.

Endemic Fluorosis (Mottled Enamel). The effects of endemic fluorosis
are of considerable dental, medical and public health interest. The absorption of minute quantities of fluorine during odontogenesis results in changes
which are recognized clinically in the erupted tooth as mottled enamel.

The dental interest in fluorine was originally occasioned by the unsightly
character of the mottled enamel on the teeth and the difficulties encountered
in their treatment. Teeth so affected have a dull, chalky-white appearance
when they erupt but they become gradually brown or at times almost black
in color. This coloring of the tooth, which is a posteruptive change, is most
conspicuous on the tooth surfaces which are exposed to the air or light—e.g.,
the labial surfaces of the anterior teeth. The exact chemical composition of
this discoloration, which is confined to the surface layers of the enamel, is
not known.

Early epidemiologic studies of individuals with mottled enamel revealed
that some constituent in the drinking water was probably responsible for the
peculiar dental lesions, since persons living in close geographic relation had
mottled enamel or were free from this disease depending on their water
supply. Furthermore, the lesions developed only when this particular drinking water was consumed during the tooth forming period, as adults using the
same water did not develop mottled enamel.

It was eventually determined and verified experimentally that minute
amounts of fluorine in the drinking water were the cause of mottled enamel.
The drinking water in some areas of endemic fluorosis contained as high as
20 p.p.m. fluorine. Concentrations of over 2 to 3 p.p.m. usually resulted in
mottling of the enamel. A few cases of mottled enamel have been reported
from non-endemic areas. These resulted from prolonged nursing by women
who were exposed occupationally to high concentrations of fluorine. Such
cases are of no public health importance.

The treatment of the unsightly mottled enamel consists of carefully re-

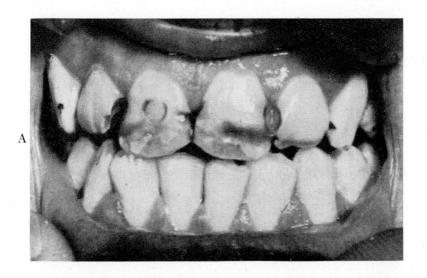

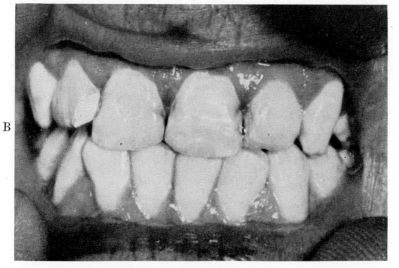

FIG. 40. (A) Patient with a moderate degree of mottling of the enamel (endemic fluorosis). (B) Patient after the teeth had been treated by the controlled application of mineral acids. The objectionable discoloration has almost disappeared. (Raper, Dent. Digest, 47:390, 1941.)

moving the superficial discolored portion of the tooth by means of grinding, treatment with strong bleaching agents or the controlled application of mineral acids.

Public Health Aspects

It was later noted that in the regions where the fluorine concentration in the drinking water approached the level which resulted in the mottling of the enamel, or around 1 p.p.m., the prevalence of dental caries was reduced markedly and at times it approached immunity. This caries protective effect was greatest when the fluorine-containing water was consumed during odontogenesis, but a lesser protective effect was present even when the fluorine-containing water was consumed after tooth eruption. Studies utilizing the fluorine radio-isotopes have demonstrated an adsorption of this element on the enamel, as well as its actual deposition in the other tooth forming tissues. This fluorine adsorption on the enamel surface explains in part the caries protective effect of this substance on the fully formed and erupted tooth.

These observations lead to an exploration of the possibilities of caries control by means of: (1) the topical application of fluorides to the fully formed tooth and (2) the addition of soluble fluorides to the municipal water supplies in sufficient amounts to exert a caries protective effect without producing mottling of the enamel.

The clinical studies of Bibby and Cheyne have demonstrated the practicability of the topical application of soluble fluorides to newly erupted teeth. The first molars so treated developed approximately 40-50% the number of new carious lesions which were observed in the untreated control molar teeth. Once the treated teeth become carious, however, the caries progresses at a similar rate in both the experimental and control teeth.

Caries control or prevention by fluorinization of the municipal water supply offers intriguing possibilities as a practical public health measure. The practicability of approach to widespread caries control must be considered on the basis of (1) the toxic effects of fluorine and (2) the existence of uncontrollable sources of fluorine intake and (3) the importance of other factors (such as diet), some of which are as yet unknown in producing fluorine intoxication. Mass caries control by fluorinization of municipal water supplies is therefore being approached with great caution, since appreciable amounts of fluorine occur in uncontrollable sources of intake and since the toxic reactions of fluorine are serious and frequently fatal. Such studies are now being conducted by the U. S. Public Health Service. Numerous technical problems arise when controlled fluorinization of the water supply of a large city is attempted.

ARGYRIA

Argyria is a permanent discoloration of the skin and mucous membranes resulting from local or systemic absorption of silver compounds. It may result from occupational exposure, but more commonly from the long continued use of silver-containing nasal drops or sprays or silver arsphenamine injections.

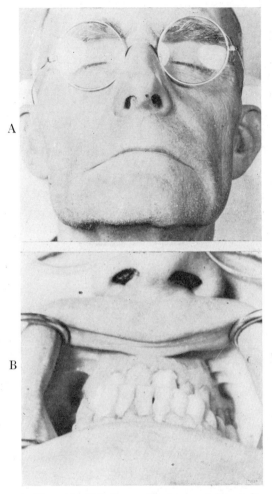

FIG. 41. (A) Generalized argyrosis resulting from the obsolete silver nitrate treatment of gastric ulcer. (B) Chronic persisting marginal gingivitis in a patient with
generalized argyrosis.

In former years argyria developed frequently in patients with gastric ulcer
who were treated with silver nitrate.

Pigmentation, Skin and Oral Mucosa

Pigmentation occurs early in the mouth but it is rarely observed by the
patient as there are no systemic or local symptoms of intolerance to the silver
preparations. The exposed body surfaces including the nail beds are usually
more deeply pigmented. This is related to the reduction of the silver com-

pounds in these tissues by sunlight. Patients with argyria appear extremely ill, although they experience few, if any, subjective symptoms.

The discoloration of the skin is slate-gray or violet in color and in marked cases there is even a suggestion of a metallic lustre. In the mouth, the pigmentation is diffusely distributed throughout the gingival and mucosal tissues. The author has observed a persistent marginal gingivitis in several patients with argyrosis, but in most instances oral symptoms other than the pigmentation are absent.

Diagnosis

The diagnosis of argyria is made on the objective findings and the history of occupational or therapeutic contacts with silver or its compounds. In doubtful cases, biopsy studies will establish the diagnosis.

In the differential diagnosis, (1) cyanosis of cardiac or pulmonary origin, (2) pigmentation due to other metals or diseases, and (3) cyanosis due to the administration of drugs, such as acetanilid and the sulfonamides, must be considered. In cyanosis of cardiac or pulmonary origin or secondary to drug therapy, the tissues are more bluish purple in color and there is a blanching of the tissue when the blood is forced out by pressure.

Treatment

Treatment consists of eliminating the source of contact with the silver compounds. Stillians has found that intradermal injections of 1% potassium ferrocyanide and 6% sodium thiosulfate result in permanent disappearance of the discoloration in the injected area.

ARSENIC

Arsenic is a toxic chemical agent. In its inorganic form, the element is a powerful poison. In certain organic combinations it is less toxic. Most cases of arsenism have their origin in industrial exposure, accidental or intentional poisoning. The varied symptoms of arsenism and their similarity to many different clinical entities have been the basis for many thrilling murder stories and the actual arsenic insurance scandal in Philadelphia. The symptoms of chronic arsenic poisoning are indefinite. Chronic gastritis and colitis are frequently the only symptoms. Keratosis of the palms and soles of the feet are commonly observed. Dermatitis, pigmentation or ulcerations of the skin may develop from long continued arsenic therapy (Fowler's solution or arsphenamine).

Oral Aspects

Oral mucosal changes due to arsenic may develop following systemic administration or the use of arsenic trioxide in pulp canal therapy. Oral mucosal reactions due to systemic arsenic therapy (usually arsphenamine) are infrequent. Stomatitis is rare compared to other arsphenamine reactions such as the nitritoid crisis. It indicates usually that the patient had a definite arsenic idiosyncrasy.

Arsenic stomatitis may be the oral mucosal manifestation of a serious desquamative dermatitis. In such cases, the symptoms are similar to those experienced in mercurial stomatitis. The oral tissues are extremely painful and they are deep red in color. In contrast to mercurialism, the mouth in arsenic stomatitis is dry. Oral lesions associated with aplastic anemia or purpura which are secondary to arsphenamine therapy resemble those described under aplastic anemia or purpura.

Arsenic trioxide is used occasionally in pulp canal therapy. The careless application of this drug, leakage due to an improperly sealed dressing or contact with the oral tissues in any manner will give rise to local lesions. A typical inflammatory reaction follows the contact of arsenic with the mucosa. A deep, penetrating, persistent and painful ulceration develops. An arsenic dressing in the pulp canal will occasionally result in an apical periostitis with necrosis of the alveolar process of the adjacent teeth. Death has occurred from swallowing improperly sealed dressings. (Prinz.) The use of the rubber dam will prevent the contact of the arsenical oxides with the soft tissues and arsenic dressings in the pulp canal should be sealed doubly as recommended by Grossman.

Friedman & Olsen reported a case of paralysis of the facial and masticatory nerves following arsenic poisoning. About 18 days after the acute effects of arsenic poisoning had disappeared the patient began to complain of inability to close her mouth, and to move any of the muscles of the face or to chew. Taste was not affected and all cranial nerves other than the 7th and the muscular portion of the 5th were normal. On the 24th day after the acute episode there was improvement in all symptoms with their eventual complete disappearance.

The treatment of arsenical burns or periostitis is unsatisfactory. Some surface anesthetic ointment can be used in the case of soft tissue burns.

AURIC STOMATITIS (GOLD STOMATITIS)

Gold salts are known to produce both chronic and acute oral symptoms. The sources of gold stomatitis are occupational and therapeutic. Auric stomatitis will increase probably with the more general use of these salts in the treatment of rheumatoid arthritis. Gold salts are also used in the treatment of certain forms of cutaneous tuberculosis, lupus erythematosus, leprosy and other dermatologic lesions which are resistant to the usual forms of treatment. Its main use is in the treatment of rheumatoid arthritis. General symptoms are uncommon. Purpura and malignant leukopenia have been reported following gold therapy but a dermatitis and stomatitis are the most commonly observed toxic reactions. They occur in from 10 to 40% of the patients who receive intensive gold therapy.

The oral lesions may be of a chronic or acute form. The chronic manifestations are similar but milder to those seen in bismuth. A faint purplish pigmentation or discoloration of the gingivae has been described with redness and congestion of the oral mucosa. The patient complains also of a metallic taste and this symptom may forewarn of more serious reactions. Vesiculation and ulceration of the oral mucosal and gingival tissues occur in the more acute reactions. Cracking and fissuring of the lips are common. The oral symptoms may be so acute as to prevent adequate nutrition. One patient who was receiving gold therapy developed whitish pea-sized patches on the gums and cheeks along the line of closure of the teeth. Pain and dysphagia were present but there was no sialorrhea.

The diagnosis of gold stomatitis is made on the basis of the history of occupational exposure or therapeutic administration of gold therapy. The

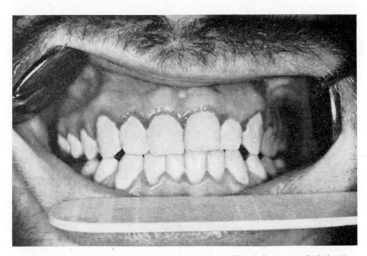

FIG. 42. Persistent gingivitis and yellowish superficial discoloration of teeth in a patient with suspected gold stomatitis. Both lesions were finally demonstrated to be due to poor oral hygiene.

treatment of auric stomatitis consists of the discontinuance of the metal therapy, the topical application of the aniline dyes and the use of a mildly alkaline mouth wash. At times the lesions are resistant to treatment.

STOMATITIS DUE TO COPPER, CHROMIUM AND ZINC

Occupational exposure to copper may result in the development of a bluish-green line on the gingivae and the teeth. The tooth discoloration is frequently permanent due to the etching of the enamel from acid fumes. Rygge reported an unusual brown discoloration of the enamel due to copper in the teeth of three children of the same family. The brown coloration of the beavers' teeth and perhaps the teeth of other rodents is due to their copper content.

The increased use of chrome compounds has resulted in frequent nasal and oral ulcerations. Chrome platers are exposed to a fine brownish spray of chromic acid which is irritating and corrosive to the mucous membranes of the nose and throat. The painful ulcerations of the nasal septum which result frequently in perforation are preceded by a burning and itching sensation. The oral lesions are usually confined to those portions of the mouth which come in contact with the chromic acid spray, but multiple ulcers may appear on the oral mucosa. They resemble fusospirochetal ulcers but the smears are usually negative for the fusospirochetal organisms. The teeth may become etched and show a persistent deep orange stain.

Burning, soreness and dryness of the mouth associated with swelling of the tongue has been reported by Lieberman. One patient stated that all foods tasted like rubber. Individuals who are sensitive to chrome compounds experience difficulty in wearing dental appliances fabricated from chrome-containing alloys. Treatment consists of proper ventilation and the use of protective masks and salves.

Zinc intoxication occurs chiefly as an occupational hazard in galvanizers, zinc oxide and molten brass workers and at times electric welders. No reports have been noted of oral or systemic symptoms resulting from the therapeutic use of this element.

The symptoms of zinc intoxication are similar in nature to an anaphylactic response with chills, fever, sweating, a rapid pulse, nausea, vomiting and dryness and burning of the upper respiratory tract. Prinz has described a stomatitis characterized by congestion and suppuration of the gingival tissues with a bluish-gray line and a metallic taste. In severe cases, the teeth may become loose due to the destruction of the alveolar process although little pain is experienced. There is painful submaxillary adenopathy and salivary gland involvement. The zinc content of the teeth has been shown to be increased in tuberculous individuals. The exact significance of this observation is not known.

RADIOACTIVE AGENTS (RADIUM X-RAYS)

Systemic Considerations

Any radioactive agent is capable of producing constitutional and local symptoms. While the immediate constitutional symptoms of malaise, nausea, slight fever and at times vomiting are distressing, they are not as serious as the radio-osteonecrosis which may follow more intensive and continued radiation. The immediate symptoms respond favorably or are lessened by the use of thiamine chloride or B complex and liver injections.

Long-continued exposure may result in sexual impotence, alopecia, brittleness of the nails, erythema, dermatitis and necrosis of the exposed areas. Pigmentation of the skin is likely to occur if cosmetics have been used on the areas irradiated, as heavy metals contained in the cosmetics cause increased absorption of the radiation. Radium or x-ray dermatitis is a serious condition which may lead to extensive ulceration and malignant degeneration.

Oral Considerations

With the increased emphasis being placed on the early diagnosis and treatment of malignancies of the head and neck region, the dentist should be cognizant of the possible dangers of ordinary dental procedures following such treatment. The irritating effect of radium acting as a heavy metal poison, its effect on the blood vessels and on the calcified structures of the teeth in addition to the possible dangers of dental roentgenography to the patient and the dentist must be considered.

Radium Poisoning. Individuals who develop symptoms of radium poisoning are rarely those receiving therapy, but the workers who are exposed to radium for long periods of time. While the whole body is affected, the oral cavity is frequently the first site where symptoms are observed. This is

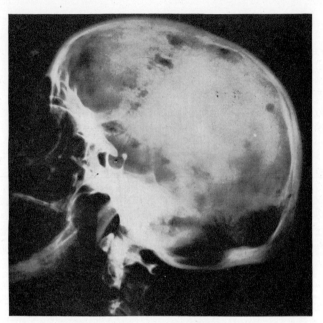

FIG. 43. Osseous defects of the skull in a patient with radium poisoning—watch-dial painter.

explained on the basis of the trauma which the oral structures experience, the high bacterial flora, the frequent presence of retained roots or periodontal disease which serve as additional sources of irritation.

Radiation of the Cervicofacial Region. Before radiation of the cervicofacial region is undertaken, all retained roots and periodontal infection must be eliminated and the best possible oral hygiene established, otherwise a serious periostitis or radio-osteonecrosis may develop. These complications are not only extremely painful but they interfere with the course of treatment. Even then the oral mucosa may become slightly irritated and painful with the development of moderate to severe xerostomia but the chances of more serious complications developing are minimized.

If heavy therapy is contemplated in elderly patients, it is usually best to extract all the remaining teeth. Watson and Scarborough recommended the removal of all teeth, irrespective of the age of the patient. Periodontal disease and other infectious lesions of the oral mucosa not only predispose to radio-osteonecrosis but the infection diminishes the radio-sensitivity of intraoral carcinoma. Caustics or strong medicaments are contraindicated in the treatment of such conditions.

Trauma of any kind, such as dental extractions, may precipitate radio-osteonecrosis long after the conclusion of therapy. Kaufman reported a fatality following a tooth extraction performed after x-ray therapy. The most

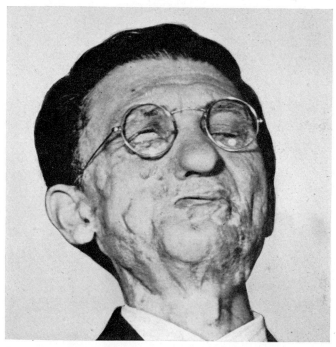

FIG. 44. Extensive scarring due to severe x-ray burns which developed following radiation therapy for a submaxillary adenitis.

conservative dental treatment is indicated following radiation, and pulp canal therapy is preferable to extractions. Loose teeth should be allowed to exfoliate. The atraumatic removal of teeth by the use of rubber bands (see hemophilia) may be applicable in some cases. Severe necrosis has followed a simple prophylaxis and deep gingival curettage is contraindicated. Partial prosthetic appliances are likely to irritate the soft tissues and in addition they place undue load on the abutments.

Patients complain frequently of thermal and touch hypersensitivity of the teeth during x-ray therapy of the head and neck. Leist reported spontaneous death of the dental pulp following radiation. The actual hard structures of the teeth appear to be involved in some manner, tending to wear away rapidly and to undergo erosion of the cervical region. Some have reported that teeth "shrink" following radiation therapy.

There is little danger to the patient in dental roentgenography. Rarely an erythema or pigmentation of the skin occurs in individuals who have been sensitized to x-rays by drugs, or those who use large amounts of cosmetics. The dentist should never attempt to give x-ray therapy with his dental x-ray equipment. (See Chapter 27.)

PHOSPHORUS POISONING ("PHOSSY JAW")

Phosphorus poisoning was at one time an important occupational disease. Today it is of little importance due to improved working conditions and the substitution of other forms of phosphorus for white phosphorus.

The outstanding symptom of phosphorus poisoning was a periostitis and osteitis of the teeth and jaws, usually the mandible. The necrotic process which usually commenced at the site of an injury, a retained root or a decayed tooth, was accompanied by pain, swelling and a fetid odor. It spread frequently to involve large portions of the jaw, including the teeth, which would become sequestrated. This process was chronic and the new callus formation at times would prevent the exfoliation of the sequestrum.

Treatment consisted of eliminating the exposure to phosphorus, establishing drainage, and preventing secondary infection.

7

Allergic Manifestations

HAY FEVER	STOMATITIS MEDICAMENTOSA AND
ASTHMA	VENENATA
SERUM SICKNESS	DENTOFACIAL ANOMALIES AND PER-
ANGIONEUROTIC EDEMA	IODONTAL DISEASES

Allergic diseases are said to affect at least 20% of the population. As a group they represent an important social, industrial and medical problem. The term allergy is used in a comprehensive sense to designate an altered reaction or response of the tissues to some substance that produces no symptoms or reactions in the normal individual under the same conditions.

The general subject of allergy can be subdivided into true allergic manifestations and those due to hypersensitivity. The altered response of sensitized individuals to animal danders (dog hair, feathers, etc.), certain foods, protein substances or plant pollens are examples of true allergy. The altered response of certain individuals to drugs, contact with metals, actinic radiations, organic substances or even thermal changes are examples of hypersensitivity. The oral mucosa is frequently the site of both true allergic and hypersensitive manifestations.

Because of the copious blood supply and the elasticity of the oral tissues, allergic manifestations in the mouth produce frequently startling lesions. Dental infections, on the other hand, may be a contributing or aggravating factor in certain extraoral allergic reactions.

The allergic manifestations of dental interest include:

(1) Allergic rhinitis—atopic coryza or hay fever.
(2) Asthma.
(3) Serum reactions.
(4) Food rashes.
(5) Angioneurotic edema.
(6) Stomatitis medicamentosa (hypersensitivity).
(7) Stomatitis venenata (contact allergy).
(8) Relation of allergy to periodontal disease, malocclusion and altered facial development.

HAY FEVER (POLLINOSIS)

Hay fever is the outstanding example of allergy. It is more common in early adult life and there appears to be a familial predisposition. The hay fever patient requires no enumeration of the distressing symptoms of his affliction. The onset and duration of the symptoms may coincide with the distribution of certain plant pollens—or the ingestion of certain foods. Individuals who are sensitive to animal danders, substances used in upholstery, and certain clothing materials experience their symptoms whenever they come in contact with the specific allergen.

The symptoms of hay fever include a marked congestion and edema of the mucous membranes, watering of the eyes and usually frequent sneezing or coughing. The affected parts itch intensely. Besides the marked inconvenience of these symptoms they interfere seriously with the best productive efforts of the individual and, more important, his rest.

The diagnosis of atopic coryza is made on the typical clinical symptoms, their time of onset and duration in respect to contact with the suspected allergens and the general background and family history of the patient. Skin testing by means of the scratch or intradermal tests will indicate the various substances to which the patient is sensitized. The nasal secretions in atopic coryza also contain a higher percentage of eosinophils and individuals with hay fever have frequently an increased number of eosinophils in the blood. The treatment of hay fever consists of desensitizing the patient by injections of minute, then gradually increasing doses of the specific allergen. This is a time-consuming and frequently unpleasant procedure, the results of which are not always successful. In acute attacks, adrenalin injections, the per oral administration of ephedrine or related compounds will give relief. Adrenalin and its related compounds should be administered only by the physician or on his recommendation. Patients with acute asthmatic attacks obtain considerable relief at the seashore and in certain mountainous climates which are relatively free from the common allergenic grasses.

ASTHMA

Asthma is an allergic disease characterized by spasms of the bronchial musculature. This obstruction of the respiratory passageways and the associated secretions gives rise to a wheezy variety of respiration when heard through the stethoscope—the music box chest. Bronchial asthma may be due to sensitivity to foods, grasses, animal emanations, miscellaneous dusts, certain vapors or odors of liquids. In about half of the cases, there is a family history of hay fever, urticaria or some other allergic manifestation.

Sensitivity to bacteria is also a causative agent. This latter type of asthma is also known as toxic asthma, indicating that some toxic agent is believed to be responsible for the clinical manifestations.

There is an impression in the south Atlantic states that both periodontal and periapical dental infection have an aggravating influence on bacterial asthma. Rarely is dental infection alone responsible for this condition, hence dramatic improvement is seldom obtained following the extraction of teeth. This remote relation between the teeth and bacterial asthma should be appreciated before extensive dental extractions are performed.

Leschke observed that in some asthmatics there was improvement following irrigation of the gingival (pyorrhea) pockets. He regarded this as clinical proof of the relation between the asthmatic symptoms and oral foci of infection. As yet no critical appraisal has been made of the importance of dental foci of infection in bacterial asthma.

SERUM SICKNESS

Certain characteristic symptoms develop occasionally in non-sensitized individuals following the injection of a foreign serum, particularly equine serum. In about 8-12 days, the patient experiences generalized body aches and pain, grippe-like symptoms and an elevation of temperature which is often accompanied or preceded by a chill. These symptoms are soon followed by an erythematous eruption which may vary from a mild papular lesion to frank urticaria. Anorexia, nausea and at times pain and swelling of the joints accompany the fever and the eruption. These symptoms which are known collectively as serum sickness subside gradually.

Patients who have previously received the same foreign serum, and who are sensitized to it, react at times in a different manner when the same serum is again injected. They are similar to those described previously, but they appear immediately, or develop within a day or two and are usually more severe.

An occasional patient may exhibit more immediate, dramatic and striking symptoms following even the initial injection of a foreign serum. This reaction is immediate and anaphylactic in character. It is for this reason that anyone who receives foreign serum is first skin tested for sensitivity by the intracutaneous injection of small amounts of the specific serum. If a positive reaction is obtained, the individual can be desensitized sufficiently to permit the administration of serum without producing dangerous reactions. Turner & Clark described temporomandibular arthropathy occurring as a manifestation of serum sickness.

ANGIONEUROTIC EDEMA (GIANT URTICARIA— QUINCKE'S DISEASE)

Angioneurotic edema may be a symptom complex rather than a distinct clinical entity. In some cases it is related to food allergy or hypersensitivity and, in others, to focal infection. Angioneurotic edema occurs also as a symptom of certain infectious diseases, endocrine disorders or emotional disturbances. In a few cases a hereditary or familial background is obtained.

The characteristic symptom of angioneurotic edema consists of a rapidly developing swelling of the affected part which may appear in 5 to 30 minutes and persist for 24 hours or several days. The site of the lesion may itch or burn, or have an uncomfortable tenseness just prior to the actual swelling.

The areas most commonly involved are the skin about the eyes and the chin, the lips and the tongue. Facial disfigurement may be marked. In the mouth,

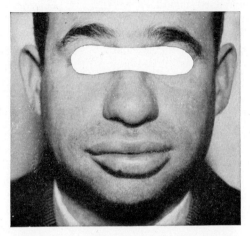

FIG. 45. Angioneurotic edema of the lips and eyes. (Haden, Allergy in Clinical Practice, J. B. Lippincott Company.)

the swellings are frequently striking due to the vascularity of the tissues and their unusual elasticity. The attacks may be infrequent or occur almost daily. At times they are precipitated by various emotional stimuli.

Strean reported an unusual case of angioneurotic edema in a patient who was wearing a full upper and a partial lower denture. The swelling occurred

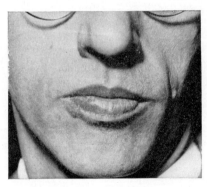

FIG. 46. Herpes labialis with canker sores following the ingestion of beef. (Haden, Allergy in Clinical Practice, J. B. Lippincott Company.)

in the upper lip and produced marked facial disfigurement. The patient's physician suspected the denture as the source of trouble but a new upper denture failed to relieve the symptoms. Nothing unusual was found in the patient's diet and she was unwilling to undergo skin tests for the foods usually eaten. On the next day a marked swelling of the lip appeared. Questioning revealed that on the previous day the patient had consumed a glass of beer in addition to her usual diet. One week later an hour after taking beer the swelling reappeared. The patient was asymptomatic for about 3 months when a glass of brandy brought on the swelling. It was concluded that the antigen to which the patient was sensitive was alcohol.

Person reported 11 cases of parotid gland swelling which were apparently on an allergic basis. Three of these patients exhibited other allergic manifestations at the same time. In one case plugs passed from the parotid gland contained large numbers of eosinophils.

The treatment of angioneurotic edema is symptomatic unless a specific allergen can be discovered, or a general disease is present which may have angioneurotic edema as a symptom. Foci of infection should be removed, not so much for a specific curative effect as for a general health measure. Adrenalin is useful in the acute episodes and in severe cases ephedrine may prevent or lessen the frequency of attacks.

The disease is of little danger to life unless the glottis is involved, in which case death may occur rapidly. There seems to be a predisposition to glottal involvement in the hereditary form of the disease which has about a 20% mortality.

STOMATITIS MEDICAMENTOSA AND VENENATA

General Considerations

Oral lesions resulting from the absorption of drugs and those due to the contact of medicaments, dentifrices, mouth washes or denture bases with the oral tissues are of particular concern to the dentist. Lesions in susceptible individuals resulting from the absorption of drugs are collectively spoken of as *stomatitis medicamentosa* while those due to contact are called *stomatitis venenata*. The important features of these two conditions are compared in Table X.

TABLE X

COMPARISON OF SOME OF THE IMPORTANT FEATURES OF STOMATITIS MEDICAMENTOSA AND VENENATA

	Stomatitis Medicamentosa (Drug Eruption or Idiosyncrasy)	Stomatitis Venenata (Contact Stomatitis)
Causative agents	Drugs—i.e., phenolphthalein barbiturates, sulfonamides.	Topical medications, dentifrices, mouth washes, denture bases, etc.
Mechanism	Due to absorption *via* the gastro-intestinal, respiratory tract or skin.	Due to contact of substance (or vapors) with the tissues.
Site of lesion	May occur in any area of body.	Lesions appear only where tissues are in contact with agent.
Site of sensitization	In the cutis. At times only in certain vascular networks as in "fixed drug eruptions" ? due to body protein being conjugated with the drug.	Result of sensitization of the epidermis.
Diagnostic aids	Withdrawal of drug. Use of small "test" dose to evoke symptoms. Patch test is negative.	Patch test usually positive. It should be performed on tissues where lesions have appeared.
Systemic manifestations	Uncommon—may be severe and even result in death.	Very rare unless secondary infection.

Stomatitis Medicamentosa (Drug Idiosyncrasy)

Causes. Any medicament may cause sensitization of the oral tissues but lesions are seen more frequently in certain groups of drugs. It may take a comparatively short time or years for the sensitization to occur but once it has developed it is usually permanent. The lesions in stomatitis medica-mentosa are not related to the chemical purity or to the toxicologic or pharmacologic action of the drug.

Eruptions reappear commonly at the same location, such as a particular area on the tongue, whenever the causative drug is taken. This is known

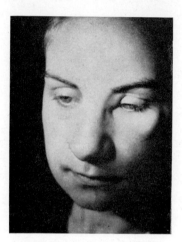

Fig. 47. Acute reaction of the "fixed type" due to acetylsalicylic acid (aspirin). (Courtesy of Dr. Thomas Meloy, Philadelphia, Pa.)

as a "fixed drug eruption," not because of the permanence of the lesion but because of its constant appearance at a given area. This clinical finding is explained on the basis of sensitization of the vascular network supplying a particular area.

Substances which result frequently in stomatitis medicamentosa are phenolphthalein, the barbiturates, the salicylates, arsphenamine, belladonna, arsenic, mercury, the bromides and iodides, quinine and the sulfonamides. While these preparations will be prescribed for most patients by the physician, the severity of the oral lesions and their localization will bring the patient to the dentist for diagnosis.

Drug eruptions are usually multiple and they have an amorphous, eroded or fungoid appearance. The lesions vary from a marked erythema to vesicle or bleb formation, an erosive or ulcerative lesion to even gangrene. The onset of the eruption is generally abrupt. A wide variety of drugs may cause similar appearing lesions or a single medicament will produce a variety of eruptions. Constitutional symptoms are rarely marked but in severe cases fever, malaise, bleeding (purpuric spots) and even death may occur.

Stomatitis medicamentosa is at times difficult to diagnose. A history of ingestion—or opportunities for absorption—of any of the drugs which commonly produce such lesions is important. If the withdrawal of the suspected drug is followed by a disappearance of the lesions, it is presumptive evidence of its causal relationship. In doubtful cases it may be necessary to give a small amount of the drug in an attempt to evoke symptoms again. The patch test will give negative results in stomatitis medicamentosa.

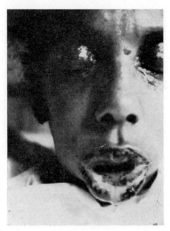

Fig. 48. Toxic eruptions due to phenobarbital (Moss and Long, Arch. of Dermat. and Syph., Sept., 1942.)

The treatment of stomatitis medicamentosa consists of the elimination of the drug responsible for the lesions. Symptomatic treatment, based on the nature of the lesions present in the mouth, should be given.

PHENOLPHTHALEIN. Phenolphthalein is the active ingredient of many proprietary laxative, liver and gallbladder preparations. This substance causes frequently an eruption in the mouth of the "fixed type." The tongue is the characteristic site of phenolphthalein eruptions, which appear as blebs, vesicles, erosions or deep ulcerations. The lesions simulate those seen in erythema multiforme or pemphigus.

THE BARBITURATE DERIVATIVES, such as nembutal, phenobarbital and sodium barbital, are prone to cause oral lesions. Gingival hyperplasia may develop following the continued administration of the barbiturates. Herpes develops frequently as the result of luminal administration. Since barbiturates are used commonly by the dentist for preoperative medication, he should be aware of their possible reactions on the oral mucosa.

ALL OF THE SULFONAMIDE DERIVATIVES have been observed to produce toxic symptoms in which oral lesions formed a prominent part of the picture.

In most instances the severe toxic manifestations have taken the form of an acute agranulocytosis. Schnee has reported a membranous inflammation of the conjunctiva, nasal, oral and pharyngeal mucosa as a toxic action to the local use of sulfathiazole.

LESIONS DUE TO THE HALOGENS, especially iodides, are characterized by cutaneous pustular reactions and at times the development of fungoid lesions. Franks & Davis observed a case of agranulocytosis which was secondary to quinine administration. Acetanilid, phenacetin, Empirin and amidopyrine may also produce oral lesions. The relation of these latter substances to malignant neutropenia is discussed in Chapter 21.

Stomatitis Venenata

Causes. Stomatitis venenata results from the contact of the causative agent with the sensitized oral tissues. The severe irritative lesions (not burns) which follow the use of sodium perborate mouth wash in some individuals are a good example of stomatitis venenata.

The more common causes of stomatitis venenata that might be encountered in dental practice are enumerated below:

(1) MEDICAMENTS USED IN DENTAL PRACTICE:
   Sodium perborate.
   Campho-phenique—chloroform.
   Aromatic oils—eugenol and eucalyptol.
   Iodine-containing preparations.
   Formalin-containing preparations—cold sterilizing solutions, etc.
(2) DENTAL FILLING OR PROSTHETIC MATERIALS:
   Metallic plastic fillings—amalgams.
   ? Mercury causative agent.
   Denture base materials.
   Vulcanite.
   Acrylic.
   Metallic alloys, Ticonium, Vitallium, etc.
(3) DENTAL OR COSMETIC PREPARATIONS USED BY THE PATIENT:
   Dentifrices—powders, pastes and liquids.
   Mouth washes—sodium perborate.
   Denture-cleaning creams or powders.
   Lip sticks, rouge, chewing gum, etc.

The symptoms of stomatitis venenata are usually local. The subjective symptoms are as a rule out of proportion to the objective lesions. The affected tissues have a fiery red color and a smooth waxy appearance due to the associated edema. The patient complains of an intense burning or itching sensation. Small shallow ulcerations are observed in mild cases while superficial necrosis of the tissue occurs in more severe reactions.

The lesions of stomatitis venenata develop less slowly than those of stomatitis medicamentosa. The reactions bear more relation to the concentration of the causative agent than in the latter condition. They may appear soon after contact with the causative agent, or develop after considerable periods of contact, during which time mucosal sensitization takes place. Sensitivity to the suspected material can be determined by means of patch testing. See Chapter 4, Laboratory Procedures.

The treatment of stomatitis venenata consists of the elimination of the causative agent and local symptomatic care depending on the nature of the existing lesions.

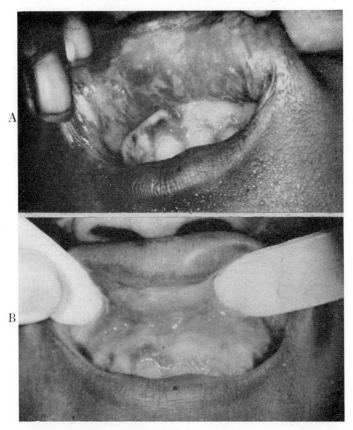

FIG. 49. (A) Acute allergic stomatitis of eight years' duration due to sensitivity to numerous foods. (Courtesy of Dr. James R. Cameron, Philadelphia, Pa.) (B) Same case following treatment with duodenal extract (experimental product).

STOMATITIS VENENATA DUE TO MEDICAMENTS USED IN DENTAL PRACTICE. The medicaments which are employed commonly in dental practice will produce lesions in sensitized individuals.

Sodium perborate is a frequent cause of these undesirable reactions. These lesions result from the use of sodium perborate in proper concentrations and they must be distinguished from those caused by too concentrated a preparation. While the former lesions are also spoken of as sodium perborate burns, they represent actually a form of stomatitis venenata. When proprietary

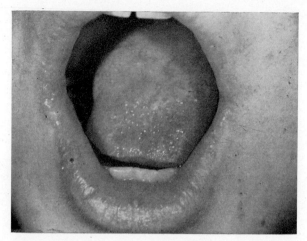

FIG. 50. Stomatitis venenata caused by the chewing of poison-ivy leaves. Numerous small ruptured vesicles can be seen on the lips.

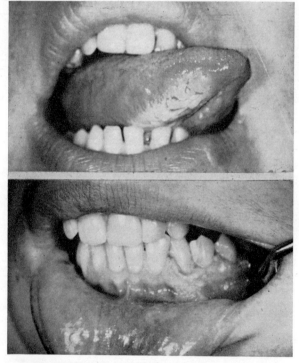

FIG. 51 (*Top*). Chemical burn of the ventral surface of the tongue due to eugenol.

FIG. 52 (*Bottom*). Chemical burn of the gum tissue in the region of the left mandibular canine and first premolar due to chloroform.

sodium-perborate-containing preparations are used, the flavoring agents may act as an additional irritant.

The aromatic oils used in dental practice such as oil of cloves or euca-lyptol will produce a slough or superficial necrosis when applied to sensitized tissues. Silvers reported an interesting case of stomatitis venenata with pur-puric manifestations, which was due to a dentifrice containing oil of cloves and oil of cassia. Chloroform and campho-phenique will also cause tissue necrosis in susceptible individuals.

Preparations containing iodine such as the strong tincture, Talbot's iodine and Lugol's solution will cause acute vesicular reactions in some individuals. Questioning will elicit usually a history of similar trouble following their use in the past.

Cold sterilizing solutions which contain formalin are a source of irritation to the patient's oral tissues. Formalin exerts a caustic action on the oral mucosa in many individuals. The effect of cold sterilization solutions on the dentists' hands is discussed under occupational hazards of dentistry.

STOMATITIS VENENATA DUE TO DENTAL FILLING MATERIALS. The mate-rials contained in plastic metallic fillings have been occasionally the cause of stomatitis venenata. Such reactions occur less frequently with silver amalgam than with copper amalgam. In some cases there appears to be a familial sen-sitivity to mercury. An unusual dryness and burning of the mouth, loss of appetite, gastric disturbances and restlessness have been reported following the insertion of amalgam fillings. These symptoms disappeared completely following the removal of the fillings. Such cases are uncommon.

Repeated swellings of the face following the insertion of amalgam fillings have been reported. In one patient, following the fourth amalgam filling, there was a marked swelling of the eyelids and oral mucosa and a dermatitis of the face, neck and shoulders. The patient gave a strongly positive patch test to a 2.5% solution of bichloride of mercury. Patch tests of the other ingredients of the amalgam fillings were not made. Traub & Holmes ob-served 2 cases of mercurial dermatitis which resulted from amalgam fillings. One patient also had a mild mercurial stomatitis. In their opinion, such cases represent contact stomatitis rather than the result of mercurial absorption.

There is no danger of chronic mercurialism developing, due to the presence of amalgam fillings, although rare reactions may develop in individuals who exhibit a sensitivity to mercury or some other metallic constituent of the amalgam. The possible dangers to the dentist from the improper manipula-tion of amalgam fillings is another matter. Gold restorations and silver amalgam fillings discolor rapidly in some mouths. The component of the saliva responsible for this change is not known.

The local oral lesions which result from the electrolytic action of saliva between dissimilar metallic fillings are discussed under galvanism. These lesions are not considered to be a manifestation of contact stomatitis.

STOMATITIS VENENATA DUE TO PROSTHETIC MATERIALS OR APPLIANCES. Every dentist has had patients who complain of pain and burning of the tis-sues beneath a denture. Soreness of the mucous membranes will occur in a certain proportion of denture patients until the tissues have time to adapt themselves to this foreign body—the denture. The increased pressure on the soft mucosal tissues, the slight movement of the denture during chewing in the highly populated bacterial environment readily explain these symptoms. Sinclair believed that these disturbances can be largely prevented with adequate C nutrition.

In a few patients, these initial symptoms persist or they develop after the denture has been worn for a while. This clinical syndrome has been called "rubber sore mouth." Speculation has existed as to whether the lesions were

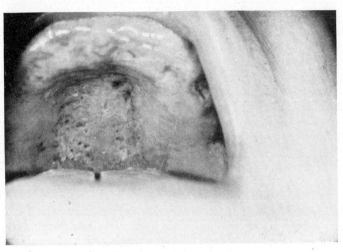

Fig. 53. Superficial necrosis of the denture-contacting area of a patient with stomatitis venenata due to an acrylic denture which was processed from inadequately refined materials. (Patient of Dr. L. Sobol, Philadelphia, Pa.)

due to mechanical or bacterial irritation or some constituent of the vulcanized rubber such as the coloring agent—which is usually mercuric sulfide.

Kaminsky *et al.* studied patients with lesions of the mouth, especially those of the tongue, who were also wearing vulcanite dentures. Patch tests of vulcanite scrapings from the denture gave violent reactions in over half of the cases consisting in some instances of a large local swelling with pustule formation. The positive reactions lasted in some patients for more than two months. Red vulcanite and that containing "metallic" granules gave the greatest per cent of positive reactions. Since patch tests of the ingredients of the rubber were usually negative before curing, it was concluded that rubber acquires its allergenic properties during vulcanization. Patients who placed their dentures in alkaline solutions, or those who alkalinized their oral cavity had less trouble with their prosthetic appliances.

Acrylic and Plastic Materials. Rattner reported the first case of stomatitis venenata associated with the wearing of a plastic denture. With the general acceptance of methyl methacrylate as a denture material, instances of stomatitis venenata have been observed due to this substance.

In the cases seen by the author the acrylic materials employed were not those which were highly purified and recommended for dental use. The irritating substance responsible for the undesirable effects was usually a constituent of the liquid monomer. An acute stomatitis venenata due to the use of an inadequately refined acrylic material is shown in the accompanying illustration. There was superficial necrosis of all the tissues in contact with the dentures. A severe glossitis was also present. Patch tests were performed using the processed acrylic denture, the polymer and the monomer. Positive reactions were obtained from both the processed denture and the monomer. Similar tests performed on a control subject were negative. A second patch

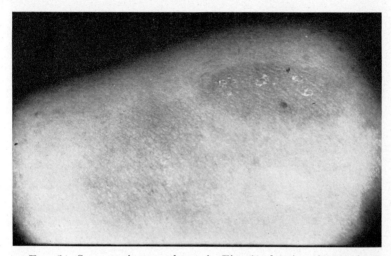

Fig. 54. Same patient as shown in Fig. 53 showing the result of a "patch test" on the patient's arm of the upper denture and a small rectangle of the acrylic denture base.

test, using the original acrylic material, an A.D.A. Council approved clear and tinted dental acrylic was then performed. A positive reaction developed only from the original inadequately refined acrylic material. These patch tests required approximately 36 hours to develop, but the erythematous and vesicular reaction remained for 4 to 5 days and well defined areas of pigmentation persisted for over three weeks. This patient has experienced no difficulty when wearing dentures processed from an acrylic which was manufactured for use in the mouth.

Moody, a dentist, experienced severe edema and dermatitis from the accidental contact with the monomer during the processing of a denture. The reaction was so severe he was compelled to remain at home under treatment for more than two weeks.

The symptoms of contact stomatitis due to acrylic materials are usually more acute than those associated with vulcanite denture bases. Symptoms appear immediately or in the course of several weeks. The patient complains of the symptoms described under "rubber sore mouth" and in acute cases there is superficial necrosis of all the denture-contacting tissues. Pain is intense and salivation is profuse. Local adenopathy may be present in cases with tissue necrosis. General symptoms of malaise are experienced by some patients.

Due to Metallic Denture Base. Stomatitis venenata may also be caused by sensitivity to any element of a metallic denture base. Allergy due to gold

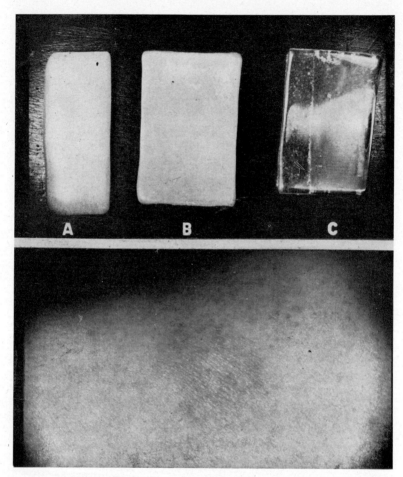

Fig. 55 (*Top*). Materials used in second patch test: (A) processed acrylic material used in patient's denture, (B) A.D.A. Council approved tinted acrylic and (C) untinted sample of the material used in B.

Fig. 56 (*Bottom*). Patch test was obtained only from sample A.

or silver is rare, but it is not uncommon to find allergy due to nickel or another of the base metals. Deisler & Sheets reported an interesting case of allergy to the nickel which was present in denture base alloys. The patient was unable to wear dentures constructed of either Ticonium or Vitallium, both of which contained this element.

Suspected allergy to a metallic denture base can be checked by covering all but a small part of the tissue-bearing denture area with a zinc oxide-eugenol or some other similar denture paste. If the mucosal reaction is observed only at that area which is in contact with the metal, it is highly probable that there is an allergy to some constituent of the metallic alloy. If a metallic denture base is still contemplated, patch tests with the particular alloy should be performed prior to the construction of the denture.

A   B

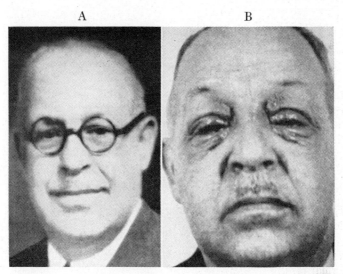

Fig. 57. Severe reaction from acrylic liquid. (A) Appearance before reaction. (B) Appearance ten days after reaction. (Moody, Dental Digest, 47:305, 1941.)

In cases of suspected stomatitis venenata due to denture bases other causes for irritation, such as bacterial or mechanical factors, should first be ruled out. The possibility of a sensitivity to the denture cream which is used for cleansing the denture or to adhesive powders should be considered. Loveman reported a case of stomatitis venenata which was eventually demonstrated to be caused by a denture cleansing cream which was not completely removed before the denture was worn. The flavoring agent, oil of anise, was the specific sensitizing agent.

The local lesions in cases of stomatitis venenata due to denture bases should be treated conservatively. Hypertonic saline mouth washes, if not painful, are beneficial. Sodium bicarbonate mouth washes are usually well tolerated. The topical application of the aniline dyes, such as a solution of 1% neutral acriflavine, to the superficial necrotic areas minimizes secondary infection and relieves the pain.

DUE TO DENTAL OR COSMETIC PREPARATIONS USED BY THE PATIENT. Stomatitis or cheilitis (inflammation of the lips) may result from a sensitization of the oral tissues to some constituent of a dentifrice, mouth wash, chewing gum, lip stick or similar preparations. Instances of sensitivity to practically all the well-known dentifrices and mouth washes have been reported. Such occurrences are no indication of the lack of purity of the product. Certain substances are more likely to give rise to these unfavorable reactions. Hexylresorcinol, the main constituent of S.T. 37, is prone to cause stomatitis venenata. Sodium perborate, especially the highly flavored variety, frequently produces undesirable reactions even when used in the proper concentration.

Teretsky reported a case of stomatitis due to sensitivity to chewing gum in which the patient complained of a burning sensation of the mouth and tongue. Numerous small vesicles in various stages of formation and degeneration were present on the palate. These symptoms coincided with the time the patient had been chewing gum and they disappeared after the patient ceased chewing gum. Tischler observed a case of gingivitis and general stomatitis due to the drinking water of a particular community. The author observed a case of aphthous stomatitis due to allergy to a municipal water supply. The stomatitis could be prevented by using bottled spring water.

ALLERGY AND ITS RELATION TO DENTOFACIAL DEVELOPMENT AND PERIODONTAL DISEASE

Allergy has been suggested as one of the causes of dental deformities and of periodontal disease. The importance of allergy as a causative or predisposing factor in these conditions has not been sufficiently determined. It is conceivable that nasal allergy during the developmental period could result in abnormal facial growth. Bowen found dental deformities five times as frequently in children suffering from nasal allergy as in a non-allergenic control group.

The possible etiologic significance of allergy in periodontal disease has received more attention abroad than in this country. Albanese believed that the sensitization of the oral tissues to certain bacterial forms is an important etiologic factor in periodontal disease. His treatment consisted of cutaneous auto-immunization, utilizing material obtained from the patient's own mouth. The results obtained by this form of treatment are considered to be superior to other forms of therapy. Hulin was also impressed with the importance of allergy in periodontal disease.

Healy, Daley and Sweet concluded that many cases of gingivitis and its end result, periodontoclasia, are related to some systemic dysfunction. They found that patients with periodontal disease could be placed in two general groups on the basis of the differential leukocyte counts of the gingival blood as compared with the finger prick blood. In the first group the differential counts were similar while in the latter there was a local eosinophilia in the gingival differential blood count, constituting in some cases 45 to 65% of the total white count. Because of this local eosinophilia these authors assumed that allergy must be an underlying etiologic factor in these patients.

Patients in the "allergic" or second group were found to have a general allergic background. Positive reactions were found to almost all foods including many of the fruits and vegetables, such as oranges and lettuce, which are generally believed to be protective to these tissues. Considering the numerous agents which come in contact with the oral mucosa, it is readily appreciated that these tissues might become sensitized to a variety of substances. Gingivitis and periodontal disease on an allergic background had in common a

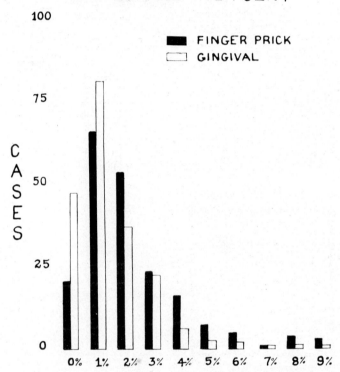

FIG. 58. Percentage of eosinophils in the finger prick and gingival blood smears. (Stine & Burket, Am. J. Orth. and Oral Surg., 30:527-30, 1944.)

gingival eosinophilia, capillary dilatation, increased capillary permeability and exudation. Such cases were treated best by the exclusion of the reagin or the offending substance. Healy *et al.* did not report the finger prick and gingival differential counts following therapy.

In an attempt to determine the significance of allergy as an etiologic factor in periodontal disease a group of clinic patients selected at random were studied by Stine and the author. Using a method similar to that employed by Healey *et al.*, the gingival and finger prick differential blood counts of 200 patients were studied.

A high eosinophil count was found in the gingival blood in 18% of the 200 cases.

The relation of the gingival to finger-tip eosinophils for each of the 200 cases is shown in the accompanying illustration. Finger-tip eosinophil percentage is represented along the base line, and gingival eosinophil percentage along the vertical line. The cases included within the heavy-lined square, 162 in number, had an eosinophil count within normal limits of 0 to 4 per cent. All the cases beyond the limits of the large square had an eosinophil count of over 4 per cent in either, or both, the gingival and finger-tip blood. The diagonal line running from the 0.0 point divides the cases, so that those lying

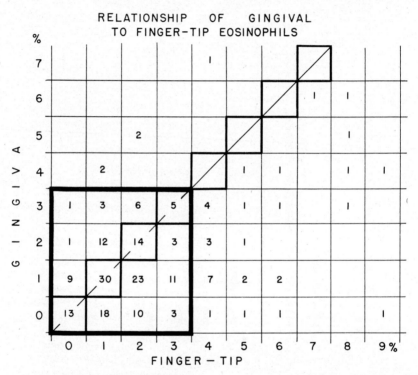

FIG. 59. The relation of the gingival to finger-tip eosinophiles for each of the 200 cases studied. Finger-tip eosinophile percentage is represented along the base line, and gingival eosinophile percentage along the vertical line. The cases included within the heavy-lined large square, 162 in number, had an eosinophile count within normal limits of 0 to 4 per cent. The cases beyond the limits of the large square all had an eosinophile count of over 4 per cent in either or both the gingival and finger-tip blood. The diagonal line running from the 0,0 point divides the cases so that those lying above the line have a higher gingival than finger-tip eosinophile count, those below the line have a higher finger-tip than gingival count, and those in the squares through which the diagonal line passes have an equal eosinophile count in both finger-tip and gingival blood. (Stine and Burket, Am. J. Orth. and Oral Surg., 30:527, 1944.)

above the line have a higher gingival than finger-tip eosinophil count, those below the line have a higher finger-tip than gingival count and those in the squares through which the line passes similar finger-tip and gingival eosinophil counts.

The gingival eosinophil count was greater than the finger-tip count in just 5 cases, and in none of these was a history of a known allergy obtained. No attempt was made to treat these 5 cases on the assumption that allergy was an etiologic factor. It appears that allergy, as evidenced by local eosinophilia, was not an important etiologic factor in the causation of periodontal disease in this group of patients. This, however, does not exclude allergy as an etiologic factor.

REFERENCES

FUSOSPIROCHETAL INFECTIONS

Albray, R. A.: Diagnosis and treatment of Vincent's disease, Dent. Items of Interest, 51:275-89, 1929.

Arnold, C. H.: Plaut-Vincent's infection of vagina, report of a case. J. A. M. A., 94:1461, 1930.

Ast, David B.: Vincent's angina—a reportable disease, New York J. Dent., 11:63, 1941.

Barenberg, L. H., & M. W. Bloomberg: Use of sulpharsphenamine in Vincent's angina and stomatitis in children, J. A. M. A., 83:25, 1924.

Barenberg, L. H., & J. M. Lewis: Vincent's (fusospirillary) infection of ear, J. A. M. A., 94:1065, 1930.

Barker, L. F., & S. R. Miller: Perforating ulcer of the hard palate resembling tertiary syphilis, J. A. M. A., 71:793-7, 1918.

Belding, P. H., & L. J. Belding: Why Vincent's infection?, J. A. D. A., 22:2114, 1935.

Benedek, T.: Fusospirochetal onychia and paronychia, Surg., 11:75, 1942.

Bennett, J. L.: Vincent's infection in psychiatric patients, Psychiat. Quart., 14:632, 1940.

Brams, J., I. Pilot & D. J. Davis: Studies of fusiform bacilli and spirochetes. Their occurrence in normal preputial secretions and in erosive and gangrenous balanitis, J. Infect. Dis., 32:159, 1923.

Britton, B. H.: Treatment of Vincent's angina with copper sulphate and glycerine, Southwestern Med., 17:28, 1933.

Broughton-Alcock, W.: Invasion of intact buccal mucous membrane by spirochetes, Proc. Roy. Soc. Med., 23:21, 1930.

Brown, R. D.: Sperm fluctuation in health and disease, Southern M. J., 36:619, 1943.

Bryant, C. K.: Blood counts in 22 cases of Vincent's stomatitis, J. Dent. Research, 9:284-85, 1929.

Burkwall, H. F.: Noma, Am. J. Orthodontics & Oral Surg., 28:394, 1944.

Cady, F. C.: Dental health in State Department of Health of U. S., Pub. Health Bull., No. 251, Wash., 1939.

Carr, M. W.: Intravenous arsphenamine in treatment of advanced fusospirochetosis, J. Dent. Research, 16:1, 1937.

Caskey, C. R.: Vincent's associated with unusual skin manifestations, Urol. & Cutan. Rev., 36:370, 1923.

Chu, Fu-Tang & Chuan Fan: Cancrum oris, a clinical study of 100 cases with especial reference to prognosis, Chinese M. J., 50:303, 1936.

Cobe, H. M., & L. G. Grace: Ulceromembranous gingivitis, Dental Cosmos, 73:461-67, 1931.

Colby, F., & H. B. Barr: Vincent's disease following bite of hand, Texas State J. Med., 28:467-70, 1932.

Council on Dental Therapeutics: Treatment of Vincent's infection, J. A. D. A., 29:461-4, 1942.

Current Comment: Dangers of sodium perborate, J. A. M. A., 110:445, 1938.

Cuthbert, S., & F. R. P. Williams: Gingivostomatitis with special reference to Vincent's gingivitis, J. Roy. Nav. M. Serv., 29:115, 1943.

Daley, F. H.: Incidence of Vincent's infection based on 3,771 smears, J. A. D. A., 18:1025, 1931.

Dalitsch, W. W.: Vincent's stomatitis and related infections, J. A. D. A., 21:1255, 1934.

Dean, R. D., & M. T. Dean: Clinical manifestation of fusospirochetal infections, J. Dent. Research, 11:747, 1931.

Devell, W. D., & J. F. Landon: Gangrenous vulvitis associated with mouth and rectal lesions in a child, J. Pediat., 9:75, 1936.

Diamond, J. S.: Noma (oral) complicating non-specific ulcerative colitis, Am. J. Digest. Dis. & Nutrition, 2:698, 1936.

Dillon, Chas.: Nutritional and other factors in trench mouth, Brit. Dent. J., 74:242, 1943.

Disraeli, I.: Compilation of fusospirochetosis statistics throughout the U. S., J. A. D. A., 19:494, 1932.

Donson, S. D.: Vincent's infection contracted during luetic treatment, Dent. Cosmos, 75:883, 1933.

Easton, E. R.: Vincent's simulating acute appendicitis, Am. J. Surg., 22:74, 1933.

Editorial: The army and Vincent's ulceration, Brit. Dent. J., 72:1-5, 1942.

Eskow, Bernard, & D. E. Berman: Conservative treatment of Vincent's stomatitis, J. A. D. A., 30:924, 1943.

Farrell, G. W., & W. A. McNichols: Efficacy of various medicaments in the treatment of Vincent's stomatitis: report of 794 cases, J. A. M. A., 108:630, 1937.

Fields, H., Jr.: Therapy of fusospirochetosis (Vincent's), J. A. M. A., 114:1073, 1940.

Filler, W., et al.: Treatment of Trichomonas vaginalis vaginitis with Negatan (Negatol), Am. J. Obst. & Gynec., 43:1057, 1942.

Firestone, C.: Tonsillectomy as a curative for oral fusospirochetosis, Northwest Med., 31:335, 1932.

Fish, E. W.: Acute ulcerative stomatitis, Lancet, 235:558, 1938.

Foote, G. B.: Dental considerations of Vincent's infection, Mil. Surgeon, 88:290, 1941.

Garson, P.: Local oral medication with sulfanilamide in lozenge form, Brit. M. J., 2:452, 1943.

Glickman, I., & B. G. Bibby: Effect of sodium perborate upon the gingival mucosa: A controlled experiment, J. A. D. A., 31:1201, 1944.

Goadby, K. W.: Diseases of the gums and oral mucous membrane, Oxford Medical Publication, 1925.

Goldberg, L., & J. M. Thorp: Nicotinic acid excretion in normal men and in cases of Vincent's gingivitis, J. So. Afric. Med. Soc., 7:85, 1942.

Goldman, Henry M.: Report of the histopathologic study of the jaws of a diet-deficient monkey, and its relation to Vincent's infection, Am. J. Orthodontics & Oral Surg., 29:480, 1943.

Goodridge, D. L.: A case of Vincent's ulceration in a patient undergoing syphilitic treatment, Brit. Dent. J., 72:12, 1942.

Hardy, N.: Vincent's ulceration, Brit. Dent. J., 70:401, 1941.

Hayden, W. Y.: Vincent's infection, J. Canad. Dent. A., 8:178-9, 1942.

Hirsch, F. G., & C. L. Spingarn: The treatment of fusospirochetal infections of the mouth and throat with sulfathiazole, Mil. Surgeon, 93:299, 1943.

Hirschfeld, I.: Vincent's infection of the mouth, J. A. D. A., 21:768, 1934.

Hudson, O. C.: Human tooth injuries, New York State J. Med., 44:1910, 1944.

Janetos, D. S.: Trench mouth aboard a United States naval auxiliary vessel, U. S. Nav. M. Bull., 43:308, 1944.

Jennings, C. W.: Vincent's developing in patients under treatment for syphilis, South. Med. & Surg., 95:496, 1933.

Jewesbury, E. C. O.: Misuse of intravenous N.A.B. for Vincent's infection, Brit. M. J., 2:360, 1943.

Joss, C. E., & H. L. Kirkpatrick: Fatal case of Vincent's angina, J. Kansas M. Soc., 34:310-1, 1933.

Jump, H. D., & S. J. Sperling: Fusospirochetal (Vincent's) infection of pleura and vagina, J. A. M. A., 98:219, 1932.

Kelly, Florence C.: Bacteriology of artificially produced necrotic lesions in oropharynx of monkey, J. Infect. Dis., 74:93, 1944.

Kent, Basil S.: Necrotic gingivitis, Lancet, 1:642, 1943.

King, J. D.: Vincent's disease treated with nicotinic acid, Lancet, 239:32, 1940.

King, J. D.: Acute ulcerative stomatitis, Lancet, 241:293, 1941.

King, J. D.: Nutritional and other factors in "trench-mouth," with special reference to the nicotinic acid component of the vitamin B_2 complex, Brit. Dent. J., 74:113, 1943.

Kline, B. S.: Experimental gangrene, J. Infect. Dis., 32:481-3, 1923.

Kramer, L. R.: Should Vincent's infection be reported? (A record of eight deaths in one year (1938) in Kansas due to Vincent's infection), J. A. D. A., 26:1569-1571, 1939.

Lapira, E.: Ulcerative stomatitis associated with an avitaminosis in Malta, Brit. Dent. J., 74:257, 1943.

Leudingham, R. S.: Sodium citrate, a spirochetocide, J. Lab. & Clin. Med., 21:922, 1936.

Lichtenberg, H. H., et al.: Pathogenicity of fusiform bacillus and spirillum of Plaut-Vincent; clinical and experimental study, J. A. M. A., 100:707-11, 1933.

Linton, C. S.: Treatment of Vincent's angina of the tonsil: Preliminary report, J. A. M. A., 123:341, 1943.

Ludwick, William E.: Observations relative to the therapeutic value of heavy metals in treating Vincent's gingivitis, U. S. Nav. M. Bull., 42:584, 1944.

Lufkin, A. W., & T. Disraeli: Vincent's infection, Pac. Dent. Gaz., 37:611, 1929.

Lyons, D. C.: Public health regulations for the control of Vincent's infection, Dent. Items of Interest, 66:15, 1944.

MacFarlane, L. H.: Cancrum oris following measles, Brit. J. Child. Dis., 33:275, 1936.

Madden, J. F.: The balanitides, J. A. M. A., 105:402, 1935.

McDonagh, J. E. R.: Acute ulceration of the vulva, Brit. J. Dermat., 36: 285, 1924.

McMillen, S. I.: Successful treatment of noma with formaldehyde, Am. J. Dis. Child., 50:1495-6, 1935.

McMillen, S. I.: Successful treatment of noma with solution of formaldehyde, Am. J. Dis. Child., 62:590, 1941.

Mead, Sterling V.: Diseases of the Mouth, ed. 5, St. Louis, Mo., C. V. Mosby Co., 1940.

Meleny, F. L.: Use of zinc peroxide in oral surgery, Internat. J. Orthodontia, 23:932, 1937.

Meleny, F. L.: The prophylactic and active use of zinc peroxide in foul smelling mouth and neck infections, Ann. Surg., 107:32, 1938.

Miller, S. C., et al.: Nicotinic acid and Vincent's infection, New York J. Dent., 10:424, 1940.

Miller, S. C., & W. M. Greenhut: Acute necrotic gingivitis (Vincent's infection); seasonal and age relations, J. A. D. A., 31:910, 1944.

Morris, M. L., & C. E. Franklin: A preliminary report on the use of nicotinic acid in the treatment of fusospirochetal disease of dogs, North Amer. Vet., 20:31-33, 1939.

Morrison, J. P.: Case of Vincent's infection associated with erythema multiforme, J. A. D. A., 28:1938, 1941.

Nizel, A. E., & Samuel Rubin: Zinc peroxide's role in treatment of Vincent's stomatitis, Mil. Surgeon, 93:49, 1943.

Pelner, Louis: Treatment of severe case of Vincent's angina with a sulfanilamide derivative, New York State J. Med., 41:1358, 1941.

Pilot I., & A. E. Kanter: Studies of fusiform bacilli and spirochetes. Further observations on their distribution about the genitalia of normal women and their significance in certain genital infections and tumors, Arch. Dermat. & Syph., 10:561, 1924.

Pincus, P.: Notes on ulcerative gingivitis in man, Brit. Dent. J., 75:309, 1944.

Pollack, J. E.: Dangers of infection due to human bites as compared to animal bites, Dent. Items of Interest, 63:1092, 1941.

Prinz, H., & S. Greenbaum: Diseases of the Mouth and Their Treatment, ed. 2, Philadelphia, Lea & Febiger, 1939.

Ronchese, Francesco: Bite and dental injury, J. A. M. A., 127:1050, 1945.

Rosebury, T.: Is Vincent's infection a communicable disease?, J. A. D. A., 29:823, 1942.

Rosenthal, S. L.: The effect of medicaments on the motility of the oral flora with special reference to the treatment of Vincent's infection, J. Periodontology, 8:71, 1937.

Rosenthal, S. L.: Sodium carbonate in the treatment of Vincent's infection, J. A. D. A., 28:972, 1941.

Rosenthal, S. L., & E. Gootzeit: Incidence of B. fusiformis and spirochetes in the edentulous mouth, J. Dent. Research, 21:373, 1942.

Schamberg, M. I.: A timely and proper estimate of the therapeutic value of sodium perborate and its compounds in the treatment of infections of the mucous membrane, Dent. Items of Interest, 65:888, 1943.

Schwartzman, J., & L. Grossman: Vincent's ulceromembranous gingivo-stomatitis, Arch. Pediat., 58:515-20, 1941.

Shallenberger, P. L., et al.: The use of penicillin in Vincent's angina, J. A. M. A., 128:706, 1945.

Shirazy, E.: Fusospirochetosis, International Clinics, Vol. II, series 3, Philadelphia, Pa., J. B. Lippincott Co., 1940.

Silber, Samuel: The treatment of tonsillitis, pharyngitis, and gingivostomati-tis with the bismuth salt of heptadienecarboxylic acid in cocoa butter suppositories, J. Pediat., 32:59, 1943.

Sinclair, J. A.: Vitamin A and B deficiency in Vincent's infection, J. A. D. A., 26:1611, 1939.

Speirs, Richard E.: The prevention of human bite infections, Surg., Gynec. & Obst., 72:619, 1941.

Spies, T. D., et al.: Use of nicotinic acid in treatment of pellagra, J. A. M. A., 110:622, 1938.

Stransky, E.: Noma in the Philippines, J. Philippine M. A., 21:501, 1941.

Stammers, A. Frank: Vincent's infection: Observations and conclusions regarding the etiology and treatment of 1,017 civilian cases, Brit. Dent. J., 76:147, 1944.

Stine, D. G.: Blood picture in Vincent's infection, Missouri State M. J., 37:277, 1940.

Strock, Alvin E.: Relationship between gingivitis and penicillin administration, J. A. D. A., 31:1235, 1944.

Tarnow, O. S.: Blood findings in Vincent's angina, Med. Klin., 17:1024, 1921.

Taylor, F. E., & W. H. McKinstry: A serological investigation of Vincent's angina, Brit. M. J., 60:231-37, 1917.

Thoma, Kurt: Oral pathology, St. Louis, C. V. Mosby Co., 1941.

Thoma, K. H.: Vincent's infections or fusospirochetosis, Am. J. Orthodontics & Oral Surg., 27:479-88, 1941.

Thompson, L. E.: A fatal case of brain abscess from Vincent's angina following extraction of tooth under procaine hydrochloride, J. A. M. A., 93:1063-5, 1929.

Tomlinson, T. H., Jr.: Oral pathology in monkeys in various dietary deficiencies, Pub. Health Rep., 54:431, 1939.

Topping, N. H., & H. F. Fraser: Mouth lesions associated with dietary deficiencies in monkeys, Pub. Health Rep., 54:416, 1939.

Valenzuela, R. H.: Therapy of noma, Revista Mex. de Pediat., 13:310, 1943.

von Haam, E.: Venereal fusospirochetosis, J. Trop. Med., 18:595, 1938.

Wagner, E. H., et al.: Laboratory diagnosis in Vincent's, J. Dent. Research, 10:591, 1930.

Webster, F. F.: Epidemic of ulcerative gingivitis treated at the Glasgow Dental Hospital, Dent. Rec., 61:319, 1941.

Wigoder, Lionel: Three unusual cases of Vincent's ulceration, Brit. Dent. J., 73:261, 1942.

Williams, R. H.: Fusospirochetosis: recovery of the causative organism from the blood, with report of two cases, Arch. Int. Med., 68:80-93, 1941,

Winograd, M. G.: A case of noma of the mouth following measles, Dental Cosmos, **68**:779-80, 1926.

METALS

Akers, L. H.: Ulcerative stomatitis following therapeutic use of mercury and bismuth, J. A. D. A., **23**:781-5, 1936.

Arnold, F. A.: Change of Water Supply and Oral Lactobacilli, Pub. Health Rep., **57**:773-80, 1942.

Artz, C. P.: Lead intoxication in children from burning of battery casings; report of 2 cases, West Virginia M. J., **37**:410-14, 1941.

Aub, J. C., *et al.:* Effects of treatment on radium and calcium metabolism in human body, Ann. Int. Med., **11**:1443-63, 1938.

Bloomfield, J. J., & W. Blum: Health hazards in chromium plating, Pub. Health Rep., **43**:2330-51, 1928.

Brittingham, J. W.: Bismuth poisoning in treatment of syphilis, J. M. A. Georgia, **22**:323, 1933.

Cecil, Russel L., *et al.:* Gold salts in the treatment of rheumatoid arthritis, Ann. Int. Med., **16**:811, 1942.

Colby, Robert A.: Radiation effects on structures of the oral cavity: A review, J. A. D. A., **29**:1446, 1942.

Costello, Maurice J.: Mercury vapor gingivitis in a glass blower working with neon lights (Wood filter as an aid in diagnosis), Arch. Dermat. & Syph., **51**:215, 1945.

Cruickshank, D. B.: Natural occurrence of zinc in teeth, variations in tuberculosis, Brit. Dent. J., **68**:257, 1942.

Danckworth, P. W., & G. Siebler: Zur Toxikologie des Bleis und seiner Verbindungen, Arch. d. Pharm., **265**:424-26, 1927.

Epstein, S., & H. M. Schamp: Sodium fluoride mouth rinse: Report of two cases, J. A. D. A., **31**:1233, 1944.

Felsher, I. M., & K. K. Jones: The prevention of Bi-gingivitis by the use of sodium hexameta phosphate, J. Invest. Dermat., **4**:135-42, 1941.

Flury, F.: Mercurial poisoning from dental fillings; comment on Stock's article, München med. Wchnschr., **73**:1021, 1926. Abst. J. A. M. A., **87**:685, 1926.

Friedman, A. P., & C. W. Olsen: Paralysis of facial and masticatory nerves following arsenic poisoning, Bull. Los Angeles Neurol. Soc., **6**:85, 1941.

Guy, C. C.: Stomatitis following injection of mercurochrome-220 soluble in tuberculosis sinus, J. A. M. A., **82**:2119, 1924.

Higgins, W. H.: Systemic poisoning with bismuth, J. A. M. A., **66**:648, 1916.

Hodges, Paul C., *et al.:* Skeletal sclerosis in chronic sodium fluoride poisoning, J. A. M. A., **117**:1938, 1941.

Holmes, G.: Dermatitis following gold injections for rheumatism, Brit. M. J., **1**:58, 1935.

Hudson, E. H.: Purpura haemorrhagica caused by gold and arsenical compounds, with report of 2 cases, Lancet, **2**:74-77, 1935.

Jones, R. R.: Symptoms in early stages of industrial plumbism, J. A. M. A., **104**:195-200, 1935.

Kehoe, R. A., *et al.:* Lead absorption and excretion in certain lead trades, J. Indust. Hyg. & Toxicol., **15**:306-19, 1933.

Kemp, F. H., *et al.:* Spondylosis deformans in relation to fluorine and general nutrition, Lancet, **2**:93, 1942.

Kety, S. S., & T. V. Letonoff: Treatment of lead poisoning by sodium citrate, Am. J. M. Sc., 205:406, 1943.

Lain, E. S.: Electrogalvanic lesions of the oral cavity produced by metallic dentures, J. A. M. A., 100:717, 1933.

LeBel, L. J. B.: Generalized argyria, J. M. Soc., New Jersey, 31:703-05, 1934.

Lederer, L. G., & F. C. Bing: Effect of calcium and phosphorus on retention of lead by growing organisms, J. A. M. A., 114:2457, 1940.

Lenartowicz, J., & B. Jaloway: Essais de production d'argyrie artificielle chez les animaux, Ann. de dermat et syph., 9:483-94, 1938.

Levine, S. A., & J. A. Smith: Argyria confused with heart disease, New England J. Med., 226:682, 1942.

Lieberman, H.: Chrome ulcerations of the nose and throat, New England J. Med., 225:132, 1941.

Linsman, J. F., & C. A. McMurray: Fluoride osteosclerosis from drinking water, Radiology, 40:474, 1943.

Machle, W.: Lead absorption from bullets lodged in tissues; report of 2 cases, J. A. M. A., 115:1536-41, 1940.

Machle, Willard, E. W. Scott, & E. J. Largent: The metabolism of fluoride, Indust. Med., 11:288, 1941.

Marchmont-Robinson, S. W.: Effect of vitamin C on workers exposed to lead dust, J. Lab. & Clin. Med., 26:1478, 1941.

Marin, J. V.: The treatment of mercurial and bismuth stomatitis by ascorbic acid, Abs. J. A. M. A., 118:1260, 1942.

Markow, H.: Urticaria following a dental silver filling, New York State J. Med., 43:1648, 1943.

Martland, H. S.: Occupational poisoning in manufacture of luminous watch dials, J. A. M. A., 92:552-59, 1929.

Mascheroni, H. A., & C. Reussi: Fluorin osteosis, Rev. méd.-quir. de pat. femi., 9:147, 1941.

Maulbetsch, A., & E. Rutishauser: La teneur des dents en plomb, Arch. internat. de pharmacodyn et de thérap., 53:55, 1936.

McKay, F. S.: Mottled enamel: The prevention of its further production through a change of the water supply at Oakley, Idaho, J. A. D. A., 20:1137, 1933.

McKhann, C. F., & E. C. Vogt: Lead poisoning in children, J. A. M. A., 101:1131, 1933.

Merenlender, J.: Zur Kenntins der Embolia cutis arterialis mendicamentosa (bismutica), Arch. f. Dermat. u. Syph., 167:708, 1933.

Moore, J. E., & A. Keidel: Dermatitis and allied reactions following arsenical treatment of syphilis, Arch. Int. Med., 27:716, 1921.

New York Inst. of Clin. Oral Pathology: Case report of radium necrosis of the jaws, Arch. Clin. Oral Path., 1:218-20, 1937.

Pandit, C. G., et al.: A study of the factors involved in the production of mottled enamel in children and severe bone manifestations in adults, Indian J. M. Research, 28:533, 1940.

Rapoport, M., & A. S. Kenney: Case of lead encephalopathy in breast-fed infant due to use of lead nipple shields by mother, J. A. M. A., 112:2040, 1939.

Rathmell, T. K., & F. L. Smith, Jr.: Toy dishes and acute plumbism, J. A. M. A., 114:242, 1940.

Rosenthal, M.: Experimental radium poisoning changes in teeth of rabbits produced by oral administration of radium sulphate, Am. J. M. Sc., **193**: 495-501, 1937.

Royster, L. T.: Argyria; report of case in patient aged 5½ years, J. Pediat., **1**:736, 1932.

Rygee, J.: Trois cas de coloration brune de l'email de toutes les dents chez trois enfants de meme famille, Acta Odontol. Scandinavica, **1**:57-74, 1937.

Schmidt, J.: Untersuchung über Bleigehalt im Zahnstein und Speichel bei Arbeitern des Bleigewerbes, Zentralbl. f. Gewerbehyg., **10**:101, 1933.

Scholtz, J. R., K. D. McEacher, & C. Wood: Sobisminol mass: clinical results with oral administration, J. A. M. A., **113**:2219, 1939.

Silber, S.: Bismuth suppositories: in throat infections: Bacteriology and pharmacology: effectiveness, absorption, excretion, toxicity, J. Pediat., **25**:244, 1944.

Smith, R. A.: Effect of x-rays on the developing teeth of rats, Am. J. Orthodontics & Oral Surg., **24**:428-36, 1938.

Society Transactions: Gold dermatitis and stomatitis, Arch. Dermat. & Syph., **42**:721-22, 1940.

Sollmann, T., & N. E. Schreiber: Chemical studies of acute poisoning from mercury bichloride, Arch. Int. Med., **57**:46, 1936.

Spiegel, L.: Discoloration of skin and mucous membrane resembling argyria, following use of bismuth and silver arsphenamine, Arch. Dermat. & Syph., **23**:266, 1931.

Spira, Leo: Chronic fluorine poisoning (fluorosis)—signs and symptoms, Edinburgh M. J., **49**:707, 1942.

Stillians, A. W.: Argyria, Arch. Dermat. & Syph., **35**:67, 1937.

Sulman, F., *et al.*: Selective bismuth melanosis of female genital tract induced by treatment with sex hormones, Endocrinology, **32**:293, 1943.

Tabershaw, L., *et al.*: Plumbism resulting from oxyacetylene cutting of painted structural steel, J. Indust. Hyg. & Toxicol., **25**:189, 1943.

Teleky, L.: Occupational diseases of bones and joints, Indust. Med., **11**:164, 1942.

Traub, E. F., & R. H. Holmes: Dermatitis and stomatitis from mercury of amalgam fillings, Arch. Dermat. & Syph., **38**:349, 1938.

Wilkie, J.: Two cases of fluorine osteosclerosis, Brit. J. Radiol., **13**:213, 1940.

Wile, U. J., & C. J. Courville: Pityriasis-rosea-like dermatitis following gold therapy; report of 2 cases, Arch. Dermat. & Syph., **42**:1105, 1940.

Williams, H. B.: Chronic lead poisoning, J. A. M. A., **112**:534, 1939.

ALLERGIC MANIFESTATIONS

Barton, R. L., & Paul A. O'Leary: Fixed drug eruption produced by diphenylhydantoin sodium, Arch. Dermat. & Syph., **48**:413, 1943.

Bass, M. H.: Idiosyncrasy to metallic mercury, with special reference to amalgam fillings in the teeth, J. of Pediat., **23**:215-18, 1943.

Cahn, Lester R.: Mouth lesions of local and systemic origin, J. A. D. A., **28**:909, 1941.

Cahn, L. R.: Denture-sore mouth, Ann. Dent., **3**:33, 1936.

Cohen, M. B.: Orthodontic problems associated with allergy, Angle Orthodontist, 7:150, 1937.

Cook, R. A.: Allergy in drug idiosyncrasy, J. A. M. A., 73:759, 1919.

Dennie, C. C.: Angioneurotic edema and dermatitis venenata-like lesions due to the oral administration of sulfathiazole, J. A. M. A., 120:197, 1942.

Deissler, K. J., & G. R. Sheets: Contact stomatitis due to a denture in a metal sensitive patient, California & West. Med., 47:354, 1942.

Fuchs, A. M.: Allergy related to dental practice, Dental Outlook, 26:10, 1939.

Gardner, E., & W. B. Blanton: The incidence of aspirin hypersensitivity, Am. J. M. Sc., 200:390, 1940.

Goldman, L., & B. Goldman: Contact testing of the buccal mucous membrane for stomatitis venenata, Arch. Dermat. & Syph., 50:79-84, 1944.

Goldstein, H. I.: Chase-Lain-Goldstein Syndrome—Galvanic batteries in human mouth, Rev. Gastroenterol., 10:206, 1943.

Greenbaum, S. S.: Stomatitis venenata and allergy, Dental Cosmos, 72:768, 1933.

Harper, P.: Idiosyncrasy to ammoniated mercury ointment, report of 2 cases, J. Pediat., 5:794-99, 1934.

Healy, J. C., F. H. Daly, & M. H. Sweet: Medical aspects of periodontoclasia and gingivitis, J. Lab. & Clin. Med., 21:698, 1938.

Hix, J. B.: Contact dermatitis from Teel, Arch. Dermat. & Syph., 43:847, 1941.

Kaminsky, A., et al.: Glossodynia and glossitis due to sensitivity to a vulcanite prosthesis, Semana med., B. Aires, 49:674, 1942.

Kasselberg, L. A.: A severe pemphigus-like reaction following administration of sulfamerazine, J. A. M. A., 123:1035, 1943.

Klatell, J. S.: Sulfonamides, Am. J. Orthodontics & Oral Surg., 29:255, 1943.

Loveman, A.: Stomatitis venenata, Arch. Dermat. & Syph., 37:70, 1938.

Miller, J.: Chellitis from sensitivity to oil of cinnamon present in bubble gum, J. A. M. A., 116:131, 1941.

Moody, W. L.: Severe reaction from acrylic liquid, Dental Digest, 47:305, 1941.

Moss, R. E., & W. E. Long: Toxic eruptions due to phenobarbital, Arch. Dermat. & Syph., 46:386, 1942.

Murray, M.: Relation of foci of infection to some allergic states, Cincinnati J. Med., 23:211-14, 1942-3.

Paul, T. M.: Prompt and permanent annihilation of sensitiveness to all allergens, Urol. & Cutan. Rev., 47:36-41, 1943.

Pearson, R. S. B.: Recurrent swellings of the parotid glands, Arch. Dis. Childhood, 10:363-76, 1935.

Prickman, L. E., & H. F. Buchstein: Acute abdominal allergy, S. Clin. North America, 17:1005-11, 1937.

Ratner, Bret: Allergy of the oral cavity in children, New Zealand Dent. J., 37:52, 1941.

Rattner, H.: Stomatitis due to sensitization to dental plates, J. A. M. A., 106:2230, 1936.

Schnee, I. M.: Membranous inflammation of oropharynx nose and conjunctiva due to sulphathiazole administration, Brit. M. J., 506, 1943.

Silvers, S. H.: Stomatitis and dermatitis venenata with purpura resulting from oil of cloves and oil of cassia, Dent. Items of Interest, 61:649, 1939.

Silvers, S. H.: Stomatitis venenata and dermatitis of anal orifice from chewing poison ivy leaves, J. A. M. A., 116:2257, 1941.
Turner, P. L., & T. W. Clarke: Temporomandibular arthropathy in serum sickness, Annals of Allergy, 1:115-19, 1943.
White, C. J.: Allergic manifestations in the oral mucosa, J. A. D. A., 24:1521, 1937.

SECTION THREE

DISEASES OF THE TONGUE AND DERMATOLOGIC DISEASES OF DENTAL INTEREST, MINOR STOMATITIDES

8

The Tongue

GENERAL CONSIDERATIONS	BLACK HAIRY TONGUE
FREQUENCY OF CLINICAL ENTITIES	GEOGRAPHIC TONGUE
DEVELOPMENTAL ANOMALIES	BURNING TONGUE
FUNCTIONAL AND PHYSIOLOGIC	PAINFUL PAPILLAE
CHANGES	VARICOSITIES OF THE LINGUAL
TRAUMATIC INJURIES TO TONGUE	VEINS

GENERAL CONSIDERATIONS

The tongue should be examined as carefully as the teeth. The amount of coating, the muscle tone, color, the relative numbers and distribution of the various lingual papillae and any lesions on the dorsum and margins of this organ should be noted. Adequate illumination, preferably daylight, is essential for this examination. The color of the tongue should not be determined when it is forcibly protruded from the mouth—a common method of examination. When the tongue is forcibly extended, the lingual veins are usually compressed by the lower incisor teeth, which results in congestion and mild degrees of cyanosis. This is also true when the examiner pulls the tongue out by grasping it with a gauze square or a towel. The color of the tongue can be appraised best with this organ lying passively in its usual location. The tongue margins should be carefully examined for indentation markings or crenations produced by the teeth or prosthetic appliances.

The examination of the tongue has been a ritual of the physician, irrespective of the location of the patient's symptoms. In spite of these numerous examinations this organ remains still one of the least understood and least carefully studied structures of the body. The tongue is an excellent index of the constitutional state but seldom of individual diseases.

117

It is both impossible and impracticable to discuss all the diseases of the tongue. The lingual lesions have been mentioned under the discussion of the oral aspects of the various disease entities. Tongue lesions in the deficiency diseases, pernicious anemia, stomatitis medicamentosa, in syphilis, tuberculosis and actinomycosis are important. The tongue lesions to be discussed in this chapter represent in most instances primary lingual diseases rather than tongue manifestations secondary to a systemic disturbance.

The physiologic mechanism of the various tongue changes, such as the coating of the tongue and the papillary atrophy, is just being appreciated. This knowledge explains why similar atrophic lingual changes are associated with many different diseases. A physicochemical analysis of the various disease entities associated with atrophic lingual changes led Wäldenstrom to the conclusion that atrophic lingual changes are due to a break or deficiency in one or more of the oxidase enzyme systems. Lack of iron or the inability to use iron would cause serious disturbances in Warburg's and the cytochrome enzyme systems while ariboflavinosis and aniacinosis would interfere with the normal function of the flavine and pyridine enzymes. These conclusions have been borne out by clinical experience.

FREQUENCY OF CLINICAL ENTITIES

McCarthy noted the frequency of the various clinical entities in the examination of 396 patients with tongue lesions.

Syphilis of the tongue..................... 65
   Atrophic glossitis.................. 45
   All other forms................... 20
Chronic glossitis....................... 61
Geographic tongue...................... 55
Congenital fissured tongue............... 50
Papillitis............................... 48
Atrophic glossitis of secondary anemia..... 32
Ulcerative glossitis..................... 20
Glossodynia............................ 16
Varicosities............................ 12
Black hairy tongue...................... 9
Atrophic glossitis of pernicious anemia..... 9
Traumatic glossitis..................... 6
Glossitis rhombica mediana.............. 5
Tuberculosis of the tongue.............. 4
Pseudo hairy tongue.................... 2
Macroglossia.......................... 1

This tabulation is a useful guide to the frequency of the various tongue lesions, if one remembers that cases of leukoplakia and tongue lesions associated with the dermatoses are omitted. The incidence of geographic tongue and congenitally fissured tongue is larger than that observed in our dental out-patient clinic, where atrophic lesions associated with the nutritional deficiencies are seen more frequently. The selection of cases from private or clinic practice will considerably affect the frequency of the various lesions.

Lesions of the tongue can be grouped conveniently into:

(1) Developmental anomalies.
(2) Functional and physiologic changes.

(3) Tongue lesions secondary to systemic disease (covered elsewhere).
(4) Traumatic injuries.
(5) Neuralgias—glossodynia and glossopyrosis.
(6) Cancerphobias and malignancies involving the tongue.

DEVELOPMENTAL ANOMALIES

The more important developmental anomalies of the tongue include: ankyloglossia (tongue-tie), bifid tongue, absence of papillae, fissured tongue, macroglossia, thyroglossal cyst, lingual thyroid and glossitis rhombica mediana.

Ankyloglossia results from an undue shortening of the lingual frenum. At one time this condition was believed to be incompatible with normal mental development and early operation was performed, at times somewhat crudely by the midwife's finger. A mild degree of ankyloglossia is of no clinical significance and, if severe, the condition can be easily corrected surgically. A bifid tongue or bifid tip of the tongue is rare and of little practical importance. It results from lack of complete fusion of the lateral halves of this organ.

Macroglossia may be real or relative. In relative types, the tongue is of normal development but there is a marked decrease in the size of the jaws. True macroglossia is a common symptom of cretinism and mongolism. An unusually large tongue in an individual with slow and thick speech and a lowering of the pitch of the voice should suggest cretinism or myxedema. Brodie *et al.* reported an interesting case of muscular macroglossia which was studied in relation to jaw development.

At times aberrant portions of the thyroid gland may persist in the tongue just anterior to the circumvallate papillae. This anomaly rarely gives rise to symptoms. A cyst develops infrequently in the lingual portion of the thyroglossal duct, which results in a cystic mass in the midline of the tongue just anterior to the apex of the circumvallate papillae. This cyst may become secondarily infected.

Median Rhomboid Glossitis

Median rhomboid glossitis, or glossitis rhombica mediana, is a developmental anomaly more likely to be seen by the dentist and one most likely to cause difficulty in diagnosis. This condition is important only insofar as recognition of its true nature is concerned. Patients with this lesion are usually the subject of much diagnostic speculation, they develop frequently a cancerphobia and at times the lesion is removed surgically because of its suspected malignant nature.

Glossitis rhombica mediana results from the failure of the lateral halves of the tongue to fuse before the tuberculum impar becomes interposed between them just anterior to the circumvallate papillae. This produces a roughly rhomboidal-shaped area in the midline of the tongue just anterior to the circumvallate papillae. The deeper red color of this area contrasts definitely with the adjacent coating of the tongue. This rhomboidal area which

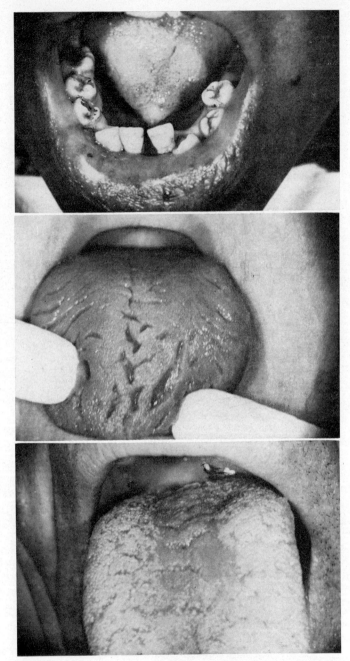

FIG. 60 (*Top*). Ankyloglossia or tongue-tie due to an abnormally short tongue frenum.

FIG. 61 (*Center*). Congenitally fissured (scrotal) tongue. In this case there was a familial history.

FIG. 62 (*Bottom*). Mild example of glossitis rhombica mediana. The central smooth area is always devoid of papillae.

is usually slightly raised from the rest of the tongue surface is devoid of papillae. It has at times a tufted appearance and it is occasionally fissured. Mild inflammatory changes are not unusual.

Subjective symptoms are rarely experienced. When this area is lobulated and fissured, mild inflammatory reactions may take place in the depths of the fissures. Surgical intervention is seldom advisable and there have been no reports of malignant lesions developing at the site of a previous median rhomboidal glossitis. Mild antiseptic mouth washes and the use of aniline dyes will control effectively the mild inflammatory symptoms.

FUNCTIONAL AND PHYSIOLOGIC CHANGES

Coated Tongue (Furred Tongue)

The examination of the tongue coating is a familiar and time-honored ritual. Considering the millions of times this organ has been examined, little factual knowledge has accrued as to the significance of a coated tongue. It was once believed that the coating of the tongue was an indication of the appearance of the gastric mucosa. This is now known to be untrue although certain atrophic changes, such as those seen in some of the nutritional deficiencies, are accompanied by atrophic changes of the gastric mucosa.

The tongue coating is composed of bacteria, small particles of food and the desquamating keratinized epithelial cells which are found on and between the filiform papillae. The degree of tongue coating which can be considered as normal varies in different individuals and during different periods of life. Ehrlich & Ehlert found the dorsum to be regularly hornified from childhood on, increasing gradually in thickness until about 65 years of age when it decreases rapidly. The anterior portion of the tongue shows more inflammatory and pathologic changes because of its lessened degree of keratinization.

The abnormally coated tongue has always been associated with disturbed function of the gastro-intestinal tract. Some theories of etiology have even inferred that the coating resulted from the retrograde movement of the gastric and intestinal contents. This has been disproved by the careful studies of Crohn and Drosd, who admit however that an "upset stomach" is usually followed in 6 to 12 hours by a coating of the tongue. They found that the vomiting associated with pyloric or intestinal obstruction is invariably accompanied by a furred tongue but that the vomiting of pregnancy or seasickness is not associated with a coated tongue. Mouth breathers and individuals who sleep with their mouths open commonly have a coated tongue.

Others believe that the tongue coating is related to constipation. In former years, the tongue coating furnished sufficient justification for purgation. Constipation has been invoked experimentally in healthy individuals for from 3 to 6 days without causing any change in the tongue coating and there is no evidence that any particular condition of the large or small intestines will result in an abnormal coating of the tongue.

The mechanism of the tongue coating can be explained by readily understood mechanical and physiologic facts. The formation of the tongue coat is a continuous process which occurs chiefly at night, when the normal cleansing mechanisms of the oral cavity are not functioning. This continuously forming coating of the tongue is normally removed by the salivary flow in conjunction with mechanical factors accompanying speech and mastication. The chewing of food is an important aid in eliminating this accumulated material, as considerable mechanical action is present during the formation of the food bolus and its passage into the pharynx. The importance of the salivary flow should not be minimized, although it has been shown that lack

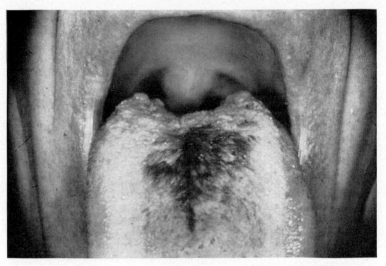

FIG. 63. Hypertrophy of the filiform papillae with secondary discoloration. Several large circumvallate papillae are visible posteriorly near the lateral margins of the tongue.

of flow alone will not result in a coated tongue. This is demonstrated in patients with xerostomia.

Any local or general condition which interferes with the above described cleansing mechanisms will permit the development of an abnormally coated tongue. In the usual febrile illness, the soft or liquid diet, the lack of normal attention to mouth hygiene, the diminished salivary flow due to the fever and the general body dehydration, all favor the retention of the coating. As the tongue coating increases, additional opportunities are available for the fermentation and decomposition of the food particles which result in the marked halitosis that is associated with a coated tongue. The coating may become stained due to ingested foods or drugs, smoking, or microorganisms.

With an understanding of the pathogenesis of the abnormally coated tongue, its proper clinical significance and a rationale of treatment become clearer. The restoration of a normal physiologic environment and function of the oral structures will result in rapid disappearance of the coating. In the case of the tongue coating associated with the use of sodium perborate, it is surprising how rapidly the coating and discoloration will disappear when this substance is no longer used. The days of tongue scraping by the individual or the professional man are past.

A coated tongue is not sufficient justification for a diagnosis of constipation or other gastro-intestinal ailments. It is not generally appreciated that the tongue furnishes a rather accurate appraisal of the state of hydration of the individual. The importance of a careful examination of the tongue should not be minimized by the altered clinical significance of the coated tongue, as the atrophic and color changes and the variations in tone of this organ are important diagnostic aids.

Atrophic Tongue Changes (Atrophy of Lingual Papillae)

Atrophic tongue changes in general are of greater clinical significance than an abnormally coated tongue. The cause of atrophic lingual changes are usually systemic in nature and the dentist should make a careful study in an effort to determine the cause. A smooth red tongue is usually due to a nutritional deficiency of some sort. Atrophic lingual changes are found in pellagra, sprue, pernicious anemia, the anemias associated with parasitic infections and the iron deficiency anemias. Atrophic tongue changes are associated with gastric hypoacidity, less frequently with hyperacidity. Atrophic glossitis forms a part of the Plummer-Vinson syndrome and it is also seen in chronic alcoholism.

In appraising atrophic lingual changes, the practitioner must consider what would be normal for the age of the particular patient. In the later years of life the tongue coating becomes normally less marked and the muscle tone of this organ decreases, so that what would be a pathologic tongue for a middle-aged individual would be a normal tongue for an aged person.

TRAUMATIC INJURIES TO TONGUE

The tongue is the frequent site of injury due to the interposition of this organ between the teeth during falls, fights, epileptic seizures, accidental biting or at times injuries received in the dental office. Copious hemorrhage is characteristic of traumatic lesions of the tongue. They are of less concern to the general practitioner than to the oral surgeon.

The tongue should be examined always for signs of scarring. The tongue is lacerated frequently during epileptic seizures, producing marked scarring and at times deformity of this organ. This one sign may suggest an epileptic background and prevent unpleasant experiences, especially if general anesthesia is to be administered.*

Traumatic injuries of this organ occur occasionally during oral surgical procedures. The forceps or elevator may slip and injure the tongue, or it may become lacerated when a tooth fractures. In most cases, these wounds heal readily because of the generous blood supply. Copps & Epstein observed a case in which carcinoma developed following an injury to the tongue which was inflicted during the extraction of a tooth.

* This scarring must be differentiated from the sclerous interstitial glossitis of late syphilis.

BLACK HAIRY TONGUE (*LINGUA NIGRA*)

True black tongue, which is a clinical entity, must be distinguished from pseudo-black tongue, which is a discoloration of the lingual coating due to fruits, candy, drugs, medicaments or the superficial pigmentation resulting from the decomposition of blood. Casper believes that if pigment-producing bacteria or fungi are not isolated from the tongue, the condition must be considered pseudo-black tongue. Black tongue in the human is not analogous to canine black tongue which is a symptom of niacin deficiency.

True black tongue is due to a superficial infection with pigment-producing bacteria, molds or fungi accompanied by certain morphologic changes of the tongue coating. Weidman isolated a Streptothrix from a case of black tongue. Kennedy and Howles reported 2 patients with black hairy tongue who developed this condition a short time after they had placed their cigarets on a moldy surface while smoking. *Monilia albicans* was isolated from the lingual lesions and the sites where the cigarets had been placed. These authors do not explain the mechanism of the discoloration. Swinburne considered the oral flora incidental rather than causal.

The "hairs" observed in this condition are hyperkeratinized, hyperplastic, filiform papillae. It is believed that there is a congenital predisposition to the long papillae, but that local irritating agents such as syphilis, tobacco or certain mouth washes may give rise to this peculiar anomaly. In Weidman's case he found the Streptothrix organisms entwined around the papillae.

Black tongue is most common in the male past middle life and it is rarely seen in young adults. The patient seldom complains of any subjective symptoms but in extreme cases the elongated filiform papillae may touch the palate or the roof of the mouth and cause gagging or a tickling sensation. It is not unusual to be able to part the hyperplastic, hyperkeratinized and discolored filiform papillae. In most cases the condition is discovered accidentally by the patient or it is called to his attention by friends or his dentist.

While black hairy tongue is harmless and disappears usually spontaneously, it is often resistant to treatment. The patient should receive some active treatment if only for psychologic reasons. Prinz suggested removing the elongated papillae by swabbing the tongue with 10 to 15% salicylic acid. This treatment is preferable to the use of escharotic agents recommended by Wise. The swabbing of the tongue with 3% hydrogen peroxide will frequently remové the discolored papillae.

GEOGRAPHIC TONGUE (*ERYTHEMA MIGRANS*, WANDERING RASH)

Geographic tongue is a clinical entity whose etiology has never been clearly established and whose pathosis is not known. This condition occurs chiefly in children but it is often seen in females, particularly those of a nervous temperament. Geographic tongue is not due to a bacterial or fungus infection. At times the lesions are present only during the menses. It has been

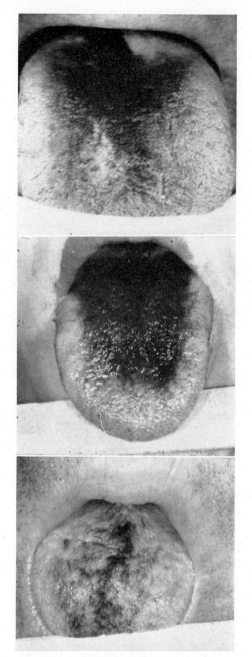

FIG. 64 (*Top*). True black tongue. The discoloration is due to pigment-producing organisms.

FIG. 65 (*Center*). Markedly discolored tongue resulting from the use of 3% hydrogen peroxide, 8% chromic acid and potassium permanganate during the treatment of a fusospirochetal gingivitis.

FIG. 66 (*Bottom*). Pseudo-black tongue. Hypertrophy and staining of the filiform papillae. Cultural results were negative for pigment-producing bacteria or fungi.

observed clinically that patients with an allergic history have a predisposition to this disease.

The initial lesions are seldom noticed by the patient as the subjective symptoms, when present, consist only of a slight burning or itching sensation. Geographic tongue is usually discovered accidentally when the tongue or oral cavity is examined for some other cause. The lesions begin as one or more non-indurated red macular spots which are devoid of filiform

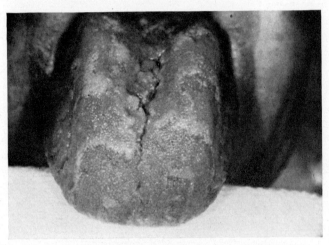

FIG. 67. Typical lesions in geographic tongue. This patient has also deep fissures of the tongue.

papillae. These macules enlarge forming circles of increasing circumference. The margins are well defined, slightly raised and yellowish in color. Just within this border the tissues are frequently bright red. The junction of several of the enlarging rings produces a map-like appearance which has given rise to the name of geographic tongue.

The diagnosis of geographic tongue presents no difficulties. It must be differentiated from simple depapillated areas which are seen occasionally on an otherwise normal tongue. Diffuse lichen planus or early leukoplakia of the tongue may present some diagnostic problems in the adult. Day-to-day observation of the distribution of the lesions on the tongue surface will permit a correct diagnosis. Mild drug eruptions appear similar to geographic tongue, but in the former, the lesions are usually painful and can be ruled out by means of a negative history of drug ingestion.

Geographic tongue requires no specific treatment. The condition is self-limiting and no serious sequellae have been reported. The apprehensive patient should be assured that the lesion is not precancerous. This type of patient will appreciate a mild mouth wash. The administration of diluted HCl U.S.P. will cause the lesions to disappear in some individuals. The usual dosage is 2 cc. which should be administered in gelatin capsules or perles to protect the teeth.

BURNING TONGUE (GLOSSOPYROSIS)

Burning tongue may be a symptom of a systemic disease like pellagra, sprue or pernicious anemia, or it may be of local origin and significance. Glossopyrosis of the latter type is discussed in this section. Burning tongue represents a symptom complex which may arise from a number of factors, among which local exciting or aggravating causes are important. In some cases, glossopyrosis represents a true neuralgia of the lingual branch of the 5th nerve while in others it is associated with disturbances of gastric secretion or psychoneurotic changes. It is impossible to determine in every case a likely cause for the glossopyrosis.

This complaint is common in the 4th to the 7th decades of life with about an equal distribution between the 2 sexes. These patients are usually of a nervous temperament. They are greatly concerned about their affection and develop often a cancerphobia. Artificial dentures, the eating of highly spiced foods, smoking, alcoholic beverages and local irritative factors such as calculus, malposed teeth, lingual bars, etc., are important aggravating factors. Fox claimed that glossopyrosis will develop reflexly in cases of gastric hypo- or hyperacidity.

The outstanding finding in these patients is the lack of any clinically observable lesion. It must be remembered that, although no clinical lesion can be detected, these patients experience pain! At times the tip of the tongue, the region usually presenting symptoms, is slightly smooth and reddened. In many cases the distribution of the pain does not follow any recognized anatomic pattern.

The diagnosis of glossopyrosis can be made only on the basis of the history. The history should determine whether the patient is taking any medicine or treatment which might give rise to these symptoms. Primary systemic causes for burning tongue, such as pernicious anemia, pellagra, sprue, nutritional deficiencies and secondary anemia should be ruled out. It is possible, based on the therapeutic response to B complex therapy, that many cases of glossopyrosis represent the first manifestation of a subclinical nutritional deficiency. Ulcerative lesions of the lingual lymphoid tissue (the lingual tonsil) may produce pain referred to the anterior portion of the tongue. Patients presenting these symptoms should have a complete blood count, a general nutritional appraisal based on readily observable physical characteristics and a nutritional history. At times more involved laboratory studies such as a gastric analysis and galactose tolerance tests are desirable.

True neuralgias of the lingual branch of the 5th nerve are commonly associated with paroxysms of pain which can be elicited by stimulating certain areas of the tongue and not the more or less continuous pain of glossopyrosis.

If no systemic background for the complaint can be found, the patient should be advised to refrain from eating highly spiced foods, smoking, and drinking alcoholic beverages. Gratifying results may follow such simple procedures. Some brands of cigarets are more frequently associated with these symptoms than others. All forms of local irritation such as salivary calculus, dental caries, and rough or irregular fillings should be eliminated.

These patients often rub the tip of their tongue against the lingual surface of the mandibular anteriors or a lingual bar "when they are nervous" or when they are concentrating. Small calcareous deposits on the lingual surfaces of the mandibular incisors will aggravate the symptoms of glosso-pyrosis and may give rise to subjective and objective symptoms similar to those characteristic of pernicious anemia.

If dentures are worn, they should be highly polished where they come in contact with the tongue and if possible they should be removed at night. All local irritative factors should be eliminated. Sodium-perborate-containing preparations are contraindicated in the treatment of these symptoms. Roentgen ray therapy, given by a competent radiologist, is at times helpful and successful. The administration of vitamin B complex on empiric grounds, either orally or better parenterally in conjunction with liver extract, is frequently beneficial and it may cause amelioration of the symptoms of glossopyrosis even in the absence of clinical signs of B complex deficiency.

After careful study, the patient should be assured that this symptom is not an indication of any serious systemic disease and that the danger of cancer is no greater than if these symptoms were not present.

PAINFUL PAPILLAE (PAPILLITIS)

Middle-aged patients complain occasionally of painful lesions on the lateral aspect of the tongue near its base. A careful examination of this area may show a hyperemic, slightly hypertrophied tissue or an enlarged circumvallate papilla.

This particular portion of the tongue rests often against the distolingual line angle and cusp of the lower third or second molar, or the posterior portion of a lower partial denture. Digital palpation may reveal a rough or sharp tooth margin. Smoothing of the tooth margins with stones and sand-paper discs and the application of a medicament such as Talbot's iodine ½ strength will often relieve the symptoms.

These patients not uncommonly develop a cancerphobia. In fear of this type of lesion they may seek treatment by the physician who applies silver nitrate to the area or advises x-ray therapy which many times results in a decreased salivary flow and an accentuation of the local symptoms. Scholtz obtained satisfactory results following the repeated electrodesiccation of these areas. This treatment seems preferable to radiation therapy.

Carcinoma may also develop at this area and if an ulcerative lesion is present it should be considered as malignant until proven otherwise. Under no circumstances should silver nitrate be repeatedly applied to such a lesion.

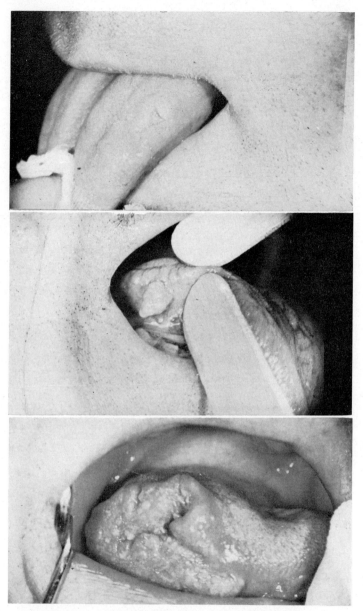

Fig. 68 (*Top*). Traumatic ulcer of the tongue due to continued irritation from a broken-down tooth. This type of lesion may become malignant if the cause of the irritation is not eliminated.

Fig. 69 (*Center*). Small fibroma of the lateral margin of the tongue. The covering mucosa is smooth and intact. There is no induration of the adjacent tissues.

Fig. 70 (*Bottom*). Squamous cell carcinoma of the right side of the tongue producing marked induration and deformity. Numerous adherent crusted areas of leukoplakia are present on the malignant growth.

VARICOSITIES OF THE LINGUAL VEINS

In middle-aged adults the lingual veins may develop varicosities and become tortuous. When first discovered, these veins have a startling appearance and they often cause undue apprehension. The practitioner should

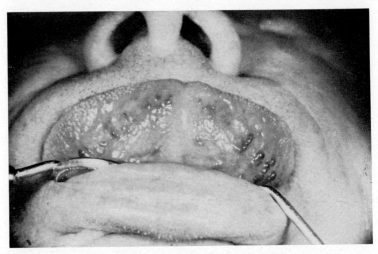

FIG. 71. Varicosities of the lingual veins. These varicosities are believed by some clinicians to be an early symptom of right-sided heart failure.

explain to the patient the nature of these lesions, using the varicosities of the lower extremities as an analogy. No treatment is indicated other than the assurance of the benign nature of the lesions.

It is stated that distension of the ranine veins is an indication of poor circulatory efficiency, and that undue prominence of these structures warrants caution in the administration of a general anesthesia.

9

The Dermatoses

GENERAL CONSIDERATIONS

Since the oral mucosa and the skin have a common embryologic origin it is not surprising that oral mucosal changes are observed frequently in various dermatologic conditions. When dermatologic lesions are present the diagnosis of the oral manifestations is not too difficult.

When the oral lesions are the only manifestation of the disease or when they precede the skin changes, diagnosis becomes increasingly difficult if not impossible. The dentist should have sufficient knowledge of the oral lesions associated with the common dermatoses to enable him to determine whether the treatment of the oral lesions is within his domain or that of the dermatologist.

The clinical appearance of the oral manifestations as a rule varies considerably from those on the skin. The appearance of the oral lesions is altered by peculiarities of their environment. The increased vascularity of the tissues produces marked changes in color and the constant moisture and warmth of the oral cavity results in early maceration of the tissues. Vesicles and bullae are of only transitory duration and they appear usually as erosions of various depths surrounded by epithelial tags. The ever-present dense bacterial population of the oral cavity results commonly in superficial infection of the lesions. For these reasons the oral manifestations of dermatologic lesions often present problems in diagnosis.

LEUKOPLAKIA BUCCALIS

Leukoplakia is a chronic disease characterized by a loss of translucency, a thickening and hyperkeratinization of the oral mucosa. Early leukoplakia rarely produces symptoms which cause the patient to seek professional attention. For this reason the dentist should make a thorough examination in every patient so that leukoplakic lesions can be diagnosed early when conservative treatment is effective. Untreated and advanced cases of leukoplakia frequently undergo malignant degeneration. While our discussion of leukoplakia is concerned primarily with oral mucosal involvement, this disease is also found in the trachea, renal pelves, bladder, cervix uteri and vagina.

The dental practitioner will probably see more cases of leukoplakia than any other serious oral lesion. The increasing frequency with which this disease is observed may be an actuality or the result of more thorough and frequent oral examinations.

Leukoplakia is a disease of middle life, occurring rarely before the age of 50. Approximately 95% of all cases are observed in males. Leukoplakia is relatively rare in the Negro in spite of numerous predisposing causes present in the members of this race. The occurrence of the disease is determined in part by the personal habits of the individual. Poor oral hygiene and neglected dental care appear to be important predisposing factors. A high incidence of leukoplakia and carcinoma is found in the natives of the Malay States, Siam and parts of India where it is the common practice to chew betel nuts.

Etiology

A number of general and local factors predispose to oral leukoplakia. General predisposing factors include individual susceptibilities, possible hormonal and nutritional factors and associated systemic disease. Individuals with a blond skin and blue eyes, those who are unusually sensitive to actinic rays or those who have a delicate skin, are prone to develop the disease. Vitamin A deficiency may predispose to the development of leukoplakia. Deficiency of this vitamin results in metaplasia and hyperkeratinization of the epithelium, producing a histologic picture similar to that associated with leukoplakia. Hormonal disturbances have also been suggested as etiologic factors (see treatment). The therapeutic evidence supporting any of these etiologic theories is inconclusive.

From ancient times, leukoplakia has been associated with syphilis or thought to be one of its protean manifestations. While leukoplakia and syphilis are found in the same individual there is no scientific basis for regarding one as the result or the cause of the other. Eichenlaub determined the incidence of leukoplakia, tuberculosis and syphilis in 16,802 World War I veterans.

LEUKOPLAKIA BUCCALIS, SYPHILIS AND TUBERCULOSIS IN 16,082
WORLD WAR I VETERANS

(From Eichenlaub)

	Number	Number with Leukoplakia	Per Cent Involved
Syphilis.	622	33	5.3
Tuberculosis.	2,408	39	1.6

A higher percentage of syphilitic patients (5.3%) as compared to (1.9%) also had leukoplakia. Considering the numbers involved, this percentage difference assumes statistical significance. The exact relationship between syphilis and leukoplakia is not known.

Local predisposing factors of importance include mechanical, chemical, thermal and electrical (chemical?) forms of irritation. Poor oral hygiene is

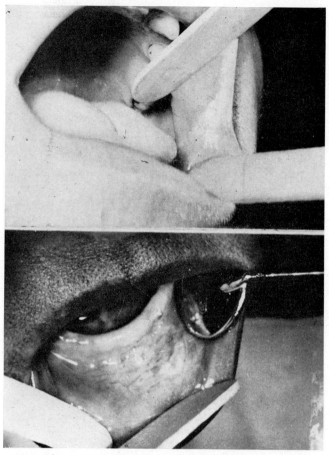

FIG. 72 (*Top*). Typical location and distribution of leukoplakia of the cheek.
FIG. 73 (*Bottom*). Leukoplakia of the mucobuccal fold due to the habit of holding snuff in this area.

a definite predisposing factor. Mild mechanical irritation over long periods of time is known to predispose to the development of this disease. Leukoplakic areas are observed occasionally in relation to broken roots, faulty crowns, malposed teeth, fractured dentures or other prosthetic appliances. The patient may be unaware of the irritation or they may be aggravating the condition unconsciously by constant pressure on the involved areas.

Tobacco, particularly when smoked, is a definite predisposing factor. All but 5 of the 327 patients with leukoplakia studied by Eichenlander used tobacco in the form of cigarets, pipe, cigars and chewing in the order named. Roffo has demonstrated the presence of carcinogenic agents in the distillation products of burning tobacco. Leukoplakia has been experimentally produced by the use of these substances. The chemical irritation is caused by the distillation products produced during the burning of the tobacco plus mechanical and thermal irritative factors in pipe smokers. Cigaret and cigar smoking are less likely to cause leukoplakia as the distillate products are filtered somewhat by the unburned tobacco before they reach the oral tissues. The curing and flavoring agents contained in chewing tobacco and snuff are also important sources of irritation, particularly if the cud is held consistently in one area.

Highly seasoned foods, condiments, alcoholic beverages all predispose to leukoplakia. Galvanism is said to be an important factor. Prinz observed an unusual case of leukoplakia of the tongue in a telephone lineman who tested the polarity of the circuits by touching the 2 wires to the tip of his tongue. Galvanism is of minor importance as a predisposing cause of leukoplakia in general.

Many factors predispose to leukoplakia. Some are general in nature such as hereditary tendencies, the complexion of the individual and possibly nutritional and hormonal derangements. Important local factors are those resulting from mechanical, thermal, chemical and possibly electrical irritation of the oral tissues. Multiple factors may be present in any given case. Clinical experience indicates that the use of tobacco, especially pipe smoking, and mechanical irritations are local factors of considerable importance. Poor oral hygiene is usually present in mouths where leukoplakia is found. It may play a more important rôle than is generally believed.

In leukoplakia there is an increased keratinization and thickening of the stratum corneum with a flattening of the rete pegs. An accumulation of small round cells is found characteristically in the papillary layer of the corium. Although irregularities of the basal cell layer may be present, this structure remains intact unless there is malignant degeneration. When ulceration is present, it is usually associated with malignant changes.

Symptoms

The lack of subjective symptoms is one of the characteristic features of early leukoplakia. The initial stage, which consists of erythema of the oral mucosa, is seen rarely. If noted, the patient ascribes generally the symptoms to too much smoking or to some local source of irritation. The normal pink, translucent color of the mucosa is replaced gradually by a whitish area or plaque. The patient complains occasionally of dryness or burning of the tissues after smoking, drinking alcoholic beverages or eating highly seasoned foods. Later there may be tenderness and soreness, but it is not unusual to find advanced lesions without any subjective symptoms.

The typical leukoplakic lesion is whitish or yellowish-white in color and has a well-defined but irregular margin. It has a leathery consistency. The location and shape of the lesion may be related to local predisposing factors. In smokers, a white area is frequently seen on the vermilion border of the lower lip. This persistent whitish plaque associated with smoking is known

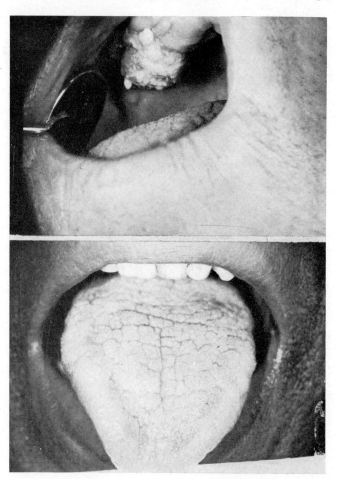

FIG. 74 (*Top*). Crusted form of leukoplakia which was associated with a squamous cell carcinoma of the right alveolar ridge in a 54-year-old man.
FIG. 75 (*Bottom*). Extensive leukoplakia of the tongue. The patient had a positive serologic test for syphilis.

as the "smoker's patch." At first this can be rubbed or pulled off, but in time the area becomes permanent and it may eventually turn into a squamous cell carcinoma before the individual considers the lesion is other than a "scab."

The location of the lesions on the oral mucosa is an important aid in diagnosis. Over 50% of all lesions are found on the cheek mucosa with the remainder being distributed on the tongue, palate, lips, sublingual space and gingiva in the order named. The typical cheek lesions extend posteriorly

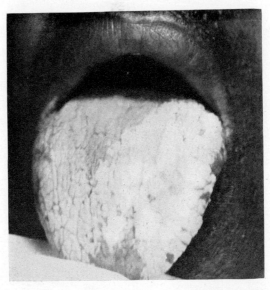

FIG. 76. Leukoplakia buccalis (Grade 4 verrucous carcinoma). (McCarthy, J. A. M. A., 116:16-21, 1941.)

from the corners of the mouth along the interdental line. The concentration of soluble irritating products in this area from smoking or chewing tobacco is believed to account for the frequent occurrence of leukoplakia in this region. The dorsum of the tongue is another common site. The mobility of this organ may be noticeably impaired, particularly when there is an associated syphilitic glossitis. The sublingual space, the buccal and labial alveolar gingivae are involved less frequently. When leukoplakia is associated with malignant lesions, it may have a frosted, crusted appearance. Whenever ulceration or fissuring occurs, the possibility of malignant degeneration should be considered seriously.

Leukoplakia of the palate presents a variety of clinical manifestations. This tissue at times has a dull white appearance with many small red depressed areas which represent the orifices of the palatal glands. The leukoplakic lesions

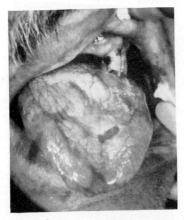

FIG. 77. Syphilitic atrophic glossitis with leukoplakia. (McCarthy, J. A. M. A., 116:16-21, 1941.)

may involve primarily the opening of palatal glands, obstructing these structures and producing characteristic nodular elevations on the palate. The leukoplakia in other cases may be limited to small raised rings on the palate

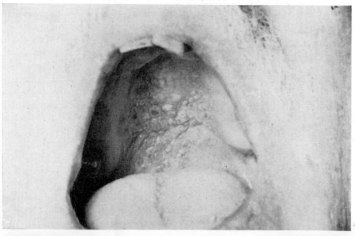

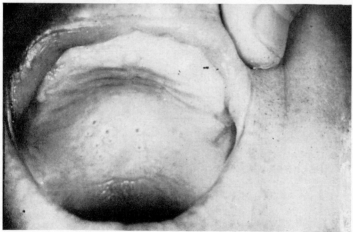

FIG. 78 (*Top*). Extensive leukoplakia of palate with enlargement of the palatal glands. (Patient of Dr. John H. Gunter, Philadelphia, Pa.)

FIG. 79 (*Bottom*). Circular areas of leukoplakia about the inflamed orifices of the palatal glands (Stomatitis nicotinus).

about the openings of the ducts. These variations in the clinical appearance result from different degrees of involvement of the various structures on the palate. Thoma called leukoplakic involvement of the palatal glands, *stomatitis nicotina,* because of the frequent history of excessive use of tobacco in these individuals.

The lymph nodes are involved rarely in leukoplakia. However, local adenopathy may be due to unrelated inflammatory lesions of the head and neck and, rarely, malignant metastases.

Some clinicians attempt to grade leukoplakia numerically (Grade I, II, III, IV) according to the severity of the lesion. This practice seems of questionable clinical value. Some benign appearing lesions tend to progress in spite of conservative treatment while some advanced lesions often regress under similar treatment. Any area of leukoplakia with fissuring or ulcerations should be regarded as malignant until proven otherwise.

Diagnosis

Leukoplakia can usually be diagnosed on the basis of its clinical appearance in conjunction with the presence of one or more general or local predisposing factors. When ulcerative changes are present the correct diagnosis becomes not only more difficult but also more imperative.

Malignancy, lichen planus, mucous patches, traumatic changes of the oral mucosa, thrush or localized areas of scarring must be considered in the differential diagnosis. Lichen planus presents the greatest difficulty. A blood Wassermann should be taken if there is any suspicion of a luetic infection, and it is a desirable procedure in all cases. A biopsy is indicated when malignant degeneration is suspected. If the lesion is small, it should be removed in its entirety. The biopsy should be taken by one experienced in this procedure and the tissue should be sent to a competent pathologist for interpretation.

Differential Diagnosis. A clinical test which aids in differentiating leukoplakia from other lesions, producing similar appearing changes of the oral mucosa, has been used by the author for some years. This consists of drying the affected area and applying Lugol's solution to the lesion. Areas of leukoplakia will not take the deep mahogany stain because the glycogen content of the involved cells is decreased. As a consequence, the involved area is outlined sharply by the brown-staining normal oral mucosa. Traumatic lesions of the cheeks will take a deeper brown stain.

Treatment

Early leukoplakia can be treated by conservative measures if the patient is co-operative. Since co-operation is so essential, the patient should be informed directly and truthfully of the possibility of malignant change, if the treatment advised is not followed implicitly. Partial co-operation will not produce results. The chronic nature of the disease should be emphasized and the patient should not look for noticeable change in the lesion in a short time.

Conservative treatment consists of the complete cessation of smoking, the use of alcohol or the ingestion of highly seasoned foods. All forms of local irritation should be eliminated. If the lesion is rubbed gently for 5 minutes, twice daily with a soft cloth moistened with water and castile soap (or other pure soap), marked improvement will take place frequently. It is not unusual to observe leathery areas of leukoplakia become softened under this treatment and at times disappear completely. The use of caustics, so commonly practiced by the medical profession, is of no value and may be harmful. Sutton & Sutton stated that "applications of silver nitrate are particularly successful in promoting the progress of leukoplakia into carcinoma." Nathanson and Weisberger obtained satisfactory therapeutic results by the injection of female sex hormones. No other reports have appeared concerning this method of treatment.

Knoof reported the successful use of the vitamin B complex. There is some doubt as to whether all the conditions this investigator treated were clinical leukoplakia. This form of therapy as well as large doses of vitamin A have not resulted in marked clinical improvement in advanced lesions.

The advisability of placing dentures over areas of leukoplakia arises often in dental practice. It is noted frequently that heavy smokers who wear dentures will develop these lesions just beyond the denture margins. Vaughn studied the effect of denture wearing on leukoplakia of the hard palate. He noted that if the denture is properly constructed, not itself a source of irritation, that it may constitute a good form of treatment. Leukoplakia disappeared completely under such dentures (vulcanite) in a relatively short time, even when there was no change in the personal habits of the patient. The time for response varied from a few weeks to months. The insulating and protective functions of the denture were believed responsible for the clinical improvement.

The treatment of advanced leukoplakia is a surgical problem.

Prognosis

The prognosis in mild cases of leukoplakia is good. The prognosis of the more advanced lesions is variable.

LICHEN PLANUS

General Considerations

Lichen planus is a chronic dermatologic disease of considerable dental interest because of its frequent occurrence on the oral mucosa.

This disease develops usually between the ages of 35 and 50 years and has a predilection for females. The specific causative agent of lichen planus has not been determined. Severe emotional upsets, nervous exhaustion or overwork frequently precede the eruption. Arsenic and gold compounds are capable of producing an attack. Barock et al. listed poorly fitting dentures and smoking as contributing causes.

The typical dermal lesions of lichen planus consist of recurrent crops of firm polygonal or angular-outlined glistening papules which have a reddish-purple or violaceous color. As they become older, they develop a deeper purple color. The lesions appear frequently along the line of a scratch or at the site of an abrasion. Ulceration occurs rarely. The lesions are commonly found on the flexor surfaces of the wrists and forearms and on the ankles. Varying degrees of pruritus, itching, accompany the skin eruption. Patients are occasionally unaware of the lesions, particularly when they are confined to the oral mucosa. Constitutional symptoms due to lichen planus are absent and spontaneous remissions and recurrences are frequent.

The diagnosis of the dermal lesions offers no particular difficulty when the characteristic violaceous, pruritic, angular eruptions are present in a patient without constitutional symptoms. The diagnosis of the oral lesions of lichen

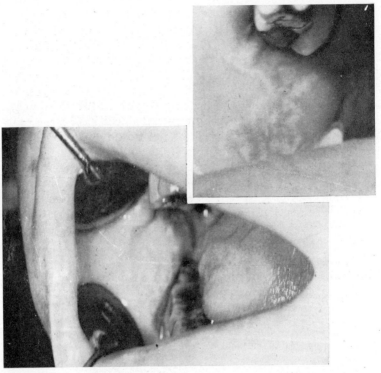

FIG. 80. Lichen planus of the cheek.

planus, which may be more difficult, is discussed under the oral aspects of this disease.

The treatment of lichen planus is not always easy or satisfactory. The time-honored Fowler's solution affects cures or remissions in some cases. Dietary regulation, ultraviolet radiation and injections of mercurial salts and bismuth preparations have all been used with success. Vitamin B complex has given promising results in other cases. Since spontaneous remissions are known to occur it is difficult to evaluate any form of therapy.

Chipman considered it important to eliminate dental foci of infection. Sutton & Sutton also stressed the importance of removing dental foci of infection as a part of the general treatment of the disease. They found cases which were unresponsive to all therapeutic efforts until appropriate dental treatment had been received. They have dental x-rays made routinely of their patients with lichen planus, and they "order" removed all pulpless and abscessed teeth and request the treatment of periodontal disease when it exists.

Oral Aspects

The dentist should be familiar with the oral lesions of lichen planus because of their frequent occurrence on the oral mucosa and at times their con-

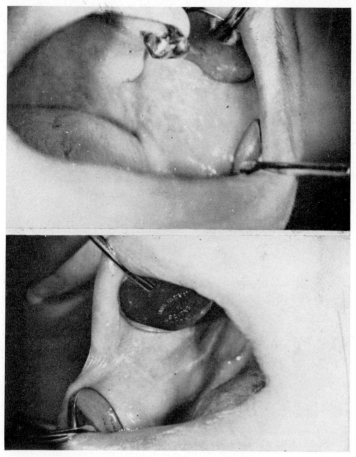

FIG. 81 (*Top*). Lichen planus of the cheek.
FIG. 82 (*Bottom*). Linear lesions of lichen planus of the cheek.

finement to the oral cavity. Oral lesions are present in over 50% of the cases. Only a small proportion of the patients seen in a dental outpatient clinic with oral lesions of lichen planus have the dermal lesions. Either the incidence of lichen planus confined to the oral cavity is much greater than is generally believed or the oral lesions precede the skin lesions more often than is commonly stated in dermatologic textbooks. In some patients, the dermal lesions have been observed to develop weeks or months after the oral lesions.

Symptoms. The mucosal lesions of lichen planus appear as a fine network of white lines (Wickham's Lines), arranged in a branching lacelike pattern

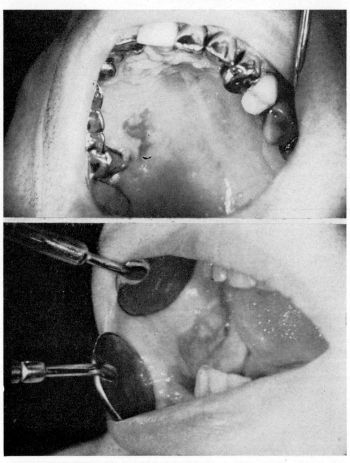

Fig. 83 (*Top*). Lichen planus of the erosive type. Note the delicate white linear lesions extending from the margin of the eroded area.

Fig. 84 (*Bottom*). Erosive form of lichen planus of the cheek. The lesions are found characteristically in the molar region.

which are found characteristically on the cheek mucosa along the interdental line in the molar region. The trauma to which these tissues are subjected during chewing may predispose to the development of lesions in this location. Small raised prominent dots are found where these lines intersect. Pearly gray or purplish angular papules are also found on the oral mucosa. Individual lesions frequently coalesce. The mucosa surrounding these lesions presents no abnormalities. Lichen planus lesions also develop on the hard and soft palate, the floor of the mouth and less frequently the gingiva. They appear as if a mild caustic had been applied to the tissues. Lichen planus may also involve the lips, particularly the lower lip. The normal pink of these structures is masked by a network of fine white lines. Like the dermal lesions, oral lichen planus shows little tendency to erosion or ulceration.

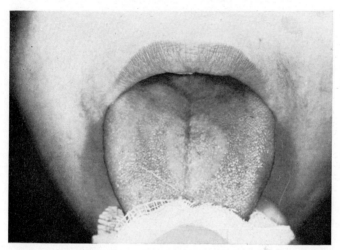

Fig. 85. Large plaque-like lesion of lichen planus on the dorsum of the tongue. The patient had extensive lesions on the buccal mucosa.

Lesions on the tongue appear usually as oval or polygonal papules and plaques 1 to 5 mm. in diameter. Frequently streak-like plaques are seen and in extensive cases the coalesced lesions involve the major portion of the dorsum of the tongue. Lingual lesions in general are less firm and less discretely outlined than those of the oral mucosa. They must be distinguished from those of erythema migrans, leukoplakia and geographic tongue. In the latter disease, the lesions vary their position from day to day, while in lichen planus they remain fixed in position.

An erosive form of lichen planus is seen less frequently. This type of lesion occasions a more acute reaction in the mucosal tissues. During their early development, the lesions are covered with a yellowish cheesy material. Later they appear as an irregularly outlined reddened, scarred area about whose margins fine radiating white lines may develop. When present, these lines afford the key to the diagnosis. These erosive lesions of lichen planus are mildly painful when highly spiced or acid foods are eaten. If doubt exists as to the nature of these lesions, biopsy study will permit a diagnosis. The specimen should be sent to a competent skin pathologist or dermatologist for diagnosis.

Diagnosis. When lichen planus is confined to the oral mucosa considerable difficulty may be experienced in the diagnosis. A careful examination of the oral tissues should be made for the characteristic white lines. Thicken-

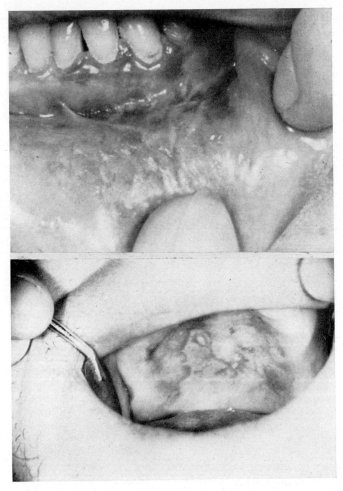

FIG. 86 (*Top*). Lichen planus of the gingiva and mucosal surface of the lower lip. (Patient of Dr. Gordon Winter, Binghamton, N. Y.)

FIG. 87 (*Bottom*). Erosive form of lichen planus of the palate. These painful lesions interfered with the wearing of an upper denture.

ing of the cheek mucosa along the interdental line due to trauma may be mistaken for early lesions of lichen planus. Differentiation of the lingual lesions from geographic tongue has already been mentioned. The oral manifestations of erythema multiforme are usually more acute and they are nearly always associated with dermal lesions which will permit a definite diagnosis. The lesions of lichen planus must be differentiated from those of leukoplakia. In some cases differentiation is almost impossible. The lesions of leukoplakia are more leathery and yellow in color and they are usually situated more anteriorly on the cheeks. A biopsy may be required to make a definite diagnosis. The following tabulation compares the more outstanding findings in traumatic lesions of the cheek, leukoplakia and lichen planus.

TABLE XI

COMPARISON OF THE CLINICAL FEATURES OF LEUKOPLAKIA, LICHEN PLANUS AND TRAUMATIC LESIONS OF THE CHEEK MUCOSA

	Leukoplakia (Oral)	Lichen Planus (Oral)	Traumatic Lesions
Sex—age	Predominantly in the male, 95% of all cases. Usually develops in the older age period 45-60 years.	Seen in both sexes, slightly more prevalent in the female. Age range 35 to 50 usually.	Either sex, usually in young patients, particularly those of nervous temperament.
Location of the lesions	Common on tongue, palate and cheeks, beginning at oral commissure and extending back on interdental line.	Most frequently on the cheek along the interdental line in the molar region.	Usually interdental line in the molar area.
Appearance of the lesion	Irregularly shaped yellowish white leathery lesions. May be related to local sites of irritation such as rough teeth, pipe stem, etc.	On cheeks, fine interlacing lines or polygonal or geometric-shaped papules. Rarely ulcerates. Purplish in color. On tongue irregularly shaped areas.	Irregularly shaped grayish areas of eroded mucosa.
Surrounding mucosa	May be slight inflammatory reaction.	Usually normal.	Usually definite inflammatory reaction about the lesions. At times small submucous hemorrhages.
Subjective symptoms	Mild irritation in early lesions. Pain or burning sensation on eating hot or highly spiced foods. Dryness of mouth, leathery feeling, no pain on pressure unless secondary infection.	Rare—may feel rough to tongue. No pain on pressure.	Pain may be marked, particularly on pressure.
Result of painting with Lugol's solution	Lesions fail to take the stain.	Early lesions stain normally. Older lesions stain slightly less readily than the normal mucosa.	Lesions take deeper stain than surrounding normal mucosa.
Progress of untreated lesions	Becomes thicker, fissured, ulcerated and at times undergoes carcinomatous degeneration.	May persist, regress or disappear.	May become ulcerated and secondarily infected with fusospirochetal organisms.

Treatment. The oral lesions require no specific treatment. They are resistant to the general treatment and they often persist long after the dermal eruption has cleared. Local sources of mechanical irritation should be eliminated. Mild astringent mouth washes give at least psychologic relief.

Prognosis. There are isolated reports of malignant growths developing on an old lichen planus lesion.

HERPES SIMPLEX

General Considerations

The various manifestations of herpes simplex are frequently encountered by the dentist. While rarely serious, the lesions are disfiguring, annoying and painful.

In 1915 Schamberg grouped "canker sores" with herpes simplex and more recent studies, particularly those of Woodburne, indicate that recurrent aphthae, herpetic stomatitis, gestationis and genitalis are all manifestations of the herpes simplex virus. Youmans produced typical herpetic lesions in humans and animals by inoculations of the vesicular fluid. Mikulicz's aphthae or *periadenitis mucosa necrotica recurrens* is probably of different and yet unknown etiology.

Oral Aspects

Many different conditions predispose to the clinical development of the herpes lesions. Herpes labialis is commonly associated with pneumococcal

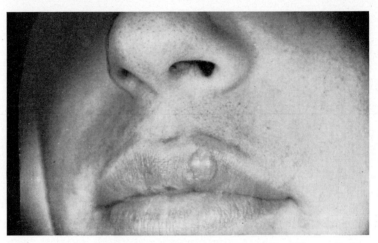

FIG. 88. Typical herpetic vesicle on the upper lip. The vesicular lesion is rarely observed in the mouth.

pneumonia, meningitis and the common cold. During the winter of 1940-41 a high incidence of oral aphthous lesions was noted with the appearance of the mild influenza epidemic on the eastern seaboard. Herpetic lesions are common during menstruation, pregnancy or in thyroid disease. They may follow dental operative procedures and the use of the rubber dam. They have been associated with allergy and focal infection.

The initial herpetic infection may be evidenced by a stomatitis in infancy or it may go unrecognized as a mild respiratory infection. Epidemic forms of herpetic stomatitis and pharyngitis have been reported by Levine. The general adult population acquires usually a high degree of immunity to the infection; however, those whose immunity is less highly developed or those whose resistance is lowered by other causes may present occasional or recurrent lesions. ·

Of some dental interest is the possibility of transmitting the infection by salivary droplets. The virus can be demonstrated readily in the saliva, as well as other body secretions during the clinical course of the disease. In recurrent herpes it is practically absent from the oral secretions during quiescent periods. Hudson considers that the transmission of the infection by salivary contamination is particularly important in infancy.

Symptoms. The patient complains frequently of itching, burning or a feeling of fullness of the tissues before the appearance of the lesion. These subjective symptoms are soon followed by localized hyperemia and vesicle formation. The irregularly disposed vesicles, which are filled with a clear yellow fluid, constitute the characteristic herpetic lesion. The individual lesions vary from the size of a pin head to a centimeter in diameter. The

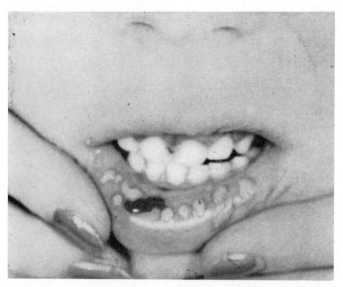

Fig. 89. Acute herpetic stomatitis in a 4½-year-old girl.
(Courtesy of Dr. L. I. Grossman, Philadelphia, Pa.)

vesicle stage is of short duration, especially in the mouth where rupture occurs early due to the trauma of mastication. Epithelial tags, remnants of the ruptured vesicle wall, may be found about the periphery of the lesion. These eroded areas are surrounded by a bright red areola. The lesions are extremely painful for their size. When multiple lesions are present in the mouth eating may be difficult. At times several aphthae will coalesce to form an irregularly shaped lesion. There is usually an accompanying increase in salivary flow.

Herpes labialis arises usually at the mucocutaneous junction and frequently at the commissures of the lips. The vermilion borders of the lips, the frenum of the upper lip and the tongue are common sites for herpetic eruptions. Large linear lesions are found frequently in the buccal sulcus. Involvement of the gums is uncommon. The lesions become covered during healing with a thick, yellowish, cheesy-appearing material. If seen at this stage, the lesions may present difficulties in diagnosis. When secondary infection occurs or when lesions develop repeatedly at the same site, slight scarring may result. Resolution takes place in 10 days to 2 weeks.

Diagnosis. The diagnosis of herpetic lesions can be made on the basis of the history of onset, and the characteristic appearance of the early lesions and their location. Healing oral mucosal lesions are confusing to those un-

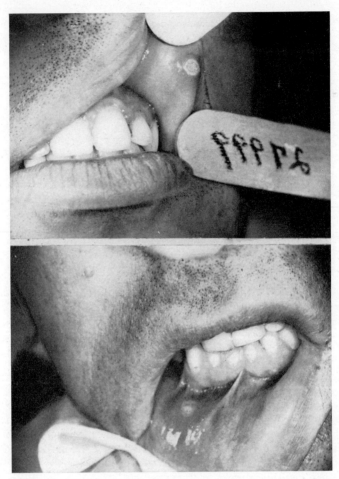

Fig. 90. Typical solitary herpetic lesions showing infiltrated base of lesion and erythematous border.

Fig. 91. Solitary herpetic lesion of the lower lip associated with the eating of English walnuts.

familiar with their peculiar thick yellowish cheesy appearance. Accompanying coryza, menstruation or a gastro-intestinal upset may aid in confirming the diagnosis.

DIFFERENTIAL DIAGNOSIS. In the differential diagnosis, one must consider herpes zoster, pemphigus, impetigo, allergic manifestations due to food or drugs and erythema multiforme. The lesions of herpes zoster are rarely bilateral and, when present, are confined to an area corresponding to a sensory nerve distribution. In pemphigus constitutional symptoms are more severe and lesions may be found on the cutaneous surfaces. In impetigo the lesions are not confined to the mucocutaneous orifices but often extend some

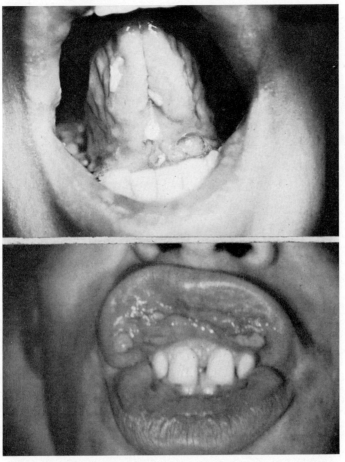

FIG. 92 (*Top*). Healing herpetic lesions on ventral surface of tongue in an 18-year-old male with acute herpetic stomatitis.

FIG. 93 (*Bottom*). Patient with acute herpetic stomatitis. Note the multiple herpetic lesions on the upper lip in various stages of development.

distance from the lips on the cheeks and they are also found on the hands, arms, and other parts of the body. Allergic reactions of a vesicular nature can be ruled out usually by the short duration of the lesions. Erythema multiforme of the oral mucosa and lips may present a problem in diagnosis. In this disease the gums are often affected. If the beginning lesions can be studied, a correct diagnosis can be made. Prinz recommended a therapeutic test with Fowler's solution in doubtful cases.

Treatment. The solitary occasional aphthae are treated commonly with local applications of zinc chloride (8%), camphorated phenol, spirits of cam-

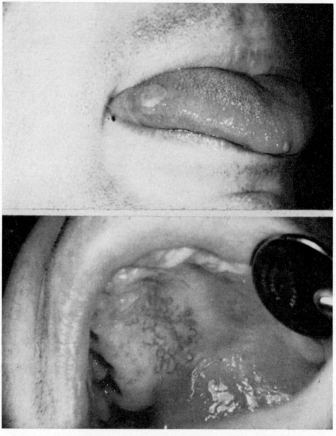

Fig. 94 (*Top*). Recurrent herpetic ulcers of the tongue of seventeen years' duration. Treated successfully with repeated vaccinations of cowpox (smallpox) vaccine.

Fig. 95 (*Bottom*). Herpes simplex lesions appearing at the area of novocaine infiltration anesthesia. Patient complained of postoperative pain.

phor, Talbot's iodine, camphor ice, sulfonamide solutions, liquified phenol or an ordinary alum pencil. These remedies give symptomatic relief rather than cure the condition.

Roentgen therapy, ¼ to ½ skin erythema dose will prevent further development of the lesions if given early. This is more satisfactory in the occasional herpetic lesions of the lips and it is not recommended for the recurrent lesions.

In recurrent herpes with extensive involvement, other forms of treatment are indicated. Because of the group immunologic relationship of the various virus diseases, recurrent herpes has been treated by Schmidt with smallpox vaccine and Frank used formolized herpes virus. It is interesting to note in this regard that many patients with recurrent herpetic infections also give a history of having difficulty in obtaining a vaccination take. At times, repeated smallpox vaccinations at 10-day intervals are necessary to control recurrent herpetic lesions. This form of treatment is effective in many patients.

An occasional patient will develop herpes labialis following the application of the rubber dam. This can be prevented frequently by prescribing therapeutic doses of vitamin B complex or thiamin chloride for several days prior to the dental appointment.

In 1923, Gerstenberger reported the successful treatment of herpetic stomatitis and herpes labialis in children with yeast. Weisberger described the pinpoint vesicles of the buccal mucosa associated with B_2 or riboflavin deficiency. The author and Hickman treated successfully cases of herpes labialis and oral aphthae of the recurrent type with the vitamin B complex. In certain cases as little as 1 mgm. of thiamin chloride per day would prevent lesions.

In one instance the development of recurrent aphthae was related to the drinking water supply. Repeated observations by this patient (a dentist) demonstrated that the usual clinical course of the various stages of the lesion and the size of the aphthae could be stopped by the administration of B complex. Small pin-head sized aphthous ulcers decreased promptly in size and disappeared within 24 hours. In another patient, the prophylactic administration of the B complex prevented the aphthous lesions developing after the eating of English walnuts.

In a severe case of herpes labialis and genitalis 50 mgm. of thiamin chloride, 50 mgm. riboflavin, 250 mgm. nicotinic acid, 250 mgm. Ca pantothenate, and 100 mgm. of pyridoxine hydrochloride per day for 3 days resulted in the disappearance of the penile lesions and all the oral lesions with the exception of 1 small ulcer. This patient's roommate had a "cankersore" a week before the acute herpetic stomatitis and genitalis.

Herpetic manifestations should not be considered a specific symptom of vitamin B complex deficiency in the same category as cheilosis or pellagra. All cases of herpetic manifestations will not show marked improvement following vitamin therapy. In stubborn cases of recurrent herpetic stomatitis, complete allergic studies and desensitization may prove beneficial. Some cases are resistant, unfortunately, to all forms of therapy.

Prognosis. The prognosis in general is excellent. In the case of secondary infection or lesions recurring at the same location, some slight scarring may result.

HERPES ZOSTER (SHINGLES)

Herpes zoster is the result of an irritation of a posterior root ganglion of the spinal nerves or an extramedullary ganglion of a cranial nerve. It is characterized by a burning and itching sensation and vesicle formation along the distribution of the involved nerve.

Any kind of inflammation of the sensory nerve ganglion may produce the symptoms of herpes zoster. A virus related closely to the chicken pox virus is believed responsible for some cases of this disease. Irritation of a posterior root ganglion due to spinal anesthesia, neoplastic metastases, leukemic cellular infiltrations or any other cause of irritation may result in the herpetic manifestations.

The disease is rare. It occurs at times in small epidemics. It is most frequently found after middle life and it is commonly associated with overwork, fatigue or malnutrition. It has a slight predilection for nervous irritable individuals. Herpes zoster lesions have developed following massive doses of thiamin chloride. Herpes zoster can be considered as a transitory sensory analogue of poliomyelitis, producing characteristic changes in the spinal fluid as well as congestion, hemorrhage and lymphocytic infiltration in the region of the posterior root ganglion.

Symptoms

Constitutional symptoms of fever, malaise and leukocytosis may precede the eruption. Cases of suspected unilateral pleurisy are many times found to be herpes zoster of the thoracic region. The herpetic eruption is usually preceded by pain of a burning or itching character which follows the distribution of a sensory nerve. The vesicles which are surrounded by a distinct erythematous base, make their appearance slowly. They rupture or ulcerate and heal gradually in 5 to 10 days. The lesions are characteristically unilateral, and are confined to the area supplied by the involved spinal ganglion. Permanent scarring of the skin takes place occasionally. Neuralgic pains with hyperesthesia of the affected area may persist long after the eruption has disappeared.

Berggren and Schuler studied the site of involvement in 2,014 cases of herpes zoster. The 5th nerve was involved in 16% of the cases, the cervical nerves in 25%, the dorsal in 48%, the lumbar in 9% and the sacral in 2%. The first division of the 5th nerve is involved most frequently. Corneal opacities may result from involvement of this branch. Herpes zoster of the maxillary and mandibular divisions of the 5th nerve result in lesions on the skin, on the oral mucosa or on both. The oral mucosal manifestations are of shorter duration than the dermal lesions. The anterior portion of the tongue, the soft palate and the cheek are the most frequent intraoral sites of herpes zoster.

Prinz and Greenbaum described a case of herpes zoster of the mental region which was believed due to a misplaced, malformed supernumerary right canine. The pain and vesiculation disappeared on the removal of the tooth. Weinberger reported 3 cases of herpes zoster, said to have been caused by decayed teeth.

The geniculate ganglion of the 7th nerve may also be involved. A syndrome of pain in the ear, dizziness and a bloody discharge from the external auditory meatus, with or without facial paralysis, is known as Hunt's syndrome. Taste fibres supplied by this nerve are also affected.

The diagnosis of herpes zoster can usually be made on the basis of the history and the characteristic distribution, location and appearance of the lesions. When the eruption is confined to the oral cavity, it must be differentiated from herpes simplex, manifestations of vitamin B_2 deficiency, pemphigus and epizoötic stomatitis.

Treatment

The treatment of dermal herpes zoster is in the province of the dermatologist. When lesions are present on the oral mucosa, the topical application of mild antiseptics such as one of the aniline dyes will prevent secondary infection of the lesions. In cases of severe pain, associated with involvement of the Gasserian ganglion, Rosewal injected novocaine in the region of the ganglion. Anesthesia is said to be obtained in about 15 minutes, with cessation of the pain and drying of the vesicles within 24 to 48 hours. High vitamin B_1 therapy has been used without remarkable success. B complex therapy gives symptomatic relief and probably shortens the course of the dermal lesions.

TABLE XII

COMPARISON OF HERPES SIMPLEX AND HERPES ZOSTER

	Herpes Simplex (Herpes labialis—fever blister, canker sore—aphtha)	Herpes Zoster (Shingles)
Causative agent	(a) Virus pathogenic for the rabbit with low pathogenicity for man.	(a) Virus believed to be closely related to varicella virus. (b) Any injury to spinal sensory ganglion, i.e., trauma, tumor.
Predisposing cause	Colds, fever, menstruation, pregnancy, emotional or gastro-intestinal upsets, exposure to actinic light, allergy.	Debilitated malnourished individuals
Incidence	Very common. Infection practically universal.	Uncommon.
Age-sex distribution	Usually adolescent or young adult. More common in females. May occur in children as acute stomatitis.	Usually in mid-adult or elderly patients.
Site and distribution of lesions	Lips, oral commissures, buccal mucosa, tongue, frenum. May appear on genitalia. Usually bilateral.	Thoracic cage most common site. 1°, 2°, 3°, div. of 5th N. in the order named. Usually unilateral, rarely bilateral.
Symptoms	Vesicular eruption which develops on an erythematous base. Burning and itching sensation preceding development of the lesion.	Vesicular eruption on an erythematous base. Intense deep burning pain which is not affected by topical medication. May interfere with rest. May be associated with malaise, mild fever and leukocytosis at onset.
Duration	Usually 10-14 days.	Several weeks or months at times.
Treatment	Topical medication gives only symptomatic relief. Application of caustics, at times B complex therapy, elimination of allergic foods. Repeated vaccination.	X-ray therapy, vitamin B complex general supportive treatment.
Recurrences	Common—may occur for many years.	Uncommon, one infection usually confers lasting immunity.

PEMPHIGUS

General Considerations

Pemphigus is a rare disease which is characterized by the formation of successive crops of bullae or vesicles on the mucocutaneous body surfaces. The oral mucosal lesions may be the first evidence of this serious disease.

Gellis and Glass stated that pemphigus constitutes about 0.8% of all dermatologic lesions, the majority of the cases occurring in the 4th and 5th decades. There is a definite predisposition for the Hebrew race, reaching over 75% of the total cases in some reports.

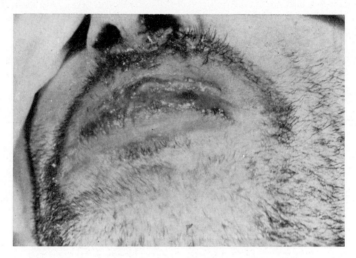

FIG. 96. Patient with generalized pemphigus. The initial symptoms were diagnosed as a fusospirochetal infection. Note how the beard growth has ceased about the lips. (Patient of Dr. L. I. Grossman, Philadelphia, Pa.)

The causative agent of pemphigus is not known but a virus or streptococcal infection or some metabolic disturbance has been suggested. A history of contact or familial association with known cases has been obtained in a few instances. The disease has been transmitted from animal to animal by inoculation of the vesicular fluid and the blood serum, but it has not been passed experimentally from one human to another. Talbot and Coombs found a decrease in the Na, Ca, and Cl levels and an increase in K levels in the blood serum in pemphigus. The decrease in Na could be correlated with the severity of the clinical symptoms. These findings are similar to those associated with adrenal cortex deficiency.

The constitutional symptoms of pemphigus include weight loss, cachexia, nervousness, anemia and general pruritus. The characteristic lesions consist of large vesicles which develop painlessly on normal appearing skin or mucosa. The bullous fluid usually turns a yellow color, due to secondary infection. The blebs break and are replaced by a hard yellow-brown crust. With the development of the lesions, the patient complains of considerable pain and severe itching. The first group of vesicles or bullae will about heal when another group makes its appearance.

Oral Aspects

Symptoms. Mouth lesions occur in most cases of acute pemphigus vulgaris, although they may be transitory and unrecognized due to their early

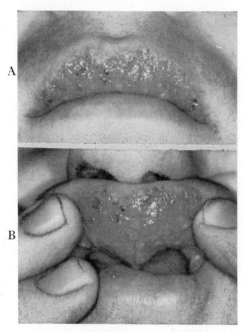

FIG. 97. Pemphigus in a 27-year-old chemist. Painful ruptured vesicles on (A) vermilion border of the lip and (B) the oral mucosa.

rupture. A reddish painful erosion is seen more frequently which represents the base of the bullae, surrounding which are the fragments of the oral mucosa from the ruptured bullae. Oral lesions are found commonly on the lips, cheeks, tongue, palatal mucosa, soft palate and less often the gums. Patients with both cutaneous and oral pemphigus complain more of the pain and discomfort of the oral lesions. Even the swallowing of fluids is painful and the resulting disturbance contributes materially to the rapid decline of the patient.

A marked sialorrhea is one of the outstanding symptoms of acute oral pemphigus. The saliva drips and runs from the mouth and it has an unusually irritating effect on the tissue with which it comes in contact. It is frequently blood-streaked from the bleeding, eroded bases of the ruptured bullae. This sialorrhea contributes to the derangement of ionic balance in the blood serum.

The oral manifestations in chronic pemphigus often give the first clue to the true nature of the disease. The patient may complain of an indefinite burning and itching sensation in the mouth or the symptoms of a chronic fusospirochetal infection, minus the typical bacteriologic findings. Preceding

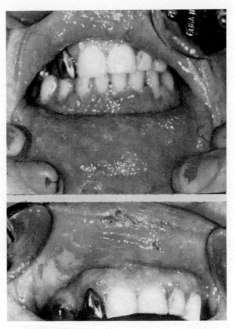

FIG. 98. Eroded vesicles in a 54-year-old woman with pemphigus. The lesions were localized to the oral cavity for six months.

the actual onset of the disease, there is often an initial dryness of the mouth similar to that experienced in herpetic stomatitis and an uncomfortable feeling when ingesting spicy and highly seasoned foods. The mucosal bullae at times precede the cutaneous lesions by weeks or months.

Hailey reported 3 cases of pemphigus confined to the oral mucosa. All his patients complained of nervousness, weakness, loss of weight, and painful sores and ulcers in the mouth. Lesions were also present in the vagina in one patient. All had received various treatments for Vincent's angina and some for syphilis and diphtheria before the diagnosis of pemphigus was established.

Diagnosis. It is not difficult to make the diagnosis in the acute form of the disease when the characteristic multiple bullae and the systemic symptoms are present. In chronic pemphigus, however, the diagnosis is more difficult. Recurring herpetic infections, the various allergic manifestations and the drug eruptions must be ruled out. An atypical "chronic Vincent's infection" at times precedes the typical manifestation of pemphigus. The presence of recurring mucosal blebs or erosions associated with loss of weight, cachexia, nervousness and pruritus should suggest pemphigus.

Nikolsky's sign is said to aid in making the clinical diagnosis. To elicit this sign, the skin or mucosa of a person suspected of having pemphigus is forcibly stroked with finger tip or a tongue depressor, where it appears perfectly normal. The formation of a small bleb or the separation of the superficial layers of the stroked tissue constitutes a positive reaction.

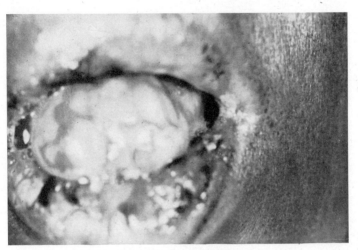

FIG. 99. Vesicles on the lips and tongue of a patient with acute pemphigus.

LABORATORY AIDS TO DIAGNOSIS. (1) The Pels-Macht test is used for differentiating between pemphigus and other skin diseases simulating it. The blood serum, the bullous fluid or even saliva can be utilized.

(2) Gellis and Glass found the erythrocyte sedimentation rate is increased to the pathologic range.

(3) Hematologic findings in pemphigus indicate a secondary anemia and an elevation of the total white count.

(4) Urbach described a complement fixation reaction using a brain extract of an experimentally infected rabbit as the antigen. It is said to be positive in 75% of the cases.

DIFFERENTIAL DIAGNOSIS. Herpetic stomatitis, secondary luetic lesions, chronic fusospirochetal infection, diphtheria, erythema multiforme, varicella, epizoötic stomatitis and allergic reactions to drugs, dentures or mouth washes must be considered in making a diagnosis of pemphigus.

Treatment. The general treatment of pemphigus is in the province of the dermatologist. Numerous remedies have been tried, including sulfanilamide, germanin, arsphenamine, adrenal cortex administration, sodium chloride, urotropin and penicillin. Transfusions and high vitamin intake aid in maintaining the nutrition of the patient. Effective therapy is not known.

Oral care consists of the treatment of the ruptured vesicles, the maintenance of good oral hygiene, and measures taken for the relief of pain. The mouth hygiene is important from the nutritional standpoint and is usually neglected because of the severe pain. Conservative measures are indicated, and tooth brushing is out of the question. Mechanical cleansing with cotton moistened with a mildly alkaline mouth wash is about all that can be done. Ruptured bullae should be treated with 1% crystal violet or 1% acriflavine to prevent secondary infection.

Anesthetic sprays or troches give relief from pain and permit the taking of nourishment. Dental prophylaxis must be done with extreme care to prevent hemorrhage aggravating still further the secondary anemia.

Prognosis. The prognosis in pemphigus is grave, as it is one of the most fatal skin diseases. In acute pemphigus, death may ensue within 3 or 4 weeks but the chronic form may run a protracted course lasting for months or years. The patient dies usually from some intercurrent infection due to his weakened physical condition.

ERYTHEMA MULTIFORME (INCLUDING PLURIORIFICIALIS)

General Considerations

Erythema multiforme is a fairly common inflammatory dermatosis which is characterized by great variation both in the appearance and the distribution of the eruption. The lesions begin usually as papules, macules or less frequently as bullae. The exact cause of erythema multiforme is not known but sensitivity to foods and in some instances drugs is known to give rise to this condition.

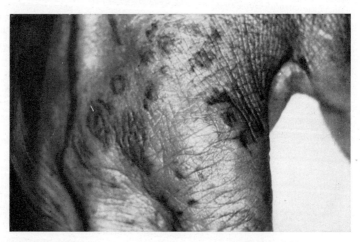

FIG. 100. Typical skin lesion in erythema multiforme.
(Patient H. C.)

The onset of the disease is rapid and symptoms of malaise, arthritic pains or even mild fever may be present, in addition to the dermal eruption. The face, oral mucosa and backs of the hands are common sites for this eruption.

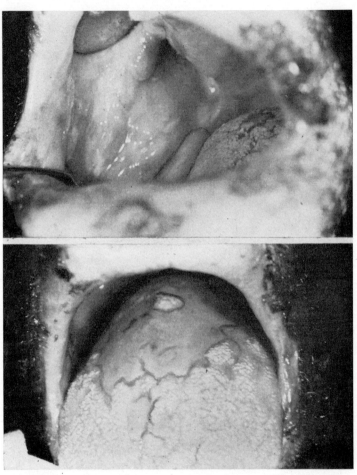

FIG. 101 (*Top*). Oral mucosal lesions in erythema multiforme. (Patient H. C.)

FIG. 102 (*Bottom*). Tongue lesions in erythema multiforme. (Patient H. C.)

The dermal lesions are at first edematous or firm, bright red in color but they gradually fade to a deep purple as they regress. The eruption persists as a rule for 10 to 14 days or even longer. Recurrences are common and they appear to be associated with a lowered general resistance.

Oral Aspects

Symptoms. The oral lesions of erythema multiforme are found on the lips, the tongue, and cheeks and at times the gums. The initial reddish areas

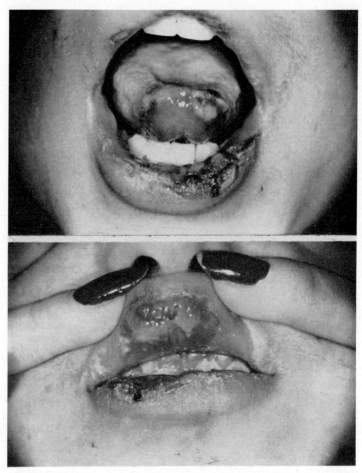

FIG. 103 (*Top*). Lip and tongue lesions in erythema multiforme. (Patient J. S., 23 years old.)

FIG. 104 (*Bottom*). Lip lesions of erythema multiforme in patient J. S. The lesions are more asymmetric and have a deeper red color than the mucous patch.

with blue borders undergo secondary changes rapidly. They become superficially eroded and they are covered later with a yellowish opaque material. On the tongue there is a loss of papillae at the site of the lesion with a regeneration of the papillae with the regression of the lesion. Intense pain is an outstanding symptom and patients with extensive oral involvement suffer acutely. A moderate sialorrhea is present. During the acute phase of the disease it may be impossible to take solid nourishment because of pain.

The diagnosis of oral erythema multiforme in the absence of dermal lesions is difficult and at times impossible. The marked variation in the size and shape of the lesions with their blue-tinged borders and the mild constitutional symptoms should favor the diagnosis. Few bacterial forms are seen on smears made from the lesions.

McEwen reported a case of erythema multiforme with extensive oral foci of infection in the gingiva (? periodontal disease). The patient succumbed later to subacute bacterial endocarditis. Other clinicians have commented on the relationship between oral sepsis and erythema multiforme. The oral hygiene has been poor in the majority of the cases seen by the author. Although oral sepsis may have no direct etiologic connection with erythema multiforme, it aggravates the local symptoms and its effect on the general resistance of the individual may render him more susceptible to recurrences.

An unusual form of erythema multiforme, occurring chiefly in children, which is characterized by a sharp febrile reaction (102° to 104° F.), headache, conjunctivitis, vesicular stomatitis and sialorrhea has been reported by Campbell et al. This condition may be a form of herpetic stomatitis. The oral and facial lesions precede the general body eruption by several days. The oral symptoms, which are acute and distressing, are accompanied by a marked increase in the flow of saliva. Stevens and Johnson have also described an eruptive fever with stomatitis and ophthalmia, which is probably similar to that described by Campbell. In the case observed by Chick and Witzberger there was an accompanying acute fusospirochetal stomatitis, while in Ageloff's case there were bleeding bullous ulcerations of the eyes, mouth and vagina.

Numerous cases with somewhat similar symptomatology with lesions on the oral mucosa, conjunctiva and urethra have been noted in adolescents, especially army camp personnel. In some instances there has been clinical evidence of the contagious nature of this symptom-complex. While the constitutional symptoms are occasionally severe the patients complain mostly of the painful mucosal lesions.

Treatment. The usual topical medicaments are of little value, but considerable relief is obtained from the use of boric acid mouth washes. The topical application of 2% aqueous proflavine will prevent secondary infection of the lesions. Substances such as sodium perborate, iodine containing preparations or caustics are contraindicated.

The prognosis of erythema multiforme is good. Complications are rare.

MINOR DERMATOSES OF DENTAL INTEREST

Lupus Erythematosus

Lupus erythematosus is a dermatosis which is characterized by irregularly shaped reddish lesions which increase in size by peripheral extension, leaving scarred areas in the central portion. They have a tendency to be bilateral. The causative agent of lupus erythematosus is not known but undue exposure to actinic rays often precipitates an attack. The bridge of the nose, the cheeks, the forehead and the ears are common sites for lupus erythematosus.

Lesions of lupus erythematosus occur on the oral mucosa in about 15% of the cases. The oral manifestations, which usually develop after the dermal lesions have made their appearance, are found on the tongue, the hard palate, the oral mucosa of the cheek and on the lips. Lupus erythematosus of the gums is rare. The oral mucosa at the site of the lesion is reddened, atrophic and easily traumatized. Well developed lesions consist of large shallow ulcerations, about whose periphery numerous whitish pin-head areas can be seen. The lesions frequently have a purplish color. After healing, the affected parts are replaced by a thin soft scar tissue.

The diagnosis of oral lupus erythematosus in the absence of skin lesions should be made with caution. The lesions closely simulate lichen planus, particularly the erosive type, and at times leukoplakia.

The treatment of lupus erythematosus is in the province of the dermatologist. Focal infection may serve as an aggravating factor. Hartzell reported a case in which the extraction of a "capped" tooth, with a periapical radiolucent area resulted in permanent improvement after numerous remedies had been tried without success.

Scleroderma

Scleroderma is a rare disease characterized by hardness and rigidity of the skin and subcutaneous tissues of the affected areas. Secondary changes due to pressure may take place in the underlying structures. The current etiologic theories are discussed in a paper by Looby and the author.

Scleroderma may exist in a generalized or a cicatrixing or "coup de sabre" form. In the latter form of the disease, the lesions approximate at times the terminal distribution of a nerve. The initial stage of edema and thickening of the skin is rarely recognized by the patient. The induration and the atrophy of the skin and subcutaneous tissues are striking. The lesion has an ivory or pale white color; rarely it is slightly pigmented. Hemiatrophy is fairly common in cases of facial involvement, sometimes being accompanied by false ankylosis of the temporomandibular joint.

The oral cavity is frequently involved. The tongue, soft palate and larynx are common sites. The tongue may become so stiff that eating is difficult and speech is much disturbed. Thoma described resorption of the alveolar bone and tilting of the teeth due to extrinsic pressure caused by the oral lesions.

Looby and the author reported a case of scleroderma of the "coup de sabre" form which developed in a 5½-year-old girl. The distribution of the dermal lesion followed the terminal facial distribution of the sensory divisions of the 5th nerve. Attention was called to the oral involvement by the failure of the maxillary left first incisor to erupt along with the maxillary right first incisor. In the region of the unerupted tooth there was a deep scarring of the gum and a depression of the alveolar process which extended some distance from the alveolar ridge to the mucobuccal fold. The tip of the upper left first incisor was just visible at the bottom of this depression. The tongue, soft palate, cheek and floor of the mouth were not involved.

In view of the chronologic development of the scleroderma in relation to tooth eruption and the peculiar location of the alveolar defect, it is believed that the retention of the maxillary left first incisor was the result of alveolar involvement associated with the linear scleroderma of the forehead, face and neck.

Stafne and Austin noted that there was a diffuse widening of the dental periosteal space in some patients with diffuse scleroderma. This change was

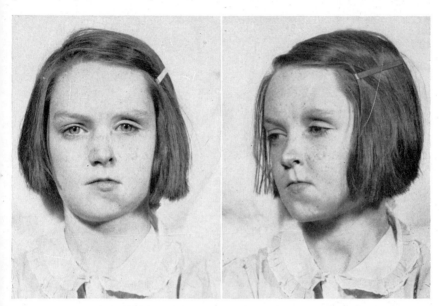

FIG. 105. Scleroderma of the face (coupe de sabre form) which follows the terminal distribution of the fifth nerve. (Looby and Burket, Am. J. Orthodontics and Oral Surg., **28**:493-8, 1942.)

always more marked in the posterior teeth. In some cases, the diagnosis of scleroderma was suggested on the basis of the roentgenologic changes. It was later verified by more complete studies on the patients.

The treatment of any form of scleroderma is difficult and unsatisfactory.

Fordyce's Disease

A symptomless condition, resulting from hypertrophic aberrant sebaceous glands in the lips, oral mucosa and the genitalia, was first described by Fordyce in 1896. The disease is rare in childhood, increasing in frequency after puberty. The lesions are less prominent in the female. About ⅘ of all adults will show some evidence of this disease. If mild cases are omitted, 39% of adult males and 14% of adult females will show well developed lesions.

The etiology of the condition is not known. The hypertrophy of the aberrant sebaceous glands is probably the result of the trauma of chewing, irritation from smoking, bacteria or a combination of these factors. The lip lesions are often marked in pipe and cigaret smokers.

The lesions consist of hypertrophic aberrant sebaceous glands of the vermilion borders of the lips, the oral mucosa and the genitalia. Some claim that the openings of the glands become plugged due to chronic irritation, but Chambers demonstrated in serial sections an opening to the oral cavity or exterior skin surface. Fordyce's disease is usually symptomless. The patient is generally unaware of the lesions until they are accidentally discovered or they are called to his attention. In marked cases there may be a slight burn-

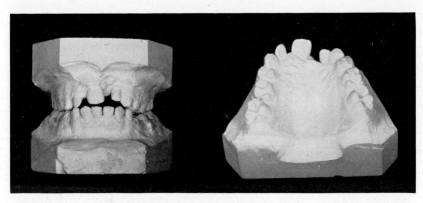

Fig. 106. Casts showing malformation of the jaws and delayed tooth eruption which was associated with the intra-oral changes associated with the scleroderma. (Looby and Burket, Am. J. Orthodontics and Oral Surg., 28:493-8, 1942.)

ing or itching sensation. Patients at times become alarmed when the lesions are discovered and they develop occasionally a cancerphobia.

The hypertrophic sebaceous glands are commonly found on the cheeks along the line of closure of the teeth, particularly in the molar region. At times, the hypertrophic sebaceous glands are limited to an area surrounding the opening of Stenson's duct. The lips are also a frequent site of involvement, and in marked cases their characteristic light pink color is replaced by the chamois-colored sebaceous glands. The upper lip is most often affected. These lesions are especially prone to occur in individuals with gummy or mucinous deposits on the lips or the corners of the mouth.

The aberrant sebaceous glands are usually flush with the surrounding mucosa or they are only slightly elevated. If the tissues are stretched, the lesions become more prominent and appear as slightly raised yellow dots or globules. Numerous glands may coalesce and form large irregularly shaped yellow plaques. This is commonly seen on the lips. The patient then complains of a symmetrical fading of the vermilion border of the lip.

Diagnosis. The diagnosis is usually made on the basis of the clinical appearance and the characteristic location of the lesions. A small biopsy will establish the diagnosis in doubtful cases. The lesions must be differentiated from milium and xanthelasma. In the former, small cysts are present, containing sebaceous material. They are found on the upper eyelid and in the malar and temporal regions. They are thought to be related to heavy milk

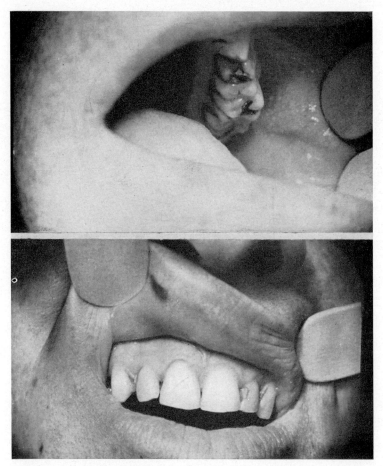

FIG. 107 (*Top*). Fordyce's granules on cheek mucosa in molar region.

FIG. 108 (*Bottom*). Fordyce's granules on upper lip. The patient was a heavy smoker.

drinking. In xanthelasma, one finds elongated chamois-colored wrinkled areas which are characteristically found in the loose tissue beneath the eyes.

Treatment. Treatment is usually not indicated. The patient should be assured that the condition is not associated with malignant disease. The individual lesions can be treated with carbon dioxide snow, fulguration, cautery or roentgen therapy by a dermatologist.

Pityriasis Rosea

Pityriasis rosea is a dermatologic condition of unknown origin which is characterized by scattered, scaly red patches of irregular shape and size. A primary lesion or "herald spot" precedes the generalized eruption by 1 to 2 weeks. The lesions which heal first in the central portion are characteris-

A   B

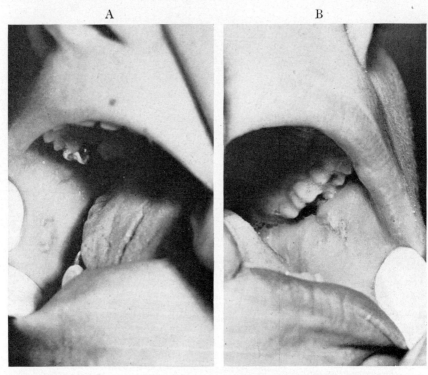

Fig. 109. Lesions on the mucous membranes in patients with pityriasis rosea. (A) An erythematous segmented or incomplete annular lesion with a definitely raised border, clear center and a ruffled scaling or desquamation rolled up posteriorly on the right buccal mucosa. (B) A punctuate hemorrhagic lesion on the left buccal mucosa. (Guequierre and Wright, Arch. of Dermat. and Syph., 43:6, 1000, 1941.)

tically associated with considerable pruritus. The disease is self-limiting and it regresses as a rule in 6 to 8 weeks.

Greenbaum, Quequierre and Wright described lesions which were limited to the oral mucosa. The deep red round macular lesions observed on the cheeks underwent early desquamation and had a dirty grayish appearance. Punctate hemorrhagic lesions were also observed.

The author experienced oral lesions in pityriasis rosea. The oral symptoms were most marked during the first week of the general cutaneous eruption. A generalized catarrhal stomatitis with sialorrhea preceded the more specific mucosal lesions. Small, round, raised, slightly painful lesions developed on the cheek mucosa, particularly in the molar region along the interdental line. Eroded areas, similar in appearance to the measles enanthem, developed in the central portion of the lesions. The oral symptoms disappeared completely within 10 days.

Treatment of the oral lesions consists of bland mouth washes and mild antiseptics such as the aniline dyes.

Lupus Vulgaris

Lupus vulgaris is a form of skin tuberculosis which may arise from exogenous inoculation or by way of the blood or lymphatics from an endogenous focus. Facial involvement occurs in about 70% of all cases. The disease develops usually in early life.

The dermal lesion begins as a small, pin-head, brownish red papule with a glistening surface which increases gradually in size. When these soft nodules are viewed under the slight pressure produced by a microscope slide (diascopic pressure) they have an "apple butter" appearance. The individual nodules may remain stationary, regress without ulceration or become larger and ulcerate. The fibrous scar which results in the healing process produces marked disfigurement. The treatment of lupus vulgaris is not too satisfactory and in spite of energetic treatment the lesions may persist and progress.

Mucosal involvement in lupus vulgaris is common. The cheeks, the soft palate, the tongue and less often the gums are usual locations. Oral lesions develop frequently at the site of local irritation. They vary from small, intensely red nodules to irregular papillomatous lesions. There is a tendency for bilateral involvement. At times fine, whitish lines surround the erythematous area. Superficial ulceration and fissuring develop in extensive lesions. The oral lesions are only moderately painful, unless they become ulcerated and secondarily infected. Merle-Beral believed that the prognosis is particularly serious when the disease involves the gums and periodontal tissues as the teeth loosen rapidly and sequestration of the alveolar process occurs. The small salivary glands are occasionally involved in lupus vulgaris as in other forms of tuberculosis.

The diagnosis of oral lupus vulgaris in the absence of dermal lesions is difficult. This disease appears often in individuals who have already had tuberculosis. Biopsy studies and animal inoculation will permit a diagnosis. The oral lesions of lupus vulgaris are treated symptomatically. Sutton and Sutton found that the oral lesions respond fairly well to superficial cauterization. If pain is a prominent symptom, anesthetic troches can be prescribed.

Galvanic Lesions

Galvanism means a discussion of the effects of a flow of electric current. The term electrogalvanism is tautological. Saliva which is a good electrolyte, and metals which occupy different positions in the electrometric series, fulfill the requisites of a galvanic cell. Thus, in the oral cavity which contains fillings, bridges or dentures of different metals, there are the essential components of a complete battery, and an electromotive force can be demonstrated under such conditions.

When metallic restorations, occupying different positions in the electrometric series, are included in an external electric circuit, a small flow of cur-

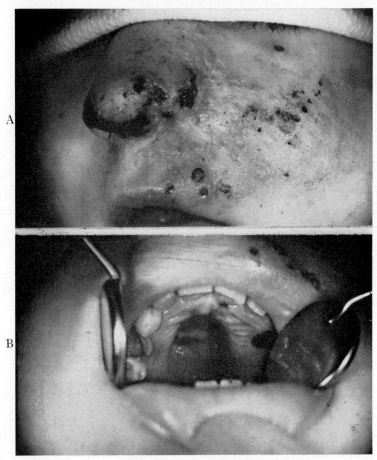

Fig. 110. (A) Lupus vulgaris showing typical nodules near vermilion border of the upper lip and marked scarring and deformity of the left nostril. (B) Lupus vulgaris of the palate. The palatal vault is composed of a nodular mass of tissue which has resulted in erosion of the hard palate.

rent can be demonstrated. This is no proof however that any current flows under normal conditions. Experimental data indicate that an electric circuit between the saliva, the restorations and the oral tissues is not present. Readings obtained between 2 different metallic fillings are initially high, but they drop rapidly to a steady value. This observation is typical of a galvanic cell which is not in use. Since these readings are obtained in a circuit which is parallel with any "natural" circuit, it can be assumed that, if a "natural" circuit does exist, no current flows.

Oral symptoms associated with galvanism include a salty, astringent or metallic taste which is most marked in the morning. The patient may complain of a burning or stinging sensation which is accompanied by an increased flow of saliva. Shallow, eroded areas or ulcers develop less frequently, in the tissues contacting or adjacent to the restorations. The ulcers are said to develop near the restoration of lower potential.

Oral leukoplakia and carcinoma have been reported due to galvanism. Prinz described a case of leukoplakia of the tongue which developed in a telephone worker who was accustomed to test the polarity of an electric circuit by touching the two wires to his tongue. The two small leukoplakic areas disappeared when this practice was stopped.

It is possible for local galvanic currents to be set up between crystals of different elements in the fillings and the saliva. These may also cause reactions in the adjacent contacting tissues. These local galvanic currents are probably more important in the production of erosive lesions of the oral mucosa than the flow of current between two different restorations. The possibility of local lesions being due to sensitivity of the oral mucosa to a constituent of the filling must not be overlooked. The various forms of metallic stomatitides should be ruled out.

Lesions ascribable to galvanism are of little practical importance. The visible signs and subjective symptoms are extremely uncommon. Their importance as the causation of malignant lesions in the mouth is of no practical significance.

Boeck's Sarcoid

Boeck's sarcoid is a benign tumor which is believed to represent a dermal tuberculous infection in an individual with high immunity and mild allergic reactivity. The dermal lesions consist of multiple, asymmetrically distributed, brownish red, cutaneous nodules or plaques.

Oral mucosal involvement is rare. Schroff reported a case of reputed Boeck's sarcoid in which oral lesions were present. The patient complained of a painless, yet tender, irregular swelling in the region of the parotid gland. The growth appeared to be within the substance of the gland, obscuring the orifice of Stenson's duct. The diagnosis was made on the basis of biopsy study. The patient was treated with large amounts of arsenicals, with satisfactory results. Boeck's sarcoid is believed to be closely related to uveoparotid fever. Biopsy studies in numerous cases of uveoparotid fever have revealed the histologic picture of sarcoidosis.

Acrodynia (Swift's Disease—Pink's Disease)

Acrodynia is a rare disease of unknown etiology which is of interest mainly to the pediatrician. At times, striking oral symptoms are present. Because of the similarity of some of the symptoms to pellagra, it is believed that acrodynia may be due to a vitamin deficiency.

The disease affects principally young children. It is characterized by redness, swelling, itching and pain of the extremities, tachycardia and hypertension, photophobia and degenerative changes of the peripheral nerves and spinal cord. Intertrigo and desquamation of the soles of the feet are common.

Oral Aspects

In acrodynia, there is marked salivation with ulceration of the gums, buccal mucosal and tongue. The teeth are described as falling out, in the absence of obvious gingival disease. Bruxism, or grinding of the teeth, is common. Spence described a case in which the child chewed his tongue off.

The general treatment in acrodynia is directed toward maintaining an adequate food intake. Numerous case reports indicate that striking results are obtained following the intramuscular administration of thiamin chloride. Durand observed patients receiving this type of treatment to grow worse when the injections were discontinued. The oral lesions are treated conservatively. The tissues are cleaned with cotton swabs moistened with hydrogen peroxide or saturated boric acid solution.

FOOT AND MOUTH DISEASE—EPIZOÖTIC STOMATITIS

Epizoötic stomatitis is an acute, contagious disease, characterized by fever, chills, malaise and the formation of vesicles on the fingers, toes, oral mucosa and lips.

Epizoötic stomatitis is caused by the smallest known virus and the one which was first demonstrated to produce disease in man. It retains its infectiousness in extremely high dilutions (1:10,000,000). The disease is rare in this country. Direct contamination from infected animal secretions such as raw milk is the common method of transmission. The hedge-hog has been found to be naturally infected and it is believed by some to be an animal vector. Guinea pigs are susceptible to the disease and it has been produced experimentally in man with the development of the classical symptoms.

After an incubation period of 3 to 4 days the patient complains of headache, lassitude, chills or fever. Pains in the neck muscles, dysphagia or a burning sensation of the palmar surfaces of the hands are common.

The primary vesicles appear at the point of entry of the virus, most often on the lips, the oral mucosa, or the fingers. The feet are rarely involved in man. The exanthem consists of various-sized vesicles which develop rapidly, break and usually heal without leaving a trace. There is a marked increase in salivation, and mandibular adenopathy develops. The disease reaches a crisis about the 10th day, but it requires 3 to 4 weeks before the eruptions cease forming and eventually heal.

The diagnosis of foot-and-mouth disease is made on the basis of the constitutional symptoms, the characteristic location and appearance of the vesicular eruption in conjunction with a history of possible contact with the virus. It can be corroborated by animal inoculations.*

* Permission to inoculate animals with suspected material is not granted to anyone other than State and Federal veterinarians who are charged with the responsibility of making diagnosis in cases where foot-and-mouth disease is suspected (Sutton & Sutton).

In the differential diagnosis, pemphigus, herpetic infections, varicella, allergic conditions and, more rarely, erythema multiforme must be considered.

The treatment of the oral lesions is largely symptomatic. The topical application of 2% aqueous crystal violet, and the use of a mild alkaline mouth wash is all that is required. The prognosis is good in adults, but in children the outcome is dependent on the maintenance of adequate nutrition in the presence of the painful mouth lesions.

10

Gingivitis

GENERAL CONSIDERATIONS

Simple gingivitis, or inflammation of the marginal gum, is one of the most common diseases of the oral tissues. Both the high prevalence of simple gingivitis and its mild symptoms contribute to personal and professional indifference. The significance of a simple gingivitis is too often underestimated by the patient as well as the dentist, with the result that this early symptom of more serious periodontal disease is all too commonly disregarded and neglected.

Because of its anatomic location and histologic structure, the marginal gingiva is more frequently involved than is the mucosa of the palate or the cheek. The gums lack the well developed, keratinized, protective layer which is found on the palate and to a lesser degree on the cheek mucosa. Thus the gums are more susceptible to all types of irritation, including that incident to chewing. These delicate, gingival tissues may manifest pathologic changes either under conditions of understimulation (function) or where the stimuli exceed the physiologic limit.

Gingivitis represents an inflammatory response to some local mechanical, bacterial, chemical or thermal irritant. Gingival changes may also be the first manifestation of a systemic disturbance such as scurvy, pregnancy, diabetes or leukemia. Even under these conditions, local predisposing factors are usually important in respect to the site and severity of the symptoms.

In most instances the exact causative agent cannot be determined and, for a consideration of the differential diagnosis, treatment and prognosis, it is convenient to group the simple gingivitides according to the general nature of the irritating agent, such as those which are due to mechanical, bacterial, chemical and thermal agents. If the exact causative agent is known, it can be used to qualify the term gingivitis, e.g., cotton roll gingivitis, staphylo-

172

coccal gingivitis. A combination of irritating agents is frequently present. For example, a secondary bacterial involvement of varying degree is the rule in mechanical, thermal and chemical injuries to these tissues.

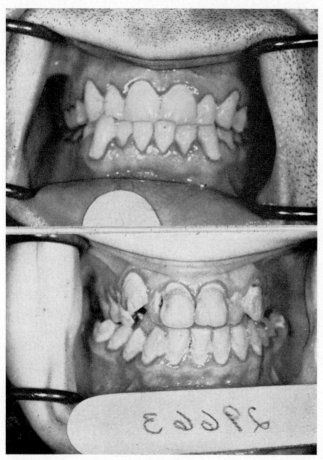

FIG. 111 (*Top*). Persistent chronic marginal gingivitis secondary to a nutritional deficiency.
FIG. 112 (*Bottom*). Simple gingivitis due to lack of oral hygiene.

BACTERIAL FORMS

A listing of all the known bacterial gingivitides would require the enumeration of most of the known pathogenic organisms. In a discussion of any gingivitis of bacterial origin, it should be remembered that the oral flora is not only dense but varied as to the organisms which are present. It is composed of a large number of the so-called "opportunists," in addition to those bacteria which are generally considered as pathogens. These "opportunists" may become locally pathogenic whenever the general or local resistance is lowered sufficiently to permit them to gain a foothold. The fusospirochetal symbiosis is an excellent example of "opportunists" organisms and recent studies suggest that the actinomycetes might be similarly regarded.

An hygienically clean mouth has a heavy bacterial population. The recognition of this complex bacteriologic picture is important when we come to consider the clinical lesions. Because of this varied flora, it is impossible in most cases to incriminate any particular organism as the causative agent. For this reason bacterial smears are frequently of only negative diagnostic value and in general bacterial cultures give still less information. When a marked predominance of any one bacterial form is present, we generally infer that this particular organism may be of etiologic importance.

In cases where the causative agent cannot be determined, it is justifiable to use a pathologically descriptive term such as catarrhal gingivitis, hypertrophic gingivitis or ulcerative gingivitis. The latter term should not be used when referring to fusospirochetal infections. This terminology is desirable from the standpoint of prognosis and treatment for, when the causative agent is not known, it is practical to treat the gingivostomatitis on the basis of the pathologic lesions which are present.

Many of the specific bacterial types of gingivitis, such as fusospirochetal, pneumococcal and gonococcal gingivostomatitis and the gingivostomatitides associated with the common childhood diseases, are discussed in other chapters. There are 2 forms of gingivitis of primary bacterial causation which are not discussed elsewhere. They include streptococcal and staphylococcal gingivostomatitis. While uncommon, both of these diseases are of considerable importance because of their confusion with fusospirochetal infections and the unfavorable clinical response which ensues if caustic agents are used in their treatment.

Streptococcal Stomatitis

Streptococcal gingivostomatitis is usually manifested clinically as a diffuse, acute or chronic inflammation of the gums and oral mucosa. In stained smears, there is a predominance of streptococcal forms which are demonstrated culturally to be alpha streptococci (*Streptococcus viridans*). Attention has been focused on streptococcal stomatitis as a disease entity by Mead. Mumford and Hepplestein described an epidemic of stomatitis and dermatitis which was apparently due to *Streptococcus pyogenes*. The general and local symptoms improved following sulfonamide therapy.

This form of gingivostomatitis is not common. It may occur simultaneously with an upper respiratory infection, or develop alone. As in other forms of stomatitis, general and local predisposing factors are more important in the causation of the clinical disease than the presence of these organisms in the mouth. The author has seen a streptococcal gingivitis develop during the treatment of an oral fusospirochetal infection in which the tissues had been overmedicated. This complication was not recognized for some time because progress smears were not made.

Symptoms. The subjective symptoms of streptococcal stomatitis are similar to, but milder in degree than, those associated with oral fusospirochetal infections. Its onset is occasionally acute, but more frequently there is a gradual development. The affected tissues are bright red and bleed readily. Ulcerative lesions are uncommon but small mucosal erosions are seen frequently. These occur usually a short distance from the marginal gingivae or on the cheek mucosa. The pain is not such an outstanding symptom as in fusospirochetal stomatitis, and the typical fetid odor is lacking.

Constitutional symptoms of fever, malaise and adenopathy may be present. A temperature of 101° F. (oral) has been recorded by the author.*

Diagnosis. The diagnosis of streptococcal gingivostomatitis is based largely on the symptomatology and the clinical and smear findings. The absence of ulcerative lesions of the marginal gingiva and of the interdental papilla, and the absence of the characteristic metallic odor, aid in differentiating this condition from fusospirochetal infection. Streptococcal stomatitis must be differentiated from the oral lesions associated with the nutritional deficiencies or hormonal disturbances. In the former, other visible signs of the nutritional deficiency can usually be observed. A careful medical history will assist in making a differential diagnosis.

Bacterial smears are of value, chiefly in ruling out the possibility of fusospirochetal infection. As in other forms of gingivostomatitis, bacteriologic cultural studies should be evaluated critically. The alpha streptococcus is a common inhabitant of the oral cavity, and it would be indeed unusual not to obtain these organisms on a culture of the gingival region or the oral mucosa. Pure cultures of alpha streptococci are obtained in some cases of streptococcal stomatitis.

Treatment. The general supportive measures discussed under fusospirochetal gingivostomatitis are also of value in this disease. Supplemental vitamin therapy is beneficial but not curative. Frequent mouth washes with hot bicarbonate of soda, 1 teaspoonful to a glass of hot water, are soothing and beneficial.

Caustics and iodine-containing medicaments for topical application should be avoided, as they seem to aggravate the symptoms. Acriflavine 1%, crystal violet 1% or tincture of metaphen 1:200 are effective medicaments for topical application. After the bacterial phase of the infection is under control, local predisposing factors in the form of inadequate dentistry, local functional disturbances or faulty contact points should be corrected.

Staphylococcal Stomatitis

Another type of gingivostomatitis is associated with a predominance of the *Staphylococcus aureus,* which is revealed in bacterial smear and culture. This form of gingivostomatitis, like streptococcal stomatitis, may follow overmedication of the oral tissues.

Symptoms. The clinical features of staphylococcal stomatitis are fairly constant. The marginal and alveolar gingival tissues have a white, cauterized appearance. The tissues are acutely painful in spite of the lack of ulcerative

* Oral temperatures in any acute stomatitis may give inaccurate readings because of the local hyperemia of the tissues. While rectal temperatures are more significant they are impractical in non-hospitalized patients.

lesions. Desquamation of the superficial tissues of the gums, oral mucosa and lips is a prominent symptom. Sialorrhea and painful, regional adenopathy are usually marked. Mild constitutional symptoms may be present.

The diagnosis of staphylococcal stomatitis can be made on the basis of the objective and subjective symptoms, the clinical findings and the indicated bacteriologic studies. The lack of involvement of the interdental papillae and marginal gingivae help to differentiate staphylococcal stomatitis from fusospirochetal stomatitis, and the whitish cauterized appearance of the tissues will aid in differentiating it from streptococcal stomatitis.

Treatment. Staphylococcal gingivostomatitis responds readily to frequent mouth washing with physiologic saline or sodium bicarbonate mouth wash. The topical application of acriflavine 1% or crystal violet 1% is beneficial. The use of sulfathiazole-medicated paraffin blocks or chewing gum will also result in prompt clinical response. All caustic drugs should be avoided.

TRAUMATIC GINGIVOSTOMATITIS (MECHANICAL GINGIVOSTOMATITIS)

A certain degree of stimulation of the gums is necessary for the maintenance of a healthy tone. Stimuli which exceed those which are physiologically essential may give rise to gingivitis. Traumatic gingivitis can arise therefore when there is a lack or an excess of the stimuli which are essential for health of the tissues.

Localized areas of gingival trauma are common in almost every mouth. They may exist due to certain intrinsic factors, such as missing teeth, eating habits or malocclusion. Faulty contact points, improperly contoured fillings or the failure to replace lost teeth satisfactorily, often result in food impaction and traumatic injury not only to the gums but also to the periodontal tissues.

Tooth Brushing

Improper brushing of the teeth results in inadequate gingival stimulation needed in view of the soft foods we customarily eat. It also allows food debris to accumulate in the gingival crevice. This not only favors calculus deposition with its mechanical gingival irritation, but it favors bacterial growth and acid production which may be important factors in the production of cervical cavities.

A more common cause of gingival irritation occurs from an improper or too rigorous tooth brushing technic. Good intentions, so many minutes' time and the expenditure of a certain amount of energy are no measure of the effectiveness of the gingival stimulation and tooth cleansing. An improper tooth brushing technic not only fails in accomplishing its intended purpose but it may result in irreparable damage to both the hard and soft oral tissues. A vigorous horizontal method of tooth brushing at times results in marked loss of tooth substance and even exposure of the pulp. The patient's desire for clean, healthy dental structures defeats his own purpose because of an improper method. If the time spent on stressing the merits of a particular dentifrice were devoted to proper tooth brushing instruction, dentistry and the patient would be benefited.

Tooth picks, tooth brush bristles, the hulls of popcorn, fish or chicken bones which become lodged in the gingival crevice, the dental periosteum or the palate will result in irritative lesions. The failure to completely remove dental ligatures or rubber dam ringlets will give rise to local areas of gingivitis and periodontitis. Orthodontic appliances, clasps, lingual or palatal bars

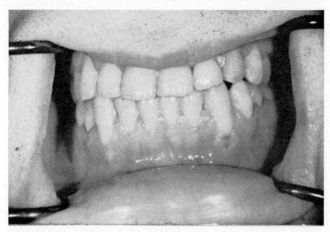

Fig. 113. Mechanical irritation and destruction of the marginal gingiva in the mandibular canine region due to a horizontal method of tooth brushing.

or wires which are used for fracture fixation also serve as mechanical irritants to the gums and oral mucosa.

Habits

Various habits such as bobby-pin biting, pen or pencil biting, the biting of the earpieces of glasses or other similar habits will result in overfunction of the involved teeth and local areas of gingivitis. It may require repeated questioning to determine the exact causative factor in these cases. Frequently these habits are a part of the individual's occupation.

Accidents

Traumatic lesions of the lips are commonly associated with falls, fights or accidents. These wounds, which are usually infected, are accompanied by considerable pain and swelling of the parts. They have a jagged irregular outline and their location and extent can be related in most instances to a particular tooth or group of teeth. In injuries of this nature, roentgenograms of the soft tissues should be taken to determine whether any foreign-body fragments can be demonstrated in the tissues. This is particularly important if portions of the anterior teeth have been fractured.

Dentures (*Decubital Ulcers Due to Denture Flanges*)

The sharp edges of fillings, crowns or prosthetic appliances, carious teeth or retained roots may result in chronic irritation to the contacting tissues. Deep painful ulcerations result at times. If the source of irritation is not eliminated or corrected, it may predispose to malignant change.

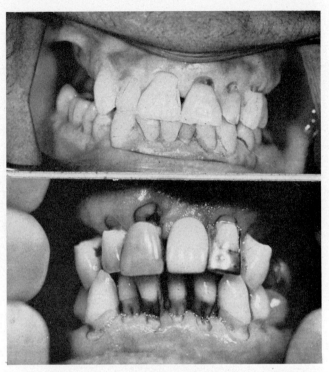

FIG. 114 (*Top*). Cervical notching of the teeth, especially on the left maxillary region, resulting from an improper method of tooth brushing.

FIG. 115 (*Bottom*). Marked abrasion of the teeth and recession of the gums due to an improper method of brushing. The region formerly occupied by the pulp canal can be seen in many of the teeth. (Courtesy of Dr. H. I. Cragin, Philadelphia, Pa.)

Traumatic irritation due to ill-fitting denture flanges often results in striking lesions. A variety of terms has been given to these irritative lesions, such as prosthetic ulcers, granuloma fissuratum and fissured epulis. They are actually decubital ulcerations occurring within the oral cavity due to abnormal pressure on the tissues. These lesions develop rarely following the insertion of new dentures because the acute pain results in immediate desire on the part of the patient for an adjustment. The more extensive decubital ulcerations occur in patients who have not received proper denture servicing.

Normally occurring alveolar resorption results in the formation of a small space between the denture flange and the mucosa. Particularly in the incisal and canine regions, a fold of the oral mucosa and the underlying connective tissue may occupy this space between the denture flange and the alveolar supporting tissues. Both hypertrophy and hyperplasia of the tissue occurs with time and the constant pressure produced by the denture flange gives rise to a depressed fissure or ulceration in the hypertrophied tissue. The initial stages of this process are not particularly painful, and it is not unusual for large masses of hyperplastic and hypertrophied tissue with a central fissure

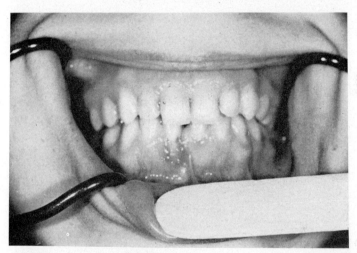

FIG. 116. Loss of alveolar gum tissue due to abnormal functional stresses being placed on the mandibular right first incisor.

or ulcerated area to develop without causing marked discomfort to the patient. In long standing cases, several fissures or folds may be formed. These fissured masses of hypertrophied tissue are most commonly observed in the anterior region. Those lingual to the alveolar ridge in the mandible give rise to particularly painful inflammatory reactions.

When ulceration is present, the pain is usually more marked. If there is secondary infection of the surrounding tissues and associated lymphadenopathy, these linear fissured granulomata can be easily mistaken for neoplastic growths. These decubital ulcers due to denture flanges have several features which aid in differentiating them from neoplastic processes. They follow closely the outline of the denture flange. A varying degree of tissue hypertrophy is usually present in some part of the lesion. In general they are cleaner, less painful and devoid of the odor which is so characteristic of oral neoplastic ulcerations. If bacterial smears are made of the decubital ulcerations, relatively few bacteria are found. The margins of these decubital ulcerations are not markedly indurated and nodules or leukoplakia are not observed.

Edema, inflammation and hypertrophy of the mucoperiosteum are often noted beneath the relief (suction) chambers of poorly fitting, upper dentures. When abnormally deep, clearly outlined suction chambers are present

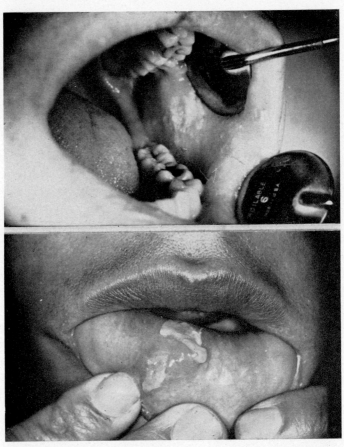

Fig. 117 (*Top*). Traumatic irritation of the cheek. This type of lesion must be differentiated from lichen planus and leukoplakia.

Fig. 118 (*Bottom*). Traumatic injury to the lip which resulted from a fall. The severe pain, the swelling and irregular margins aid in differentiation from syphilitic lesions.

in the denture, rather than true relief areas, the changes are most marked. Again, the lesions are associated with dentures that have not been adequately serviced. The slight movement of a poorly adapted denture during chewing results apparently in sufficient irritation to the tissue approximating the relief chamber, probably through negative pressures which are produced, to stimulate tissue hypertrophy.

The hypertrophied tissue has a well-defined outline which coincides with that of the relief chamber. In unusual cases, the tissue hypertrophy becomes so marked that it exerts enough pressure to induce absorption of the palatal bones.

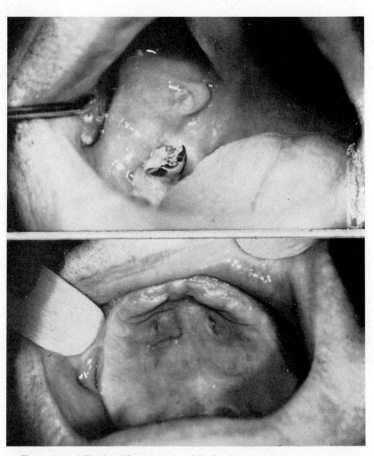

Fig. 119 (*Top*). Chronic decubital ulcer and hypertrophy of cheek due to the sharp distal lingual margin of lower right second permanent molar. This type of lesion may become malignant.

Fig. 120 (*Bottom*). Bilateral traumatic ulcers of the palate resulting from pressure of a full denture over two unerupted maxillary canines.

A less common mucoperiosteal change is occasionally noted beneath suction chambers. This consists of relative degrees of irritation and hypertrophy of the small palatal glands beneath the relief areas. This gives rise to a roughened nodular area in the palate which coincides in location and extent with the suction chamber. An edematous, granular surface which is prone to bleeding, results at other times. The firm, nodular lesions produce few if any symptoms. These tissue changes are frequently mistaken for early neoplastic lesions by the physician and the patient. They cause the patient more mental disturbance than actual physical discomfort or danger.

The treatment consists of the removal of the denture and the use of a mild saline or bicarbonate of soda mouth wash. If the tissue hypertrophy is

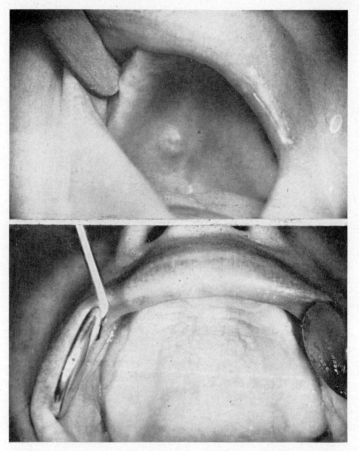

FIG. 121 (*Top*). Traumatic lesion of the palate due to a small fishbone which was imbedded in the tissues. The patient did not wear dentures.

FIG. 122 (*Bottom*). Hypertrophy of the palatal glands due to irritation from a "suction chamber" in all ill-fitting upper denture. These lesions were incorrectly diagnosed as a malignant growth of the palate.

marked, a minor plastic operation will be required before a new denture is made which should be correctly relieved over this area.

These traumatic injuries associated with the wearing of dentures can be markedly reduced by regular denture servicing and rebasing when indicated.

The dentist has neglected to educate his patient of the importance and the need for regular denture servicing. A good denture, like a pair of shoes, requires frequent inspection and professional attention for best service. Full

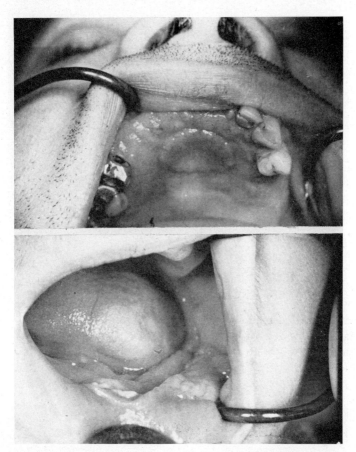

FIG. 123 (*Top*). Hypertrophy of the palatal tissues resulting from irritation of an ill-fitting upper denture which contained a large suction chamber.

FIG. 124 (*Bottom*). Hypertrophied tissue and decubital ulcer caused by the buccal flange of an ill-fitting lower denture. This type of lesion is also called a prosthetic ulcer, granuloma fissuratum or fissured epulis.

and partial denture-wearing patients require periodic professional attention to check that the original intermaxillary space and occlusal relations are maintained and in the case of partial dentures to determine that the abutment teeth are not being subjected to abnormal strains and stresses. Too many patients regard a denture as a permanent accessory to the body, rather than a prosthetic appliance which is fashioned with consideration for its biologic functions and which is still dependent upon the living supporting tissues for satisfactory fulfillment of this function.

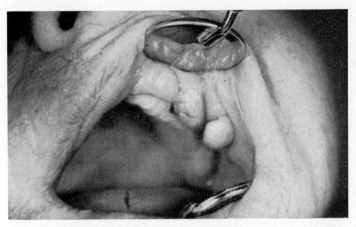

FIG. 125. Hypertrophied and hyperplastic tissue reaction due to flange of an ill-fitting upper denture. The dark object in the central portion of the lesion is a retained root.

CHEMICAL CAUSES

Gingival and oral mucosal lesions result frequently from chemical sources of irritation. This form of gingivitis should not be confused with stomatitis medicamentosa or stomatitis venenata which are allergic manifestations, representing an altered individual reaction to some substance. Chemical gingivostomatitis arises from the therapeutic use of irritating drugs in the office or

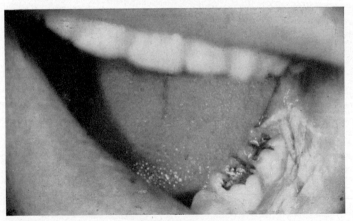

FIG. 126. Typical location and appearance of an acetylsalicylic acid (aspirin) burn of the buccal mucosa.

home, various forms of occupational exposure, tobacco, snuff, alcohol and substances which may be taken accidentally or with suicidal intent.

The common topical therapeutic agents which often result in a gingivo-stomatitis, are chromic acid, phenol, beechwood creosote, silver nitrate, tri-

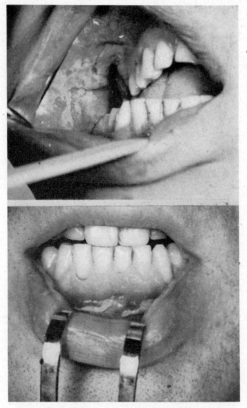

FIG. 127 (*Top*). Acetylsalicylic acid (aspirin) burn of the oral mucosa resulting from placing a crushed aspirin tablet in the mucobuccal fold opposite the molars.
FIG. 128 (*Bottom*). Typical appearance of acetylsalicylic acid (aspirin) burn of mucobuccal fold.

chloracetic acid and formalin. Drugs which are used by the patient for home medication are a common cause of gingival and oral mucosal irritation. Aspirin burns will occur when acetylsalicylic acid is applied locally for the relief of a pulpitis or a periapical abscess. Where the acetylsalicylic acid touches the gum or the buccal mucosa, irregularly shaped white plaques develop. The entire mucobuccal fold may have an opaque white appearance. These chemical burns are painful and they require 5 to 7 days to heal. If acetylsalicylic acid is used for odontalgia, it should be taken internally and not applied topically. Aspirin burns are treated by the topical application

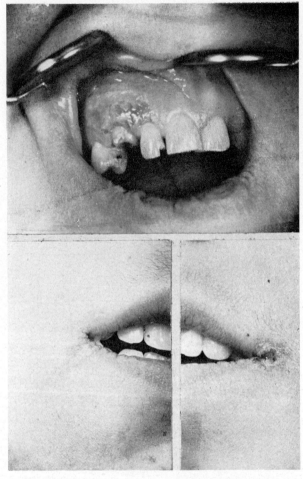

Fig. 129 (*Top*). "Cotton-roll stomatitis." The removal of the epithelium from the buccal gingiva in
the upper right second incisor-premolar area resulted from the rapid removal of a cotton roll.
Fig. 130 (*Bottom*). Phenol burn of the corners
of the mouth. When irritating drugs get under the
rubber dam they produce marked lesions.

of one of the aniline dyes to prevent secondary infection of the area by the common mouth organisms.

The toothache "drops" or "gums" which are on sale at most drug stores contain creosote or other phenol derivatives which have a caustic action on the oral mucosa. Since these substances are rarely confined to the carious lesion, gingival and mucosal burns are the rule when these toothache "drops" or "gums" are used by the patient. Other proprietary preparations which are advocated for the relief of pericementitis, contain counterirritants which often result in sloughing of the contacting tissues. The popular poultice-type of pad is a familiar example of this type of preparation.

Occupational exposure to a variety of agents will result in irritation of the oral mucosa. Workers in acid-manufacturing establishments commonly experience mucosal irritation. Chrome platers, storage battery workers and the workers in any occupation in which acid fumes are present, will experience

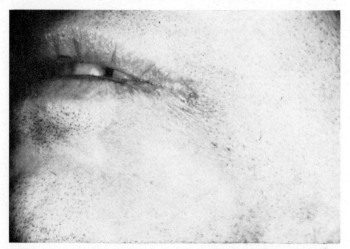

FIG. 131. Chemical burn due to creosote-containing "toothache drops" which were used by the patient.

mucosal irritation or burns. Cement workers frequently experience a dermatitis and inflammation of the oral mucosa, due to the high alkalinity of the cement dust. Likewise highly alkaline chemical reagents which might come in contact with the oral tissues, will result in superficial maceration and necrosis. In the case of strong alkalies the action of the chemical is not limited to the more superficial layers of the tissues like other types of caustic agents, *i.e.*, silver nitrate.

A diffuse form of chemical irritation or burn of the gums and oral mucosa has been noted within recent years in welders. The irritation is due apparently to the fluxes contained in the welding rods. The metallic oxides which are formed during the welding operation, usually electric arc welding, are the irritating agents. These lesions are associated frequently with a fusospirochetal infection. Clinical cure is not possible unless the individual will take the proper precautions to prevent exposure to the fumes.

Substances which may be taken with suicidal intent, such as Lysol, iodine, phenol, lye and caustic potash, will produce severe chemical burns of the oral tissues. A concentrated solution of mercuric bichloride will also produce a chemical burn. The author observed a patient who had taken this substance with suicidal intent. The oral tissues presented a severe irritation due to the contact with this substance. Several days later an acute necrotic stomatitis developed. The large sloughing lesions which were present throughout the mouth, particularly on the gums in the molar regions, were the result of systemic absorption of the mercury compound from the intestinal tract. At necropsy histopathologic studies of the jaws revealed that the gum capillaries were plugged with a black, flocculent material which was demonstrated to be a mercurial salt.

THERMAL BURNS

Severe burns of the oral mucosa are uncommon. Mild burns of the oral tissues arise from the accidental ingestion of hot foods or beverages. These

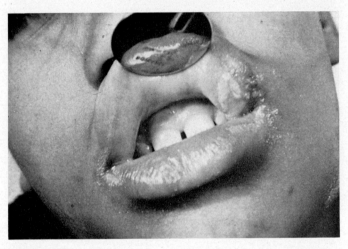

Fig. 132. Thermal burn resulting from the use of hot dental forceps for the extraction of a lower left first permanent molar under general anesthesia.

are of little consequence, as they are of relatively short duration and they involve a comparatively small area. The common site of burns due to foods is the anterior third of the tongue and the palate. There is considerable individual variation in the reaction of the tissues to heat.

Severe thermal burns of the mouth occur occasionally as an occupational accident (steam, etc.). Severe burns of the oral tissues may also occur due to carelessness in the conduct of dental practice. The common causes of accidental burns of the mouth which occur in the practice of dentistry are (1) a hot instrument (heated plastic instrument) and (2) impression materials which are too hot. The latter agents are more serious because of the extent of the tissue damage which may occur.

The burned tissues are very sore for approximately 10 days. An analgesic ointment such as butescin picrate will aid in controlling the pain. The affected tissues can be painted at frequent intervals with an aqueous solution of one of the aniline dyes to minimize the possibility of secondary infection by the mouth bacteria.

DESQUAMATIVE GINGIVOSTOMATITIS

Desquamative gingivitis is an uncommon oral disease. There is some doubt as to whether it is a symptom or a definite clinical entity. It is characterized by a diffuse inflammation of the marginal and alveolar gingiva, the dorsum of the tongue and at times the cheek mucosa. This disease occurs most fre-

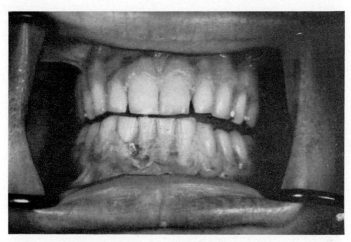

FIG. 133. Thermal burn of the mandibular gum tissue due to hot hydrocolloid impression material.

quently after the menopause or in women with an irregular menstrual history or gynecologic disorders. Desquamative gingivitis is also observed in the male.

Symptoms

The patient complains of a persistent dry or mild burning sensation of the involved tissues, which is aggravated by the ingestion of hot or highly spiced foods. The fiery red and at times purplish red color of the involved tissues are clearly demarcated from the uninvolved oral mucosa. Small water-filled blisters may precede the desquamative lesions in which the superficial epithelial tissues become separated from the deeper layers and slough off. This desquamation of the superficial epithelial layers is most marked on the labial and buccal alveolar gingivae. Slight trauma results in bleeding because the tissues lack the usual keratinized epithelial covering. This disease is characterized by its chronicity and its frequent exacerbations.

Diagnosis

The diagnosis of desquamative gingivitis can be made on the basis of the duration of the disease, the clinical appearance and distribution of the lesions in association with the medical history and at times biopsy studies. Bacterial smears usually reveal numerous epithelial cells and few bacterial forms. The gingival and mucosal changes which result from sensitivity to ingested drugs, may simulate the lesions of desquamative gingivitis. The former are properly considered under stomatitis medicamentosa. They are usually more acute and transitory.

Treatment

Desquamative gingivitis is resistant to the usual forms of topical medication. Caustics of all kinds should be avoided. Within recent years sex hormone therapy has been used in the treatment of desquamative gingivitis. Richmond and Abarbanel and Ziskin reported success with this form of therapy. The former authors obtained the best therapeutic response by injection of estradiol dipropionate locally into the buccal mucosa although gingival massage with diethyl stilbestrol ointment was found to be effective also.

Miller *et al.* were not favorably impressed with this form of therapy. Female sex hormone therapy seems to benefit some cases but this type of therapy is still in the experimental stage. Since a general response may be obtained from this form of therapy, it should be administered only by the physician.

ENLARGEMENT OF THE GUMS

An increase in size of the gums is often seen by the dentist. A wide range of causative factors may produce gingival enlargement. In many cases it is related to local conditions, such as poor oral hygiene, food impaction, mouthbreathing or occlusal hyperfunction. A systemic background is present in many patients. Frequently the gingival hypertrophy will be manifested only in those areas where local irritations are present. With the possible exception of dilantin hyperplasia and diffuse fibromatosis of the gum, enlargement of the gum should be considered as a symptom and not a disease.

Gingival enlargement is common if one considers the instances of isolated hypertrophy of one or more interdental papillae or the enlargement of the tissue about one or more teeth. The more extensive and generalized types of this condition are seen less often but they are encountered by every practicing dentist.

An outline of the various causes of gingival enlargement may aid in determining those factors which are important in a given case.

It is well to differentiate between (1) hypertrophy of the gums, which consists of an increase in the size of the cellular elements making up the gingiva, and (2) hyperplasia which consists of an actual increase in the number of the cellular elements. Varying degrees of hypertrophy and hyperplasia may be found together. It is not unusual for a simple hypertrophy of long standing to be associated with some degree of hyperplasia. The treatment-planning and prognosis of any case of gingival enlargement depend on the relative amounts of hypertrophy and hyperplasia.

Both gingival hypertrophy and hyperplasia are found commonly in children, the adolescent or the young adult. They are found only after the eruption of the deciduous or permanent teeth. At times a history of an hereditary

TABLE XIII

Causes of Gingival Enlargement (Hypertrophy and Hyperplasia)

(A) LOCAL INFLAMMATORY AND TRAUMATIC FACTORS.

    (1) Poor oral hygiene, accumulations of calculus.
    (2) Malposed teeth, faulty contact points.
    (3) Unusual tooth brush habits.
    (4) Occlusal overfunction.
    (5) Irritation from ill-fitting crowns, clasps, prosthetic or orthodontic appliances.
    (6) Mouth breathing.

(B) SYSTEMIC PREDISPOSING FACTORS.

    (1) Endocrine.
        (a) Puberty.
        (b) Menstruation and pregnancy.
        (c) Hypothyroidism and pituitary dysfunction.
        (d) Diabetes.
        (e) Gonadal disturbances.
    (2) Nutritional.
        (a) Scurvy.
        (b) Subclinical nutritional deficiencies of mixed types, including B complex.
    (3) Blood dyscrasias.
        (a) The leukemias—particularly monocytic and myelogenous.
        (b) Polycythemia vera.
        (c) Cooley's anemia.
    (4) Drugs.
        (a) Dilantin.
        (b) The barbiturates.
    (5) Idiopathic forms.
        (a) Diffuse fibromatosis of the gums.

TABLE XIV

Comparison of the Clinical Features of Gingival Hypertrophy and Gingival Hyperplasia

	Hypertrophy of the Gingiva	*Hyperplasia of the Gingiva*
Age and frequency....	More common. Usually in children or adolescents.	Less common. Usually in adolescents.
Histopathology.......	Increase in the size of the usual cellular elements. Interstitial edema, hyperemia, chronic and acute inflammatory reaction in corium. The keratinized epithelial surface is usually deficient.	Increase in the number of the cellular elements which may be also accompanied by increase in size. Inflammatory changes and edema less common. Frequently there is an increase in thickness of the epithelial surface.
Symptoms...........	Swelling of the interdental papillae and the marginal gingivae. Reddish or reddish purple color to the tissues. Edema of the tissues with ready bleeding.	Usually a diffuse enlargement of the tissues which are light pink in color, firm in consistency with little tendency to bleed.
Response to treatment.	Usually responds satisfactorily to local treatment and the proper tooth brush regime. Surgical treatment may be required at times.	Response to local conservative treatment generally unsatisfactory. Surgical treatment is usually required.
Prognosis...........	Good.	Fair. At times it may be necessary to remove the teeth.

or familial background is obtained. There also appears to be a definite individual susceptibility to gingival enlargement. The normal growth stimulus which is present during adolescence, may be an important factor in the frequent appearance of hypertrophy at this age.

The histopathologic findings in the simple irritative forms of hypertrophic gingivitis consist of the usual acute and chronic inflammatory changes in the subepithelial connective tissue. The keratinized layer may be thinner than normal and entirely lacking at the sites of erosions or of acute inflammatory reactions. Marked irregularities in the length and arrangement of the rete pegs are common. This results in a histologic picture which is somewhat similar to that seen in malignant neoplasms except that the basal cell layer of the epithelium remains intact in hypertrophic gingivitis. In the gingival hypertrophy associated with hormonal disturbances, there is also a decrease in the thickness or a loss of the keratinized epithelial layer of the gums. A mild inflammatory reaction is present in the subepithelial connective tissue and varying degrees of hyperplasia are observed.

In dilantin hyperplasia there are marked variations in the thickness of the epithelial tissues with proliferations extending deep within the connective tissue. The increased number of nuclei are evidence of the marked hyperplasia. In fibromatosis of the gums, the connective tissue hyperplasia is the outstanding finding. The thick, keratinized epithelium which is seen in these forms of gingival enlargement, accounts for the marked freedom from hemorrhage.

Gingival Hypertrophy. SYMPTOMS. Hypertrophy of the gums is more commonly encountered by the dentist than hyperplasia of the gums. It is found most often on the interdental papillae, the buccal or labial gingiva and the lingual gingiva in that order. It begins in most instances as a localized process which is related to an area of poor oral hygiene, food impaction or other mechanical irritation which can be readily eliminated or controlled by the dentist. The interproximal gingivae, which are usually involved first, bulge out between the teeth, producing more favorable sites for food impaction and secondary infection. They are glossy, smooth and edematous, pitting on pressure. They bleed readily. Pain is usually not a prominent symptom but the protruding masses of purplish red tissue detract considerably from an otherwise pleasing appearance. The hypertrophy tends to spread and involves gradually the entire labial or buccal gingiva and at times the lingual gingiva.

The numerous pseudo pockets which are formed by the gingival hypertrophy, make the maintenance of the proper oral hygiene difficult. As a result, these tissues become susceptible to secondary infection with the oral flora, including the fusospirochetal organisms. A fetid odor results from the decomposition of food debris in these inaccessible areas.

Drifting and spacing of the teeth occur in long standing cases of extensive hypertrophy. The pressure of the enlarged tissues on the alveolar process and on the interseptal bone results in resorption of these tissues. Long continued edema of the gums predisposes to the formation of new connective tissue fibres and the gradual transformation of the gingival hypertrophy into a hyperplasia.

THE DIAGNOSIS of gingival hypertrophy should present no difficulty. The edema of the tissues, their bright red or purplish-red color and their tendency to hemorrhage should permit differentiation from hyperplasia of the gums. Instrumentation in some forms of hypertrophic gingivitis which are secondary to systemic diseases, e.g., leukemia, may result in undesirable complications. These systemic factors should be ruled out before any instrumentation is begun.

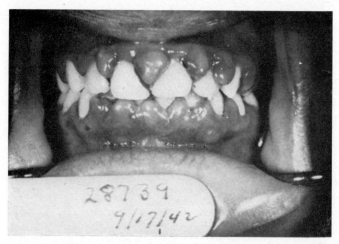

FIG. 134. Hypertrophy of the gingiva with secondary fuso-spirochetal infection in a 15-year-old girl.

A gingival enlargement, affecting primarily the maxillary anterior teeth, is frequently seen in mouth breathers. These patients also commonly have a severe Class II malocclusion. The gingival enlargement consists mainly of hypertrophy of the tissues but, as in all cases of long standing hypertrophy, some hyperplasia develops.

Several theories have been offered to account for the gingival enlargement in mouth breathers. It is believed that the alternate moistening and drying of the gums result in mild inflammatory changes which give rise to a hypertrophic reaction. As in other forms of gingival enlargement, local irritative factors are important predisposing causes. In some patients a co-existing endocrine background may be responsible for the abnormal dentofacial development and the gingival changes. Secondary bacterial infection of the pseudopockets formed by the gingival hypertrophy at times produces more acute inflammatory reactions.

Treatment. The successful treatment of this form of gingival enlargement is chiefly dependent on the correction of the mouth breathing. The patient should be referred to an otolaryngologist to see if there is some obstruction of the upper air passages, such as adenoids. Many times orthodontic treatment will be required to correct the malocclusion and permit the normal closure of the lips during sleep.

All local irritative factors such as calculus, the margins of cervical cavities or areas of food impaction should be corrected. Some clinicians advocate the use of a protective ointment on the gums or the wearing of a facial mask during sleep to protect the tissues from drying. The latter forms of treatment at best only ameliorate the condition. If frank malocclusion does not preclude normal closure of the lips, they can be taped together during sleep to prevent irritation to the soft tissues. Cellophane or "Scotch" tape is as satisfactory as the regular adhesive tape; it is lighter and easier to remove.

The treatment of hypertrophic gingivitis consists of (1) establishing excellent oral hygiene, (2) the elimination of all local predisposing factors, (3) the elimination of as many of the recognized systemic predisposing causes as is possible and lastly but most important (4) proper home care by the patient. The treatment of hypertrophic gingivitis is usually difficult and many times it is not entirely successful. The lack of a satisfactory result may be due to the failure to discover all the causative factors or it may not be possible to eliminate them. Much of the success of the treatment of hypertrophic gingivitis rests with the patient who, because of his age or indifference to the condition, cannot always be impressed with his role in treatment. The chances of obtaining a satisfactory clinical result by means of conservative treatment will decrease with the increase in the amount of hyperplasia.

When the diagnosis of gingival hypertrophy has been established and the more important systemic predisposing factors have been ruled out, the first step in the treatment is the careful removal of all hard and soft deposits about the teeth. This may be difficult because of hemorrhage from the edematous congested tissues. The packing of the pseudopockets with a zinc oxide-eugenol surgical pack prior to the instrumentation will reduce the pain and the hemorrhage and furthermore it will permit the operator to proceed more quickly and efficiently with less discomfort to the patient. Daley advocated the use of acetone base-plate gingival packs in the treatment of the hypertrophic form of gingival enlargement. After careful instrumentation has removed the hard and soft deposits from the teeth special attention should be given to instructing the patient in the proper method of tooth brushing and gingival stimulation. A mouth wash is desirable for no other reason than to get the patient oral hygiene conscious. Local predisposing factors such as poor dentistry should then be corrected.

Strong astringent agents are theoretically beneficial in the treatment of the hypertrophic edematous tissues. While such agents may aid in the treatment of hypertrophy, due to edema, they are secondary in importance to thorough instrumentation and the elimination of all local predisposing factors. Both Talbot's iodine and zinc chloride 8% have mild astringent properties and they rarely cause tissue damage. Glycerite of tannic acid or a paste of zinc chloride 8% and powdered copper sulphate can be used if stronger astringent agents are desired. Wisps of cotton moistened with the former are packed beneath the hypertrophied tissue. The zinc chloride copper sulphate paste is packed beneath the gum margins and allowed to remain for 5 to 7 minutes. A hypertonic saline solution is of some value in reducing the tissue edema.

The patient's diet should be checked and changes suggested when they are indicated. The administration of large quantities of orange juice, 8 to 16 oz. per day, often proves beneficial. Supplemental vitamin C, 150-300 mg. per day, may also be tried if the fresh fruit juice cannot be obtained or if it produces undesirable reactions of any kind.

In cases of extensive gingival hypertrophy or where undesirable hyperplasia is present the affected tissues must be removed surgically. Electrosurgery offers an easy and effective way of eliminating this tissue.

Local treatment is often of value even when the gingival hypertrophy or hyperplasia is associated with systemic disease. While systemic factors should be removed whenever possible, the elimination of local irritative factors may be all that is necessary to obtain a satisfactory clinical result. Gingival enlargements are commonly found in children with hypothyroidism or pituitary dysfunction. In such cases the response to local treatment is likely to be unsatisfactory.

The gingival changes which are associated with puberty, menstruation and pregnancy may resist all forms of local treatment. The gingival enlargement which is so common during adolescence will at times regress spontaneously after 15 to 17 years of age. If the gingival hypertrophies and hyperplasias associated with adolescence are removed surgically, a satisfactory and permanent result is usually obtained.

Accurate studies might reveal more frequent hypertrophic gingival changes at the menstrual period and during pregnancy. As a rule the hypertrophy or bleeding is so slight and of such a short duration and produces so few symptoms that the dentist is not consulted. Hypertrophic changes are also observed in other tissues related to the oral cavity. Premenstrual swelling of the salivary glands is not rare.

A 25-year-old patient was recently treated, who experienced a marked hypertrophy of the gum flaps about the partially erupted mandibular third molars at each menstrual period. The gum flaps would remain symptom-free until about 2 to 3 days prior to menstruation when a marked swelling of these tissues would take place. The hypertrophy was so extensive that the tissues were traumatized by the opposing teeth. They would bleed freely and occasionally become secondarily infected. These symptoms, which had persisted for 8 years, were finally relieved by the surgical removal of the gum flaps. The treatment of the gingival changes associated with menstruation and pregnancy are discussed in the sections devoted to these subjects.

Slight hypertrophic changes which fail to respond to local treatment and a proper tooth brushing regime, frequently have a nutritional background. The oral findings in frank scurvy with the purplish red, hypertrophied, bleeding gums are rarely seen in the child and especially in the adult. The subclinical nutritional deficiencies are much more common and important. The gums will present a variety of appearances. The marginal 2 to 3 mm. of these tissues are often edematous and reddened or at other times they are rose-pink. Such lesions fail to respond satisfactorily or permanently to the usual forms of local treatment, whether given at the dental office or by the patient at home. These patients are susceptible to recurrent non-specific forms of gingivitis and fusospirochetal infections.

These slight, persistent, hypertrophic changes may be found in individuals of a good economic status, who are eating what is considered to be a satisfactory, if slightly unbalanced, diet. This type of patient requires a careful nutritional study with special investigation of the absorptive function of the gastro-intestinal tract. While the gingival lesions may be the main concern of the patient and the dentist, these cases are primarily medical in nature. If

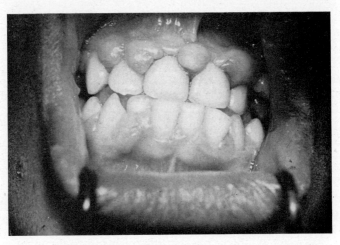

Fig. 135. Hyperplasia (fibrosis) of the gingivae secondary to long-standing hypertrophy.

there is an abnormal absorptive function, oral supplemental vitamin therapy or dietary change will prove of little value.

The oral changes associated with the blood dyscrasias are described in detail in the sections devoted to this subject. A generalized gingival hypertrophy is often the earliest symptom of these diseases. A complete history in such cases will usually reveal symptoms of gradually increasing weakness, malaise, loss of weight and adenopathy which should suggest the systemic basis for the oral manifestations. The characteristic gingival ulceration and necrosis may not develop for some time after the hypertrophy has appeared.

Hyperplasia of the Gums. In the proliferative type of gingival lesions, the tissues have the normal pink color or at times they are slightly paler than normal. The tissue is firm, hard and fibrous in consistency, due to the increase in the fibrous connective tissue. It does not bleed readily and it does not pit on pressure. Typical examples of gingival hyperplasia are found in the gingival enlargements which are associated with the administration of dilantin or phenobarbital and in diffuse fibromatosis of the gums. A moderate degree of hyperplasia is found in the gingival enlargement which is associated with gonadal disturbances.

Dilantin gingival hyperplasia and the gonadal gingival hyperplasia are discussed under epilepsy and diseases of the urogenital system respectively.

DIFFUSE FIBROMATOSIS. Diffuse fibromatosis of the gums is an uncommon form of marked gingival hyperplasia. The exact cause of this peculiar change

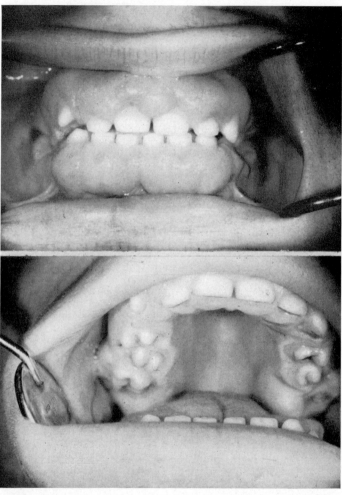

FIG. 136. Diffuse fibromatosis (hyperplasia) of the gums in a 19-year-old boy. There was recurrence of the gingival hyperplasia following surgical removal.

is not known. Ruggles suggested that it is neoplastic while Hertzler likened it to a keloid reaction resulting from mild irritation of the marginal gingiva.

This marked hyperplasia of the gums begins usually with the eruption of the permanent dentition, less commonly with the eruption of the deciduous dentition. A familial history has been obtained in some instances. In severe cases the dense firm gum results in spacing of the teeth, alveolar resorption and marked changes in the profile and general facial appearance. This mass of hyperplastic tissue not only interferes with speech but it gives rise to difficulty in chewing food and prevents the normal closure of the lips.

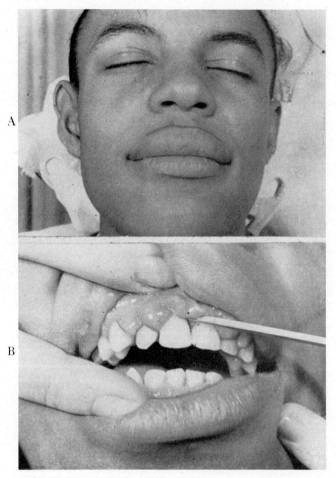

Fig. 137. (A) Negro boy aged 15 years with enlarged lips (macrocheilia) due to repeated streptococcal infections of these tissues. (B) Unusual form of gingival hypertrophy and hyperplasia in same patient. No systemic basis could be found. The enlarged gingival tissues contained numerous small amorphous calcified masses.

The surface of the hyperplastic tissue often has a nodular appearance due to the thickened, hyperkeratinized epithelium. There is no difficulty in differentiating between simple hypertrophy of the gums and diffuse fibromatosis. The medical history will enable one to rule out the possibility of barbiturate or dilantin hyperplasia. In dilantin hyperplasia there is a clear-cut line of demarcation between the hyperplastic tissue and the normal gum tissue which is not present in gingival fibromatosis.

The treatment of gingival fibromatosis is unsatisfactory. Conservative treatment by instrumentation is of little value. Gingivotomy of the hyperplastic tissue is usually followed by regrowth. In the case reported by Ball the gingivotomy was followed by radiation of the tissues. A satisfactory clinical result was obtained.

Prinz believed that in cases of extensive diffuse fibromatosis the most successful form of treatment consisted of extraction of the teeth which were associated with the gingival enlargement and the surgical elimination of all of the hyperplastic tissue. When there is generalized involvement of both dental arches, this is rather a formidable undertaking which must be done in several stages. It would seem desirable to try gingivotomy and radiation before the more radical form of treatment is undertaken in which the teeth are sacrificed.

GINGIVAL HYPERPLASIA DUE TO THE BARBITURATES. Gingival enlargement may follow the long continued administration of the barbiturates as sedatives. Gable observed gingival enlargement in epileptic patients who were given either phenobarbital, dilantin or both drugs. Veterinarians have also noted hyperplasia of the gums of small animals receiving this group of drugs. The gingival enlargement which is so commonly observed in the epileptic patient is usually, perhaps incorrectly, attributed to poor oral hygiene.

HALITOSIS

Bad breath or halitosis should be considered a symptom and not a disease. An abnormal breath odor is objectionable, whether it arises from the lungs, the respiratory passages or the mouth. Since many of the causes of bad breath are due to oral pathosis, the dentist should be familiar with the various local and systemic factors which may be responsible for this condition.

A faint, slightly sweetish odor on the expired air is normal. This may undergo slight variations depending on the time of day, the rate of salivary flow, the bacterial population of the mouth and such physiologic processes as menstruation. The breath is always slightly heavier in the morning. The usual odor is readily modified by disease and characteristically so in some clinical entities.

Abnormal odors of the breath may arise from (1) local disease processes in the mouth, the lungs and the respiratory tract and (2) odors which are imparted to the expired air by substances which are liberated from the blood stream in the lungs. These include abnormal chemical constituents which are found in some diseases or substances which are normally present in the blood following the absorption of certain foods.

Odors arising from sources other than the mouth are of less interest to the dentist than to the physician, as they cannot be appreciably altered by the establishment of good oral hygiene. Since abnormal odors from the lungs or the lower respiratory tract may be detected on the expired air, it is necessary to separate odors from these sources from odors arising in the mouth. Brening *et al.* devised a technic for separating lung from mouth odors. While this method is applicable for research studies, it is not practical for clinical use. Sulser *et al.* devised an instrument, the osmoscope, which permits objective measurement of the intensity of breath odors.

Extra-oral Causes

Bad breath, secondary to disease processes of the lungs and respiratory passage, is less common than that due to oral causes. It is often referred to as true halitosis. Any open suppurative lesion of the lungs will result in a foul breath. The breath of a patient with a lung abscess is putrid and sickening. Similar in nature but milder in degree is the odor associated with bronchiectasis. Chronic sinusitis, particularly of the maxillary sinus, or the associated postpharyngeal discharge, will result in an abnormal odor to the breath.

The most common extra-oral cause of bad breath results from the transfer of odoriferous substances dissolved in the blood stream. These may consist of substances derived from foods or beverages (garlic, alcohol), substances produced during the abnormal or incomplete metabolism of food (acetone) or waste substances which are not properly eliminated through normal channels (urea-ammonia).

There are some conflicting explanations for the production of halitosis due to substances such as onions and garlic. At one time the odor was believed due to small particles of these substances which had become lodged between the teeth or in the gums—thus modifying the breath. While some odor may be imparted to the breath by these retained food particles within ½ to 1 hour after ingestion, this source of odor is soon exhausted.

The careful and ingenious studies of Crohn and Drosd gave us much information about the production of halitosis of this type. They demonstrated that the prolonged breath odor which persists following the eating of garlic or the drinking of alcoholic beverages is not derived from material which remains in the mouth. It results from the absorption of this material, usually from the gastro-intestinal tract, and its gradual elimination through the lungs. This was established by inserting a test substance, garlic for instance, in a jejunostomy opening or a colostomy stoma. Within a few hours the substance could be noted on the breath, where it persisted for hours, although the portion of the intestinal tract used had been completely severed from the stomach. They found that unless there is belching or vomiting, the stomach contents are not detected on the breath. Alcohol is a possible exception, since it can be absorbed from the gastric mucosa.

Oral Causes

Anything which interferes with the normal physiology of the oral cavity is likely to give rise to an abnormal or offensive breath. The decreased salivary flow which is associated with dehydration states, whether they arise from fever or from the ingestion of alcoholic beverages, will give rise to a malodorous breath. Persons consuming a liquid diet, particularly those on a milk or cream diet, are prone to develop an offensive breath due to the tongue coating which favors the lodgement of food debris and bacterial action.

Poor Hygiene. Failure to maintain proper oral hygiene will permit food particles to collect and undergo bacterial decomposition. This is particularly true when the interdental papillae have been lost through recession or ulceration. The pseudopockets or gum flaps associated with erupting teeth, particularly mandibular third molars, favor the accumulation of food debris and secondary bacterial decomposition in spite of attempts to maintain proper oral hygiene. They are a common and important oral cause of abnormal breath.

Sulser *et al.* determined by means of the osmoscope the relative importance of dental decay, periodontal disease and gingivitis in producing breath odors. Periodontal disease, gingivitis and dental decay, in the order named, were found to be important in giving rise to a bad breath. Individuals with periodontal disease, particularly the type associated with suppuration, have frequently an offensive breath. At times, the odor is due simply to poor oral hygiene but in other cases it is present in spite of the frequent use of mouth washes and the usual methods of oral hygiene. The numerous pockets and interdental areas, with their contained debris, bacteria and at times pus cannot be effectively cleansed by the usual methods of oral hygiene. Highly flavored or scented mouth washes and proprietary breath sweeteners only substitute another odor for the objectionable one. They are effective but for a short time.

Dentures. Denture-wearing patients have frequently a malodorous breath. This occurs when proper attention is not given to cleansing the dentures. Dentists all too commonly fail to instruct adequately the patient in the care of the denture, particularly partial appliances with their numerous food impaction areas. Artificial dentures require at least the same attention as natural dentures to prevent offensive breath. The appliances can be effectively cleansed with brushes specially made for this purpose and any good denture cream, dentifrice or soap and water. It is desirable to brush the denture after each meal, but when this is impossible the appliance should at least be washed in running water.

Artificial dentures should be removed at night, except in special instances. This rests the supporting tissues, eliminates the possibility of accidental dislodgement and also aids in preventing an objectionable breath. When dentures are allowed to remain in place during sleep there is a tendency to neglect the proper oral hygiene. The appliances can be placed overnight in ordinary tap water to which have been added a few drops of mouthwash.

Extractions and Oral Surgery. A fetid breath is a common occurrence, following dental extractions or oral surgery. This is due to a lack of normal chewing, the consumption of a soft diet, slight bleeding and the increased bacterial population of the mouth. Mild gingival bleeding or oozing is not unusual in simple gingivitis and in many of the blood dyscrasias. Bacterial decomposition of this blood gives rise to a particularly foul odor.

Ulcerative lesions of the oral cavity are accompanied by a malodorous breath unless special precautions are taken. Noma, which is a massive gangrenous process of the oral tissues, is characterized by a putrid and offensive odor. Ulcerated malignant growths of the oral cavity likewise have a bad odor. Necrotic lesions in the blood dyscrasias, particularly leukemia, are accompanied by putrid odor.

The mechanical cleansing action of frequent mouth washings whether of water, saline solution or half-strength ($1\frac{1}{2}\%$) hydrogen peroxide is valuable for reducing the odor. Meleny called attention to the value of zinc peroxide in controlling and eliminating the odor of gangrenous lesions of the oral cavity. An aqueous paste of zinc peroxide, not zinc oxide, is a most valuable preparation for controlling offensive odors which are associated with necrotic lesions of the mouth.

TABLE XV

BAD BREATH

(A) EXTRA-ORAL CAUSES (True halitosis).
    (1) Gangrenous processes in the lungs and respiratory passages.
    (2) Elimination of odoriferous substances from the blood stream.
        (a) Obtained from ingested foods and beverages, *i.e.*, garlic, onions, alcohol.
        (b) Abnormal accumulation of normal or abnormal constituents in the blood stream, *i.e.*, acetone breath in diabetes, ammoniacal odor in uremia.
(B) ORAL CAUSES.
    (1) Areas of food impaction and decomposition.
        (a) Gum flaps associated with erupting teeth.
        (b) Loss of the interdental papillae due to:
            (1) Fusospirochetal infection.
            (2) Abnormal gingival recession.
    (2) Periodontal pockets.
    (3) Improper or inadequate artificial denture hygiene.
    (4) Ulcerative, necrotic or bleeding lesions in the mouth: benign or malignant.

The metallic odor of the breath in fusospirochetal and metallic stomatitis is one of the outstanding symptoms of the disease. Prinz believed that it is the most important and characteristic clinical symptom of fusospirochetal stomatitis. It is readily controlled by any of the agents which have been discussed for the treatment of this disease but zinc peroxide is particularly effective.

The oral causes of bad breath can be benefited by proper dental care and patient co-operation. The dentist can treat the diseased tissues, eliminate local factors which may favor the accumulation of food debris and instruct the patient in the proper oral hygiene, but the final success of overcoming this objectional symptom rests with the patient who must conscientiously follow the treatment which the dentist prescribes.

REFERENCES

TONGUE

Abelson, S. M., *et al.*: Muscular macroglossia, Am. J. Dis. Child., **62**:624, 1941.

Anderson, Douglas: The tongue in medical diagnosis, Med. J. Australia, **1**:308, 1944.

Beder, O. E., & D. E. Ziskin: Case report of hemangiomas of tongue and cheek treated with radium, Am. J. Orthodontics & Oral Surg., **30**:73, 1944.

Binkowitz, B.: Blood supply of the tongue—early sign of cardiac decompensation, Med. J. & Record, **137**:426, 1933.

Boucher, R.: Burning sensation of the tongue as a sign of gastric ulcer, Union Med. du Canada, **61**:1000, 1932.

Comroe, Bernard I.: Diagnostic importance of the tongue in internal medicine, Am. J. M. Sc., **194**:661, 1937.

Cook, T. J.: The tongue, Am. J. Orthodontics & Oral Surg., **27**:1, 1941.

Cooper, G. W.: Laboratory method in false or pseudo black tongue, West Virginia M. J., **28**:126, 1932.

Copps, L. A., & S. Epstein: Traumatic cancer of the tongue, Arch. Otolaryng., **34**:1023, 1941.

Dummett, C. O.: Pertinent facts about the tongue and breath as aids in the diagnosis of disease, Am. J. Orthodontics & Oral Surg., **30**:57, 1944.

Ehrich, W., & F. Ehlert: Mucous membrane of the tongue at different periods of life, Deutsche. monat. Zahnheil., **51**:865, 1933.

Engman, M. F., Sr.: Lingual tonsillitis, Arch. Dermat. & Syph., **1**:137, 1920.

Gilpin, S. F.: Forty-eight cases of glossodynia, J. A. M. A., **106**:1722, 1936.

Gregg, L. A., & F. B. Utley: Tongue in nutritional disorders, Pennsylvania M. J., **46**:933, 1943.

Hardgrove, T. A.: Surgical case histories, J. A. D. A., **26**:126, 1939.

Heidingsfeld, M. L.: Hairy or black tongue, J. A. M. A., **55**:2117, 1910.

Isaacs, R., C. C. Sturgis, & M. Smith: Treatment of pernicious anemia, J. A. M. A., **91**:1687, 1928.

Jeghers, Harold: Nutrition: The appearance of the tongue, as an index of nutritional deficiency, New England J. Med., **227**:221, 1942.

Katzenellenbogen, I.: Nicotinic acid in the treatment of endemic glossitis, Dent. Rec., **60**:34, 1940.

Kennedy, C. B., & J. K. Howles: Black hairy tongue, Arch. Dermat. & Syph., **42**:566, 1940.

Little, Raymond D.: Lingua nigra, U. S. Nav. M. Bull., **43**:360, 1944.

Martin, H. E., & M. E. Howe: Glossitis rhombica mediana, Ann. Surg., **107**:39, 1938.

McCarthy, F. P.: A clinical and pathologic study of oral lesions, J. A. M. A., **116**:16, 1941.

McEnery, T. E., & F. P. Gaines: Tongue-tie in infants and children, J. Pediat., **18**:252, 1941.

Means, J. H.: Observations of the tongue and what it teaches us about the patient's general condition, Internat. Clinics, **4**:1, 1935.

Michaelson, N. M.: Tongue wounds, Am. Rev. Soviet Med., **1**:216, 1944.

Nelson, A. W.: Transient benign plaques of tongue—(geographical tongue), J. Med., **8**:293, 1927.

Pagano, A.: Relation of varices at base of tongue to pharyngeal disease, Morgagni, 73:1945, 1931.

Prinz, H.: Wandering rash of the tongue, Dental Cosmos, 69:272, 1927.

Rose, B. T.: Lingual tonsillitis, Lancet, 2:14, 1927.

Scholtz, M.: Painful papillae, Arch. Dermat. & Syph., 32:801, 1935.

Schroff, J.: Burning tongue, Rev. Gastroenteral, 2:347, 1935.

Schütt, F. E.: Lingua nigra cured with nicotinic acid amide, Rev. Odontologica, 29:758, 1941.

Schwindt, L. W.: Specific tongue conditions noted in peptic ulcer cases, Med. Times & Long Island M. J., 60:242, 1932.

Sluder, G.: Lingual tonsillitis, Am. J. M. Sc., 156:248, 1918.

Waldenstrom, J.: Is the condition of the papilla on the tongue a mirror of cell oxidations?, Upsala lak. foren. for., 46:215, 1941.

Weidman, Fred. D.: The affinities between black tongue and trichomycosis, Arch. Dermat. & Syph., 18:647, 1928.

Whittle, C. H.: Geographic tongue, Proc. Roy. Soc. Med., 25:919, 1932.

Yates, A. L.: Fungus infection of the mouth and throat and nose and ear, Canad. M. A. J., 50:540, 1944.

Zeisler, E. P.: Monilia infection of the tongue, Arch. Dermat. & Syph., 15:171, 1927.

THE DERMATOSES

Leukoplakia Buccalis

Becker, W. S.: Review of the leukoplakia problem as related to the mouth, J. A. D. A. & Dent. Cosmos, 24:1453, 1937.

Bogen, E., & E. N. Loosmis: Tobacco tar—an experimental investigation of its alleged carcinogenic action, Am. J. Cancer, 16:1515, 1932.

Burke, E. T.: Treatment of severe lingual leukoplakia, Brit. M. J., 2:113, 1935.

Cahn, L. R.: A note on the histopathology of leukoplakia of the palate, Am. J. Orthodontics & Oral Surg., 27:35, 1941.

Eichenlaub, F. J.: Leukoplakia buccalis, Arch. Dermat. & Syph., 37:590, 1938.

Friedell, H. L., & L. M. Rosenthal: The etiologic role of chewing tobacco in cancer of the mouth, J. A. M. A., 116:2130, 1941.

Garb, J., & G. Rubin: Dyskeratosis congenita with pigmentation, dystrophia ungium and leukoplakia oris, Arch. Dermat. & Syph., 50:191, 1944.

Grace, E.: Influence of a carcinogenic compound in cancer of the oral cavity, J. A. D. A., 30:1358, 1943.

Martin, H., & C. E. Koop: Precancerous mouth lesions of avitaminosis B; their etiology, response to therapy and relationship to intra-oral cancer, Am. J. Surg., 57:195-225, 1942.

McCarthy, F. P.: Etiology, pathology and treatment of leukoplakia buccalis, with report of 316 cases, Arch. Dermat. & Syph., 34:612, 1936.

Nathanson, I. T., & D. B. Weisberger: Treatment of leukoplakia buccalis and related lesions with estrogenic hormone, New England J. Med., 221:556, 1939.

Orr, H.: Peculiar papular eruption of the hard palate, Brit. J. Dermat., 42:436, 1930.

Quick, D.: Leukoplakia and allied mouth conditions, Canad. M. A. J., 40:234, 1939.

Roffo, A. H.: Carcinome developpe chez un lapin apres trois ans, par l'effect du tabac, Neoplasmes, 11:77, 1932.

Roffo, A. H.: Der Tabak als krebserzeugendes Agens Deutsche med. Wchnschr., 63:1267, 1939.

Roffo, A. H.: Ueber die Prinzipien der Krebserzeungenden Wirkung des Tabaks, Schweiz. med. Wchnschr., 71:549, 1941.

Ronchese, F.: Leukoplakia and tobacco, Arch. Dermat. & Syph., 36:1222, 1937.

Savill, A.: Treatment of pruritus vulvae leukoplakia and kraurosis, Brit. J. Dermat., 52:321, 1940.

Simpson, F. E.: Cancer and precancerous lesions of the lip, Illinois M. J., 79:459, 1941.

Swift, B. H.: Relation of vitamin A to leukoplakia, J. Obst. & Gynec. Brit. Emp., 43:1053, 1936.

Thoma, Kurt H.: Stomatitis nicotina and its effect on the palate, Am. J. Orthodontics & Oral Surg., 27:38, 1941.

Touraine, A., & A. Baudonin: Trois observations de leucoplasie electrogla-vanique, dont une avec cancer, Bull. Soc. f. de dermat. et syph., 44:2066-71, Dec. 1937.

Vaughn, H. C.: Leukoplakia—relation to vulcanite dentures, J. A. D. A., 22:65, 1935.

Herpes

Alvarez, W. C.: Canker sores (Editorial), Minnesota Med., 20:602, 1937.

Arnold, D. G.: Herpes zoster as sequel of spinal anesthesia, J. Internat. Coll. Surgeons, 4:66, 1941.

Bartels, H. A.: Some notes on the etiology of herpes simplex, Dent. Items of Interest, 53:30, 1931.

Basch, J.: Treatment of aphthous stomatitis with neoarsphenamine, Deutsche med. Wchnschr., 54:1206, 1928.

Beecher, W. L.: Canker sores in mouth-specific hypersensitiveness or allergy as a cause, Clin. Med. & Surg., 35:903, 1928.

Berggreen, P., & E. G. Schuler: Zur Kenntnis der Lakalisation des Herpes zoster, Dermat. Wchnschr., 106:216, 1938.

Berlin, C.: Behcet's syndrome with involvement of the central nervous system, Dent. Rec., 64:75, 1944.

Black, W. C.: Acute infectious gingivostomatitis, Am. J. Dis. Child., 56:126, 1938.

Breese, B. B.: Aphthous pharyngitis, Am. J. Dis. Child., 61:669, 1941.

Burnet, F. M.: Herpes stomatitis and herpes virus, Proc. Cong. Australian Dent. Soc., 249, 1939.

Burnet, F. M., & D. Lush: Herpes simplex—studies on antibody content of human serum, Lancet, 1:629, 1939.

Denny-Brown, D., R. D. Adams, & P. J. Fitzgerald: Pathologic features of herpes zoster: note on "geniculate herpes," Arch. Neurol. & Psychiat., 51:216, 1944.

Dodd, K., L. M. Johnston, & G. J. Buddington: Herpetic stomatitis, J. Pediat., 12:95, 1938.

Elford, W. J., & I. A. Galloway: Centrifugation studies; viruses of foot-and-mouth disease and vesicular stomatitis, Brit. J. Exper. Path., 18:155, 1939.

Fisher, A. A.: Treatment of herpes simplex with moccasin snake venom, Arch. Dermat. & Syph., 43:444, 1941.

Foster, P. D., & A. B. Abshier: Smallpox vaccine in treatment of recurrent herpes simplex, Arch. Dermat. & Syph., 36:294, 1937.

Frank, S. B.: Formalized herpes virus therapy and neutralizing substance in herpes simplex, J. Invest. Dermat., 1:267, 1938.

Gerstenberger, H. J.: Etiology and treatment of herpetic (aphthous and aphtho-ulcerative) stomatitis and herpes labialis, Am. J. Dis. Child., 26:309, 1923.

Goeckerman, W. H., & L. F. X. Wilhelm: Herpes zoster and herpes simplex: report of case in which both appeared simultaneously; analysis of their etiology, Arch. Dermat. & Syph., 35:868, 1937.

Greenfield, Lt. H.: Labial sunburn in the tropics, Mil. Surgeon, 96:355, 1945.

Hall, W. C.: Radiation treatment of herpes simplex, Am. J. Roentgenol., 39:393, 1938.

Hastings, H.: Herpes zoster oticus, with report of 2 cases, Ann. Otol., Rhin. & Laryng., 44:899, 1935.

Hill, F. T.: Herpes zoster oticus: report of 3 cases, Ann. Otol., Rhin. & Laryng., 45:666, 1936.

Holt, L. E.: Diseases of Infancy and Childhood, New York: Macmillan Company, 1922.

Hudson, N. P., E. A. Cook, & F. L. Adair: Relation of herpes antiviral property of human blood to sex, pregnancy and menstruation, J. Infect. Dis., 59:60, 1936.

Kampf, M. B.: Herpes gestationis, Arch. Dermat. & Syph., 42:982, 1940.

Kelly, R. J.: Treatment of herpes simplex with moccasin venom, Arch. Dermat. & Syph., 38:599, 1938.

Lane, J. L., & P. P. Vinson: Sulfanilamide in treatment of aphthous stomatitis, Virginia M. Monthly, 66:528, 1939.

Leonard, Pohl: Aufreten von herpes simplex au der Wangerschleimhaut und lippe im anschluss au eine Mandibularisinjektion, Zeitschrift für Stomatologie, 25:763, 1927.

Levaditi, C., P. Harvier, & S. Nicolau: Experimental study on encephalitis, Ann. de l'Inst. Pasteur, 36:63, 1922.

Levine, H. D., S. O. Hoerr, & J. C. Allanson: Vesicular pharyngitis and stomatitis; unusual epidemic of possible herpetic origin, J. A. M. A., 112:2020, 1939.

Lewis, G. M.: Herpes gestationis—successful treatment with sulfathiazole, Arch. Dermat. & Syph., 46:841, 1942.

McCombs, P., A. Tuggle, & C. M. Guion: Roentgen-ray therapy in treatment of herpes zoster, Am. J. M. Sc., 200:803, 1940.

McDowell, M. M.: The use of cobra venom for the relief of pain in herpes zoster, Med. Rec., 153:173, 1941.

Nagler, F. P. O.: Specific cutaneous reaction in persons infected with virus of herpes simplex, J. Immunol., 48:213, 1944.

Negus, V. E., & N. C. Crabtree: Herpes zoster of the seventh, ninth and tenth cranial nerves, J. Laryng. & Otol., 58:192, 1943.

Neve, C. T.: Paralysis of the facial nerve with herpes zoster, Dental Cosmos, 65:221, 1923.

Nicolau, S., & L. Kopciowska: La morphologie de l'inframicrobe herpetique, dans le tissu des animaux infectes experimentalement et le mecanisms de la formation des inclusions qu'il engendre dans les cellules, Ann. de l'Inst. Pasteur, 60:401, 1938.

Rosenberger, H. C.: Herpes zoster with facial paralysis and acoustic symptoms, Ann. Otol. Rhin. & Laryng., 50:271, 1941.

Schmidt, F. R.: Vaccination for herpes, Arch. Dermat. & Syph., 32:106, 1935.

Scott, McT. F.: Herpetic stomatitis in infants and children, Proc. Royal Soc. Med., 37:310, 1944.

Smith, S. F.: Regional injection of thiamine chloride in herpes zoster, J. M. Soc. New Jersey, 38:396, 1941.

Templeton, H. J.: Is aphthous stomatitis due to virus of herpes simplex?, Arch. Dermat. & Syph., 14:439, 1926.

Thomas, C. C.: Herpes simplex, Arch. Dermat. & Syph., 43:817, 1941.

Van Rooyen, C. E., A. J. Rhodes, & A. C. Ewing: Herpes labialis after sulphapyridine and T.A.B. therapy, Brit. M. J., 2:298, 1941.

Vitamins in Prevention of Pellagra, foreign letters (Paris), J. A. M. A., 112:2075, 1939.

Wagener, K.: Pathogenicity of vesicular stomatitis virus, Cornell Vet., 21:344, 1931.

Weinberger, W.: Herpes zoster nach Zahnextraktion, Ztschr. f. Stomatol., 31:1441, 1933.

Woodburne, A. R.: Herpetic stomatitis, Arch. Dermat. & Syph., 43:543, 1941.

Weisberger, D.: Lesions of the oral mucosa treated with specific vitamins, Am. J. Orthodontics & Oral Surg., 27:125, 1941.

Youmans, J. B.: Herpetic fever with stomatitis; report and discussion of case in which virus was isolated, South. M. J., 25:228, 1932.

Zahorsky, J.: Herpetic sore throat, South. M. J., 13:871, 1920.

Ziskin, D. E., & Margaret Holden: Acute herpetic gingivostomatitis, J. A. D. A., 30:1697, 1943.

Minor Dermatoses

Abramowitz, E. W.: Oral lesions on hard palate and gums of Darier's disease, Arch. Dermat. & Syph., 45:976, 1942.

Ageloff, H.: Erythema multiforme bullosum with involvement of the mucous membranes of the eyes and mouth, New England J. Med., 223:217, 1940.

Anderson, N. P.: Lichen planus of the gums, Arch. Dermat. & Syph., 49:84, 1944.

Artom, M.: Progressive facial hemiatrophy in a case of scleroderma, Arch. ital. di. dermat., sif., 13:458, 1937.

Ayres, S., Jr., & W. D. Anderson: Focal infection in dermatology, Arch. Dermat. & Syph., 34:421, 1936.

Barock, J. J., et al.: Lichen planus of the oral mucosa, Urol. & Cutan. Rev., 46:187, 1942.

Barber, H. W.: Circumscribed scleroderma of the buccal mucosa, Proc. Roy. Soc. Med., 37:73, 1944.

Barber, H. W.: Pustular psoriosis of the extremities, Guy's Hosp. Rep., 86:108, 1936.

Barcoglia, A.: Hemilateral scleroderma with hemiatrophy and vitiligo in a boy 4 years of age, Pediatria, 45:533, 1937.

Beerman, H., & J. H. Stokes: Rosaceae complex and demodex folliculorum, Arch. Dermat. & Syph., 29:874, 1934.

Bernard, F. J.: Acrodynia; report of case, J. A. D. A., 24:1858-60, 1937.

Burch, G. E.: Pathology and symposium. Etiology and abnormal physiology of scleroderma, New Orleans M. & S. J., 92:6, 1940.

Butler, J.: Erythema multiforme confined to mucous membranes, Arch. Dermat. & Syph., 6:1, 1922.

Cannon, A. Benson: Dermatologic diseases frequently encountered by oto-laryngologists, N. Y. State J. Med., 44:1661, 1944.

Carr, M. W.: Pemphigus; clinico-pathological study, Ann. Dent., 4:129-48, 1937.

Case report: Lichen planus of the gums, Ann. Dent., 2:158, 1944.

Chambers, S. O.: Structure of Fordyce's disease as demonstrated by wax reconstruction, Arch. Dermat. & Syph., 18:666-72, 1928.

Chick, F. E., & C. M. Witzberger: Erythema multiforme exudativum accompanying oral Vincent's infection, Am. J. Dis. Child., 35:572, 1938.

Chipman, E. D.: Etiology of lichen planus, J. A. M. A., 71:1276, 1918.

Clements, F. W.: Pink disease: consideration of 3 aetiological possibilities, M. J. Australia, 2:430-32, 1940.

Crawford, S.: Cicatrizing morphea with ankylosing arthritis and osteoblastic change, Arch. Dermat. & Syph., 33:506, 1936.

Crawford, S.: Juvenile acrodynia; report of 11 cases, Arch. Dermat. & Syph., 26:215-37, 1932.

Culver, G. D.: Lupus erythematosus of the mucous membrane, J. A. M. A., 65:773, 1915.

Denzer, B. S., & S. Blumenthal: Acute lupus erythematosus disseminatus, Am. J. Dis. Child., 53:525, 1937.

Dlugasz, Henryk: Foot and mouth disease in man, Brit. M. J., 189:1943.

Durand, J. I., V. W. Spickard, & E. Burgess: Acrodynia treated with intra-muscular injections of vitamin B_1, J. Pediat., 14:74-78, 1939.

Ellis, F. A.: Reactions to nirvanol, phenytoin sodium and phenobarbital: report of a case of ectodermosis erosiva pluriorificialis following ingestion of phenytoin sodium, South. M. J., 36:575, 1943.

Erger, Benjamin D.: Erythema multiforme pluriorificialis, Mil. Surgeon, 95:308, 1944.

Exchaquet, L.: Un cas d'acrodynie avec perte des dents et ostéomyelite du maxillaire, Rev. méd. de la Suisse Rom., 50:543-46, 1930.

Feit, H., et al.: Rosacea interpreted as a bacterid from focal infection, J. A. M. A., 105:1738, 1935.

Fox, Howard: Lichen planus confined to mouth, Arch. Dermat. & Syph., 24:1071, 1931.

Fordyce, J. A.: A peculiar affection of the mucous membrane of the lip and oral cavity, J. Cutan. & Genito-Urinary Dis., 14:413-20, 1896.

Gahan, E.: Lupus erythematosus clinical observations in 443 cases, Arch. Dermat. & Syph., 46:685, 1942.

Gareau, U. J.: Acrodynia, Canad. M. A. J., 46:51-54, 1942.

Garfield, W. T., et al.: Lupus erythematosus disseminatus acutus haemor-rhagicus, Arch. Dermat. & Syph., 30:772, 1934.

Ginandes, G. J.: Eruptive fever with stomatitis and ophthalmia; atypical erythema exudativum multiforme, Am. J. Dis. Child., 49:1148, 1935.

Goldstein, Hyman I.: Chase-Lain-Goldstein syndrome—galvanic batteries in the human mouth, Rev. Gastroenterol., 10:206, 1943.

Greenbaum, Sigmund S.: Oral lesions in pityriasis rosea, Arch. Dermat. & Syph., 44:55, 1941.

Guequierre, J. P., & C. S. Wright: Pityriasis rosea with lesions on mucous membranes, Arch. Dermat. & Syph., 43:1000, 1941.

Hartley, L. P., & Chas. F. Nelson: Erythema multiforme pluriofacialis, Army Dent. Bull., 14:119, 1943.

Hartzell, M. B.: Lupus erythematosus and focal infection, Arch. Dermat. & Syph., 2:441, 1920.

Hay, J. Duncan: Pink's disease treated by intramuscular B₁—report of eight cases, Practitioner, 146:264, 1941.

Herz, L. F.: Acrodynia, its symptoms and possible causes: with review of literature, Urol. & Cutan. Rev., 44:388-94, 1940.

Hollander, Lester: Galvanic burns of the oral mucosa, J. A. M. A., 99:383, 1932.

Howles, J. K.: Scleroderma. The dermatologic aspects, New Orleans M. & S. J., 92:6, 1939.

Hunter, F. T.: Hutchinson-Boeck's disease—historical note and report of case with apparent cure, New England J. Med., 214:346, 1936.

Immenkamp, A.: Clinical and pathological picture of lupus of the oral mucosa with special consideration of lupus of the gums, Deutsche Zahnartzl. Wchnschr., 39:377, 1936.

Kight, H. M.: Acrodynia (oral manifestation), J. Periodontology, 7:52-54, 1936.

Lever, W. F.: Severe erythema multiforme: report of two cases of the type ectodermosis erosiva pluriorificialis, with development of cicatricial conjunctivitis and keratitis in one case, Arch. Dermat. & Syph., 49:47, 1944.

Looby, J. P., & L. W. Burket: Scleroderma of the face with involvement of the alveolar process, Am. J. Orthodontics & Oral Surg., 28:493, 1942.

Margolies, A., & F. Weidman: Statistical and histologic studies of Fordyce's disease, Arch. Dermat. & Syph., 3:723, 1921.

McEwen, E. L.: Erythema multiforme; report of case with necropsy findings and deductions, Arch. Dermat. & Syph., 13:331, 1926.

Merle-Beral, J.: Contribution à l'étude du lupus primitif des gencines, La Semaine, Dentaire, 16:861-72, 1934.

Michelson, H. E.: Uveo-parotitis; sarcoid reaction, Arch. Dermat. & Syph., 39:329, 1939.

Monash, Samuel: Oral lesions of lupus erythematosus, Dental Cosmos, 73:511, 1931.

Montgomery, D. W.: Lichen planus of the lips, Arch. Dermat. & Syph., 38:401, 1938.

Montgomery, D. W., & G. D. Culver: Lichen planus in two brothers, J. Cutan. Dis., 37:242, 1919.

Morrison, J. P.: A case of Vincent's infection associated with erythema multiforme, J. A. D. A., 28:1938, 1941.

Murphy, R. C.: An eruptive fever involving the mouth and eyes, New England J. Med., 230:69, 1944.

New York Inst. of Clin. Oral Pathology: Case history of pemphigus vegetans, Arch. Clin. Oral Path., 2:65, 1938.

O'Leary, P. A.: A clinical study of 103 cases of scleroderma, Am. J. M. Sc., 180:95, 1930.

Reinhard, M. C., & H. A. Soloman: Electric currents from dental materials as etiologic factor in oral cancer, Am. J. Cancer, 22:606, 1932.

Ruppe, C., L. LeBourg, & J. Guerin: L'osteo-thorio-nécrose tardive des maxillaires, Rev. de stomatol., 37:456-65, 1935.

Sagall, B.: Pemphigus, Am. J. Orthodontics & Oral Surg., 22:1271, 1936.

Schroff, Joseph: Oral manifestations of skin disease, J. Dent. Research, 10:219, 1930.

Smith, R. C., E. A. Meyers, & H. D. Lamb: Ocular and oral pemphigus; report of case with anatomic findings in eyeball, Arch. Ophth., 11:635, 1934.

Smith, T.: Mucous membrane lesions in lupus erythematosus, Brit. J. Dermat., 18:59, 1906.

Soicher, Irving: Ulcer of the lip following local anesthesia, J. A. D. A., 31:368, 1944.

Spence, J. C.: Child with Pink's disease who chewed his tongue off, Newcastle M. J., 12:39, 1932.

Stafne, E. C., & L. T. Austin: A characteristic dental finding in acrosclerosis and diffuse scleroderma, Am. J. Orthodontics & Oral Surg., 30:25, 1944.

Stevens, A. M., & F. C. Johnson: Eruptive fever with stomatitis, conjunctivitis, etc., Am. J. Dis. Child., 24:526, 1922.

Stokes, J. H., & H. Beerman: Effect on the skin of emotional and nervous states, Arch. Dermat. & Syph., 26:478, 1932.

Templeton, H. J.: Localized scleroderma with bullae, Arch. Dermat. & Syph., 43:360, 1941.

Thompson, W. C.: Uveoparotitis—6 cases in negresses, Arch. Int. Med., 59:646, 1937.

Townend, B. R.: Pink's disease—Report of case in which extensive exfoliation of deciduous and permanent teeth occurred, Brit. Dent. J., 58:514, 1940.

Wagener, K.: Die Maul- und Klauenseuche als medisinisches problem, Med. Klin., 34:173, 1938.

White, C. J.: Fordyce's disease, J. Cutan. Disease, 23:97, 1905.

Zakon, S. J., M. Dorne, & E. A. Skolnik: Pemphigus of the mouth improving with acetarsone therapy, Arch. Dermat. Syph., 48:457, 1943.

GINGIVITIS

Ball, E. I.: Case of gingivoma or elephantiasis of the gingiva, J. Periodont., 12:96, 1941.

Blakenhorn, M. A., & C. E. Richards: Garlic breath odor, J. A. M. A., 107:409, 1936.

Brening, Robt. H.: The determination of halitosis by use of the osmoscope and the cryoscopic method, J. Dent. Research, 18:127, 1939.

Buchner, H. J.: Diffuse fibroma of the gums, J. A. D. A., 24:2003, 1937.

Coolidge, E. D.: Hypertrophic gingivitis, J. A. D. A., 28:1381, 1941.

Glickman, I., & B. G. Bibby: Effect of sodium perborate upon the gingival mucosa: A controlled experiment, J. A. D. A., 31:1201, 1944.

Haggard, M. A., & L. A. Greenberg: Breath odors from alliaceous substance, J. A. M. A., 104:2160, 1935.

Haley, P. S.: Treatment of paradentosis and hypertrophic gingivitis by the use of acetone, J. A. D. A., 27:511, 1940.

Henry, T. C.: Atypical ulcer-membranous stomatitis, Brit. M. J., 2:273, 1942.

Langille, J. A.: Acute membranous stomatitis and conjunctivitis (report of 3 cases), Canadian Med. A. J., 50:141, 1944.

MacDonald, A. C.: Bleeding gums and gingivitis in naval ratings, Lancet, 245:697, 1943.

Miralli, A.: Familial elephantiasis of the gingivae, Arch. ital. chir., 29:401, 1931.

Mumford, P. B., & A. G. Heppleston: An epidemic in children characterized by diversity of lesions in skin and mucous membranes, probably caused by streptococcus pyogenes, Brit. J. Dermat. & Syph., 55:143, 1943.

Murphy, Albert B.: A pharyngeal syndrome probably of virus origin, Ann. Otol. Rhinol. & Laryng., 52:391, 1943.

Newby, C. D.: Hypertrophied gingival tissues, J. Canad. Dent. A., 6:183, 1940.

Orban, B.: Discussion of the "case of gingivoma or elephantiasis of the gingiva," J. Periodont., 12:100, 1941.

Ruggles, S. D.: Primary hypertrophy of the gums, J. A. M. A., 84:20, 1925.

Rushton, M. A.: A case of general hyperplasia of the gums, J. Brit. Dent. A., 70:338, 1941.

Schnee, I. M., Membranous inflammation of the oropharynx, nose and conjunctiva due to sulfathiazole administration, Brit. M. J., 24:506, 1943.

Shane, S. J.: Oropharyngeal ulceration with conjunctivitis and skin lesions, Canad. M. A. J. (Montreal), 49:309-10, 1943.

Smith, W. J.: A hemolytic streptococcal stomatitis, Brit. Dent. J., 73:234, 1942.

Stenstrom, T.: Die Klinik der Maul- und Klauenseuche beim menschen im Lichte der Jüngsten Forschung (experimental foot-and-mouth infection in humans), Acta. med. Scandinav., 107:372, 1941.

Stern, Leo., Leon Eisenbud, & K. Klatell: Analysis of oral reactions to dilantin-sodium, J. Dent. Research, 22:157, 1943.

Strock, A. E.: Relationship between gingivitis and penicillin administration, J. A. D. A., 31:1235, 1944.

Tempestini, O.: Gingivite ipertrofica da disormonismo sintona patologico di puberta, Stomatol., 30:723, 1932.

Walton, C. H. A., A. M. Graham, & L. P. Lansdown: Acute ulcerative stomatitis, 3 unusual cases, Lancet, 2:214-16, 1941.

Ziskin, D. E., & Edw. Zegarelli: Idiopathic fibromatosis of the gingivae, Ann. Dent., 2:50-55, 1943.

11

The Respiratory System

THE COMMON COLD	ASTHMA
OZENA	LUNG ABSCESS
SINUSITIS	PULMONARY FOREIGN BODIES
OTITIS MEDIA AND MASTOIDITIS	PNEUMONIA
TONSILLITIS	VIRUS PNEUMONIAS
PERITONSILLAR ABSCESS	INFLUENZA
LARYNGITIS	PLEURISY
HICCOUGH	EMPYEMA
BRONCHITIS	ACUTE PULMONARY EDEMA
FUSOSPIROCHETAL TRACHEOBRON-	SILICOSIS
CHITIS	

THE COMMON COLD (ACUTE RHINITIS-CORYZA)

The common cold is an acute catarrhal inflammation of the upper respiratory passages. While usually not serious, it is an important disease because of its almost universal prevalence and because it predisposes to more serious respiratory infections. It has great economic importance when one considers the total man days lost due to this illness.

The cause of the common cold remains one of the future conquests of medicine. A virus is thought to be the etiologic agent. Fatigue, wet feet, overheated rooms, rapid and unequal changes of temperature, anatomic abnormalities of the nasal passages as well as poor ventilation are important predisposing factors.

The initial symptoms of the common cold consist of dryness or tickling in the nose and throat, sneezing, and a feeling of chilliness, then the characteristic mucopurulent nasal discharge develops. Herpetic eruptions of the lips are common. Malaise, fever and gastro-intestinal symptoms of varying severity may accompany the above symptoms. The nasal discharge gradually becomes less copious and heavier as the constitutional symptoms disappear. The average cold lasts 5 to 7 days. The individual with a severe cold rarely considers the possibility of passing his infection to others, either unavoidably or by means of indiscriminate sneezing or coughing in crowded places.

The treatment of the common cold is mainly preventive and symptomatic. Bed rest is desirable in the acute stage. Fluids should be given in large quantities and the diet should be easily digested and rich in vitamins. The intranasal use of vasoconstrictor agents will lessen the probability of sinus involvement. Aspirin gr. X q. 3 hrs. is thought to be beneficial by some. The prophylactic use of cold vaccines (not the oral variety) and supplemental poly-vitamin therapy during the cold months are of value in some cases.

Oral Aspects

A catarrhal stomatitis and gingivitis frequently accompany an upper respiratory infection. The oral tissues may feel hot, be painful and appear hyperemic and edematous. Like other forms of catarrhal stomatitis, these symptoms require no specific treatment.

An upper respiratory infection interferes seriously with a dentist's professional duties. He should not operate on patients during the acute stage of the infection unless an appropriate mask is worn. Even then some patients think they are being exposed unnecessarily. While a dentist can hardly refuse to work on a patient who has a cold, he can tactfully suggest that the dental work be done at a later date. A considerate dentist or patient will not run the risk of giving the other a cold.

OZENA

Ozena is an atrophic condition of the nasal tissues which is frequently accompanied by necrosis of the bone. Bacterial putrefaction of the nasal secretions and the necrotic bone produce a foul odor. Ozena must be differentiated from *fetor ex ore*.

SINUSITIS

Sinusitis is an acute inflammation of the mucosa of the nasal accessory sinuses. It is often a complication of an upper respiratory infection. The maxillary sinus is most frequently involved.

Symptoms

In acute sinusitis there are headache, severe pain localized in the region of the involved sinus, an elevation of temperature and malaise. Edema and redness of the malar eminence and beneath the eyes are common objective signs of maxillary sinusitis. The location of the swelling and the referred pain in the teeth may cause the patient to seek dental treatment. A common symptom of chronic sinusitis is the morning headache which disappears gradually during the day due to better drainage of the sinuses in the upright position. A post-pharyngeal discharge is an annoying symptom.

Diagnosis

The diagnosis of maxillary sinusitis is made on the basis of the history, the physical and x-ray findings and transillumination. Firm pressure over the region of the sinus may give rise to severe pain. The percussion note of an infected maxillary sinus is dull as compared with the more resonant note of an aerated sinus. While a suggestion of sinus involvement can be obtained from the regular intraoral dental films, occlusal films or better AP plates are required to make the diagnosis. Transillumination which can be performed in the dental office will give valuable information.

The treatment of maxillary sinusitis is in the province of the otolaryngologist. If free drainage of the infected sinus is not established through normal or artificial channels, necrosis of the bony walls of the sinus will occur which may result in septicemia, meningitis and often death depending on the sinus involved. Modern methods of sinus treatment do not require or sanction the removal of a tooth to establish drainage.

Oral Aspects

The roots of the upper premolars and molars and the nerves supplying these structures are in close proximity to the maxillary sinus, many times being separated only by the sinus mucosa. This relationship explains the dental symptoms which are associated frequently with sinus disease.

Alveolar dental abscesses of the premolars and molars open occasionally into the maxillary sinus and produce a sinusitis. Some clinicians believe that infected teeth are only the cause of maxillary sinus infection when a granuloma of an upper molar or premolar involves the floor of the overlying antrum. It is difficult by means of bacteriologic studies to prove an etiologic relation between periapical dental infection and maxillary sinusitis.

Maxillary sinusitis is more frequently the cause of dental symptoms. The teeth in close anatomic relationship to the sinus ache. They feel elongated and they are frequently sensitive to percussion. Pain in the upper premolars and molars which is unaccounted for by local lesions may be due to a maxillary sinusitis. Apparently healthy teeth should not be removed until the patient has been examined for sinus infection.

A root fragment is forced occasionally during extraction into the maxillary sinus. When this occurs, the patient should be informed of the complication. If the operator has not had experience with similar cases, it is best to refer the patient to a competent oral surgeon or otolaryngologist for removal of the root fragment.

Following the removal of a tooth near the maxillary sinus, normal healing of the socket fails occasionally to take place. A polypoid mass of friable, often bleeding tissue fills the alveolus and extends into the mouth. If the extraction has been complete, the dentist should suspect the existence of a polyp or possibly a new growth in the sinus. The patient should be referred to an oral surgeon or otolaryngologist.

Dental root cysts of the upper premolars and molars may encroach on the sinus and almost obliterate this structure. When infected, these cysts are at times diagnosed incorrectly and treated (unsuccessfully) as acute sinus infections. Special x-ray studies will permit a correct diagnosis and successful treatment.

Furuncles of the external auditory canal, particularly those on the anterior wall, may give rise to painful symptoms during chewing which are referred to the region of the temporomandibular joint. The differentiation of these furuncles of the external auditory canal from lesions of the temporomandibular joint proper are discussed under the latter disease.

OTITIS MEDIA AND MASTOIDITIS

Infections of the middle ear, otitis media, and of the mastoid air cells, mastoiditis, are common in childhood. They occur frequently in association with acute tonsillitis, scarlet fever, measles, influenza, mumps and upper respiratory infections. A marked irritability and an unexplained temperature rise in children may be the first evidence of an otitis media. Severe pain, fever and at times nausea and vomiting are present. Otoscopic examination of the ear drum establishes the diagnosis. It may be necessary to incise the ear drum (myringotomy) to obtain adequate drainage. Otitis media must be differentiated from a furuncle of the external auditory meatus.

Middle ear infections may extend to the mastoid air cells. Symptoms of mastoiditis include those present in otitis media plus tenderness on pressure over the mastoid process. X-ray studies of the mastoid air cells aid in making a diagnosis. Before the advent of the sulfonamides, mastoiditis was a common surgical emergency in children but now many of these cases are successfully treated without surgery by chemotherapy.

In long standing cases of otitis media or mastoiditis permanent facial paralysis may develop as a result of damage to the facial nerve.

TONSILLITIS

Inflammations of the various collections of lymphoid tissue in the throat and pharynx are common, particularly in childhood. The faucial tonsils are most frequently involved, then the pharyngeal tonsils (adenoids) and lastly the lingual lymphoid tissue.

The importance of tonsillar infections may have been overemphasized in the past. Certainly mankind has not been correspondingly bettered in proportion to the number of tonsils that have been removed. It is well known that tonsillar infections may be an important foci of infection. The relationship of tonsillar infections to rheumatic heart disease will be discussed under this disease.

Acute follicular tonsillitis in children or young adults has all the characteristics of an acute infection. In addition to the local symptoms of swelling, pain and dysphagia, there are headache, chilly sensations and general muscular aches. Marked swelling of the cervical lymph nodes is usually present. There are fever, a rapid pulse and leukocytosis. Acute follicular tonsillitis is usually due to a streptococcal infection. The acute symptoms regress in 3 to

5 days under suitable nursing care and chemotherapy; or otitis media, acute nephritis, arthritis or peritonsillar abscess may follow. The treatment of tonsillitis is in the province of the otolaryngologist.

Oral Aspects

Chronic tonsillar infection may be an important focus for recurrent stomatitis and fusospirochetal infection of the mouth. Similarly, poor oral hygiene may serve as a focus for chronic tonsillitis. Tonsillar infections due to the fusospirochetal organisms (Vincent's angina) will be discussed under fusospirochetal disease.

PERITONSILLAR ABSCESS (QUINSY)

Peritonsillar abscess, or quinsy, is usually a complication of acute tonsillitis. In peritonsillar abscess there is a marked systemic reaction with extreme pain, dysphagia and a high leukocytosis. This condition is serious, as there is always the possibility of extension of the infection to the deeper structures of the neck, erosion of a large artery or the spontaneous rupture of the abscess during sleep with aspiration of the infected material. The abscess is usually incised under local anesthesia as soon as definite fluctuation is noted. Recurrences are not uncommon.

LARYNGITIS

Acute

Acute laryngitis results usually from abnormal use of the vocal cords (cheering, public speaking), irritation due to excessive smoking, drinking of alcoholic beverages or the extension of an inflammatory process from the nose and throat. The condition is far less serious than the marked symptoms would indicate. With rest of the voice it usually clears up in a few days.

Chronic

Chronic laryngitis is frequently secondary to chronic sinusitis or periodontal infection. Treatment should be directed to the elimination of these foci. Persistent hoarseness is at times the first manifestation of a more serious disease. The dentist may be the first to notice a gradually developing hoarseness as he has the opportunity of seeing and hearing his patients periodically. Serious causes of chronic laryngitis include tuberculosis or syphilis (secondary or tertiary), carcinoma of the larynx and, more rarely, hoarseness resulting from pressure on the recurrent laryngeal nerve due to aortic aneurysm or intrathoracic tumor.

A slowly developing hoarseness may precede by many months the more typical symptoms of these diseases. In tuberculous laryngitis the patient usually experiences acute pain and dysphagia. Carcinoma of the larynx should always be considered in cases of persistent hoarseness in individuals of the "cancer age." The dentist should refer these patients to a competent otolaryngologist for examination. Should any surgery be necessary, strict attention should be given the oral hygiene prior to the operation.

HICCOUGH

Hiccoughs are caused by spasmodic contractions of the diaphragm, as a rule due to some form of vagal irritation. They occur frequently following rapid eating. Epidemics of hiccoughs have been reported in which the etiologic agent was thought to be a virus. The transitory hiccoughs are of little significance, but continuous hiccoughs for several hours or days are a serious problem. Reed reported a case of hiccoughs of a week's duration which was cured following the removal of infected teeth.

The common methods of treatment aim to increase the CO_2 content of the blood, thereby producing a more normal respiratory stimulus. A simple method is to have the patient breathe into a paper bag for several minutes. A more effective method consists of placing a 4-inch square piece of dry ice in 2 oz. of water in a #10 paper bag and instructing the patient to breathe the gases in the bag for several minutes. General anesthesia may be helpful in controlling severe attacks.

BRONCHITIS—BRONCHIECTASIS

Bronchitis is an inflammation of the mucosa lining the bronchi. Acute bronchitis is associated frequently with an upper respiratory infection. Chronic bronchitis is common in damp moist climates where it is often secondary to some chronic infection of the upper respiratory tract. Bronchiectasis is a localized saccular dilation of the smaller bronchi which occurs usually in the lower lobes of the lungs. It may be congenital or secondary to other respiratory diseases such as influenza or chronic bronchitis. Poor oral hygiene serves as a focus for recurrent attacks of bronchitis and bronchiectasis.

FUSOSPIROCHETAL TRACHEOBRONCHITIS

Secondary infection of suppurative pulmonary lesions with the fusospirochetal organisms is not unusual in patients with poor oral hygiene. The clinical symptoms simulate those observed in pulmonary tuberculosis with chronic cough, night sweats and occasionally hemoptysis. The breath odor of patients with fusospirochetal tracheobronchitis is similar to that found in acute oral fusospirochetal infections.

While the usual oral fusospirochetal forms are generally considered to be saprophytes, they may assume a pathogenic role especially when associated with suppurative processes in which necrosis is present. In both monkeys and man a suppurative tracheobronchitis can be experimentally produced by the intratracheal inoculation of material scraped from the gums and teeth of patients having pyorrhea or fusospirochetal stomatitis. Moreover, the fusospirochetal organisms are present in such numbers in these lesions that they must be considered as being of etiologic significance. Evidence of this nature tends to substantiate the belief that fusospirochetal infections of the oral cavity are infectious and can be contagious.

Holinger and Rigby treated this form of tracheobronchitis by the administration of small doses of arsenicals, the administration of vitamin C, the use of autogenous vaccines and at times the bronchoscopic aspiration of collected material.

Oral Aspects

The establishment and the maintenance of good oral hygiene will go far to prevent the development of fusospirochetal infection of suppurative pulmonary lesions. The general treatment of this disease, once it has developed, should always be preceded by the necessary oral treatment to minimize the chances of a recurrence of the infection.

ASTHMA (BRONCHIAL ASTHMA)

Asthma is considered to represent an allergic response which is characterized by a spasmodic contraction of the smooth muscles of the bronchi. This may result from contact with certain foods, pollens, dusts, animal emanations, bacterial toxins or unknown causes. Asthma is usually a progressive disease which becomes more severe with age.

The symptoms of asthma are those associated with deficient pulmonary ventilation. The greatest difficulty is encountered in the expiratory phase of respiration. Death occurs occasionally during an acute asthmatic attack. Secondary cardiac changes follow asthma of long duration.

In certain geographic areas, bacterial allergy is considered to be an important cause of asthma. If the asthma is believed due to bacterial allergy, oral foci of infection in the periodontal and periapical tissues should receive serious consideration. (See Chapter 7.)

LUNG ABSCESS

A lung abscess is a localized area of suppuration and necrosis of the parenchymal tissue. They are the sequellae of acute bronchitis, bronchiectasis, the aspiration of infected material during anesthesia or pyogenic infections of tuberculous cavities. Pulmonary abscesses due to the fusospirochetal organisms produce a particularly foul lesion. Foreign bodies in the lung such as buttons, peanuts, or tooth fragments also cause lung abscesses.

The symptoms of lung abscess include an irregular fever, expectoration of large quantities of putrid sputum, a progressive weight loss and at times amyloidosis. The diagnosis is made on the basis of the past history, the physical findings and x-ray studies.

Stern believed that the aspiration of infected material from tartar encrusted teeth and purulent gums during sleep is a likely explanation for the lung abscesses of "unknown etiology." The extremely poor oral hygiene presented by these patients could not be accounted for on the basis of age, sex, illness or social status. The incidence of oral sepsis in the "unknown etiology group" was 7 times greater than that in the "posttonsillectomy" group. In another study Stern found that 12 of 70 consecutive and unselected patients with pulmonary abscess gave histories strongly suggestive of causes traceable to dental operations. Abscesses may occur without the aspiration of pieces of the filling or tooth.

Oral Aspects

Good oral hygiene is an important prophylactic against lung abscesses. It is also of definite value in preventing pyogenic infections of tuberculous cavities or recurrent attacks of bronchitis or bronchiectasis. In fusospirochetal abscesses of the lungs it is believed that the organisms come originally from the oral cavity as they both have similar morphologic characteristics. The unsuspected aspiration of a tooth or tooth fragment during extraction or the aspiration of a small dental instrument have been known to produce lung abscesses.

PULMONARY FOREIGN BODIES

Foreign bodies occluding or obstructing a main respiratory passage will produce marked symptoms of cyanosis and asphyxia. Sudden and violent attacks of coughing, accompanied by shortness of breath and chest pain are classical symptoms of a foreign body in the lungs. These symptoms are particularly significant if they follow dental extractions or operations. Small foreign bodies at times produce few if any symptoms and they may be discovered accidentally during chest radiography or following the development of a lung abscess.

Oral Aspects

Most of the cases of dental foreign bodies result from operations performed under general anesthesia where no, or inadequate, throat packs are used. Occasionally a tooth or filling fragments find their way into the respiratory passages during extraction under local anesthesia. The proper functioning of the pharyngeal reflexes will assist in preventing such accidents and for this reason bilateral mandibular injections should not be given at the same sitting.

Root canal therapy without the rubber dam is to be condemned both in respect to the root canal technic and the risk of the aspiration or swallowing of a small root canal instrument. Inlays, crowns, pieces of amalgam or inlay wax are all potential foreign bodies. When one considers the great number and variety of dental operations performed without the rubber dam, it is to the credit of the dentist's technic and the patient's quick pharyngeal reflexes that more accidents of this nature do not occur. The risk of respiratory tract foreign bodies can be almost entirely eliminated by the use of the rubber dam and proper throat packs.

While many individuals customarily sleep with their dentures in place, this practice is not without danger. Small partial dentures or removable appliances should be removed from the mouth before retiring. Because of their small size these appliances are more easily swallowed or aspirated than full dentures and in addition the numerous clasps which they contain make removal difficult if they should become lodged in the air passages.

PNEUMONIA

Pneumonia is an inflammation of the lung parenchyma. The pneumococcus is the most frequent bacterial cause of pneumonia although the staphylococcus, the streptococcus, Friedländers bacillus, and viruses also cause pneumonia.

Pneumococcal pneumonia occurs at all ages. The mortality of the disease, particularly in the aged, has been reduced markedly by the use of penicillin therapy and the "sulfa" drugs. At least 35 different strains of pneumococci are known to produce the disease. Pneumococcal pneumonia may follow an upper respiratory infection, influenza, chilling or exposure to cold, fatigue or anything which lowers the body resistance. It occurs most frequently in the male.

The typical attack of pneumonia is ushered in by a stabbing knife-like pain in the chest, a chill, shortness of breath, fever (often to 104° F.), and the characteristic blood-streaked or "rusty" sputum. There is a marked increase in the respiratory rate which may increase until it bears a 1:2 ratio to the pulse. Varying degrees of cyanosis are common and characteristic. The physical signs are those associated with consolidation of the lung tissue.

One of the characteristics of pneumococcal pneumonia is the resolution by crisis which occurs as a rule within 5 to 7 days after the onset of the disease. Within a few hours the ausculatory signs of consolidation disappear, the temperature drops to normal and the physical appearance and mental activity of the patient change dramatically.

Diagnosis

Pneumonia is diagnosed by means of the history, the physical findings, x-ray and bacteriologic studies. The type of pneumococcus is determined usually by serologic studies of the organisms obtained from the sputum or pharynx. Rapid methods of pneumococcal typing are now available. The treatment of the disease is in the province of the physician. Chemotherapy and specific serum therapy have resulted in a marked lowering of the mortality and a reduction of the complications.

Oral Aspects

Pneumococcal infections of the oral mucosa and the tongue have been reported in the absence of pulmonary involvement. These conditions occur mostly in children and debilitated adults. Constitutional symptoms of fever, vomiting, anorexia and dehydration are present. The oral mucosa is covered with small silver flecks which resemble the lesions of moniliasis. These flecks, which are present on the buccal mucosa, the anterior portion of the palate and beneath the tongue, are actually colonies of pneumococci. Engman and Weiss described a pneumococcal infection of the tongue which was characterized by pain, soreness and burning sensation with fiery red, raised circinate patches covering the entire surface of this organ. Grayish white spots were also seen on the cheeks and the hard palate.

Pneumococcal infections of the oral mucosa are diagnosed by means of bacteriologic smears and cultures and the characteristic flecks on the mucosa. The lesions must be differentiated from thrush, diphtheria and fusospirochetal infection. Treatment consists of the local application of sulfapyridine or the use of penicillin lozenges.

The author observed a common and characteristic change within the dental pulp of patients succumbing to pneumonia. There were numerous areas of hemorrhage in the odontoblastic layer with localized areas of atrophy and destruction of this tissue. Hemorrhages were also common throughout the pulp. The histopathologic changes were similar to those seen in vitamin C deficiency. It is possible the dental changes were secondary to a lowered vitamin C nutrition resulting from the pneumonia.

VIRUS PNEUMONIAS—"Q" FEVER

Pneumonias may be caused by infectious agents other than bacteria, such as viruses and chemical irritants. The common form of virus pneumonia is known as "Q" fever because of its prevalence in Queensland, Australia. A similar if not identical form of virus pneumonia is found in the western states and to a lesser extent throughout the United States. Here it is known as Nine Mile Fever or American "Q" fever.

There is a close relation between the virus of influenza, psittacosis and "Q" fever. The American variety of "Q" fever is caused by *Rickettsia diaporica* which has been demonstrated in dogs, animal ticks and rodents. Individuals having this virus infection do not have agglutinins in their blood for Proteus X19 and XR as is the case with typhus and Rocky Mountain Spotted Fever.

In the United States the virus pneumonias produce clinical features similar to bronchopneumonia with symptoms of pain, malaise, anorexia and drowsiness and a fever of 102° to 104° F. which lasts for a week or more. The incidence of pulmonary infections of viral etiology is increasing, or at least they are being recognized more frequently. They are becoming a distinct clinical problem in medical treatment since they are not responsive to sulfonamide therapy and as yet no specific therapeutic measures have been discovered. Following the acute episode the convalescence is slow and the individual experiences frequently a chronic cough for some time.

A severe ulcerative stomatitis has developed in an occasional patient convalescing from virus pneumonia. This may represent a specific lesion due to the same virus which was responsible for the pneumonia or a secondary complication due to the lowered resistance of the tissues.

INFLUENZA

Influenza is an acute tracheobronchitis accompanied by marked symptoms of toxemia. Secondary complications are frequent and serious. In pandemic influenza, the disease spreads rapidly. The morbidity may be from 2% to 30% with a low mortality, less than 1% in the Army in the 1918-19 epidemic. Influenza is now known to be a virus disease with the influenza bacillus being a secondary invader. Two strains of virus, A and B, have been identified and a third infectious agent has been reported by Horsfall.

Symptoms

Typical influenza (epidemic) is characterized by the abruptness of onset and the extreme severity of the toxemia. The marked prostration cannot be accounted for on the basis of the objective findings. Nausea, vomiting and nosebleed are common symptoms. There is a catarrhal inflammation of the conjunctiva, nose, pharynx and trachea. The pharynx is intensely red. The temperature may reach as high as 105° F. in severe cases. The pulse is slow in relation to the temperature. The blood count reveals usually a leukopenia.

The diagnosis of influenza may be difficult in sporadic cases but during an epidemic it is easy. There is no practical diagnostic test.

Treatment of influenza consists of absolute rest and the forcing of fluids. Return to activity should be cautious. Complications due to secondary bacterial infection can be reduced in frequency and severity by the use of the sulfonamides. Recovery may be rapid, but more often it is marked by protracted weakness and the development of complications. Bronchopneumonia and lobar pneumonia are the most frequent and fatal complications. Acute sinusitis, mastoiditis, pleurisy, lung abscess and cardiac involvement are common. Bronchiectasis is a late but serious sequella. Because of the marked epithelial metaplasia in the bronchi, some authorities think that influenza may predispose to primary neoplasms of the lung.

Brown showed that the use of vaccines, prepared from chick embryos inoculated with both influenza A virus and X strain of canine distemper virus, reduces the incidence of the disease about 50 per cent.

Oral Findings

Oral manifestations are encountered rarely except during epidemics of this disease. Under such conditions oral lesions have been noted in 5 to 25% of the cases. In influenza the oral mucosa is particularly susceptible to secondary infection and postinfluenzal fusospirochetal stomatitis, noma, parotitis and osteomyelitis have been reported.

Benjamin Rush, writing of the influenza epidemic in 1790, described the oral lesions as follows: "They [the patients] complained of a soreness in their mouth, as if they had been inflamed by holding pepper in them. Some had swelled jaws and many complained of toothache." These observations were accurate. Harris noted edema and a bluish red color of the gums and oral mucosa in the influenza epidemic of 1919. Pain was a prominent oral symptom. Shallow ulcers covered with grayish yellow areas of fibrin were observed frequently along the margins of the tongue and at the commissures of the lips. Odontalgia due to the congestive pulpitis was experienced in teeth without cavities or large fillings. Infection and hemorrhage in the pulps of some of these teeth were observed.

During the mild 1940 influenza epidemic characteristic changes of the fungiform papillae of the tongue were noted. These changes, which included various degrees of swelling and inflammation, were considered a reliable diagnostic sign of the stage of the influenzal infection. The oral lesions require no special treatment aside from the use of a bland mouth wash. Zinc chloride, 8%, applied topically to the ulcers will relieve the pain.

PLEURISY

Inflammation of the serous membrane lining the pleural cavities, the pleurae, is known as pleurisy. Pleurisy may be the first clinical symptom of a tuberculous infection or represent a complication of some other respiratory or pulmonary infection.

The characteristic clinical symptom of pleurisy is pain on breathing. There is usually a mild temperature reaction and an accompanying cough. On auscultation a friction rub, produced by the rubbing together of the roughened pleural surfaces, can be heard. When an effusion (fluid) is present, the friction rub may be absent.

Pleurisy with effusion can be demonstrated by physical examination but preferably by x-ray. This type of pleurisy is associated usually with a tuberculous infection, although pneumococcal and streptococcal forms of parenchymal infection result occasionally in pleural effusion. In pleurisy with effusion, dyspnea and pyrexia may be prominent symptoms. The treatment of pleurisy is a medical problem. The oral aspects of this disease are remote.

EMPYEMA

Empyema refers to a suppurative infection of some body cavity. The term should be qualified by the name of the affected organ, i.e., empyema of the pleural cavity.

Pleural empyemas result often from secondary infection of a pleural effusion or occur as a complication of a pneumococcal or streptococcal pneumonia. The leukocyte count and the temperature are elevated in pleural empyemas. The treatment of a pleural empyema is both medical and surgical. The use of the sulfonamides and penicillin have improved the prognosis in both the medical and surgical forms of treatment.

. Oral Aspects

Pleural empyema with a predominance of the fusospirochetal forms is recognized clinically. It may be secondary to fusospirochetal bronchitis or the rupture of a fusospirochetal abscess. The pus from such an empyema has a foul odor similar to that associated with any other fusospirochetal infection. The maintenance of good oral hygiene will go far to prevent the initial fusospirochetal pulmonary infection.

ACUTE PULMONARY EDEMA

Acute pulmonary edema is one of the common cardiac emergencies due to left ventricular failure in hypertensive heart disease. This symptom may arise during sleep in a mild form—nocturnal dyspnea. In acute pulmonary edema the patient has great difficulty in breathing. He is literally drowning in his own body fluids.

Some relief can be obtained by placing the patient in an upright position, limiting the return of blood to the right heart by tourniquets about the extremities or phlebotomy. Morphine sulphate $\frac{1}{4}$ gr., atropine sulphate $\frac{1}{100}$ gr. are the usual remedies. Oxygen inhalation, if available, is of value.

SILICOSIS

Silicosis is a chronic pulmonary disease characterized by fibrosis and atelectasis of the pulmonary parenchyma. The slightly soluble silica is irritating to the pulmonary tissues, rendering them susceptible to infection, particularly tuberculous. Silicosis is an important occupational disease in rock drillers, sand blasters and foundrymen. The early diagnosis of silicosis can be made only by means of the x-ray, but in the more advanced disease the symptoms are similar to those of tuberculosis.

Pumice contains a small percentage of silica but the dentist's or the patient's exposure to this material is so brief that no untoward results have been observed. Some of the substitutes for pumice which are widely used in dental laboratories, because of their cheapness, contain from 70-90% free silica. Kramer reported a case of silicosis which developed in a dental technician who had been polishing dentures with such a compound for several years without proper exhaust or ventilating system.

12

The Cardiovascular System

INTRODUCTION	PERIARTERITIS NODOSA
ANGINA PECTORIS	SYNCOPE
CORONARY OCCLUSION	SHOCK
SUBACUTE BACTERIAL ENDOCARDITIS	PAROXYSMAL TACHYCARDIA
RHEUMATIC HEART DISEASE	SOLDIER'S HEART
CHOREA	CONGESTIVE HEART FAILURE
HYPERTENSION	VENOUS THROMBOSIS AND THROM-
CONGENITAL HEART LESIONS	BOPHLEBITIS
COARCTATION OF THE AORTA	

INTRODUCTION

The common occurrence of cardiovascular disease in the older adult group and the many dental relationships in these diseases emphasize their importance to the dental practitioner. These interrelationships have been dramatically called to the attention of the profession by Darlington's "Death & Dentistry." Although fatal cardiac accidents are uncommon in dental practice, this does not minimize the need for a thorough understanding and appreciation of the potential dangers that these patients present to the practicing dentist. Dental infections may cause or aggravate heart disease. Removal of foci of infection may precipitate a relapse in certain cases of heart disease, and in others any operation or anesthesia is full of risk.

The dentist is in an unique position to perform a real health service to his patient by being watchful for objective and subjective symptoms of early cardiac decompensation. The average patient rarely seeks medical care unless he is ill, but he has formed the habit of visiting his dentist "twice a year." Thus the dentist has an unusual opportunity of detecting early signs of cardiac failure and referring these individuals for medical supervision at a time when the results of conservative methods of therapy will be most effective.

Comroe stressed the importance of the health service that the dentist can render his patient by taking a brief general history of the patient once or twice a year. He suggested the following questions relative to the cardiovascular system.

(1) When was your last physical examination?
(2) Was your blood pressure normal at that time?
(3) Do you become short of breath on climbing one flight of stairs? Must you pause halfway up to catch breath?
(4) Do your ankles swell during the day?
(5) Have you had any discomfort or pain over your heart?
(6) Have you ever had rheumatic fever?
(7) Has any one of your ancestors or of your present relatives had high blood pressure?
(8) Are you extremely nervous?

Much of this information can be obtained in an indirect manner during the twice-yearly dental visits. Such an evaluation of the cardiovascular and general health status of the patient is essential before the administration of a general anesthetic. It is no less important in certain forms of heart disease even when local anesthetics are used. It is our professional responsibility to perform our specialized duties and at the same time to take reasonable precautions that our patient's well-being, or life, is not jeopardized. Physicians referring cardiac patients to the dentist should acquaint him with the diagnosis and assist in the choice of the anesthetic and supervise any prophylactic measures such as sulfonamide therapy.

ANGINA PECTORIS

Symptoms

Angina pectoris is a symptom complex characterized by severe substernal pain, frequently accompanied by a sense of impending death, which is usually precipitated by physical exertion or emotional stress.

The exact etiology of angina pectoris is not known, but anoxemia of the cardiac muscle is probably the basic lesion. The symptoms occur when the blood supply of the heart is inadequate for the needs of the moment. It is associated with coronary artery disease and certain drugs or tobacco may precipitate an attack due to their vasoconstrictor action on the coronary vessels.

Angina pectoris comprises about 25% of all forms of heart disease. It is most common in the age range from 45 to 65 and males are more frequently involved than females. Individuals whose occupation is associated with mental stress—the so-called high pressure business and professional man— are frequently affected. This syndrome may precede typical coronary artery disease.

Symptoms in the typical anginal attack usually follow physical exertion or emotional stress. The individual is seized with a vise-like, crushing pain in the substernal region. There is an associated fear of impending death. The pain radiates characteristically to the left shoulder and down this arm to the finger tips but it may radiate to other areas including the neck region and even the jaws. This painful seizure lasts seconds or a few minutes, seldom longer. It is relieved in most cases almost immediately by the cessation of exertion. For this reason, and because of the intense pain, the individual com-

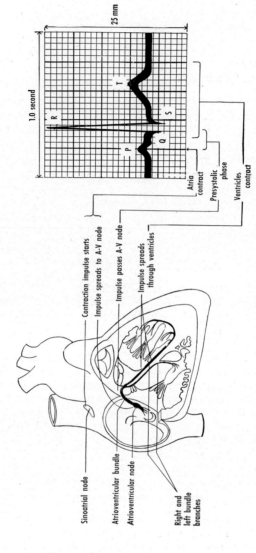

Fig. 138. Illustrating the phases of the cardiac cycle as reflected in the electrocardiogram. (Permission to reproduce the above was granted by the editors of the Roche Review, Hoffmann-LaRoche, Inc., Nutley, N. J.)

monly maintains a fixed position during an attack. Severe pain following the ingestion of a hearty meal may represent mild anginal attacks rather than "acute indigestion." During the anginal seizure, there is little variation in the pulse rate, temperature or blood count. (Compare coronary occlusion.) If the pain persists for more than a few minutes, coronary occlusion or some acute abdominal condition should be considered.

The diagnosis of angina pectoris or anginal pain rests almost exclusively on the patient's history. In some instances electrocardiographic (E.K.G.) recordings may be of assistance.

The treatment of angina pectoris consists of: (1) the use of drugs for the relief of the acute attack and as a means of increasing coronary flow; (2) limiting the demands on the heart to a degree commensurate with its blood supply; and (3) surgical procedures for eliminating pain pathways and methods of increasing the blood supply to the heart by establishing collateral circulation. Death may occur during the initial attack, at a subsequent attack, or as a result of coronary occlusion. In some chronic cases cardiac failure ensues.

Oral Aspects

Acute anginal attacks may occur as a result of nervous reaction associated with dental work, particularly extractions. Anginal attacks have been experienced when the patient was sitting in the dental chair before any work had been started. The pain of angina pectoris is occasionally referred to the jaws and teeth, causing the patient to seek dental attention. If the dental practitioner fails to take a careful history, there may be not only unnecessary extraction of teeth but a considerable risk to the patient. Anginal jaw pain is characterized by its extreme severity, its onset following exertion and its disappearance with rest. These characteristics will serve to differentiate it from the usual pain of dental origin. A brief medical history should reveal other characteristic symptoms of angina pectoris. One patient observed experienced bilateral pain in the lower premolar region on the slightest exertion. It was felt that this represented an anginal equivalent.

When working on patients with known angina pectoris, all precautions should be taken to reduce the painful stimuli as these may give rise to an increase in blood pressure and an anginal attack. The patient should not be permitted to become nervous or excited. A calm and assured attitude on the part of the practitioner will do much to put the patient at ease. One of the short acting barbiturates such as pentobarbital (Nembutal N.N.R. 1½ gr.) or Ipral N.N.R. 2 gr. should be taken 30 minutes before the appointment. It is advisable to consult the patient's physician regarding any pre-operative medication and consultation should be routine when extractions are contemplated.

Procaine hydrochloride 1½ or 2% without adrenalin is the anesthetic of choice for dental extractions. Adrenalin accelerates the heart rate, increases the blood pressure and possibly causes constriction of the coronary arteries— conditions which favor anginal attacks.

Not more than 2 teeth should be removed at a sitting. If precordial or chest pain is experienced during dental extractions or cavity preparation this symptom should be considered seriously and no further work attempted.

Any general anesthetic that might cause anoxemia of the cardiac musculature is contraindicated. For this reason, ethyl ether or divinyl ether are preferred to nitrous oxide. A general anesthetic should not be administered without the attendance of the patient's physician, preferably with the patient hospitalized.

If the patient experiences an anginal attack while in the dental chair, a $\frac{1}{150}$ or $\frac{1}{100}$ gr. nitroglycerine tablet should be placed immediately in the sublingual space or an amyl nitrite pearl should be inhaled. Both of these measures will afford prompt relief. Amyl nitrite may cause such a marked lowering of the systemic blood pressure as to decrease the coronary flow. Consequently there is some question whether it should be used in angina pectoris.

CORONARY OCCLUSION

Coronary occlusion results from the closure of one of the coronary arteries or its branches as a result of thrombus formation, arteriosclerotic changes involving these vessels or their openings, and more rarely embolism. The painful symptoms and the often fatal sequellae result from the impaired nutrition of the cardiac musculature due to a diminished blood supply.

Coronary occlusion affects all classes and social groups without discrimination. It is most common past middle life (50 to 70 years) but it occurs frequently in the 4th decade. Males are affected at least 3 times as often as females. Coronary occlusion may be the initial evidence of serious cardiovascular disease, or it may represent a sequella of hypertension, angina pectoris, localized or generalized arteriosclerosis or rarely diabetes.

Slow occlusion of the coronary arteries may result from arteriosclerotic changes in the coronary arteries or rapid diminution in blood flow may result from thrombus formation. Prolonged vascular spasm is also a possibility as clinical attacks of coronary occlusion are not always associated with demonstrable pathologic changes. Physical exertion or emotional excitement, the use of tobacco or alcohol, do not appear to be exciting factors. A history of preceding anginal attacks, hypertension and arteriosclerosis or a hereditary background is common.

Symptoms

Severe, squeezing, persisting pain localized in the cardiac region is the most outstanding symptom in typical coronary occlusion. This pain lasts for hours or days. In some cases it radiates in a manner similar to that observed in angina pectoris, involving the left shoulder, arm, neck region and along the jaws. The pain is not associated with physical exertion or excitement; in fact, it occurs usually during rest and frequently while the patient is asleep. Symptoms of shock may appear, with pallor and a cold sweat. Nausea and vomiting are not uncommon. There may be evidence of pulmonary edema resulting from partial failure of the left heart. Amyl nitrite, nitroglycerin or other vasodilating agents which are so effective in relieving the pain in angina pectoris are of no avail in coronary occlusion.

There is a marked fall in blood pressure, the pulse is feeble, rapid and irregularities may be noted with the development of cardiac arrhythmias. The temperature is elevated usually on the second or third day and there is a polymorphonuclear leukocytosis. The erythrocyte sedimentation rate is elevated. The EKG shows changes which at times permit a diagnosis of coronary occlusion when the clinical findings are doubtful. It affords some information as to the location of the myocardial damage and its severity.

The treatment of coronary occlusion consists of the relief of pain in the early stages of the disease (morphine sulphate) and absolute mental and physical rest during the prolonged convalescence.

Prognosis

Coronary thrombosis may be immediately fatal, or myocardial rupture in the infarcted area may occur during the first week or 10 days. If the patient survives this period, the chances of surviving the acute attack are good. Cardiac function gradually returns, depending on the rapidity with which collateral circulation is established. Chronic cardiac failure may develop; the individuals may be required to lead a restricted life while a few regain almost normal cardiac function. Regardless of the clinical findings, varying degrees of myocardial fibrosis persist and subsequent attacks are likely. Some individuals survive several attacks but the life expectancy of patients with coronary occlusion is around 5 years.

Oral Aspects

Sudden death in the dental office due to coronary occlusion is not likely, as is the case with angina pectoris. Substernal pain, whether due to a mild coronary attack, angina pectoris or gastro-intestinal disturbances, during dental treatment should contraindicate further work until the cause and the exact nature of the complaint can be determined by the patient's physician. All dental treatment is contraindicated during the acute stage of coronary occlusion. Pain of dental origin, if present, will be relieved by the general sedatives that are so essential. During convalescence the most conservative local treatment may be permitted. Excitement and pain from any cause should be prevented as this increases the blood pressure and places an additional strain on the weakened heart.

Many patients who have survived coronary attacks will require dental treatment. A short medical history will almost invariably permit a correct diagnosis by the dentist or the patient. History of a severe attack of "acute indigestion" may warrant further inquiry from the patient's physician. With pre-operative medication and the careful control of pain by a proper operating technic, all needed dental work can be performed for these patients without undue risk.

While the actual risk in performing the usual dental treatment in these patients is small, it nevertheless is real. Steps taken to minimize this risk are appreciated by the patient and his physician, and they afford the dentist peace of mind if unfortunate complications should develop.

When extractions or minor oral surgery are necessary, the patient's physician should be consulted as a precautionary measure. Local anesthesia with procaine hydrochloride without adrenalin is recommended. If general anesthesia is necessary, nitrous oxide is contraindicated because of the marked increase in blood pressure associated with its administration, the longer excitement stage and the tendency for anoxemia. The remarks made under angina pectoris concerning the choice of general anesthetic and the precautionary measures which should be taken when it is administered apply equally well in coronary occlusion.

There are no life-saving measures in cases of coronary thrombosis or occlusion, but the dentist can take certain precautions in the selection of the anesthetic and in eliminating prolonged operations and shock as much as possible.

TABLE XVI

COMPARISON OF ANGINA PECTORIS AND CORONARY OCCLUSION

	Angina Pectoris	Coronary Artery Occlusion
Etiology...........	? Anoxemia of the cardiac musculature.	Closure of the coronary vessels by arteriosclerotic changes or by a thrombus or embolus.
Incidence..........	50 to 70 year age group. Males predominate.	45 to 65 year age group. Males predominate.
Predisposing causes.	Nervous and mental strain, the so-called "high pressure" modern life. Usually professional men and business executives. Aggravated by smoking or the use of alcohol.	Associated with hypertension, angina pectoris, arteriosclerosis, etc.
Symptoms.........	Severe pain, frequently following physical exertion, emotional or nervous stress. Pain of squeezing constricting nature which characteristically radiates down the left arm— may be referred to the jaw. Pain of short duration. Relieved by the cessation of exertion or the use of vasodilators such as nitroglycerine or amyl nitrite.	Pain not related to physical exertion. Occurs frequently during sleep or rest. Severe pain which persists for hours or days. Pain is not relieved by vasoconstrictors.

SUBACUTE BACTERIAL ENDOCARDITIS (SBE)

Subacute bacterial endocarditis is a highly fatal disease which is caused in the majority of cases by the *Streptococcus viridans*. This disease has a marked predisposition for individuals who have rheumatic valvular lesions and those with congenital cardiac or vascular defects. The immediate exciting factors are frequently difficult to determine but upper respiratory infections, surgical trauma and dental extractions are commonly related chronologically to the onset of the clinical symptoms.

Subacute bacterial endocarditis may occur at any age but it is most common in mid-adult life. The disease is so insidious in its development that the symptoms may not be recognized for several months. The patient experiences progressive weakness, loss in weight, dyspnea, anorexia and vague aches, pains and grippe-like symptoms. A low grade fever is usually present.

Once the fibrinous vegetative lesions (thrombi) have developed on the cardiac valves, they serve as a focus for the continuous dissemination of bacteria throughout the body. The bacteria are present in the deeper portions of the vegetations where they are less susceptible to chemotherapy. These vegetative lesions are friable and small pieces break off occasionally and form emboli. These showers of emboli cause varied symptoms depending on their size and their site of lodgement. The petechial hemorrhages in the conjunctivae and the oral mucosa represent phenomena associated with minute emboli. Larger emboli lodge occasionally in the spleen, kidneys, lungs and the brain where they produce symptoms referable to the structures and organs involved.

The clinical diagnosis of subacute bacterial endocarditis is made frequently by the elimination of other conditions which might produce mild febrile symptoms, weakness and loss of weight such as brucellosis, tuberculosis or a malignancy. The final diagnosis is made on the physical findings and the demonstration of a positive blood culture.

The treatment of subacute bacterial endocarditis is generally ineffective, with recovery occurring in less than 1 case in 100. The combined use of sulfanilamide and heparin (to prevent thrombus formation) has been followed by an occasional cure, but this form of treatment is not without its dangers.* In rare cases, where the vegetative lesions have been localized to a vascular anomaly which could be eliminated surgically, i.e., patent ductus arteriosus, recovery has occurred following operation. The *Streptococcus viridans,* the common etiologic agent, is not particularly susceptible to the sulfonamides, penicillin or vaccine therapy.

Oral Aspects

While it is almost impossible to determine with certainty the origin of the bacteria which give rise to subacute bacterial endocarditis, there is considerable laboratory and clinical evidence pointing to the importance of an oral focus. The alpha Streptococcus or *Streptococcus viridans* is a common inhabitant of the oral cavity and it is also recovered in a high frequency from the periapical tissues.

In their study on the etiology of subacute bacterial endocarditis, Okell and Elliot made blood cultures before and following the extraction of teeth under nitrous oxide anesthesia. They demonstrated the presence of a transient bacteremia, usually of *Streptococcus viridans,* in 76% of the cases. The percentage of positive cultures was related to the state of the oral hygiene. These investigators demonstrated that the organisms responsible for subacute bacterial endocarditis were disseminated commonly through the blood stream, following dental extractions. The author, with Burn, carried on similar studies except that the teeth were removed under novocaine anesthesia. The percentage of positive cultures was lower (17%) than those reported by Okell and Elliot (76%) which could be accounted for in part by the local vaso-

---

* Penicillin therapy has shown some promise as a therapeutic agent.

constrictor action of the adrenalin in the local anesthetic. By the use of a non-pathogen, *Serratia marcesens,* it was demonstrated later that the gingival crevice is an important site from which the bacteria gain entrance into the blood stream. Topical antiseptics were found to be ineffective in rendering this field sterile. Fish showed that actual cauterization of the gingival crevice prior to extraction markedly reduced the percentage of transient bacteremias.

Taran found that the bacteremias following dental extractions in rheumatic fever patients persist much longer than those occurring in control subjects. These transient bacteremias are of little significance in a normal individual, but in a person who has experienced a previous rheumatic infection and who has "lodgement foci" on the heart valves, they may mark the beginning of a fatal infection.

Poor oral hygiene and periodontal disease may be even a greater hazard in such patients. Murry and Moosnick demonstrated a transient bacteremia following the chewing of paraffin cubes in 55% of the 336 patients with varying degrees of caries and "pyorrhea." The organisms recovered were small diplococci (not classified further) in 84% of the positive cultures and a slow growing *Staphylococcus albus* in the remaining 16% of the cultures.

Evidence of a clinical nature is more difficult to assess. Many of the case reports are inconclusive as far as a direct relation between dental extractions and subacute bacterial endocarditis are concerned, although a suggested chronologic relation exists in most instances. Libman stressed the causal relationship between dental infection and subacute bacterial endocarditis. Geiger analyzed 50 cases of subacute bacterial endocarditis selected at random from the records of the New Haven Hospital. The symptomatic beginning of the fatal infection was mentioned specifically in 12 cases in which it followed closely dental extractions, and in 5 others there was suspicion of infection from a dental focus. Four of the 6 cases seen by Doane had extractions 3 to 6 months before the onset of symptoms. In each case a known rheumatic valvular disease had existed some years, yet in spite of this fact the mouth hygiene had been neglected and the patient was referred to the dentist without any prophylactic measures. Kempf and Smith and Clagett reported cases in which dental operative procedures were the likely precipitating cause. Schwartz and Salman however did not experience a single case of subacute bacterial endocarditis in 100 rheumatic patients who had multiple extractions.

Regardless of the inconclusive proof of an etiologic relationship between dental extractions or oral sepsis and subacute bacterial endocarditis, it is apparent when one considers the unfavorable course of the disease that every known prophylactic measure should be taken to preclude the possibility of transient bacteremias occurring in patients with known valvular lesions— particularly those on a rheumatic basis. As Geiger brought out, while it is acknowledged that the sulfonamide drugs are not actively bacteriocidal against *Streptococcus viridans,* it is possible that they possess sufficient bacteriostatic properties to allow the natural defense mechanisms of the body to dispose effectively of the bacteremias.

With this in mind, Poston and Orgain tested the inhibitory effect of the various sulfonamides on 25 strains of *Streptococcus viridans* isolated from the blood stream of patients with subacute bacterial endocarditis and rheumatic fever. The growth of 17 strains was inhibited by one or more of the drugs. These authors believed it important to test the bacteriostatic action of the various compounds *in vitro* against the specific organism, before the institution of chemotherapy. If this is not possible, their studies indicate that sodium sulfapyridine has the most marked inhibitory effect on the greatest number of strains of *Streptococcus viridans*.

Northrop and Crowley demonstrated the effectiveness of the prophylactic use of sulfathiazole in reducing the transient bacteremias following the extraction of teeth. In the 97 untreated, control cases, 13% positive blood cultures were obtained, while in 50 cases in which the sulfathiazole level ranged from 3.0 to 5.6 mg./100 cc. of blood, only 4% positive blood cultures were obtained. The patients were given 6 Gm. of sulfathiazole and sodium bicarbonate before operation, 1 Gm. of each being given every 4 hours, starting at 4 o'clock the day before the appointment and terminating at noon. The extractions were carried out early in the afternoon, 1 to 2 hours after the last administration of the 2 drugs.

Taran's report emphasized the value of the prophylactic use of the sulfonamides prior to dental extractions. He experienced 18 (10%) cases of subacute bacterial endocarditis following extractions in 165 rheumatic fever patients, when no prophylactic measures were taken, and only 1 (1.2%) case in 80 patients, when prophylactic sulfonamide therapy was instituted prior to extraction.

Until more effective methods of treatment of subacute bacterial endocarditis are available, it would seem desirable to take certain prophylactic precautions when performing extractions on individuals with old rheumatic valvular lesions. Furthermore the oral hygiene of these individuals should be maintained in the best possible state.

Suggested Prophylactic Procedures for the Reduction of Post-extraction Bacteremias and the Possible Development of Subacute Bacterial Endocarditis. The following suggestions are simple, they contain no risk to the patient and, if subacute bacterial endocarditis should develop, one has the satisfaction of knowing that prophylactic procedures had been taken.

(1) The patient should be questioned about a past history of rheumatic fever or chorea or a known history of "heart disease" with valvular involvement.

(2) If a positive history is obtained, the patient's physician should be consulted. If valvular lesions are known to be present, he should be asked to supervise the administration of one of the sulfonamides—sulfathiazole or sulfadiazine—in such amounts as to attain a definite therapeutic blood level at the time of extraction and for 12 to 24 hours thereafter.

(3) Local anesthesia is the anesthetic of choice.

(4) The gingival crevice should be gently cleansed mechanically and then treated with medicaments. Fish has demonstrated clearly that cauteri-

zation by chemicals or heat is the only satisfactory method of rendering this area sterile.

(5) The surgical procedures should be as atraumatic as possible. Following extraction, a normal blood clot should be allowed to form or the wound can be packed with one of the sulfonamides.

RHEUMATIC HEART DISEASE—RHEUMATIC FEVER

Rheumatic fever is an infectious disease producing lesions in the nervous system, the subcutaneous tissues, the joints and most frequently in the heart. The causative agent has not been determined but indirect evidence suggests that the rheumatic manifestations are due to a hemolytic streptococcus.

Acute rheumatic fever is mainly a disease of childhood or early adolescence. The "growing pains" of childhood at times may be symptoms of rheumatic infection. It is particularly common in New England and the mid-Atlantic states. Cold damp weather, rapid changes in temperature, recurrent upper respiratory infections and attacks of tonsillitis predispose to the disease. There appears to be a family predisposition. Rheumatic infection in general, particularly the cardiac lesions, are characterized by recurrences.

Chorea, acute carditis, rheumatic arthritis or the typical subcutaneous nodules may be the initial symptoms of rheumatic fever. The child often complains of a sore throat, is listless and has a temperature of 100° to 102° F. At times an erythematous skin eruption, erythema multiforme, is present during the acute attack. Rheumatic arthritis is characterized by involvement of successive joints which are red, tender and painful. Even the weight of the bed clothes causes severe pain. The rheumatic nodules, small oval fibrous subcutaneous masses, are common on the extensor surfaces of the wrists and on the ankles. They are moderately painful.

Varying degrees of acute carditis occur in most cases of rheumatic fever, with permanent cardiac lesions resulting in over 50% of the cases. While a pancarditis is frequently present, the usual cardiac lesions are situated in the endocardium and the myocardium. The valvular lesions affect the mitral valve in 97% of the cases with cardiac involvement, resulting in varying degrees of insufficiency and stenosis. Valves so involved are frequently the site of subacute bacterial endocarditis. The myocardial lesions, resulting from the so-called Aschoff's bodies, produce fibrosis of the myocardium and lessened cardiac reserve. The adhesive pericarditis, which develops occasionally as a sequel to rheumatic pancarditis, interferes further with cardiac function.

The diagnosis of rheumatic fever is made on the history, the physical findings of cardiac murmurs or hypertrophy in conjunction with x-ray studies, the erythrocyte sedimentation rate and the fibrinolysin test. The leukocyte count is elevated. In doubtful cases, the clinical response following salicylate administration—the therapeutic test—is observed.

The treatment of rheumatic fever consists of rest and sedation during the acute episode. Salicylates are almost specific for the pain of rheumatic fever. The general regime of the individual with cardiac lesions often requires a restriction of the normal physical activity. Mild respiratory infections are serious, as they may result in an exacerbation of the rheumatic symptoms. The prophylactic use of the sulfonamides in preventing exacerbations of this disease is being studied.

Oral Aspects

Although recurrent tonsillar infections are believed to predispose to exacerbations of rheumatic symptoms, no direct relationship has been established between oral disease and rheumatic fever. Taran noted that the extent and amount of dental caries in a group of rheumatic children was much greater than in the nonrheumatic siblings of the rheumatic patients. This finding is probably causal rather than causative, as children with congenital heart disease also had an increased number of dental defects. It was probably difficult for members of both groups to receive dental treatment. Not infrequently the physician will become concerned about diseased tonsils and at the same time disregard numerous abscessed deciduous or permanent teeth. More attention should be given to dental treatment and the elimination of oral infections in these patients.

Individuals with rheumatic fever, or those with a past history of rheumatic cardiac damage, should have certain prophylactic measures taken when teeth are extracted. Heart valves which are the seat of past rheumatic processes are particularly susceptible to *Streptococcus viridans* infections—subacute bacterial endocarditis. The frequent occurrence of bacteremias of this organism following dental extraction has been well established and, while these bacteremias are transient in normal children, they have been demonstrated to persist for months in some rheumatic patients.

Schwartz and Salman found no greater incidence of subacute bacterial endocarditis following dental extractions in rheumatic than in nonrheumatic patients but Taran's experience was quite the opposite. In 195 consecutive cases of rheumatic heart disease on whom dental extractions were performed, 18 children developed subacute bacterial endocarditis. After sulfonamide therapy was instituted 24 hours before extraction and for 3 days afterward, only 1 out of 80 children developed subacute bacterial endocarditis, other factors remaining essentially similar. These data suggest strongly that the sulfonamides are of prophylactic value. Physicians having patients with rheumatic fever or chorea under their care should inform them of the need of prophylactic treatment whenever dental extractions become necessary. The sulfonamide therapy should be given under the supervision of the physician.

Draper *et al.* observed what they considered to be a typical dental change in patients with rheumatic heart disease. This consisted of protruding canine teeth and an asymmetric development of the palate. The rheumatic disease group of patients had the widest jaw angle of any of the groups studied and a skewed dental arch form.

Holtz and Friedman described a hemorrhagic eruption of the mouth and throat occurring in patients with rheumatic fever. The lesions consisted of circular, deep red spots varying in size from a pin point to 2 mm. in diameter. They are seen most often on the cheek mucosa in the region of Stenson's duct opening, but they are also common on the soft palate, sublingual region, uvula and the sides of the tongue. These lesions were not related to embolic phenomena. At first they have a bluish hue and at times erosion of the central portion of the lesion results in a white center.

CHOREA (SYDENHAM'S CHOREA, ST. VITUS' DANCE)

Chorea is considered a manifestation of rheumatic fever. The affected child makes more or less continuous, purposeless, irregular movements of the head, arms and legs. He is extremely irritable. Muscular weakness may be so pronounced that the child cannot walk or even feed himself. Speech at times is impossible because of the inability to control the tongue and lip muscles.

HYPERTENSION (HYPERPIESA—HIGH BLOOD PRESSURE)

The term hypertension may indicate a disease entity, essential hypertension, or a symptom which is commonly associated with cardiovascular-renal disease, or arteriosclerosis.

Essential hypertension is increased blood pressure of unknown etiology. This disease is uncommon before 30 years of age. It is found commonly in those whose occupation is associated with considerable nervous tension and worry. There is a familial predisposition. The exact mechanism of the increased blood pressure and the particular organ systems involved are not known. Evidence is pointing to the existence of a pressor substance, angiotonin, which acts on the musculature of the blood vessels. An antagonistic substance is believed to be normally present, which prevents the action of the angiotonin.

Hypertension may be present for months or years before symptoms referable to this condition are manifested or recognized. Frequent recurring and persisting headaches, shortness of breath, general malaise, nosebleeds and dizziness are common symptoms. The deep pink flush of the cheeks and lips of a patient should arouse suspicion of hypertension which can be verified or excluded by blood pressure studies. Loss of weight and appetite, vomiting, ocular complaints, and persisting headaches are other symptoms of hypertension. Ophthalmoscopic examination will reveal edema of the optic discs, new and old retinal hemorrhages and scarring. Symptoms of cardiac failure develop often after varying intervals of time, and the development of generalized arteriosclerosis is not unusual. These patients may succumb to cerebral hemorrhage, coronary thrombosis, cardiac decompensation or renal failure. A systolic pressure of over 150 mm. Hg is suggestive of hypertension, and in severe cases, systolic pressures of over 250 mm. Hg are not unusual.

The treatment of essential hypertension is temporizing and symptomatic rather than curative. Surgical operation on the autonomic nervous system, the use of drugs, such as the thiocyanates, are common methods of treatment. Attempts are made to lower the blood pressure to a degree which will minimize the symptoms.

Oral Aspects

The oral considerations of the patient with essential hypertension or hypertension associated with cardiovascular-renal disease are similar. Both hypotension and hypertension have been ascribed to oral foci of infection. Many of the data on this subject are based on isolated case reports and studies which were inadequately controlled. Meade listed hypo- and hypertension among 23 diseases of the circulatory system which may be caused by oral infections. The most extensive study was made by Frankel who compared the blood pressure findings of 17,000 patients with "heavy dentistry" (suggestive of oral sepsis) insured by the Metropolitan Life Insurance Company with suitable controls. No significant differences were found in the hypertensive group. It is more than likely that oral infection is coincidental rather than causative.

Broderick attempted to correlate the state of the teeth to the blood pressure. The patients with very good teeth had a B.P. of 116/79; those with very carious teeth a B.P. of 114/73 and those with "pyorrhea" a B.P. of 121/77. When one considers the age relationship of the various groups of patients, it is evident that there is little correlation between the state of the teeth and the blood pressure.

Anything which results in an elevation of blood pressure or causes nervousness, should be avoided in hypertensive patients. Premedication will materially allay nervousness. A minimum amount of vasoconstrictor agents should be used. Cobefrin results in a higher and more prolonged elevation of blood pressure than epinephrin. Schwartz and Soloman considered the extraction of teeth in hypertensive patients a fairly safe procedure and, if cerebral accidents should follow dental extractions, they may as well be attributed to the natural course of events in this disease as to the extraction. No increase in postoperative hemorrhage is encountered in hypertensive patients. Vasoconstrictors may be omitted entirely in the usual case. Nitrous oxide anesthesia is accompanied usually by an elevation of blood pressure, even when mild asphyxial states are avoided. Regardless of the anesthetic which is used, the patient should not be permitted to struggle. The dentist should consult with the patient's physician before proceeding with extractions or extensive oral surgery in hypertensive patients. Adequate premedication is desirable.

Odontalgia has been occasionally reported in patients with hypertension for which no local cause could be discovered. Hyperemia of the dental pulp, or congestion of this tissue resulting from the increased blood pressure, could account for the symptoms.

CONGENITAL HEART LESIONS

Common congenital cardiac anomalies include: (1) a persistent ductus arteriosus; (2) persistent defect of the interauricular septum; and (3) stenosis of the pulmonary veins in association with other complex anomalies which are known as the tetralogy of Fallot.

The clinical manifestations of these anomalies in infancy and childhood are those associated with insufficient oxygenation of the blood. In later life they may serve as a site for subacute bacterial endocarditis.

COARCTATION OF THE AORTA

Coarctation of the aorta is a developmental anomaly of some dental interest. This condition is characterized by a marked diminution in the calibre of the aortic arch just distal to where the common carotid arises. Because of the altered vascular hydrodynamics, the blood pressure in the upper extremities and the head is much higher than that in the lower extremities. The main collateral circulation around this deficiency is through the intercostal arteries, resulting in a marked hypertrophy of these vessels. Because of their increased size, they produce defects in the lower borders of the ribs which can be demonstrated roentgenologically.

Oral Aspects

The abnormal vascular pressure in the head and neck during early development results in a marked increase in size of the mandibular arteries and the arteries leading to the individual teeth. These structures are unusually conspicuous in the jaw roentgenograms. Healy and Daley tentatively diagnosed 4 cases of coarctation of the aorta on the basis of the dental roentgenologic changes. They were verified later by chest x-rays and other clinical findings.

All these patients presented 2 consistent dental findings, (1) prominence of the circulatory canals in the dental x-rays and (2) prognathism.

The chief complaint in the first case diagnosed was hemorrhage following tooth extraction. The hemorrhage was of an arterial nature and it was so severe that pressure over the bleeding socket was ineffective. The patient was under the physician's care for intermittent hemorrhage for 2 days.

PERIARTERITIS NODOSA

Periarteritis nodosa is an uncommon inflammatory disease affecting the small arteries, which is rarely diagnosed clinically. The causative agent is not known. The histopathologic findings in periarteritis nodosa are similar to those occurring in temporal arteritis. Symptoms referable to the temporomandibular joint have been reported in the latter disease.

In the reported cases of temporal arteritis, tenderness over the region of the temporomandibular joints and along the distribution of the temporal arteries was noted. Many of the patients complained of pain and difficulty in opening their mouths. The symptoms referable to the temporomandibular joint and jaws disappeared gradually. Diagnosis was made by means of biopsy study.

SYNCOPE (FAINTING)

Syncope is a sudden, transient benign circulatory insufficiency. Fear, profound emotional disturbances and pain are important predisposing factors.

Fatigue, hunger or prolonged standing among crowds or convalescence from a long illness are other causes.

The physiologic mechanism responsible for the temporary loss of consciousness is a lowered pulse pressure which produces the cerebral anemia. A feeling of uneasiness, giddiness or light-headedness may precede the actual syncope. The patient often will complain of gastric distress or pain in the precordial region but at other times fainting occurs without warning.

The clinical picture in syncope is startling. The skin is deathly pale. The pupils are usually dilated and the pupillary reflex is absent. Both the pulse and respirations are slow and feeble. There may be profuse perspiration and at times involuntary urination or defecation.

Oral Aspects

Syncope is common in dental practice. It is often associated with the removal of teeth or other painful operative procedures. Since fear and emotional disturbances predispose to syncope, adequate premedication will many times avert fainting attacks in susceptible individuals ($1\frac{1}{2}$ gr. pentobarbitol). The operator should be confident that there is satisfactory anesthesia before attempting extractions.

When a patient experiences premonitory signs of syncope, the head should be placed immediately well down between the knees. Any constricting clothing about the neck should be loosened. If fainting has already occurred, the back of the dental chair should be placed immediately in a horizontal position. In fact this position of the chair is more comfortable for the semiconscious patient than the head-between-the-knees position. Either of these postural changes will result usually in increased cerebral circulation, and a corresponding improvement in the general condition of the patient. Peripheral stimulation in the form of cold applications to the face and forehead or the inhalation of aromatic spirits of ammonia vapors are also useful. CO_2-oxygen mixture, if available, is of aid. The patient should remain in a supine position until fully recovered. Under no consideration should operative procedures be continued or performed during syncope.

If a satisfactory response is not obtained, artificial respiration and thoracic massage should be instituted. Stimulants which are injected subcutaneously are of little value because of their poor absorption due to the circulatory inefficiency. When consciousness is regained, a decided stimulating effect can be obtained by giving the patient 8 to 10 drops of aromatic spirits of ammonia in half a glass of water. In a few minutes, the physical condition of the patient will usually permit the completion of the operative procedures.

SHOCK (TRAUMATIC SHOCK)

Traumatic shock is due to an insufficiency of the circulating blood. Its initial phase is not unlike benign syncope. True shock may result from the loss of blood due to surgical operation or injury, marked peripheral vasodilation, or the loss of blood plasma such as occurs in severe crush injuries or burns.

The predisposing factors discussed under benign syncope are also important in true shock. The psychic make-up of the individual, the extent of the injury and the severity of the pain are important considerations.

In typical shock the pulse is slow and full and the blood pressure is low. In cases of severe hemorrhage the pulse may be weak, rapid and irregular. The skin is pale, cold and clammy. The mucous membranes, lips, nail beds and ear often are cyanotic. All reflexes, including the pupillary reflex, are absent or markedly diminished. The patient may respond to questioning but consciousness is of a low level.

Oral Aspects

Shock is rarely seen by the dentist. The hemorrhage encountered in dental practice is seldom severe enough to give rise to symptoms of shock. Dentists treating patients with severe facial injuries may be confronted with shock but these cases are usually out of danger of true shock before an attempt is made to treat the facial lesions. Prolonged bleeding of dental origin in hemophiliacs may give rise to shock.

PAROXYSMAL TACHYCARDIA

Paroxysmal tachycardia is characterized by a marked increase in the rate of the heart beat without alterations in its normal rhythm. Individuals prone to develop this condition have frequently a neurotic background. A diagnosis of paroxysmal tachycardia can usually be made when there is a regular pulse rate of 180 to 200.

Paroxysmal tachycardia can often be controlled by vagal stimulation. Firm pressure on the eyeballs, pressure over the carotid sheath, gagging or assuming the knee-chest position will frequently slow the rapid heart beat. If these simple procedures are ineffective a physician should be summoned.

SOLDIER'S HEART (EFFORT SYNDROME—IRRITABLE HEART)

Certain functional cardiac arrhythmias develop occasionally under nervous or emotional stress in individuals with otherwise clinically normal hearts. The frequent occurrence of these symptoms in candidates for military service has given rise to the terminology. The symptoms include heartache, palpitation, excessive perspiration, easy fatigue, nervousness and marked breathlessness on exertion. The successful treatment of soldier's heart requires both time and experience, as many of the patients have a well-developed neurosis. Parsons-Smith listed focal sepsis, gastro-intestinal disorders and respiratory infections as complicating factors.

CONGESTIVE HEART FAILURE (CARDIAC DECOMPENSATION)

Congestive heart failure is a symptom rather than a disease. It is an indication that the cardiac reserve of the individual has been exceeded and that cardiac decompensation has occurred. Under normal circumstances the functional potentiality of the heart far exceeds the work it is called upon to perform, there being a considerable cardiac reserve. This cardiac reserve may be diminished due (1) to degenerative changes in the cardiac musculature resulting from rheumatic infection or coronary artery occlusion or (2) to increased work demanded of the heart due to cardiac valvular lesions and hypertension.

GRAPHIC REPRESENTATION OF CARDIAC RESERVE

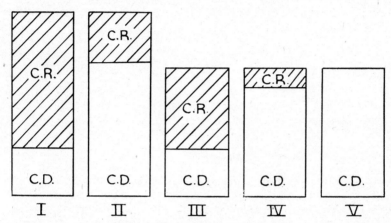

FIG. 139. The vertical columns I to V represent diagrammatically the work potentiality of the cardiac musculature in health and in various disease states. The clear areas, C.D., represent the demands made upon the cardiac musculature and the hatched areas, C.R., the cardiac reserve. In I, a normal balance between C.D. and C.R. is depicted. In II, there is increased work demanded of the heart due to early hypertension or cardiac valvular lesions with a resultant diminished C.R. In III, the C.D. is normal, but the entire work potentiality of the heart is decreased due to old rheumatic lesions or coronary occlusion with a resultant diminished C.R. In IV, we have an increased C.D. in the patient depicted in III with still further reduction of the C.R. In V, the C.D. equals or exceeds the work potentialities of the heart, in which case cardiac decompensation ensues.

This cardiac reserve becomes gradually diminished until it is no longer sufficient to fulfill the demands made upon the heart. The concept of cardiac reserve can be graphically depicted.

Congestive heart failure is common in hypertensive heart disease, coronary artery disease and rheumatic heart disease. It is associated less frequently with hyperthyroidism and syphilitic heart disease. The majority of the cases occur in the 5th and 6th decades. There is a predisposition in the male, probably because of their greater activity.

Increasing breathlessness following moderate exertion is an early symptom of congestive heart failure. Interference in pulmonary circulation is manifested by varying degrees of cyanosis and pulmonary edema. Mild pulmonary edema is associated with a chronic productive cough which is accompanied occasionally with blood-tinged sputum. Pitting edema of the lower extremities, hepatic enlargement, generalized edema and congestion of the large veins of the neck are symptoms of advanced cardiac decompensation. In severe cases the patient is short of breath unless he is in a sitting position (cardiac asthma) and such patients sleep with 2, 3 or more pillows in order to obtain rest. Normal renal function is impaired seriously because of the circulatory failure. Anorexia, vomiting and functional disturbances of the gastro-intestinal tract are common symptoms.

Treatment

The immediate treatment of congestive heart failure consists of rest, limitation of the fluid intake, the administration of diuretics and digitalis. After cardiac compensation has been established, attempts should be made to alter the living regime of the patient so that the work demanded of the heart will fall within the work potentiality of this organ.

Prognosis

The prognosis of cardiac decompensation and congestive heart failure of a rheumatic origin is much better than in syphilitic cardiac decompensation. The former patients, and at times those with hypertensive heart disease may survive several episodes of cardiac decompensation, each episode diminishing still further the remaining cardiac reserve.

Oral Aspects

The dentist should be watchful for early signs of congestive heart failure in his patients. Cyanosis of the lips, tongue and oral mucosa is readily detected in mild states of cardiac decompensation. Binkowitz described a clinical test which he claimed is indicative of early cardiac decompensation. The patient is asked to place without pressure the tip of the tongue on the palatal surface of the upper incisors. A marked distension of the ranine veins is indicative of cardiac decompensation. This organ also becomes markedly cyanotic when it is protruded from the mouth and held in a dependent position.

Patients with low cardiac reserve are poor subjects for extractions, irrespective of the anesthetic used. If dental treatment is required in patients with cardiac decompensation, it should be of a palliative nature. If extractions are indicated, they can be performed later with less risk to the patient. Local anesthetics are preferred.

VENOUS THROMBOSIS AND THROMBOPHLEBITIS

Thrombosis of the veins is not common. It may occur when there has been injury to the intimal lining of the vessels, when infection is present, or when there is abnormal venous stasis. Because of the relative venous stasis of the lower extremities, thrombosis and thrombophlebitis of the femoral and iliac vessels are most common. Venous thrombosis is produced intentionally in the injection treatment of varicose veins and hemorrhoids, and it occurs accidentally in association with intravenous therapy.

Thrombosis of the large veins of the lower extremities is a frequent *post partum* complication, due partly to venous stasis resulting from the increased intra-abdominal pressure and the actual extension of thrombi from the uterine vessels into the common iliac veins. *Post partum* thrombophlebitis of the lower extremities is called "milk leg." The thrombosed veins are painful on pressure and there is rapid development of a marked pitting edema of the affected part. It is cool to touch.

Thrombosis may be a serious and often fatal sequella of abdominal operations. Progressive thrombophlebitis may develop until a crucial vessel is involved or small portions of the thrombus break off and circulate as emboli which produce a variety of symptoms, depending on their size, number and the location of their lodgement. Strict adherence to asepsis, good surgical technic and postoperative care will minimize the possibility of postoperative thrombophlebitis and embolism.

CAVERNOUS SINUS THROMBOSIS (THROMBOPHLEBITIS)

Cavernous sinus thrombosis is a serious condition which results from septic thrombus formation in the cavernous sinus and its numerous communicating branches. It results usually from an extension of a thrombophlebitis of the veins which empty in this sinus.

Because of the extensive venous anastomoses of the head and neck region and the frequent reversal of venous flow due to the few valves in these structures, facial infections and those of the mouth may give rise to cavernous sinus thrombosis. The direct extension of antral infections may also give rise to this disease.

The classical symptoms of cavernous sinus thrombosis include exophthalmos, edema and chemosis of the eyelids and sclerae, a septic type of temperature reaction, papillo-edema and edema of the conjunctivae. Headache and vomiting may be prominent symptoms. Paralysis of the external ocular muscles is commonly present. The patients die usually of pyemia, sepsis, brain abscess or meningitis. A few cases are amenable to surgery. The general prognosis is better since the advent of the sulfonamides and penicillin.

Oral Aspects

Cavernous sinus thrombosis is of interest to the dentist because infectious processes of the face, jaws and associated parts may give rise to this serious condition.

Infections of the upper lip, face and nares can reach the cavernous sinus through the communicating angular veins. Infection from the teeth or the surrounding tissues may reach the cavernous sinus by way of the pterygoid plexus and the emissary veins from the pterygomaxillary space. Septic processes involving the parotid gland are also known to give rise to cavernous sinus thrombosis.

The majority of the reported cases of cavernous sinus thrombosis of suspected dental origin arise from infections in the upper and lower third molar regions. This is due possibly to the intimate relationship of these tissues to the pterygoid plexus, anatomic considerations which favor the direct extension of infection and mechanical factors associated with the related musculature. Many of these cases have followed surgical procedures which were

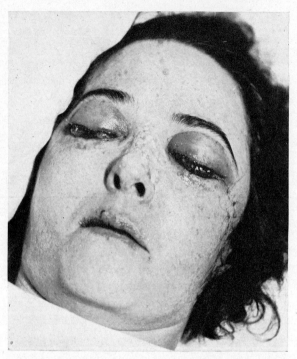

Fig. 140. Patient with cavernous sinus thrombosis which followed a mandibular injection and extraction of a lower right third molar. At necropsy the thrombophlebitis was demonstrated to extend from the area of injection along the pterygoid plexus to the skull.

performed during the acute stage of infection. In other instances it was believed that infection was carried into the deeper tissues during the injection of the local anesthetic. Cases have been recorded, however, where cavernous sinus thrombosis developed following an abscessed deciduous tooth which was removed without anesthesia.

The following case history illustrates the clinical course of a patient with cavernous sinus thrombosis which followed the extraction of a lower third molar. The pathway of the thrombophlebitis was demonstrated at necropsy.

The patient, a 35-year-old white woman, was admitted to the hospital on 2/11/35 complaining of earache and headache following the extraction of a lower left third molar ten days previously. The patient remembered that 4 or 5 syringefuls of anesthetic solu-

tion were required to produce anesthesia. The following day the patient experienced difficulty in opening her mouth and she also had a severe headache and pain in the left ear.
These symptoms persisted and treatment by 3 different physicians was ineffectual. The
day prior to admission she received 3,000 units of tetanus antitoxin.

On admission, the patient appeared acutely ill. Her temperature was 100.4° F., the cardiac and respiratory rates were 106 and 24 respectively, and the blood pressure was
125/55. The jaws could be opened only about one-half an inch. There was no evidence
of infection about the site of the extraction. There was some tenderness of the neck
muscles and over both maxillary sinuses. Soon after admission the tenderness in the
jaw disappeared but the eyeballs became painful. The left one was sore even without
pressure. The following day chemosis and conjunctival edema of the right eye were
noted. By this time the temperature varied between 103° and 105° F. Similar signs
developed in the left eye and a marked proptosis of both eyeballs became the outstanding symptom. The patient died 6 days after admission.

Laboratory findings: R.B.C. 5,330,000 c. mm., Hgb. 76% (100% = 15.6 Gm.) and the
W.B.C. varied from 12,800 to 17,850 cu. mm. with 92% polymorphonuclears, 5% lymphocytes and 3% large mononuclears. The urine was essentially negative. The blood Kahn
was negative. Lumbar puncture findings were within normal limits. Blood cultures taken
on 2 different occasions at the temperature peak were negative. A smear from the tooth
socket showed no organisms resembling tetanus bacilli.

Clinical diagnosis: Cavernous sinus thrombosis.

Pathologic diagnosis: Suppurative thrombophlebitis of the left pterygoid plexus and
cavernous sinuses, cellulitis of the peri-orbital tissues, osteomyelitis of the sphenoid and
temporal bones, multiple focal abscesses in the lungs. Microscopic examination of the
left pterygoid plexus and the surrounding connective tissues demonstrated a thrombophlebitis extending from the region of the inner surface of the ramus of the mandible to
the cavernous sinus. The adjacent connective tissue was extensively infiltrated with polymorphonuclears and lymphocytes.

While cavernous thrombosis is a rare complication which might be related
to dental procedures its seriousness justifies consideration whenever acute
infections, particularly in the molar region, are encountered.

It can be prevented largely by the exercise of good surgical judgment and
caution in the treatment of certain types of dental infections.

13

Gastro-intestinal Disease

THE MOUTH

The mouth and its contained structures comprise the first part of the gastro-intestinal tract. Acute inflammations of the oral mucosa and gums interfere seriously with the normal ingestion of food. This is particularly important in the infant and the child. In the adult, nutritional deficiencies are a common predisposing cause of gingivostomatitis, and the resulting inability to take adequate nourishment completes a vicious circle.

Because of the close relation of the oral tissues to the external environment, and the various habits peculiar to man, these tissues are unique in respect to the variety of chemical, thermal and bacterial irritants to which they are subjected. For this reason, the oral tissues show frequently the sole or the first evidence of a decreased general resistance. Thus the oral mucosa can be regarded as a sensitive indicator of the general health status of the individual, which at times is of specific diagnostic value. Because of his familiarity with the normal appearance of the oral mucosa, the dentist can play an important role in the early recognition of altered body function, as it may be manifested in subtle changes in the soft tissues of the mouth.

Diseases of the teeth or periodontal structures result not only in an impaired masticatory function, but the swallowed exudate from the gums may interfere with the normal digestion and aggravate any local infectious process that may be present in the gastro-intestinal tract. The lack of normal chewing arising from malposed teeth or uncompensated edentulous areas may interfere seriously with normal food partitioning. In the young adult, the remaining portions of the gastro-intestinal tract can compensate effectively for this lack of proper food partitioning, but in the older patient who has frequently chronic gastro-intestinal disease, this decreased ability to chew may be an important clinical consideration.

Aside from the purely biologic aspects of healthy teeth and supporting structures, they are important from both a personal and social standpoint. They give a sense of health and well-being to the individual that is in keeping with the external appearance of health which is so frequently artificially acquired.

THE SALIVARY GLANDS

Pathologic conditions affecting the salivary glands are of dental interest because the location of the symptoms brings the patient to the dental practitioner for diagnosis and treatment. The disorders of the salivary glands can be grouped as follows.

(1) Developmental defects—absence of one or more pairs of salivary glands.
(2) Functional disorders of the salivary glands.
    (a) Increased secretion—sialorrhea.
        (1) Physiologic in infancy and childhood.
        (2) Stimuli from special senses, sight or smell of food, etc.
        (3) Acute forms of stomatitis including herpetic and fuso-spirochetal infection, the metallic stomatitides and pemphigus.
        (4) Drugs.
        (5) Wearing of dentures.
    (b) Decreased secretion—asialorrhea—xerostomia.
        (1) Physiologic in the aged.
        (2) Psychic stimuli such as emotion or fright.
        (3) In dehydration states and systemic diseases resulting in or associated with dehydration states.
        (4) Disturbances in the innervating mechanisms of the salivary glands.
        (5) Drugs and irradiation of the head and neck region.
        (6) Changes associated with the wearing of dentures.
(3) Obstruction to normal salivary flow due to
    (a) Calcareous masses or inspissated mucus in the salivary ducts.
    (b) Collapse of the duct due to pressure of adjacent structures or growths.
(4) Acute pyogenic infections of the salivary glands
    (a) Occurring as a postoperative complication of abdominal surgery or during the course of debilitating or dehydrating diseases.
    (b) Secondary to blockage of the salivary duct or resulting from attempts to canulate the duct.
(5) Specific infectious processes of the salivary glands.
    (a) Epidemic parotitis—mumps.
    (b) Uveoparotid fever.

(c) Mikulicz's disease.
(d) Tuberculosis, actinomycosis and syphilis of the salivary glands.
(6) Tumors of the parotid gland.
(a) Mixed tumors of the parotid.

In rare instances, one or more of the salivary glands fails to develop. Thoma reported a case in which the sublingual glands were absent. The author studied a nine-year-old girl who had no parotid glands or ducts. Occasionally there is an accompanying absence of lachrymal glands. Children and adolescents who lack salivary glands or who have a markedly decreased salivary flow have early and rampant dental decay. Cox demonstrated experimentally in rats that a lack of salivary flow will predispose to an increased prevalence of dental decay.

Normal salivary flow is important because of its mechanical cleansing action. In addition, saliva has general bacteriostatic properties and it may also contain bacteriolytic enzymes. The CO_2 combining capacity of the saliva may be a factor in caries susceptibility or immunity. Trimble et al. found that there was an inverse relationship between the rate of salivary flow and dental decay.

Steggerda studied a university student who had complete absence of the composite salivary glands and their ducts from the standpoint of the thirst production mechanism and water metabolism. While the dry mouth necessitated the taking of a few mouthfuls of water every hour or so, the total fluid intake in 24 hours was 2,783 cc. as compared with 2,615 cc. for a control group of individuals. If the normal subjects were made thirsty by artificial means, such as NaCl consumption, they consumed more water to moisten the mouth than the experimental subject habitually drinks. While the salivary glands are essential for keeping the mouth moist and comfortable, they are not the sole factors in governing thirst. It was found that a person without salivary glands may have a normal water and NaCl metabolism.

Increased Salivary Secretion—Sialorrhea

The salivary flow in infancy and early childhood is characteristically increased. Lourie found that the parotid flow in children before the age of 3 years varied between 0.7 and 0.5 cc./5 min. while the salivary flow after the age of 7 approached the normal adult rate of .02 to 0.12 cc./5 minutes. Excessive salivary flow is particularly marked during "teething." In the acute form of generalized aphthous stomatitis, sialorrhea is a striking symptom. Children with macroglossia are commonly annoyed by excessive salivary flow.

The sight or smell of food will give rise in some individuals to a copious flow of saliva as well as gastric juice. Most acute stomatitides are accompanied by an increased flow of saliva. In a few, such as fusospirochetal stomatitis, mercurial stomatitis and pemphigus the excess salivary flow is an outstanding symptom of the disease. Excessive salivary flow is commonly seen in epileptics and mentally deficient children.

Drugs having the ability to stimulate salivary flow are known as sialogogues, of which pilocarpine is the outstanding example. Many sialogogues act by stimulation of the central nervous system centers governing salivary flow. Iodides, ammonium and mercurial salts and lobelia are also sialogogues.

Following the insertion of prosthetic appliances, especially full dentures, most patients are inconvenienced by abnormal salivary flow. This annoying symptom disappears gradually within 1 or 2 weeks as the patient becomes accustomed to the dentures. Excessive salivation may cause drooling from the lips with secondary skin changes which simulate angular cheilosis and the dermatitis associated with nutritional deficiencies. These changes are seen particularly in denture-wearing patients in which the intermaxillary space has not been properly maintained. The swallowing of excessive saliva may cause nausea and at times vomiting.

Decreased Salivary Secretion—Xerostomia—Asialorrhea

Decreased or absent salivary flow may be accompanied by annoying and painful symptoms. If the oral mucosa and the tongue become irritated, and secondary mucosal changes occur, this condition is spoken of as xerostomia. Xerostomia is not a disease entity but rather a group of symptoms which may result from a variety of causes.

A decreased salivary flow as well as a decrease in the ptyalin content of the saliva occurs usually in the aged. Psychic stimuli such as profound emotion or fear result commonly in temporary asialorrhea. Such forms of temporary cessation of salivary flow are of little clinical significance.

Any systemic disease which is accompanied by a high temperature or dehydration will result in diminished salivation. A dry mouth is a characteristic clinical finding in the uncontrolled diabetic patient, the typhoid patient and the patient ill with pneumonia. Richman and Abarbanel noted a decreased salivary flow in post-menopausal patients which disappeared following estradiol or diethylstilbestrol therapy.

Disturbances in the innervating mechanism of the salivary glands will also give rise to diminished salivary flow. The break in the nerve reflex mechanism may be due to traumatic injury to the nerves carrying the secretory fibres or a central nervous system injury. Dry mouth is a common symptom in epidemic encephalitis and some brain tumors. It may be necessary to determine whether the asialorrhea is due to actual dysfunction of the salivary gland, or some break in the nerve pathways controlling salivation.

If salivary flow can be stimulated by a centrally acting sialogogue such as pilocarpine, but not by a peripheral acting one such as lemon juice, it indicates a defect in the taste bud-salivary center pathway and the integrity of the salivary center-salivary gland pathway as well as the secretory ability of the salivary glands. Certain neurologic findings suggest that the parotid glands do not have bilateral innervation.

Belladonna, atropine, ephedrine and related drugs have a marked effect on secretory function. They cause asialorrhea. In some instances the therapeutic effect of the drug is judged by the decrease in salivary flow. Irradiation of the cervicofacial region results commonly in diminished salivation or a cessation of salivary flow. The mucosal inflammation caused by the radiation and the mechanical irritation secondary to the decreased flow of saliva produce a persistent, painful stomatitis.

In marked vitamin A deficiency states, metaplastic changes occur in the salivary glands which limit their secretory function. Because of the rarity of this condition it is of little clinical importance. Patients with a nutritional deficiency of the B complex type, especially nicotinic acid deficiency, often complain of a dry mouth.

In an occasional patient there is a temporary decrease in the flow of saliva when artificial dentures are first worn. Xerostomia in denture-wearing patients is particularly annoying because of the lack of retention of the dentures and the irritation to the denture-supporting tissues.

The oral mucosa becomes glossy, dry and roughened in xerostomia. Painful cracks and fissures which bleed easily may develop. The tongue at first is abnormally coated but later almost complete atrophy of the papillary layer takes place.

The exact cause of the decreased salivary flow must be determined before effective therapy can be instituted. If the dry mouth is associated with a nutritional deficiency, vitamin therapy should be beneficial. Saphir obtained good results following the administration of nicotinic acid 50 mg. t.i.d. The author found nicotinamide of value in stimulating salivary flow in patients with nutritional deficiency and those with temporary asialorrhea following non-specific forms of parotitis. This form of treatment is of no value if the secretory function of the glands has been lost.

Pilocarpine hydrochloride will stimulate salivary flow if the nerve pathways between the central nervous system and the salivary glands are still intact and the glands still possess secretory ability. Prinz recommended the following for this purpose:

> Rx Pilocarpine hydrochloride   0.3 cc.
>   Distilled water   15.0 cc.
>   Sig.   Five drops in a little water 3 times a
>   day after meals. Increase the dose every 3rd
>   day by 1 drop until 8 to 10 drops per dose are
>   taken.

Since it is rare that xerostomia results from disturbances of innervation, pilocarpine administration is not a panacea.

Symptomatic relief can be given the patient with xerostomia. Ordinary paraffin oil (Nujol), or 50% glycerine flavored with lemon oil, will relieve many of the annoying symptoms. Denture-wearing patients with xerostomia should coat their dentures with petrolatum or one of the many lubricating jellies or a denture powder. These agents will assist in retention of the denture and reduce the mechanical irritation of the denture-supporting tissues. Petrolatum, almond oil or cold cream are useful on the lips.

Obstruction to Normal Salivary Flow

Salivary calculi or stones within the salivary ducts are a common cause of decreased salivary flow. Calculi are found most often in the duct of the submaxillary gland (Wharton's duct), although their occurrence in the parotid duct is not unusual. Pelner called attention to the importance of uncalcified material, such as inspissated mucus or cellular debris, as a cause of obstruction. Pressure on the salivary ducts from pathologic processes of the surrounding tissues results at times in partial or complete blockage of salivary flow. A large ranula may prevent the flow of saliva from Wharton's duct and give rise to secondary symptoms in the submaxillary gland.

The symptoms of obstruction of a salivary duct are similar, regardless of the cause of the obstruction. The firm capsules surrounding the salivary

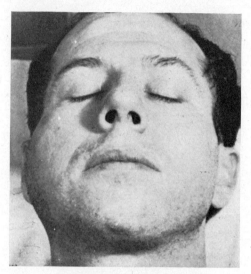

FIG. 141. Swelling associated with stone in parotid duct.

glands prevent enlargement of these organs with the production of painful symptoms. The patient experiences periodic painful swellings of the salivary gland whose duct is obstructed. The painful swellings develop at times at the thought or sight of food and they are always more marked after eating. The swellings appear rapidly when the stoppage of the salivary flow is complete and the secretion of saliva is copious. When there is only partial blockage of the duct, the pain and swelling are not such prominent symptoms. There is no evidence of inflammation unless secondary infection of the gland has developed.

Following a period in which the periodic salivary swellings are experienced, the symptoms may gradually disappear, due in part to compensatory changes occurring within the gland such as pressure atrophy. In chronic cases of obstruction, calcified material may be found in the salivary gland itself.

When there is stasis of salivary flow, the salivary gland itself is predisposed to infection. Chronic inflammation occurs most often in the submaxillary gland. In chronic cases of inflammation, surgical removal of the gland is indicated. This procedure is difficult because of the close proximity of important anatomic structures.

The diagnosis of obstruction of a salivary duct can usually be made on the basis of: (1) the relation of the swelling to eating; (2) the result of bidigital or bimanual palpation; (3) roentgenologic studies; and (4) the stimulation of salivary flow by means of citric acid (2%) for diagnostic purposes.

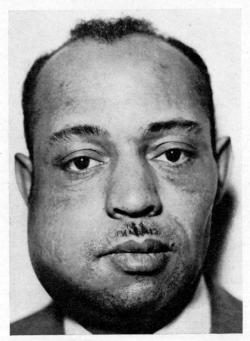

FIG. 142. Swelling in a patient with acute circumcoronitis of an erupting lower third molar. This type of swelling must be differentiated from that present in epidemic parotitis, or a stone in the parotid duct. This swelling is lower and more diffuse in outline.

Bidigital or bimanual palpation is useful in demonstrating large calculi in Wharton's duct, but the smaller deposits cannot be so readily detected by this method. Roentgenograms are a great aid in revealing the presence and location of the calcareous material particularly when it is small. X-rays should always be taken to determine whether calcified material has been deposited in the gland proper. A more difficult method of visualizing the location of the obstruction consists of canulating the salivary duct, carefully injecting some radio-opaque material and then taking x-rays. This procedure requires skill and involves a slight risk of introducing infection.

The treatment of salivary calculi is chiefly by means of surgery. Pelner reported success in the treatment of parotid duct obstruction due to inspissated mucus by the hypodermic administration of 1 cc. of 1:2,000 prostigmine methylsulfate.

Postoperative Parotitis

Postoperative parotitis is a pyogenic infection of the parotid glands which develops following abdominal operations and particularly those involving the

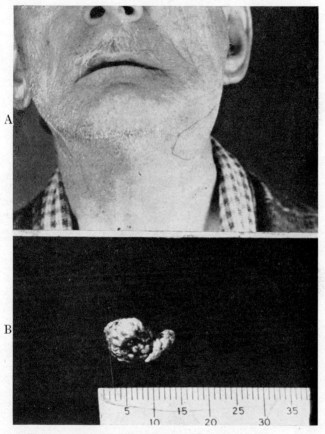

FIG. 143. (A) Swelling of the left submaxillary gland due to a stone in Wharton's duct. (B) Stone removed from above patient. (Patient of Dr. Henry A. Miller, Philadelphia, Pa.)

gastro-intestinal tract. It is one of the many complications that can occur when major operations are performed on patients with unhygienic mouths.

Postoperative parotitis is believed to result from an ascending infection by way of Stenson's duct as the bacteria isolated from the involved glands do not correspond to the type found at the site of the operation. Mucin exerts an inhibitory effect on staphylococci and the lack of this substance in the parotid secretion may explain in part the frequent involvement of the parotid glands. Postoperative parotitis is uncommon in individuals with good oral hygiene. Poor oral hygiene, decreased salivary flow due to diminished glandular function, medication (atropine) or dehydration are important predisposing factors.

The glandular symptoms develop usually 5 to 7 days following the operation. The patient complains of pain and swelling of the involved gland. The swelling may appear first just in front of the lobe of the ear where the parotid

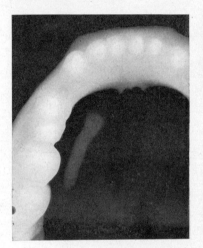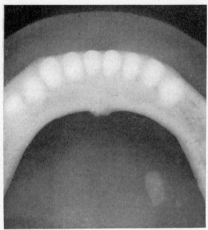

Fig. 144. (*Left*) Roentgenogram demonstrating a long oval calcareous obstruction in Wharton's duct.

Fig. 145. (*Right*) Roentgenogram demonstrating nodular calcareous deposit in Wharton's duct.

capsule is less dense. Pus can be observed flowing from the opening of the duct, or it can be produced by a slight milking action. Frank abscess formation in the gland occurs rarely.

The treatment of postoperative parotitis requires the establishment of free drainage through the duct. This can be accomplished by gentle massage or the careful passage of a filiform ureteral sound. The sulfonamides and penicillin should be effective chemotherapeutic agents.

Roentgen-ray irradiation is an effective form of treatment, once drainage is established. Gum-chewing, sucking hard candy and drinking sour beverages are used to stimulate salivary secretion. External incision is rarely required.

Inflammation of the salivary ducts and glands due to pyogenic organisms is likely when there is interference with the normal flow of saliva. Acute pyogenic infections may follow attempts to canulate the ducts of the gland or the injection of radio-opaque substances. In addition to the painful swellings the patients exhibit local and systemic signs of an acute inflammatory process.

Mumps (*Epidemic Parotitis*)

Mumps is an acute highly contagious virus disease which is characterized by painful enlargement of the parotid or other salivary glands. It is regarded as a systemic rather than a local disease as the testicles, the ovaries, the pancreas and the brain may be affected.

Mumps is most common between the ages of 4 and 14 but it represented an important military problem in World War I, ranking among the three most frequent causes of hospitalization. The disease occurs in endemic and epidemic fashion. It is believed to be transmitted by salivary droplets with the greatest infectivity occurring just before and during the onset of symptoms. The virus is present in the saliva during the first 48 hours of the disease. One attack confers usually a lasting immunity.

Symptoms. The general symptoms of mumps include increased irritability, anorexia, headache, malaise, muscle aches and at times gastro-intestinal disturbances and a fever of 101° to 102° F. A moderate lymphocytosis may be present.

Regional pain usually precedes the characteristic parotid swelling. In mumps, the pain is intensified by external pressure, jaw movements or the stimulation of salivary flow. The glandular swelling follows in a short time. While bilateral parotid involvement occurs in approximately 70% of the cases one side frequently precedes the other by several days. A more generalized unilateral swelling occurs when both the parotid and submaxillary glands are involved. The sublingual glands are rarely affected.

The characteristic swelling in mumps occurs just anterior to and below the ear. The anterior border of the enlarged parotid can often be palpated from within the mouth. Erythema of the opening of Stenson's duct is a common clinical finding. In severe cases it may be impossible to separate the teeth, to chew or to swallow without difficulty. If the affected parts remain at rest the pain is not severe—an important point in differential diagnosis.

The extra-oral complications of mumps, such as orchitis, ovaritis and encephalitis, are of little dental interest. The dental practitioner is concerned with differentiating mumps from other lesions which might give rise to similar subjective and clinical symptoms.

Enders *et al.* have developed a skin test which is useful in determining immunity to mumps. The antigen used is a heat inactivated suspension of the parotid gland of a monkey infected with the virus of mumps. An erythematous area greater than 10 x 10 mm., with rare exceptions, means immunity against the mumps virus. This test is of no value as an aid in diagnosis since as long as three months following the onset of the disease is required to develop the hypersensitivity.

Differential Diagnosis. There is no specific laboratory test for the diagnosis of mumps. The following conditions may also cause swellings in the parotid region.

(1) Acute dento-alveolar abscess. A careful inquiry as to previous dental symptoms or treatment of posterior teeth is helpful. X-rays are important aids. In a dento-alveolar abscess the pain is not intensified by stimulants to

salivary flow and it persists even with the parts at rest. The anterior border of the parotid cannot be palpated. The skin temperature of the swelling may be increased. In mumps the swelling is more anterior and closer to the ear than that found in swellings of dental origin.

Unilateral parotid and submaxillary involvement in mumps may be confused with a dento-alveolar abscess, particularly if a diseased molar is also present on the affected side.

A   B

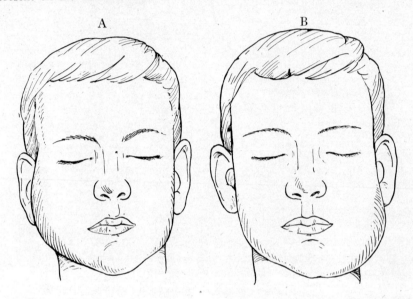

FIG. 146. (A) Typical location and configuration of swelling associated with epidemic parotitis. (B) Usual location and configuration of swelling associated with abscessed mandibular molars.

(2) Septic parotitis. Glandular enlargement secondary to salivary calculus or some other obstruction of the duct system is characterized by intermittent, painful swellings which are usually related to the ingestion of food or other stimulation of salivary flow. Both intra-oral and extra-oral palpation of the ducts is helpful. Careful probing of the duct, x-ray studies with or without lipiodol injections will usually permit a diagnosis.

(3) Mikulicz's syndrome, uveoparotid fever, tuberculosis of the parotid gland, parotid cysts and mixed tumors of the parotid are rarer possibilities which must also be considered.

Uveoparotid Fever—Uveoparotitis

Uveoparotitis is a syndrome characterized by parotitis, uveitis (inflammation of the uveal tract of the eye), and a low-grade fever which is thought to be due to a filtrable virus. It is most commonly found in the 2nd and 3rd decades. Pulmonary tuberculosis is an associated finding in some cases. There may be some relation between this disease and Boeck's sarcoid.

The parotid glands often become enlarged, hard and tender before there are any other manifestations of the syndrome. The swelling may last for months or even years. The overlying skin does not become adherent to the swollen glands and suppuration is rare. Nausea and vomiting are often present. The pupils are sluggish, dilated or irregular. Fever is a variable find-

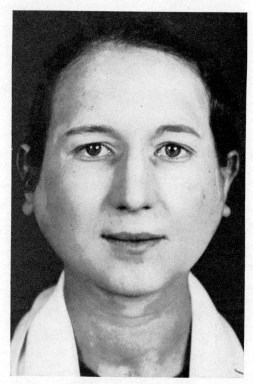

FIG. 147. Bilateral swelling in uveoparotitis. (Michelson and Becker, Arch. Dermat. and Syph., 39:329, 1939.)

ing. There is no specific treatment for this disease, which is usually self-limited.

More rarely, the salivary glands are involved as a part of a generalized disease process such as tuberculosis, actinomycosis or syphilis. Unless the more common symptoms of these diseases are manifested, the definitive diagnosis of the salivary gland enlargement is difficult. Tuberculosis of the parotid gland may present a real diagnostic problem.

Mikulicz's Disease

Mikulicz's disease consists of a symmetrical, noninflammatory swelling of the lacrimal, orbital glands and one or more pairs of the salivary glands. At times the accessory glands in the tongue and hard palate are also enlarged. The swellings are not adherent to the surrounding structures. The multiple swollen glands produce a gargoyle-like appearance to the patient. There is little if any constitutional reaction associated with the multiple glandular swellings. The causative agent is not known. The disease runs usually a protracted course.

True Mikulicz's disease should be distinguished from Mikulicz's syndrome in which the enlargement of the glands is due to some disease such as leukemia, Hodgkin's disease, uveoparotid fever, syphilis or tuberculosis. Submaxillary gland swellings must also be differentiated from adenitis of this region.

Schaffer and Jacobsen classified these conditions as follows:

CLASSIFICATION OF MIKULICZ'S DISEASE BY SCHAFFER & JACOBSEN

I. MIKULICZ'S DISEASE.
   (a) Familial type.
   (b) Mikulicz's disease proper.
II. MIKULICZ'S SYNDROME.
   (a) Leukemia.
   (b) Tuberculosis.
   (c) Syphilis(?).
   (d) Lymphosarcoma.
   (e) Toxic reactions to lead, iodides, etc.
   (f) Gout(?).
   (g) Febris uvero-parotidea subchronica.

Miller and Eusterman reported a case of Mikulicz's syndrome which was due to a lymphosarcoma of a low grade of malignancy with involvement of the stomach and the lungs. Walker found arsenic and potassium iodide therapy of benefit in the treatment of Mikulicz's disease. In some cases the affected glands had to be removed surgically.

Tumors of the Salivary Glands

Tumors of the salivary glands are of interest to the dental practitioner because of their location. Most of the neoplasms of the salivary glands are referred to as "mixed tumors" of the salivary glands because of the many tissue types present in these growths. Cartilage, bone, fibrillar connective tissue, adipose, muscle, lymphoid tissue, glandular and squamous epithelium may be present. Dockerty & Mayo found that the mixed salivary tumors occurred 4 to 5 times as often as adenocarcinoma of the cylindroma type.

Mixed salivary tumors are common between 25 and 50 years of age with about an equal distribution in the two sexes. They appear in general at an earlier age than the adenocarcinomas. These mixed tumors have a predilection for the parotid region; in the submaxillary area, the mixed tumors are only about one-tenth as common.

Mixed salivary tumors are characterized by their slow growth and the general lack of pain and tenderness. Tumors involving the soft and hard palates are usually recognized earlier by the patient, due to interference with chewing and swallowing. The tumors metastasize rarely but they may become locally destructive. Rarely they show true malignant tendencies.

The treatment of these growths is by surgery. McFarland found that recurrences were more common when the growth was removed while it was still small. Salivary fistulae or facial paralysis are possible complications following the removal of large extra-oral tumors. Postoperative recurrences of a mixed tumor are common.

PLUMMER-VINSON SYNDROME

Plummer and Vinson described a group of patients, chiefly women, who had dysphagia, anemia and atrophy of the mucosae of the upper gastro-intestinal tract. The tongue was smooth, enlarged, bright red and dry. The rest of the oral mucosa had a dull color. The oral commissure was small and inelastic with frequent fissuring at the corners. Some of these patients had lost their teeth early in life and many were completely edentulous. In common with other patients with secondary anemia, they often complained of sore mouths and their inability to wear dentures comfortably. Relative degrees of achlorhydria were also present.

Pharyngeal and intra-oral carcinoma are common in individuals presenting the above symptoms. Ahlbom analyzed 250 cases of carcinoma of the mouth and upper respiratory tract occurring in women and found that 70% of the patients had the Plummer-Vinson syndrome. Cahn has reported such a case in detail.

Since the oral symptoms in this syndrome are similar to those observed in B complex deficiency, we must consider the possibility of a common, perhaps nutritional, underlying background. The dentist should be on the alert for patients with these symptoms and see that they have the benefit of good medical care.

GASTRIC ULCER (PEPTIC ULCER—STOMACH ULCER)

Gastric ulcer is a fairly common complaint of middle life, occurring less frequently in the adolescent. It is prone to develop in males, particularly those of a nervous and emotional temperament and it is claimed by some that there is a definite "ulcer habitus."

The various theories of ulcer formation include trauma, localized vascular changes in the form of infarcts or spasm and infection from various foci. Another theory suggests that the ulcers are the result of a pre-existing hyperacidity. Extensive skin burns and certain cerebral lesions produce large ulcerations of the stomach walls by a mechanism not clearly understood.

Symptoms

The usual ulcer patient complains of pain and discomfort when the stomach is empty. The pain is localized to a fairly small area on the anterior abdominal wall. The pain in gastric ulcer is related to the acidity of the gastric contents. It is relieved by foods, particularly proteins, which combine with large amounts of acid. The patient on his own may become accustomed to frequent feedings or to the use of antacids to relieve the pain.

At times hemorrhage from the ulcer or frank hematemesis may be the presenting symptoms. Ulcer patients experience frequently a considerable loss of weight. The most serious complication of gastric ulcer results from perforation and subsequent peritonitis. Periods of quiescence and exacerbation of symptoms are characteristic. Gastric ulcers do not predispose to malignancy of the stomach. In the typical ulcer case the diagnosis can be made on the basis of the history and the symptoms with the characteristic localized pain which is relieved by food or antacids. Gastric analysis reveals usually a hyperchlorhydria. Roentgenologic studies will indicate the actual site and the approximate depth of the ulcer when it is located on a favorable area for examination. In such cases repeated roentgenologic study is of value in following the response to treatment.

The correct management of the ulcer patient is a widely discussed subject. Early cases are essentially a medical problem, whereas a perforated gastric ulcer is a surgical emergency. Surgery is also indicated in cases that fail to respond to medical treatment.

The usual medical treatment consists of bed rest, frequent feedings of liquids and soft foods containing large quantities of cream and milk. Gradually other foods are added, avoiding rough ones or those which are active in stimulating gastric secretion. Since saliva hastens the clotting of blood Hunter recommended that the salivary flow be stimulated in patients with bleeding gastric ulcer, by chewing.

Antacids are given to neutralize the hyperacidity, relieve the pain and promote healing. The time-honored Sippy powders are familiar. The various amphoteric gels, aluminum hydroxide, magnesium hydroxide and trisilicate gels are effective neutralizing agents and in addition they do not tend to cause alkalosis.

Oral Aspects

The oral aspects of gastroduodenal ulcer can be grouped as follows:

(1) The possible etiologic role of dental foci of infection.
(2) The importance of dental foci of infection or faulty chewing as aggravating or perpetuating factors of gastric ulcer.
(3) Associated oral changes in patients with gastroduodenal ulcer.

The Possible Etiologic Role of Dental Foci of Infection. The etiologic role of periapical or periodontal infection in the "ulcer patient" is difficult to assess, as much of the evidence is based on laboratory studies which are open to some question. Rosenow, Haden and others demonstrated that the organisms isolated from the tooth apices of patients with gastric ulcer have an elective localizing faculty for the gastric mucosa of the experimental animal. Montier and others were unable to confirm these findings and Miloslavich claimed that the lesions produced by Rosenow et al. were not ulcers, but multiple pyemic abscesses of the gastric mucosa. Holman pointed out that spontaneous ulcers were prone to develop in the pylorus and duodenum of dogs and he questioned whether the lesions in the experimental animals were of exogenous origin.

The clinical evidence supporting the etiologic importance of oral infection is equally inconclusive. Numerous bacteriologic studies have demonstrated similar organisms in the ulcer (usually the stomach contents), and in the oral focus. This is no evidence of an etiologic role. Alvarez, a clinician of considerable experience and reputation, was not impressed by the infectious theory of ulcer formation and consequently the part oral foci may play. The infection theory for instance fails to explain the predominance of gastroduodenal ulcers in males. The proper assessment of any etiologic relation between dental infection and ulcer formation must await more complete knowledge as to the actual etiology of the gastric ulcer.

Dental Foci of Infection or Faulty Chewing as Aggravating or Perpetuating Factors. The importance of oral foci of infection or a deficient masticatory apparatus as aggravating or perpetuating factors is more clearly understood. The gastric secretion is supposed to sterilize infected material which may be swallowed. If pus, from periodontal foci, is swallowed with the food, it may be protected from the gastric juice and by its action on the ulcer delay healing.

Montonari believed that some stomach ulcers are due to actual bacterial vascular emboli. Chewing is followed frequently by transient bacteremias when periodontal disease is present. These bacteria may localize in the region of the ulcer due to an anachoretic effect and aggravate the existing pathologic process.

Individuals with diseased gums, and especially those with a dysfunctional masticatory apparatus, have difficulty in adequately comminuting their food prior to swallowing. This large particle size has an adverse effect on the ulcer as well as the digestive function as a whole. This is shown clearly by the gain in weight and improved general condition of the edentulous "ulcer patient" after the insertion of dentures. It has also been observed that the presence of oral foci favors ulcer recurrence after operation. Jaenisch stressed the importance of the elimination of oral foci if one is to achieve permanent results in the treatment of this type of patient.

Associated Oral Changes in Patients with Gastroduodenal Ulcer. The general physical form of the individual bears an important relationship to disease. Draper *et al.* found that the usual anthropometric measurements including those of the palate, jaws and teeth differed significantly in the "ulcer" and the "gallbladder" patient, and both were apart from the normal findings. The jaw indexes were particularly significant. The comparison of the gonial angle (the angle formed by the ascending and horizontal rami of the mandible) and the anterior jaw index (the relation of the anterior jaw breadth to posterior jaw breadth) is shown in the accompanying illustration.

The incisor teeth in the "gallbladder" patient were noted to be shorter, broader and heavier than those of the "ulcer" patient. In the former, the first incisors were squarer and both second incisors were almost as broad as the first incisors and worn to a greater degree. In the "gallbladder" patient, the incisors were straight or in lingual version as contrasted to a tendency toward labioversion in the "ulcer" patient.

Gastro-enterologists are well acquainted with the poor oral conditions in this group of patients who commonly have widespread dental caries, periodontal disease and numerous missing teeth. Langstroth showed that oral sepsis is more frequent in these patients than in suitable control subjects. Schwindt described oral mucosal changes which are observed commonly in patients with gastric or duodenal ulcer. They consisted of multiple, round

A   B

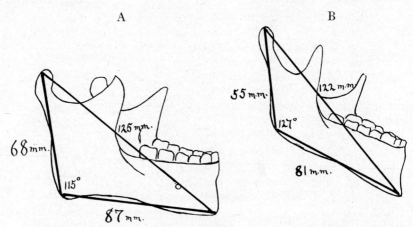

Fig. 148. Diagram showing differences in the mandibles of gallbladder type (A) and ulcer type (B). (From Draper, Dupertuis and Caughney, Human Constitution in Clinical Medicine, Paul B. Hoeber, Inc.)

or oval, confluent epithelial defects (depapillation) of the tongue which disappeared on the healing of the ulcers. These lesions were frequently multiple, often symmetrical and non-painful.

Gastric ulcer patients treated with the Sippy regime have a heavily coated tongue and a notoriously foul breath. This results from the soft milk and cream diet which favors the formation of a heavy coating on the tongue. Bacterial decomposition of food particles retained in the tongue coating accounts for the breath. When the original Sippy formulae were used which included bismuth subcarbonate, it was not unusual for these patients to develop oral symptoms of bismuth intolerance.

Vomiting occurs frequently in the gastric ulcer patients. Over a period of years this persistent vomiting, or rumination, will result in a loss of tooth substance due to the acid-containing material. Loss of tooth substance due to such causes is called perimolysis.

THE LIVER AND BILIARY SYSTEM

The liver is an important organ which can be regarded as a chemical refinery, a storehouse for important foods and as a place where numerous waste

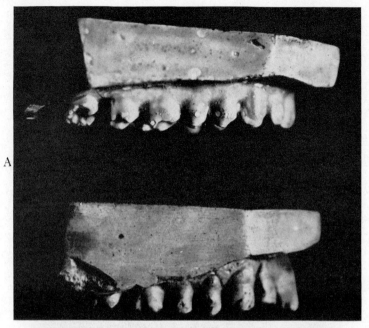

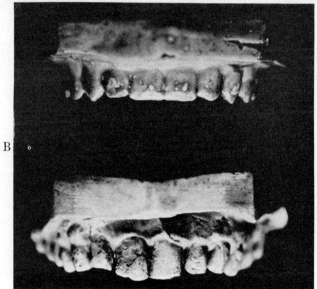

Fig. 149. Casts of upper jaws. (A) Seen from in front. Upper cast: gallbladder type. Lower cast: ulcer. (B) Seen in profile. Upper cast: gallbladder. Lower cast: ulcer. (From Draper, Dupertuis and Caughney, Human Constitution in Clinical Medicine, Paul B. Hoeber, Inc.)

products are broken down or detoxified so that they may be eliminated easily from the body. Many important substances which are concerned with the defense mechanisms of the body are elaborated in this organ.

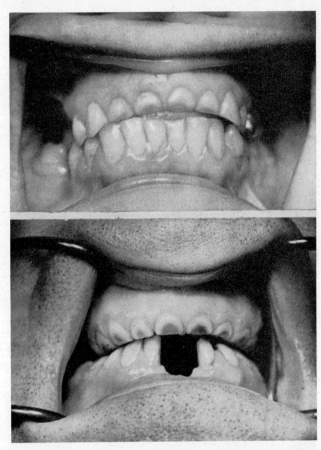

FIG. 150. Perimolysis or disappearance of tooth substance due to persisting vomiting over a period of three years in a 54-year-old woman with duodenal ulcer. The loss of tooth substance was most marked on the palatal surface of the maxillary anteriors.

FIG. 151. Unusual disappearance of tooth substance. No systemic disease, occupational or personal habits were discovered which could explain this peculiar loss of tooth substance.

The gallbladder and the biliary system are closely related both anatomically and functionally to the liver. The biliary system and the gallbladder function as a collecting duct system and a storage place for the bile which is elaborated in the liver. Since these organs function more or less as a unit the diseases of the liver and biliary apparatus will be considered together.

Jaundice

Jaundice or icterus is a symptom rather than a disease which results from an excess of bile pigment in the circulation. This excess bile pigment may be due to the failure of the liver cells to excrete the bile or to a blockage of the biliary system. The forms of jaundice of interest to the dentist are: (1) icterus gravis (see dental diseases in infancy), (2) catarrhal jaundice, (3) obstructive jaundice and (4) non-obstructive jaundice.

Catarrhal (Infectious Jaundice). Catarrhal jaundice occurs commonly in children and young adults—mostly males. In some cases there is evidence of an infectious agent but the exact cause is rarely determined. Catarrhal jaundice follows severe emotional disturbances, mild gastro-intestinal upsets or temporary obstruction of the bile ducts.

While not serious, catarrhal jaundice produces rather profound symptoms. The patient experiences first malaise, lack of normal appetite, nausea and, at times, vomiting. As the disease progresses, pruritus becomes marked and the individual feels miserable. The typical greenish-yellow color of the skin, which does not lessen the subjective symptoms, furnishes objective evidence of the deranged liver function. A mild elevation of temperature is commonly experienced during the acute stages of the disease. The treatment is symptomatic and dietary. Catarrhal jaundice is rarely fatal.

ORAL ASPECTS. The tongue is coated and the increase in bile pigments in the circulating blood is manifested by the yellowish-green color of the oral mucosa, particularly at the junction of the soft and hard palates.

In all jaundiced patients there is danger of prolonged hemorrhage following dental extractions or any surgical procedure. If surgery is necessary in jaundiced patients, they should receive prophylactic administration of vitamin K before the operation. This applies to all forms of jaundice.

Obstructive. Most cases of jaundice are of the obstructive type. In this form of jaundice, the bile is formed by the liver cells but its elimination is impeded. This may be due to stoppage within the duct system resulting from stones or inspissated bile, muscular spasm or to external pressure on the biliary passages associated with infectious or neoplastic lesions in the vicinity of the biliary system. Common bile duct blockage due to gallstones and pressure from new growths, particularly carcinoma of the head of the pancreas, are common causes of obstructive jaundice.

The symptoms of obstructive jaundice consist of greenish yellow discoloration of the skin and mucosae, pruritus, nausea, anorexia, clay-colored stools which are frequently associated with constipation, and the light yellow to green color of the urine and other body excretions. Obstructive jaundice is diagnosed on the clinical symptoms and the laboratory studies of the stools and urine. The van den Berg reaction is said to differentiate obstructive from nonobstructive forms of jaundice.

The treatment of obstructive jaundice requires the elimination of the cause of obstruction.

Nonobstructive (Hemolytic Jaundice). Nonobstructive jaundice results from an excessive hemolysis or destruction of the erythrocytes due to:

(1) an inherent abnormality in the cells (familial hemolytic icterus); (2) some acute disease; or (3) certain drugs or poisonous agents.

Acquired hemolytic jaundice is usually secondary to some acute infectious disease such as malaria, dysentery or syphilis. It is associated with a markedly enlarged spleen, abdominal and general symptoms similar to those experienced in catarrhal jaundice with the exception that they are less marked. Certain drugs also have a marked hemolytic effect. The nitrobenzene derivatives and also neo-arsphenamine may result in hemolytic jaundice (anemia). This property of phenylhydrazine is utilized in the treatment of polycythemia vera.

The diagnosis of hemolytic anemia is based on the clinical findings, the blood count and the erythrocyte fragility test which is characterized by a decreased resistance of the erythrocytes to hemolysis. Splenectomy is followed usually by prompt and permanent regression of all symptoms.

Liver Necrosis

Necrosis of the liver parenchyma results at times as a part of the syndrome of "toxemia of pregnancy" or intoxication due to drugs such as chloroform, cinchophen or neo-arsphenamine.

Hepatic Abscesses

Because of its relation to the portal and venous circulations, the liver may be the seat of pyogenic or parasitic abscesses. The pyogenic liver abscesses result from a generalized septicemia or from infected emboli derived from a pyelophlebitis in the pelvic region or from a suppurative process in the gastro-intestinal tract. Solitary liver abscesses due to the *Entamoeba histolytica* are not uncommon in patients with amebic dysentery. Echinococcal (hydatid) cysts are also prone to localize in the liver. Hepatic abscesses rupture frequently through the diaphragm into the lung or into the peritoneal cavity or bowels. Treatment is surgical.

DISEASES OF THE GALLBLADDER

Gallbladder disease may be functional or anatomic or both. The failure of this organ to empty properly following the usual stimulus retards the normal digestive processes. Chronic gallbladder infection (cholecystitis) not only interferes with normal fat metabolism but it predisposes to the development of gall stones (cholelithiasis).

Over 50% of the cases of cholecystitis are infected with the colon-typhoid group of organisms. This indicates probably a retrograde infection from the gastro-intestinal tract, but gall stones and other sources of infection, including oral foci, are known to be important etiologic factors. The chronically infected gallbladder may itself be a primary focus of infection. It is the common primary focus in typhoid carriers.

The symptoms associated with gallbladder and biliary tract disease consist of recurrent attacks of severe abdominal pain which is localized to the right upper quadrant of the abdomen, nausea and at times vomiting. These attacks follow frequently some dietary indiscretion, particularly the ingestion of fried foods or those containing large amounts of fat. In some cases only a vague discomfort and flatulence after the eating of fatty foods are experienced.

The diagnosis of gallbladder disease is based on the clinical history, the results of duodenal intubation studies and roentgenologic examinations which utilize radio-opaque materials which are secreted in the bile and concentrated in the gallbladder (cholecystography). These examinations are made following the ingestion of a test meal containing large amounts of fats. Thus it is possible to visualize the biliary secretion and its concentration in the gallbladder.

The treatment of gallbladder disease is both medical and surgical.

Oral Aspects

The early reports dealing with the association of periodontal disease and gallbladder disease were concerned chiefly with the effect of oral infection on the development of gall stones or cholecystitis. Rosenow showed that organisms recovered from dental and tonsillar infection in patients with gallbladder disease had an elective localizing property for this organ when injected in animals. As in other diseases, scattered reports of cure of cholecystitis following the removal of oral foci of infection have appeared in the literature. Oral infection may serve as a focus for cholecystitis but its clinical significance is certainly difficult to assess.

The detailed clinical studies made by Kelly, Gunter and Churchill on patients with periodontal disease, which failed to respond to the usual forms of local treatment, revealed an infected gallbladder or faulty gallbladder function in the majority of the cases. This study suggests that the oral lesions so frequently encountered in patients with gallbladder disease may be the result of disturbed nutrition due to the cholecystitis rather than the cause of the cholecystitis.

BANTI'S SYNDROME OR DISEASE

Banti's syndrome is characterized by splenomegaly, hepatic cirrhosis and anemia. Its etiology is unknown. The latest etiologic theory suggests that Banti's syndrome results from a variety of conditions which produce a chronic splenic hypertension. Important secondary symptoms are those associated with portal cirrhosis, such as esophageal varices and other manifestations of collateral portal circulation. Peroral hemorrhage has been reported.

HEMOCHROMATOSIS (BRONZE DIABETES)

Hemochromatosis is characterized by an abnormal deposition of hemosiderin, an iron pigment, in the skin and mucosae, including those of the mouth and the viscera. The skin pigmentation results in a coppery or bronze coloration which is particularly prominent on the exposed portions of the face. Cirrhosis of the liver and pancreas occur early, the involvement of the pancreatic insular tissue supposedly giving rise to the symptoms of diabetes mellitus.

Diagnosis is made on the clinical findings and the demonstration of hemosiderin in large quantities in the skin. While this disease is uncommon, it may be the cause of oral mucosal pigmentation.

APPENDICITIS

Appendicitis or inflammation of the vermiform appendix is probably the most frequent surgical emergency occurring in man. It is common in the urban population, less so in the rural population and rare in primitive groups. It occurs most often between the 10th and 35th years of age.

The exact causative agent is not known. Numerous local anatomic and mechanical factors may predispose to appendicitis, but it is believed that in most cases the clinical onset results from the passage of infected material from the cecum into the appendix. Fecal matter, fruit seeds, foreign bodies, including a tooth, have been found in removed appendices but their etiologic importance is small. Streptococci and the colon bacilli are most frequently cultured from the appendix.

The classical symptoms of appendicitis consist of sudden cramp-like pains appearing first throughout the abdomen but later becoming localized to the lower right quadrant. Nausea and vomiting are common. Pain, tenderness and muscular rigidity over the region of the appendix are characteristic. Fever may be moderate.

The diagnosis of appendicitis is made on the history of the attack and a careful physical examination. Leukocytosis is present in most cases and many surgeons consider it an important diagnostic aid.

Early surgical intervention will minimize the development of complications. The rupture of a gangrenous appendix with generalized peritonitis is the most common complication. This may result from the indiscriminate administration of cathartics. Recent advances in chemotherapy have lessened the danger of many of the complications, but even now many people still die of appendicitis or its complications.

Oral Aspects

Evidence associating oral disease with appendiceal infection is mainly of the case-history type in which an acute appendicitis has followed an attack of angina or tonsillitis. Rosenow showed that the organisms commonly isolated from the appendix have elective localizing properties when injected intravenously in animals. The anatomic relation and physiologic function of the appendix in the animals he used are not comparable to man.

Billings described a case of acute appendicitis following an attack of Vincent's angina in which fusospirochetal organisms were demonstrated in the appendix. Repeated attacks of appendicitis have also been described which occurred after root canal therapy. The organisms found commonly in the mouth, including the fusospirochetal organisms, have been isolated by Goadby and others from the diseased appendix.

Recent etiologic theories of appendicitis, which place less emphasis on the hematogenous route of origin and more on the enterogenous source of infection, minimize still more the significance of oral infection in appendicitis.

INTESTINAL TRACT DISEASES

Many of the diseases of the intestinal tract have few, if any, dental implications. They are mentioned briefly merely to acquaint the dentist with their existence.

Intestinal Obstruction

Intestinal obstruction is of considerable importance in both medicine and surgery. While it is always of immediate seriousness, the eventual prognosis is dependent on the cause of the obstruction. In the later decades of life, neoplastic growths in the intestinal tract or in the adjacent structures are common causes. Specific infectious processes such as tuberculosis, the ulcerations associated with dysentery or typhoid fever, or regional ileitis, may result in adhesions which give rise to intestinal obstruction.

In the middle decades, a loop of the gut occasionally becomes twisted (volvulus) and causes obstruction. Swallowed foreign bodies may become lodged in the intestinal tract. Cases of obstruction due to swallowed dental appliances have been reported. In young children, a portion of one segment of the intestine occasionally telescopes within a more distal part of the gut (intussusception), resulting in obstruction.

The diagnosis of intestinal obstruction is made on the basis of the history, the typical clinical and physical findings and x-ray studies. The treatment usually consists of early surgical intervention before gangrene and rupture of the intestine have occurred. The ultimate prognosis is dependent on the amenability of the obstruction to surgical treatment or removal.

Diverticulitis

Small sac-like portions of the intestines may develop, especially in the sigmoid and descending colon, during middle life. The accumulated fecal material and bacteria in these outpouchings give rise to inflammatory changes and a variety of symptoms which may simulate much more serious diseases. Pain and tenderness are usually noted in the region of the involved bowel, usually in the lower left quadrant. Diarrhea or constipation may be present. When small abscess formation occurs, partial intestinal obstruction may result. Diagnosis can only be made by means of gastro-intestinal x-ray studies.

Hirschsprung's Disease (Congenital Megacolon)

This rare disease represents a developmental or congenital anomaly which is characterized by a marked increase in size of the descending colon. A wide variety of secondary gastro-intestinal symptoms may be experienced, but persistent constipation is the outstanding symptom. At times surgery is indicated. Patients with this disease who reach maturity are often able to carry on almost normal activities. The case reported by Collins is of a practicing dentist.

TYPHOID FEVER

Typhoid fever, like diphtheria, once the scourge of city and country alike, is now mainly of historical interest. Typhoid fever is an outstanding example of a disease which has been controlled effectively by public health measures. This disease is caused by the *Eberthella typhosa*. It is transmitted by means of contaminated water supplies or food. Typhoid carriers serve as reservoirs of the disease.

Patients experience headache and anorexia with a gradually increasing fever which may exceed 104° F. By the 10th day, the typical rose-colored spots appear over the abdomen and back. The fever subsides usually by the 4th week unless complications arise. The more serious complications in typhoid fever include intestinal hemorrhage and at times perforation from ulcerated Peyer's patches, secondary pulmonary or renal infections and typhoid osteomyelitis. The diagnosis of typhoid fever is made on the basis of the history, the clinical and laboratory findings. Leukopenia with an absence of the eosinophils is a characteristic of typhoid fever. Blood cultures are commonly positive during the first week of the disease after which time the Widal reaction (agglutination test) is significant.

The treatment of the acute disease consists of good nursing care and the maintenance of adequate nutrition in the presence of the debilitating fever. An active watch should be kept for complications. Prophylactic, active immunization against typhoid, and paratyphoid A & B is an effective measure in the control of the disease.

Oral Aspects

The oral symptoms associated with typhoid fever are both specific and those due to impaired nutrition, lowered resistance and dehydration resulting from the protracted fever.

Ulcerations of the tongue, palate or oral mucosa are the most common oral complication of typhoid fever. A brown furry tongue is a characteristic finding. Orgaz believed that these lesions occur mainly in individuals who have poor oral hygiene before the onset of the fever. The ultimate prognosis of patients developing such lesions is grave. Noma has been reported by Egi during the 5th week of typhoid fever. Dental abscesses and suppuration of the submaxillary lymph nodes, from which the *Eberthella typhosa* have been isolated have also been reported.

The author recovered the typhoid bacillus from the apices of 4 out of 7 teeth at necropsy although the blood and other organ bacteriology did not reveal this organism. The past history of the patient relative to typhoid fever was not known. This finding is not surprising in view of Pickworth's isolation of the typhoid bacillus from beneath the denture of a patient 4 years after the clinical disease. The denture was not removed in the interim. Chimenti isolated *Eberthella typhosa* from the pulp of an abscessed tooth.

Suppurative parotitis is another oral complication of typhoid fever. It results probably from the diminished salivary flow and lowered resistance of the tissues associated with the fever. Osteomyelitis of the mandible and the maxilla have been reported. Full or partial dentures should be removed from stuporous patients to prevent their aspiration or swallowing.

TYPHUS FEVER

Typhus fever is a highly communicable rickettsial infection which is transmitted to man by the body louse. The disease is uncommon in the United States, being most prevalent in the Balkan countries, parts of North Africa and Ireland. During epidemics the disease is transmitted from man to man through body lice infected with *Rickettsia prowazeki*. Endemic (murine) typhus fever, the form experienced commonly in the United States, is transmitted usually by infected rat fleas.

After an incubation period of 1 to 2 weeks, the patient experiences symptoms of toxemia and prostration, headache, vomiting and a marked febrile reaction—104° to 105° F. By the 5th day of the fever, the typical "rose-spot" eruption appears in which hemorrhagic points develop frequently. These spots undergo a series of successive color changes through purple to brown, before their disappearance. The high fever results in a white, furred tongue. A characteristic tremor of this organ has been described.

Diagnosis is made by the Weil-Felix agglutination reaction using the patient's serum against Proteus X-19. Prophylactic typhus vaccination is effective. The usual course of the disease is about 3 weeks if complications do not develop.

Infections of the parotid and submaxillary glands are not infrequent complications of typhus fever. They should be guarded against by careful cleansing of the mouth.

BACILLARY DYSENTERY

Bacillary dysentery is an infectious disease of considerable importance in the tropics and in localities where adequate public health precautions are not taken. It is caused by the *Shigella dysenteriae* (Shiga or Flexner strains). The symptoms vary from diarrhea in the mild cases to severe abdominal colic and the frequent passage of stools containing blood, pus and mucus. These symptoms are often accompanied by toxic manifestations of varying severity. Diagnosis is made by culture of the causative organism.

Secondary parotitis is a frequent complication in bacillary dysentery. This results probably from the lowered general resistance of the individual and the decreased salivary flow which permit retrograde infection of the gland by the mouth organisms.

BOTULISM

Botulism is caused by contamination of imperfectly cooked meats, vegetables and other foods with the *Clostridium botulinum* or its exotoxins. The symptoms of botulism rarely develop later than 18 hours after the ingestion of the contaminated food. Ocular symptoms develop early. They vary from strabismus, mydriasis and loss of pupillary reflexes to dimness of vision and at times actual blindness. Dizziness, nausea and vomiting are present frequently. Paralysis of the muscles of deglutition may develop and the patient may experience difficulty in talking and swallowing.

Diagnosis is made on the basis of the history, the cultivation of *Clostridium botulinum* from the suspected food or demonstration of the exotoxin by means of guinea pig inoculations. Antitoxin is ineffective in the treatment of acute botulism. After the stomach and intestinal tract have been evacuated, general nursing care and the watch for complications, respiratory failure, are the usual treatment.

TETANUS

Tetanus is caused by the anaerobic *Clostridium tetani*, which is widely distributed in the soil and in the intestinal tract. The incubation period of the disease varies, depending on the site of infection. The more peripheral the infection the longer the incubation period.

Early symptoms of tetanus include an anxious expression, severe headache, local or generalized sweating and temperature abnormalities. There is tremor when the tongue is protruded. A sore throat is a frequent symptom which is often followed by dysphagia, sialorrhea and a spasmodic cough. Opisthotonus and spasms of the intercostal muscles are common. Fever is rarely present. In cases of cephalic tetanus there is paralysis of the hypoglossal and facial nerves. It may occur in spite of energetic treatment.

The prophylactic treatment of tetanus consists of the injection of 1,500 units of tetanus antitoxin following injury. The injection of 1 cc. of tetanus toxoid on 3 occasions usually produces an active immunity. The treatment of clinical tetanus taxes the resources of the physician, particularly to maintain an adequate nutrition.

INFECTIOUS MONONUCLEOSIS (GLANDULAR FEVER— PFEIFFER'S DISEASE)

Infectious mononucleosis is a benign communicable disease of unknown etiology which is characterized by fever, swelling and tenderness of the lymph nodes, a marked lymphocytic reaction in the blood and frequently lesions of the oral mucosa. In spite of its name, infectious mononucleosis is a self-limited condition.

This disease has a high morbidity among physicians, students, nurses and other institutional groups where it may occur either sporadically or in small endemics. It is recognized infrequently in private practice.

The onset of infectious mononucleosis is as a rule sudden, with malaise, headache, nausea, vomiting, prostration and frequently a sore throat. In 2 to 3 days the adenopathy develops. This adenopathy, which is most marked in the cervical triangle, is moderately painful and out of all proportion to any visible oral or pharyngeal lesion. The duration of the fever is rarely more than 5 to 7 days after which time the lymphadenopathy subsides gradually. Splenomegaly and gastro-intestinal symptoms are also common.

Conditions which may also cause cervical adenopathy and which may be accompanied by oral or pharyngeal lesions, must be considered in the diagnosis. Hodgkin's, acute follicular tonsillitis, malignant neutropenia, diphtheria, and leukemia may simulate infectious mononucleosis.

Laboratory studies: The leukocyte count which is often normal at the onset of the disease runs between 10,000 and 25,000 with large mononuclear cells comprising 40 to 80% of the total leukocyte count. This mononucleosis outlasts the clinical symptoms and may persist in mild degrees for weeks or months. The hemoglobin and erythrocytes are usually normal.

The Paul-Bunnel or heterophilic antibody test utilizing sheep erythrocytes is positive in approximately 90% of the cases. When an ox erythrocyte absorption method is used this test is believed to be specific for infectious mononucleosis.

There is no specific treatment for this disease other than rest and good nursing care. Convalescence is slow.

Oral Aspects

In about 50% of the cases, anginal symptoms are present. Paul reported that a reddened throat, petechiae of the soft palate, patches on the tonsils and stomatitis with Vincent's organisms were common during the 1st to 3rd weeks of the disease. Kilham and Steigman described tender irregular raised papules on the palate. Herpetic lesions are often present. Bernstein believed that if the Paul-Bunnel test were used more routinely, certain cases of Vincent's infection, aphthous stomatitis and granulopenia would be diagnosed as infectious mononucleosis.

The oral lesions are treated symptomatically.

TULAREMIA (RABBIT FEVER)

Tularemia is an infectious, highly contagious disease caused by *Pasteurella tularensis*. The incidence of the infection is increasing. The majority of human infections, aside from those contracted in the laboratory, are the result of contact with infected animals, especially wild rabbits, ground squirrels, pocket gophers, woodchucks and chipmunks. Insect vectors such as the horsefly and the wood tick can also transmit the disease to man.

The clinical manifestations of tularemia vary, depending on the site and mode of inoculation. A primary nodule or papule develops characteristically at the site of inoculation and later breaks down and ulcerates. This is accompanied by a fever of 102° to 103° F. There is painful adenopathy of the regional lymph nodes with occasional suppuration. In the "typhoid" type of infection the fever is the main clinical symptom.

Diagnosis is made on the clinical findings, the history of possible exposure to infection and specific agglutination tests. Treatment consists of antiserum early in the course of the disease and later general nursing care. Convalescence is slow and protracted.

Oral Aspects

Oral lesions in tularemia are infrequent. Pessin observed a patient who had a severe stomatitis and ulcerative glossitis accompanied by blood-tinged saliva which began about a week after the onset of the infection. The tongue was particularly painful. The specific nature of the lesions was not established but suggestive bacterial forms were seen at necropsy. Steigmann reported a case of facial tularemia in which the primary lesion developed below the left mandibular ramus. This was accompanied by marked submental adenopathy.

Huschultz treated a case of tularemia in which the chief clinical manifestation was a necrotizing ulceration of the entire pharynx, tongue and oral mucosa. It was felt that the ulcerated areas represented the point of origin of the disease. Tularemia with lesions confined to the tonsils produces a clinical picture simulating the blood dyscrasias.

BRUCELLOSIS (UNDULANT FEVER—MALTA FEVER)

Brucellosis is a chronic disease caused by the *Brucella melitensis* or related organisms. The causative organisms are known to be relatively widespread in the cattle in this country. Infection occurs through the ingestion of raw milk products from infected cows or more rarely from contact with the animals.

Typical symptoms include fever of a remittent type, sweating, loss of weight and general bone aches. The chronic form of the disease, when febrile symptoms are minimal, is a diagnostic problem. All cases of weakness with low-grade fever without apparent basis for these symptoms should make one think of brucellosis. Diagnosis can be made only by the cultivation and identification of the organism. An agglutination test and an intradermal cutaneous reaction are useful aids in diagnosis.

Oral Aspects

Poston & Menfee reported a case of brucellosis which was characterized by oral lesions. The patient was a 31-year-old physician who complained of sore throat, chills and fever. Four weeks previously he had been in Bermuda where large amounts of raw milk were consumed. The patient's gums were red and edematous. Throughout the mouth were small grayish elevated patches surrounded by hyperemic areas. They were most prominent on the pharynx, under the tongue and on the lips. The clinical appearance of the lesions resembled those seen in thrush, but they were more grayish and they were more difficult to remove. The anterior cervical and submental lymph nodes were enlarged.

B. melitensis was isolated from the blood stream on the 2nd and 3rd hospital days and also from the mouth lesions on 3 occasions. Cultures for monilia and fungi were negative. It was believed that the primary focus was in the mouth, since the organisms were isolated from the oral lesions and there was local adenopathy.

The oral lesions were treated initially with gentian violet and neo-arsphenamine intravenously but the organisms were grown from the mouth after the use of these drugs.

General treatment consists of injections of immune serum, vaccines, brucellin and non-specific protein therapy. In the case cited, prompt response followed the injection of immune serum. The value of the sulfonamides in brucellosis is not yet established.

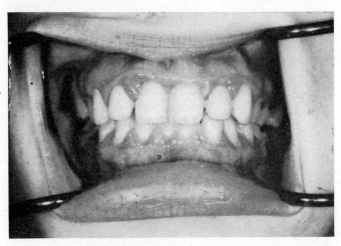

FIG. 152. Gingival changes in a patient with brucellosis. The unusual purplish rose color of the gums with hypertrophy of the interdental papillae and marked alveolar destruction were the non-specific symptoms which led eventually to the diagnosis of brucellosis.

HEMORRHOIDS (PILES)

The term hemorrhoids includes any vascular tumor (swelling) of the rectal mucosa, consisting of dilated, thrombosed and at times bleeding veins of the hemorrhoidal plexus. They are grouped as external or internal hemorrhoids, depending on whether they originate outside or within the anal sphincter.

Mild forms of the disease are common. Pregnancy, chronic constipation or any condition which interferes with normal circulation may give rise to hemorrhoids. Occupations or habits which result in congestion of the rectal vessels favor the development of hemorrhoids. Truck drivers, policemen, bookkeepers and dentists are predisposed to hemorrhoids.

External hemorrhoids appear as small purplish raised areas which become more prominent when the patient strains. They may be symptomless or itch slightly. When they become thrombosed, the pain may be intense during defecation. Internal hemorrhoids are frequently symptomless until they become thrombosed, prolapsed or ruptured and bleed. The persistent hemorrhage associated with bleeding hemorrhoids results often in secondary anemia.

The diagnosis of external hemorrhoids can usually be made by inspection. The diagnosis of the internal variety requires rectal or proctoscopic examination. It is imperative that accurate diagnosis be made of any bleeding lesion of the rectum to rule out the possibility of malignant disease.

The treatment of hemorrhoids consists of the elimination of as many of the predisposing factors as is possible. While medicated suppositories will give some symptomatic relief, the treatment of hemorrhoids is chiefly surgical. Some types of internal hemorrhoids may be treated successfully by injection with suitable sclerosing solutions.

14

The Urogenital System

GENERAL CONSIDERATIONS

Renal disease and the frequently associated cardiovascular changes constitute an important group of diseases for the medical practitioner, representing about the third most frequent cause of death. Their treatment has not been modified greatly by recent advances in chemotherapy. The kidneys aid in the elimination of the nitrogenous wastes of the body, in maintaining the normal fluid and electrolyte balance of the body and in maintaining the proper level of the plasma proteins. Derangement of renal function will thus produce a variety of symptoms.

Renal disease may be grouped conveniently for purposes of discussion into:

(A) Congenital or developmental anomalies.
    (1) Congenitally missing kidney.
    (2) Horseshoe kidney—congenitally fused kidney.
    (3) Congenital polycystic kidney.
(B) Functional renal changes.
    (1) Uremia—due to many causes.
    (2) Anuria—due to certain drugs.
(C) Inflammatory renal changes.
    (1) Acute glomerulonephritis. ⎤
    (2) Chronic glomerulonephritis. ⎬ "Bright's disease"
    (3) Nephrosis. ⎦
(D) Renal lithiasis and diseases of the renal pelves, ureters and bladder.
(E) Neoplasms of the renal tissue.

CONGENITAL OR DEVELOPMENTAL ANOMALIES

The common renal developmental anomalies consist of (1) a single kidney, (2) fusion of the upper poles of the developing kidneys to form the so-called

279

"horseshoe kidney" and (3) the congenital polycystic kidney which results from failure of the secreting and tubular elements of the forming kidney to unite properly. These lesions, while important to the patient, the physician and the surgeon, have little interest for the dentist.

UREMIA

Uremia results from the retention of urinary constituents due to (1) primary renal disease (chronic nephritis—mercury poisoning) or (2) obstruction of the urinary excretory apparatus (prostatic hypertrophy). It is an indication of severely impaired renal function, just as congestive heart failure is an indication of seriously impaired cardiac function. The symptoms of uremia are due in part to the physicochemical derangement resulting from the retained nitrogenous substances and to certain "toxic" manifestations which are difficult to explain.

Dehydration and acidosis with retention of nitrogenous compounds in the blood stream are the result of the altered blood chemistry. There is an increase in the blood urea as well as the non-protein nitrogen but the concentration of the former bears no relation to the clinical symptoms. Muscular irritability, twitching and at times actual tetany occur.

Weakness, anorexia and vomiting, headache and pruritus are some of the toxic symptoms associated with uremia which cannot be easily explained on the basis of the altered blood chemistry.

Oral Aspects (Uremic or Nephritic Stomatitis)

A membranous or ulcerative stomatitis is associated occasionally with uremia. Black considered these lesions a chemical stomatitis caused by the caustic action of ammonium carbonate which is formed from the salivary urea. The general body dehydration, the lowered resistance of the oral tissues to infection, the inability of the patient to maintain normal nutritional requirements because of the nausea and vomiting, and local irritative factors cannot be overlooked as important predisposing causes.

Bliss's experimental studies on nephrectomized dogs lends credence to the ammonium carbonate theory. He produced typical stomatitis on the inner surface of a normal dog's lip by applying to this area saliva from an experimental animal which contained 105 mg. urea 100 cc. The mucosal lesions produced in the experimental animals occurred where the mucosal tissues contacted the teeth. He demonstrated that ammonia is formed from the urea secreted in the saliva by the action of urease contained in the salivary calculus. The pH measurements and the chemical analysis of the saliva made by Black of a patient with uremic stomatitis lends support to this ammonium carbonate theory. The salivary pH was 7.4 to 7.8, salivary ammonia 40.8 mg./100 cc. and salivary urea 68 mg./100 cc.

A marked uriniferous odor is characteristic of these patients, even in the absence of oral lesions. The oral mucosa lacks the normal stippling and has a dry, pasty, yellowish appearance. Shallow red-rimmed ulcers of the oral mucosa and tongue margins, which develop first at the site of local areas of irritation or trauma, are common. The lesions become covered with a yellowish or a whitish colored material. The oral lesions are seen mostly in severely ill patients in which the prognosis is unfavorable.

Local treatment consists of the maintenance of good oral hygiene and the use of mild antiseptics such as the aniline dyes. Black treated his patient with a thorough prophylaxis and used a 1% HCl mouth wash to neutralize the ammonia. The lesions cleared up under this treatment before death. If

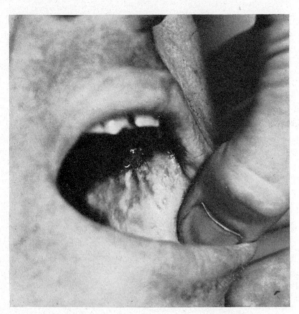

FIG. 153. Nephritic stomatitis. (Black, Urol. and Cutan. Rev., 46:75, 1942.)

alkaline pH values are obtained, a one-half strength hydrogen peroxide solution (pH 3.9) would be an excellent mouth wash and it would be preferable to the diluted mineral acid.

Anuria

Anuria is a symptom rather than a disease. It refers to the lack of urinary output or to defective excretion of urine. Common causes of anuria are obstructive lesions of the renal pelves, ureters, bladder or urethra. Pressure on the urinary tract due to new growths, adhesions, kinks or twists of the ureters, or the lodgement of urinary calculus are other causes.

INFLAMMATORY RENAL CHANGES

Acute Glomerulonephritis

Acute glomerulonephritis is not as frequent as the chronic form of the disease. This form of nephritis is commonly a sequel to an infection associated with a hemolytic streptococcus, although other organisms may be involved including alpha streptococci. Cold and wet weather and fatigue predispose to the infection.

Acute glomerulonephritis occurs commonly in childhood, developing within several weeks after an upper respiratory infection, tonsillitis or scarlet fever. The onset of the disease may be insidious or acute. In the latter instance the symptoms consist of headache, nausea or vomiting, fever, pain in the back and diminished urinary output. Cases with more insidious onset do not present such striking symptoms and a general feeling of malaise, loss of appetite accompanied by a mild fever may be all that is present. A urinary examination often gives the first clue to the diagnosis. Edema of the face, particularly the suborbital tissues, is characteristic. The edema in nephritis does not develop first in the dependent parts of the body. Acute glomerulonephritis is associated frequently with increased blood pressure, hemorrhage and edema of the eye grounds.

The diagnosis is made on the basis of the history and the characteristic urinary and laboratory findings. The urine is turbid or smoky in color due to the contained erythrocytes, albumen is $+$ to $+++$, cellular and granular casts are numerous and both erythrocytes and leukocytes are seen in the urine. The blood urea nitrogen (BUN) may be slightly elevated.

The treatment of acute glomerulonephritis consists of bed rest, chemotherapy, kidney-sparing diets, good nursing care and frequent checks on the urinary and blood chemistry findings.

Oral Aspects. Clinical evidence of the case history type, which emphasizes the close relation between oral infections and the various nephritides, is abundant. Billings was impressed with the frequency with which infections of the teeth, the tonsils or pharyngeal tissues preceded the acute nephritic episode. Haden isolated a *Streptococcus viridans* from a pulpless tooth, the blood and urine of one patient who was later cured following the removal of the pulpless tooth. Hela also stressed the significance of pulpless teeth in the etiology of nephritis. Kramer and Crocket reported a case of renal infection which was cured by the removal of pyorrhetic teeth. The actual importance of oral infection in nephritis is difficult to evaluate. Healthy periapical and periodontal tissues should be of considerable importance in renal disease due to the intimate relation of the kidneys to the vascular system, which makes bacteremias potentially dangerous.

Rosenow and Haden demonstrated, to their satisfaction, that organisms isolated from infected teeth of patients with renal disease have a particular predilection for the kidneys. Experimental nephritic lesions have been produced with alpha streptococci which were obtained from "pyorrheal" pockets. The question arises as to whether these experimental renal lesions are not embolic phenomena. (See gastric ulcer, Oral Aspects.)

It is a clinical observation that the symptoms of acute glomerulonephritis will develop occasionally following an oral or pharyngeal infection. The author observed several cases of acute nephritis which developed within 10 to 14 days following an acute alveolar abscess with rapid recovery following the elimination of the abscessed tooth. While it is impossible to establish with certainty the etiologic relationship of the dental focus to the renal lesions, the chronologic relation was strongly suggestive.

While surgical elimination of foci of infection is contraindicated generally in the patient with acute nephritis, if an acute dento-alveolar abscess is present, it had best be removed immediately. This will eliminate a potential focus from which organisms may continually gain entrance into the blood stream and aggravate and prolong the process. The continuance of such an easily removed focus may result in increased or irreparable renal damage and further diminish the renal reserve. If the patient is not receiving already the sulfonamides, one of these preparations should precede and follow the extraction.

Chronic Interstitial Nephritis

Chronic interstitial nephritis is believed to result from the incomplete resolution of acute glomerulonephritis. In some cases the acute renal episode, if present, is never recognized but these individuals are often susceptible to colds, tonsillitis and sinus infections. The symptoms of chronic interstitial nephritis develop usually during the 4th and 5th decades. The results of a routine urinary examination may be the first indication of the existence of the disease.

The symptoms of chronic interstitial nephritis are similar to those of acute glomerulonephritis, but they are milder. Hypertension is more prominent and persistent. Edema may be due to decreased amounts of plasma proteins as well as to an associated myocardial failure. Uremic symptoms are more common in chronic nephritis. The characteristic ocular and retinal changes are important aids in the diagnosis of chronic nephritis.

The urinary findings in chronic glomerulonephritis include: (1) polyuria, especially at night; (2) consistent low specific gravity to the urine; (3) albuminuria and (4) deficient renal function tests, such as the phenolsulphonephthalein test (PSP).

Oral Aspects. The oral aspects of chronic nephritis are similar to those discussed under acute glomerulonephritis. The elimination of foci of infection may assist materially in the prevention of chronic nephritis but their elimination after the establishment of the disease is less beneficial. Their removal under these circumstances is more for their beneficial effect on the general resistance. Foci of infection should be removed during a period of remission.

The Nephroses

The nephroses include a group of renal disturbances which are characterized by edema, albuminuria and a decrease in the serum albumen associated with inconspicuous inflammatory renal changes. Included in the nephroses are: (1) lipoid nephrosis (true); (2) amyloidosis of the kidney and certain stages of glomerulonephritis.

Lipoid nephrosis is essentially a childhood disease whose etiology is not clearly understood. It is characterized by the gradual development of generalized edema. Recovery after an indeterminate time is frequent unless the patient succumbs to secondary infection, particularly pneumonia.

RENAL LITHIASIS AND DISEASES OF THE RENAL PELVES, URETERS AND BLADDER

Nephrolithiasis (Renal Calculus)

There are many types of renal calculus such as uric acid calculus, calcium oxalate and calcium phosphate calculi. They are common causes of obstruction in the renal pelves. Smaller calculi (renal sand) may become lodged in the ureter during their passage to the bladder and cause not only exquisite pain but also anuria.

Oral Aspects. Renal calculi were produced in dogs by Rosenow and Meisser by the injection of bacteria obtained from the teeth of patients with nephrolithiasis. In spite of this evidence clinical experience fails to reveal an important relation between oral foci of infection and urinary calculus formation.

Pyelitis

Pyelitis or inflammation of the renal pelves occurs chiefly in the female, probably because of the greater ease of ascending urinary infections in this sex. It is found in young children and it is associated frequently with pregnancy. The usual infecting agent is the colon bacillus, but streptococcal and staphylococcal infections are common. Blood-borne infections from more distant foci, such as the teeth, are also important etiologic causes. Obstruction of urinary flow, overexertion, fatigue or undue exposure are known predisposing causes. Extension of the inflammation to the renal parenchyma is called pyelonephritis.

The symptoms of pyelitis vary greatly in severity. They consist of chills, fever, pain and tenderness in the groins and digestive disturbances, with pain and discomfort in the abdomen. Pain, burning and frequency on urination are present when there is an associated infection of the bladder, cystitis.

Oral Aspects. Oral foci of infection should be eliminated in cases of pyelitis. Danforth and Carlens considered the elimination of these foci of infection the initial step in treatment. Evidence of the beneficial effect of eliminating oral foci of infection on the diseases of the urinary tract is large. Rueck reported a case of pyelitis, cystitis and urethritis which cleared up following the removal of infected teeth. McFarlane and Fetterman reported that 65% of the urinary tract infections they studied were due to infected teeth.

DISEASES OF THE PROSTATE

The prostate gland is found in the male surrounding the neck of the bladder and the vesical third of the urethra. Its exact function, if any, has not been determined. Diseases of the prostate can be divided for purposes of discussion into acute and chronic infections, prostatic hypertrophy and malignancy of this organ.

Acute prostatitis results usually from bacterial infection, which reaches the organ by extension from the urethra. The gonococcus is the common cause of acute prostatitis. "Non-specific" prostatic infections also occur. Chronic prostatitis may be a sequal to an acute infection or develop as a result of urethral stricture, chronic cystitis or as a metastatic process from a more distant focus of infection such as the teeth. The non-specific forms of chronic prostatitis are resistant to treatment. In many instances, they represent a metastatic infection from a more distant infection. Urologists are impressed with the frequent relation between oral foci of infection and chronic prostatic involvement. Gingival and periodontal foci deserve at least as much attention as the periapical lesion.

Prostatic hypertrophy is a disease of late adult life, usually after 55 to 60 years of age. There is some evidence to indicate that this enlargement may represent a decreased endocrine activity associated with senescence. The symptoms of prostatic hypertrophy are those which are associated with urinary retention and the accompanying changes. The treatment of prostatic hypertrophy is chiefly surgical. Draper *et al.* noted marked changes in the form of the mandible in patients with prostatic hypertrophy. There was a broad gonial angle with a long horizontal ramus and a broad ascending ramus to this bone.

Malignant change in the prostate gland is not unusual. Carcinoma of the prostate is serious, as the growth in its early stages manifests few if any symptoms. Since it has a tendency to metastasize early to the skeletal system, bone pains and symptoms related to the bones are frequently the first evidence of prostatic malignancy.

15

The Reproductory System

THE OVARIES	PREGNANCY—GESTATION
VULVITIS—VAGINITIS	TESTES
MENSTRUATION	BALANITIS

THE OVARIES

The ovaries produce ova and the hormones estrin and folliculin. The hormones govern the development of the breasts, uterus, vagina and the secondary sexual characteristics. They are concerned with the changes that occur in these organs during menstruation and pregnancy.

The estrogenic hormone has a marked effect on the vaginal mucosa and a less definite one on the oral mucosa. Estrin production is normally greatest during puberty, just preceding the menses and during pregnancy. Estrin is essential for the normal development and keratinization of the vaginal epithelium. A deficiency results in lack of keratinization, an increase in the amount of mucus, debris, leukocytes and bacteria in this tissue. The vaginal changes due to estrin are so characteristic that vaginal smears are used as a clinical means of determining estrin incretion.

Ziskin, Blackenberg and Slanetz found that the injection of estrogenic hormone in castrated monkeys produced a well-keratinized gingiva which was resistant to infection and which was devoid of inflammation in the corium. Estrin was observed to stimulate cell activity as well as cell specialization. The opposite results were obtained with follutein.

Hyper- and Hypo-ovarianism

Hyperovarianism results usually from an overactivity of the anterior lobe of the pituitary. It is characterized by the rapid development of the secondary sexual characteristics, an early menarche and general precocious skeletal development.

Hypo-ovarianism results from pituitary hypofunction or a quantitative or qualitative deficiency of ovarian tissue. The menstrual flow is absent, scanty or irregular. Sterility is common.

Oral Aspects. The relationship between ovarian hyperfunction and gingival and oral mucosal changes is somewhat confusing. While it is generally

286

true that excess estrin incretion in association with local factors may result in gingival enlargement, the opposite may also occur. Ziskin and Silvers observed 2 cases of proliferative gingivitis in young girls who had low estrin output as measured by oral and vaginal smears. The gingival enlargement did not permanently respond to various forms of treatment until topical estrogen

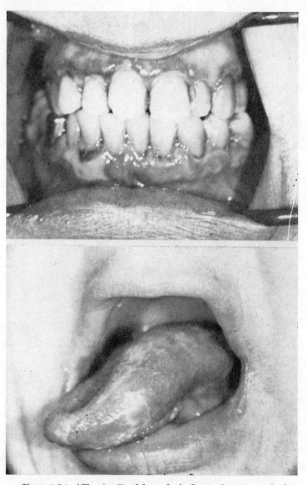

Fig. 154 (*Top*). Reddened, inflamed areas of the gingiva and irregular plaque formation which was associated with gonadal disturbances in the female. Patient had an artificial menopause. Estradiol therapy beneficial.

Fig. 155 (*Bottom*). Yellowish-white plaque-like lesions on the tongue which were associated with gonadal changes in the female. These lesions resemble those found in vitamin B complex deficiency, but they were not benefited by vitamin therapy.

therapy was used. The author saw a 27-year-old patient with purplish-red enlarged gingival tissues who had only menstruated 2 times in her life. Local treatment was of little value until ovarian function with regular menstruation was established through medical treatment.

In patients with gynecologic disorders or following the menopause, it is not unusual to find sore and tender mouths. Climacteric patients commonly

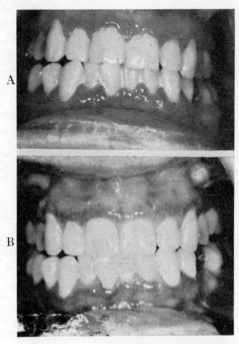

FIG. 156. Desquamative gingivitis of nine years' duration associated with ovarian dysfunction. (A) Before treatment and (B) after treatment with estrogenic hormone.

complain of a dryness or burning sensation in the oral cavity. The cheek mucosa at times has a milky appearance and irregular grayish-white areas which can be mistaken for leukoplakia. There is a diminished keratinized protective covering of the tissues. These patients may have a symptomatology similar to that described under desquamative gingivitis. The gums are raw-red, painful and bleed on the slightest provocation. Irregularly shaped grayish-yellow plaques are common on the alveolar gingivae and the oral mucosa. At times the plaques are associated with painful, shallow eroded areas which have reddish margins. The clinical findings are similar to those observed in vitamin B complex deficiency but the response to this form of therapy is limited and transitory.

Biopsy studies of the tissues removed from the lesions associated with the menopause or gynecologic disorders will reveal atrophy of the epithelium, especially of the keratinized layer. Ziskin successfully treated this form of stomatitis by means of an ointment containing estradiol benzoate, 1,000 R.U. per Gm. This was applied twice daily to the oral tissues and allowed to remain. About 25 Gm. of this ointment are used per week. Arbabanel and Richmond also obtained satisfactory clinical results using estrogenic hormone. They found that, while some effect was obtained on the oral tissues from general medication, the injection of the hormone preparations in the region of the involved tissues produced more satisfactory results. The author observed cases which responded satisfactorily to estrogenic therapy. Others, including Miller and Seidler, were not impressed with this form of treatment for desquamative gingivitis. Nathansen and Weisberger used estradiol in the treatment of leukoplakia buccalis. Males were observed to respond to this form of treatment as well as females.

Estrogenic therapy may have a still wider use in the treatment of oral mucosal lesions because of its ability to produce a well-keratinized mucosa which is resistant to infection. The consent and co-operation of the patient's physician should be obtained before any form of hormonal therapy is instituted.

VULVITIS—VAGINITIS

The vulva and the vagina are frequently the site of inflammatory changes due to irritating vaginal discharges, chemicals used in douches, infections with the *Trichomonas vaginalis,* gonococcus, diphtheria or monilial organisms and the fusospirochetal organisms. Vaginal and vulval lesions due to these organisms are discussed under the respective diseases. Special attention should be given to the oral relationship of monilial and gonococcal vulvovaginitis.

Leukoplakia also affects the vulva where it produces lesions similar to those seen in the mouth. The thickened sclerosed tissues have a dense white appearance which at times are interspersed with red cracks. Savill noted marked regression of the lesions following estrin treatment.

MENSTRUATION

Menstruation is a manifestation of puberty in the female. Its onset varies with the climate and racial characteristics. There is a cessation of the menses during pregnancy, lactation, debilitating diseases, at times during acute infectious diseases and at the menopause which normally occurs between 40 to 50 years of age.

Menstruation occurs every 3 to 4 weeks and the flow usually lasts 3 to 5 days. It is controlled through hormonal activity residing in the ovaries. There is a wide variation in the menstrual cycle as well as the duration of flow. The menstrual flow consists of cast off uterine mucosa, mucus, endometrial fragments and blood. An anticoagulant substance was believed to exist in the uterine tissue which prevented clotting of the flow. Recent studies indicate that the menstrual flow represents blood which is already chemically clotted. Bleeding from other body sites is often prolonged during this period.

Ovulation in the human is not co-incident with menstruation. It occurs usually 10 days to 2 weeks prior to the menses. In animals, especially the rat, marked cyclical changes take place in the vagina during menstruation. Similar but less marked vaginal changes are observed in the human at the time of puberty and at each successive menstrual period. Ziskin showed that the vaginal and the oral mucosal changes are governed by the same hormonal mechanism.

Oral Aspects

The first mention of the relationship of menstruation and the teeth is found in the 18th century. Reports of oral hemorrhages during the menses are common. Oral sepsis has even been suggested as an aggravating factor in menstrual difficulties. French reported an unusual case of dysmenorrhea of long standing which was cured by scraping of the tongue.

While oral changes during menstruation are not uncommon, they are rarely of sufficient magnitude to warrant professional attention. The actual incidence of the different oral symptoms and changes associated with menstruation are not available because of the lack of careful studies. The oral tissues of 80 women studied during and after menstruation revealed changes in the oral tissues in the mouths of 27 and in 20 definite inflammatory processes were noted. Capillary microscopy has demonstrated a changed distribution and an increased vascularity of the gums at this time.

The common oral changes accompanying menstruation are: (1) hyperemia, pain, swelling and hemorrhage from the marginal gingivae and interdental papillae, most marked on the labial surface; (2) herpes labialis or oral aphthous lesions; (3) dental periostitis or pulpitis; (4) prolonged hemorrhage following dental surgery; (5) swelling of the salivary glands; and (6) periodic mucosal ulcerations which are at times associated with an agranulocytic blood picture.

Gingival hyperemia and swelling of the gums with an increased tendency to hemorrhage precedes frequently or accompanies the menses. The clinical appearance is identical to that seen in pregnancy. Oral herpetic lesions are associated commonly with menstruation. At this time there is increased cellular metabolism and a general lowering of resistance which might explain the development of the lesions.

Odontalgia in the female may be the consequence of menstruation. The "menstrual toothache" consists of periodic pain in sound or filled teeth which appears and disappears coincident with the menses. A few women experience a periodontitis localized to a single tooth or a group of teeth at each menstrual period. The periostitis and pulpitis are explained on the basis of the hyperemia and capillary dilation present during menstruation.

Postoperative hemorrhage occurs more frequently during menstruation than at other times. Such cases have terminated fatally. Birbaum and Fagnani reported a case of severe postoperative dental hemorrhage in a patient known to have no blood dyscrasia. Questioning revealed that the patient was menstruating. The same authors observed small hemorrhages within the root canals of teeth under treatment, and hemorrhages following electrocoagulation performed during the menses. Patients will not elect ordinarily to have dental surgery performed at this time. In emergency cases it is well to question the female patient.

Salivary gland swelling immediately preceding and during menstruation has been reported. Racine observed this symptom in a group of women who also presented gynecologic complaints. He believed the salivary gland swelling resulted from a deficiency of the corpus luteum. His cases were treated successfully with progesterone.

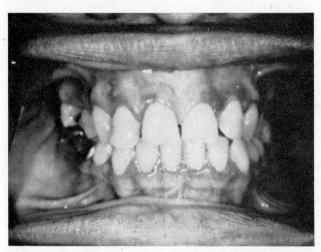

FIG. 157. Recurrent gingival hyperemia, erosive lesions and bleeding which occurred at each menstrual period in a 28-year-old female.

Mucosal ulcerations associated with menstruation are well known. Rappworth reported a series of cases with familial relationship, in which oral mucosal ulcerations developed at each menstrual period for many years. The ulcerations were not accompanied by a lowering of the granulocyte count. The exact etiology could not be determined and treatment in general was ineffective. Ziserman and later Jones reported similar lesions, which on the basis of the therapeutic response were shown to be related to some ovarian disturbance.

PREGNANCY—GESTATION

There is a legacy from antiquity to the effect that pregnancy produces serious damage to the mother's teeth. Sufficient experimental and clinical evidence has accumulated to refute the old adage "for every child a tooth."

The duration of the average pregnancy is about 275 days. It is divided classically into trimesters of approximately 3 months each. In the first trimester, the patient's symptoms are mostly subjective. The cessation of the menstrual flow is the most striking symptom. Nausea or vomiting, as early as the first month, is experienced in approximately 50% of all pregnancies.

Pigmentation of the nipples, with tingling and enlargement of the breasts are other common signs. By the third week the Aschheim-Zondek test is usually positive.

In the second trimester objective evidence becomes more manifest and the nausea and vomiting, if present earlier, usually disappear. The breasts and abdomen become enlarged and fetal movements are felt by the mother. Near the end of this trimester, the fetal heart sounds can be heard with the stethoscope and the fetal skeleton can be demonstrated by the x-ray. During the third trimester mammary and abdominal enlargement, the fetal movements and heart sounds become more prominent. The position and size of the fetal skeleton in respect to the mother's pelvis can be shown by x-ray studies.

Labor is ushered in by painful periodic uterine contractions which increase in frequency and severity until they occur every 2 or 3 minutes with a duration of approximately 1 minute. The first labor lasts usually 18 to 24 hours and subsequent ones are of shorter duration.

If the labor is long and the birth canal constricted, considerable distortion of the head may take place. Ramaker believed that this distortion of the head accounts for many cases of malocclusion, this being particularly true if the finger of the obstetrician is placed within the mouth for traction during delivery. He stressed the importance of immediate manipulation of the mouth parts into their proper relationship.

Complications of pregnancy include abortion, pyelitis, chronic nephritis, hypertensive toxemia or low reserve kidney and less commonly pernicious vomiting and eclampsia. Pyelitis, chronic nephritis, and abortion accompanying pregnancy have been studied in relation to oral foci of infection.

Oral Aspects

The oral aspects of pregnancy require a consideration of the effects of gestation on: (1) the teeth; (2) the supporting tissues; (3) the soft tissues of the mouth and (4) the importance of oral foci of infection as predisposing causes to certain of the complications of pregnancy.

Effect of Gestation on the Teeth and Alveolar Process. The belief that decalcification of the maternal skeleton and teeth occurs during pregnancy to supply minerals for the growing fetus had its origin in ancient times. Text books still stress the increased incidence of dental caries during pregnancy and suggest or infer that this is the result of mineral abstraction. Erupted teeth are not a mobilizable source of minerals in dietary deficiencies, osteomalacia, hyperparathyroidism or pregnancy, as they lack a method and mechanism whereby salts can be removed. Deakins found that the chemical composition of the dental enamel of teeth extracted during pregnancy reveals no significant departures from normal findings. There is no histologic, chemical or x-ray evidence that calcium or phosphorus can be removed from erupted teeth during pregnancy, although demineralization of the alveolar process is possible.

Caries. Increased dental caries during pregnancy can result only through changes in the external environment of the teeth, enabling those factors normally responsible for caries to act at an accelerated rate. Variations in the salivary pH or in the oral bacterial flora during pregnancy and the possible effect of the vomiting of pregnancy are factors to be considered.

The salivary pH in pregnancy has been determined by Friesell, Ziskin and others. Ziskin reported a mean pH of 6.61 in the pregnant group as compared with a mean pH of 6.72 in the non-pregnant group (normal 6.6 to 7.1). Tooth decalcification is not believed to occur until a pH 5.5 or 5.0 is reached.

Oral flora studies in pregnancy, with particular interest in the aciduric forms, have not been reported. The salivary pH studies do not suggest a

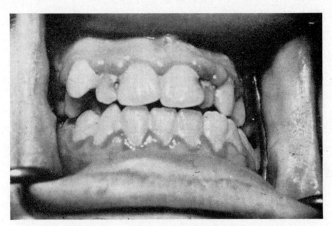

FIG. 158. Gingival hypertrophy associated with pregnancy. The lesions are most prominent in the interdental areas where the oral hygiene is poor.

marked increase in the number of acid-producing organisms. Binet showed that the incidence of caries is not increased in women experiencing "morning sickness." Furthermore the vomiting occurs in the morning, usually before food is taken, and it is not of high acidity.

Studies have been made to determine whether an increase in dental caries occurs during pregnancy. Klein noted the incidence of caries in the molar teeth of 350 female rats pregnant from 1 to 8 times, and an equal number of male animals of the same age. No difference in the caries rates was observed for the different sexes.

Some of the clinical studies of dental decay in pregnancy are based on so few observations or utilize such questionable methods of determining the caries experience that they are of little significance. Adequate controls are lacking in many of the earlier studies, and they do not consider the regular yearly increment of dental decay.

The more comprehensive clinical studies, with few exceptions, do not show an increased incidence of caries during pregnancy. Ziskin and Hotelling studied the effect of multiple pregnancies on the same dentition and their conclusions warrant quotation. "Pregnancy, *per se,* is not a cause of dental caries, while the saliva is slightly more acid during pregnancy, the degree of acidity is not sufficient to produce tooth decay, some factors operating during pregnancy actually prevent tooth decay to a significant extent."

This review of the subject of caries in pregnancy indicates: (1) that calcium salts are not abstracted from the fully formed erupted tooth in preg-

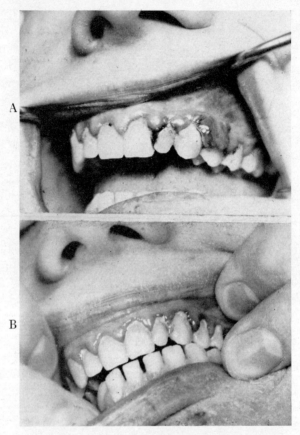

Fig. 159. (A) Pregnancy tumor in a 21-year-old woman who was seven months pregnant. The growth in the left canine and premolar region bled easily. (B) Same patient two months after delivery showing regression of gingival hypertrophy and pregnancy tumor without treatment. (Courtesy of Dr. John P. Looby, Philadelphia, Pa.)

nancy; (2) that the salivary pH of pregnant mothers is within the normal range and (3) that experimental and clinical evidence indicates that there is the normal age increment of new cavities during this period.

Gingivitis and Tumors. Gingival changes occur most frequently in individuals with poor oral hygiene. Looby studied the incidence of pregnancy gingivitis and tumors in a group of young women at the time of their first pregnancy. Of the 475 cases studied he observed a slight gingivitis in 40%, hypertrophic gingivitis in 10% and pregnancy "tumors" in 2% of the total.

Hormonal and vascular changes plus infection are the etiologic mechanisms which are believed to be responsible for the gingival changes in pregnancy. The hormonal theory finds confirmation in both the clinical and experimental observations of Ziskin and Blackenberg. Marked congestion and actual rupture of the capillaries of the interdental papillae were observed by capillary microscopy studies. Local predisposing factors such as malocclusion, local areas of poor hygiene or trauma are important determining causes.

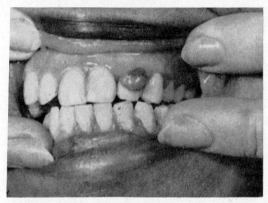

FIG. 160. Pregnancy tumor which remained after parturition six months previously. The lesion was removed surgically.

SYMPTOMS. Pregnancy gingivitis develops usually during the second trimester. It is characterized by a peculiar raspberry color of the marginal gingiva and ready bleeding. The hypertrophic changes involve particularly the interdental papillae. These tissues have a characteristic bluish-purple color and a turgid edematous appearance. Pain is not a prominent symptom, even in advanced cases. Ulceration is uncommon unless there is an accompanying fusospirochetal infection.

The "pregnancy tumors" are localized areas of extensive gingival hypertrophy. They arise usually from the gums in the vicinity of an interdental papilla or other area of irritation or infection. They vary from a purplish-red color to a deep blue, depending on the vascularity of the lesion, the amount of venous stasis and the size of the pedicle. Hemorrhage is the most frequent and important symptom. When ulceration occurs, it is usually the result of trauma incident to chewing. Bone destruction is rarely observed in "pregnancy tumors." The growths are both disfiguring and annoying.

TREATMENT. Mild cases of pregnancy gingivitis will respond to conservative treatment and the maintenance of good oral hygiene. The patient should be instructed in the proper manner of brushing the teeth and stimulating the interdental tissue. The topical application of mild astringents, such as 8%

$ZnCl_2$, are of some value. Conservative treatment is indicated until after parturition in the expectation of spontaneous regression.

Cross suggested that pregnancy tumors and gingivitis gravidarum may be related to ascorbic acid deficiency in pregnant women who require 100 to 300 mg. daily as compared with the 50 mg. for the healthy non-pregnant woman. He found that the administration of 100 to 300 mg. ascorbic acid daily in addition to dental prophylaxis was desirable. If chewing results in hemorrhage or ulceration of the growths they should be removed surgically. This is accomplished best under local anesthesia with the electric cautery which will control the bleeding.

Oral Foci of Infection in Relation to Complications of Pregnancy. A causal relation has been established between oral foci of infection and the complications of pregnancy. Galloway made a thorough study on this subject. Dental roentgenographic study revealed periapical infection (radiolucent areas) in 125 or 14.8% of the 843 cases studied. In the group with evidence of periapical infection, 85 patients had their teeth extracted and the remaining 40 retained their infection. The incidence of abortion, pyelitis and hypertension were studied in these 2 groups. Galloway's observations are summarized in Table XVII.

TABLE XVII

RELATION OF ORAL FOCI OF INFECTION TO THE COMPLICATIONS OF PREGNANCY

	Focal Infection Removed (40)	Focal Infection Not Removed (85)	No Evidence Focal Infection (618)	Incidence Total Cases (843)
Pyelitis	2.35%	17.5%	3.16%	3.5%
Abortion	4.7%	20.0%	4.43%	5.6%
Hypertension		5.0%	3.32%	3.32%

Failure to remove foci of infection in the teeth and tonsils resulted apparently in an increased incidence of abortion and pyelitis. The fear of possible abortion resulting from extraction or removal of teeth or tonsils should not be a deterring factor.

Dental Treatment in Pregnancy. The dentist is questioned frequently concerning the advisability of giving dental treatment during pregnancy. Necessary dental work including extractions should be performed unless the patient's obstetrician advises to the contrary.

The maintenance of good oral hygiene is the best protection against developing soft tissue lesions and dental caries. It is desirable for the dentist to see the expectant mother frequently, but the appointments should not last more than half an hour. Extensive restorations or tiring procedures (plugged gold foil) are not recommended during the latter months of pregnancy. Painful stimuli should be avoided as much as possible. The use of local anesthesia for operative procedures lessens the nervous strain and fatigue and has a favorable psychologic influence on the patient.

There is unjustifiable fear of extractions during pregnancy. Local anesthesia is to be preferred, unless local acute swellings contraindicate its use. If N_2O-oxygen anesthesia is indicated, the dentist should obtain the consent of the patient's obstetrician. There is an unwarranted fear of abortion associated with the administration of general anesthesia to the pregnant woman.

Solis-Cohen recommended that only 1 tooth be extracted at a time with pre-operative autogenous vaccine therapy and the administration of a sulfonamide for 3 days before and 3 days following operation. Such treatment did not cause an increase in the number of expected miscarriages, abortions or still births. It can be performed during any month of pregnancy without ill effects. The use of an autogenous vaccine is of doubtful value.

Dental care is neglected too frequently until the 8th or 9th month of gestation. It may be necessary at this time to insert temporary (cement) rather than permanent fillings. Only necessary extractions should be done.

Proper dental care during pregnancy is most essential. It should be a part of the patient's routine prenatal care. At this time the patient is keenly aware of her responsibilities as a mother and she usually welcomes information relative to pedodontic problems. The necessity of caring for the deciduous teeth, the importance of thumb-sucking, lip-biting, and other habits predisposing to malocclusion can be discussed effectively at this time.

Lactation. Lactation produces a more prolonged and severe drain on the calcium reserves of the mother than does pregnancy. The experimental studies (rats) of Klein indicate that lactation and pregnancy do not predispose to an increased incidence of caries. While Ziskin's studies showed that successive pregnancies are not associated with an increased increment of dental caries, no statements were made in his reports to indicate the percentage of the subjects who nursed their offspring or the duration of lactation. No increase in caries was noted after 6 months' lactation in 3 women studied by Hunscher. The dental aspects of prolonged lactation require further study.

The literature reports deficient lactation resulting from oral focal infection, and the secretion of organisms in the mother's milk of the same type as those present in the oral lesions. Breast abscesses have failed to heal until the removal of oral foci of infection. While these observations are of interest, they are of little present-day importance.

TESTES

The testes, or the male gonads, produce spermatozoa and one and possibly more hormones. The function of the spermatozoa is self-evident. The main testicular hormone, testosterone, is concerned with the development of the secondary sexual characteristics, the seminal vesicles, the prostate and skeletal growth.

The relationship between the oral structures and the testicles is highly circumstantial. Goadby reported cases of impotency which followed the removal of teeth. It is possible that the condition responsible for the loss of the teeth was also responsible for the impotency. Precocious dental and skeletal development has been observed in male hypergonadism and the reverse in hypogonadism. These dental changes are better explained on the basis of hyper- or hypopituitary function. Testosterone propionate (male sex hormone) has been used on a limited scale in the treatment of atrophic forms of gingivostomatitis and leukoplakia buccalis in the male. The therapeutic results have not been spectacular.

The seminal vesicles may be the seat of inflammatory processes which are secondary to foci of infection in other body areas including the oral cavity. The elimination of the oral sepsis has been known to result in a subsidence of the seminal vesiculitis.

BALANITIS

Balanitis or inflammation of the glans penis is usually due to the fuso-spirochetal or pyogenic organisms. (See extra-oral fusospirochetal infections.) Penile ulcerations are commonly found in syphilis, chancroid and lympho-pathia venereum. The lesions of herpes simplex and erythema multiforme pluri-orificialis are found occasionally on the foreskin.

16

Endocrines

GENERAL CONSIDERATIONS

The endocrine glands are an important group of organs with diverse functions which empty their secretions (preferably, incretions) into the blood stream. The incretions of the endocrines are called hormones. The hormones usually exert their action some distance from their site of production. Because of the widespread dissemination of these hormones they have an important co-ordinating action as well as a regulatory action on cellular growth, differentiation and metabolism.

The endocrine glands are of considerable interest to the dentist as they are important in the calcification of the bones and the teeth, in facial growth and dental development. Their effect has been carefully studied experimentally by Schour and others. A knowledge as to how dental development is altered by the various endocrine dysfunctions may enable the dentist to recognize an important systemic background as the cause of an oral disturbance. Endocrine dysfunction is believed to play an important role in certain forms of stomatitis and periodontal disease. This field of medical-dental relations has not been too thoroughly explored. Hormone therapy has been used on a limited scale in the treatment of diseases of the oral cavity.

The following structures are considered to be a part of the endocrine system: (1) pineal body; (2) the pituitary gland; (3) the thyroid gland; (4) the parathyroid glands; (5) the thymus gland; (6) the pancreas; (7) the adrenals; (8) the ovaries and (9) the testes. There is some evidence of an endocrine activity of the parotid gland.

THE PITUITARY BODY OR GLAND

The pituitary body is one of the most complex of all the endocrine glands. It is concerned mainly with the regulation of growth but it also is important in nitrogen and water metabolism. In addition to these main functions, it governs and co-ordinates the varied activities of many of the other endocrine glands. All the many functions of the pituitary gland cannot be discussed. The dentist is concerned primarily with the growth-promoting hormone of the anterior lobe.

The pituitary gland is divided into (1) the anterior lobe, (2) the posterior lobe and (3) the infundibular stalk. The known hormones of the pituitary and their main functions are tabulated below. Only a few have been isolated and prepared in crystalline form.

Anterior Lobe

The hormones produced by the anterior lobe act slowly and involve particularly the structural elements of the body.

(a) Growth hormone. This is produced by the eosinophile cells of the anterior lobe. This hormone acts particularly on epiphyseal growth.

(b) Gonadotropic hormones. These are produced by the basophile cells of the anterior lobe. There is a follicle-stimulating hormone (prolan A) and a luteinizing hormone (prolan B). A hormone is also increted which produces the growth and the development of the male accessory sexual characteristics.

(c) Thyrotropic hormone.

(d) Adrenotropic hormone.

(e) Lactogenic hormone.

(f) Diabetinogenic hormone.

FIG. 161. (A) Composite drawings of male patients. (1) Normality; (2) hypopituitarism, and (3) congenital untreated hypothyroidism (cretinism). The smaller size but symmetrical proportions are to be noted in (2) and the dysplasia in (3). (Composite drawings of figures in Wolf's Endocrinology, Zondek's Diseases of the Endocrine Glands, and photographs supplied by I. P. Bronstein.) In (1) the chronologic age is 13 years; statural age, 12 years; height, 5 feet. In (2) the chronologic age is 13 years; statural age, 8 years; height, 4 feet 2 inches. In (3) the chronologic age is 13 years; statural age, $2\frac{1}{2}$ years; height 3 feet 1 inch.

(B) Composite tracings of handplates taken of patients and similar to those shown in (A). (1) Normality; (2) hypopituitarism, and (3) congenital untreated hypothyroidism (cretinism). In (1) the chronologic age is 16 years; carpal age, 16 years. In (2) the chronologic age is 16 years; carpal age, 7 years. In (3) the chronologic age is 16 years; carpal age, 2 years.

(C) Effect of deficiency in secretion of growth hormone from anterior pituitary. (1) Drawings of lateral roentgenograms of skulls of albino rats. (2) Enlarged drawing of rat incisors in sagittal section. (3) Enlarged drawing of rat molars in mesiodistal section. The albino rats from which these sections and drawings were made were 300 days old at the time they were killed, but the ones on the right were hypophysectomized at 40 days. (4) Drawing from intra-oral roentgenograms from normal and hypopituitary males aged 16 years. The effect of hypopituitarism upon the growth of bone and the eruption of the teeth is to be noted. (Schour and Massler, J. A. D. A., 30:595, 1943.)

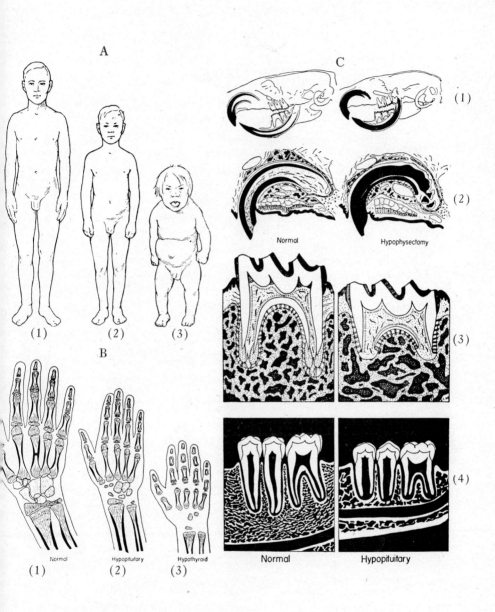

A
(1) (2) (3)

B
(1) Normal (2) Hypopituitary (3) Hypothyroid

C
(1)
(2)
Normal Hypophysectomy
(3)
(4)
Normal Hypopituitary

Posterior Lobe

The hormones of the posterior lobe have a rapid or immediate action.

(a) Pitressin. This is an antidiuretic hormone which regulates the flow of water through the kidneys, stimulates the intestinal musculature and causes contraction of the peripheral blood vessels.

(b) Pitocin. This hormone causes contraction of the uterine musculature following labor.

Hypopituitarism

Pituitary deficiency in the early years of life results in dwarfism. There is a harmonious diminished development of all the hard and soft tissues in pituitary dwarfism. This condition is rarely manifested before 6 years. Diagnosis is made on the basis of the clinical and roentgenologic findings. There is some question as to whether the favorable clinical results which have been observed following therapy represent a therapeutic response or a spontaneous cure. Pituitary hypofunction in adult life results in striking changes. The individual becomes sleepy, listless, thin and may die of inanition. This syndrome is called Simmond's disease.

Oral Aspects. Hypopituitarism has a marked influence on the development of the teeth, jaws and the face. The dental and facial development of the pituitary dwarf corresponds with the general skeletal development as determined by the degree of carpal and metacarpal development and ossification. The teeth may appear later than normal and fail to erupt completely. The crowns of the teeth are usually normal. They show frequently incomplete formation of the roots and a wide apical foramen on the roentgenogram.

The underdevelopment of the lower half of the face results commonly in crowding and malocclusion of the teeth. Markus *et al.* did not find any particular type of malocclusion in their cases of pituitary dwarfism although there was a lack of development in the facial width and the depth of the lower half of the face. They did not observe any evidence of delayed eruption of the teeth.

Hyperpituitarism—Acromegaly

The effects of excessive pituitary function (growth hormone) is dependent on the age of the individual when the hyperfunction occurs. Early in life, a harmonious general overdevelopment occurs which results in gigantism. After 6 years of age the excessive growth is limited to those parts which are still engaged in active development. These individuals have disproportionately large hands, feet, face and increased stature. The disharmonious enlargement of the palmar osseous and soft tissues as compared with the fingers, produces the "spade-shaped" deformity of the hands which is characteristic of acromegaly. These changes usually become manifested about the 30th or 40th year of life. Women at times develop hyperpituitarism following a pregnancy.

In later adult life, when most of the active growth of the body has ceased, hyperpituitarism results in less striking changes which are confined to the hands, feet, face and to a less extent the spine and clavicles. There is little if any increase in height. Symptoms of severe headache, photophobia and at times a reduction in bitemporal vision due to pressure on the optic chiasm are experienced when the pituitary hyperfunction results from a tumor of this gland.

The diagnosis of hyperpituitarism is made on the clinical and roentgenologic findings. An enlargement of the *sella turcica* and at times complete destruction of this landmark are demonstrated by means of skull x-rays. Treatment is both by surgery and x-ray radiation.

Oral Aspects. Early in life the face and the jaws participate as the other body organs in the precocious and abnormal growth. After approximately 8 to 12 years of life, the changes associated with hyperpituitarism are confined

A   B   C   D

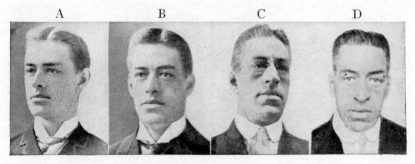

FIG. 162. A case of acromegaly. (A) The patient at age 24, before the onset of the malady; (B) at age 29, at the time of onset; (C) at age 37; and (D) at age 42, when outspoken acromegalic changes are evident. (Reproduced by permission from Cushing, The Pituitary Body and Its Disorders, J. B. Lippincott Company.)

chiefly to the lower jaw and to a lesser degree to the maxilla. The sinuses are enlarged. X-ray studies reveal a marked thickening of the calvarium and the cortical bone of the mandible. At times, periosteal ossifications are seen where muscles and tendons attach. This marked over-development of the mandible and the face produces the striking acromegalic facial expression which is characteristic of adult hyperpituitarism. These overdeveloped osseous structures are of poor quality with large bony trabeculae and poor calcification.

The lips are greatly enlarged in acromegaly. The nose is also increased in size and localized areas of hyperpigmentation are often seen along the nasolabial folds. The mandible is markedly enlarged. The angle of the jaw becomes flattened, which further increases the disproportionate relation between the jaws. There is a fanning out and a spacing of the teeth which appear to be erupted more than normal. This is probably due to an overgrowth of the alveolar process. The size of the teeth is unchanged but increased cementum deposition, which is normally a continuous process, is a common finding. The palatal arch is usually flattened. The lateral margins of the tongue have a crenated outline where this enlarged organ comes in contact with the teeth.

Simmonds Disease is a rare disease of the pituitary gland which is characterized by loss of weight, low basal metabolic rate, loss of axillary and pubic hair and amenorrhea in the female. It results usually from a tumor of the pituitary gland. It may be confused with anorexia nervosa.

THE THYROID GLAND

The thyroid gland is derived from a downgrowth of the pharyngeal wall between the first and second pharyngeal pouches. The thyroglossal duct formed by this downgrowth normally becomes obliterated. Its origin remains as a closed depression, the *foramen caecum*. If portions of the thyroglossal

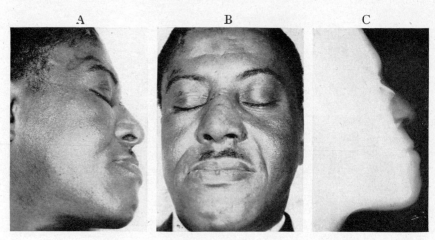

Fig. 163. Acromegalic features showing the abnormal development of the mandible. (A) profile; (B) front; (C) profile roentgenogram of the same patient.

duct fail to become obliterated, thyroglossal cysts develop. These cysts are occasionally seen within the mouth. Persistent portions of thyroid tissue near the base of the tongue may give rise to a lingual thyroid gland.

Acute thyroiditis is an acute inflammation of the thyroid gland which occasionally follows an upper respiratory infection. The gland is swollen, tender and painful. It usually develops in thyroid glands with existing benign hypertrophy.

Carcinoma of the thyroid is not rare. This tumor metastasizes early and frequently to bone. In carcinoma, the thyroid gland is hard and fixed with enlargement of the regional lymph nodes. Carcinoma frequently arises from pre-existing thyroid adenomas.

Simple Colloid Goiter

To the layman all thyroid enlargements are "goiters." "Goiter" represents a symptom, thyroid enlargement, rather than a disease and it should always be appropriately qualified.

Simple colloid goiter is a benign compensatory enlargement of the thyroid due to a lack of iodine in the drinking water or the food. Endemic colloid goiter occurs in mountainous countries and areas remote from the sea. The "goiter belt" in the United States is the Great Lakes region and parts of the Northwest. With the prophylactic methods now in use, the prevalence of endemic goiter has dropped markedly.

Simple colloid goiter most commonly appears during adolescence and it has a marked predisposition for the female. It usually disappears spontaneously after the 25th year. The thyroid hyperplasia is characteristically symmetric in form, soft and without nodules or irregularities. Thyroid enlargement may follow any period of physiologic or psychic stress such as adolescence, pregnancy, etc. Occasionally there are symptoms related to pressure on adjacent structures but constitutional symptoms are absent. Basal metabolic rate determinations fall within normal range.

The treatment of colloid goiter consists of the prophylactic administration of iodine in the water supply or the use of iodized salt in endemic areas. The therapeutic administration of iodine, desiccated thyroid or surgery are indicated in some cases.

Nodular Goiter (Adenomatous Goiter)

Nodules appear frequently in enlarged thyroid glands where they produce a conspicuous asymmetry. This form of goiter is important because of its undesirable appearance and the occasional development of toxic symptoms or malignancy.

Thyrotoxicosis—Hyperthyroidism—Exophthalmic Goiter (Toxic Thyroid—Grave's Disease—Basedow's Disease)

Hyperthyroidism or hyperactivity of the thyroid gland produces marked systemic effects. It is common in the young and middle-aged adult and, like colloid goiter, it shows a marked predilection for the female. In most instances the disease follows some psychic or emotional crisis in the individual's life. The cause of the thyroid hyperfunction is unknown. The most likely explanation is an excess of pituitary thyrotropic hormone. Focal infection may be responsible for a small percentage of the cases.

Marked nervousness, emotional instability, characteristic eye and cardiovascular symptoms, loss of weight (in spite of a hearty appetite), shortness of breath, weakness, inability to sleep, marked perspiration especially of the face and hands, a silky quality to the hair, and disturbances of the gastrointestinal tract are characteristic symptoms. Intolerance to heat is a prominent and significant finding.

Marked functional and organic changes occur in the circulatory system, which may overshadow all other symptoms. There are tachycardia, palpitation, increased pulse pressure, hypertension and cardiac enlargement. Thrills or bruits are often present over the thyroid gland. In advanced cases there are signs and symptoms of cardiac decompensation.

The eye symptoms are at times striking. The eyeballs are often protruded from their sockets (exophthalmos) and the upper lid fails to follow smoothly the vertical movements of the eye. The palpebral fissure is enlarged, producing a peculiar "staring" expression.

Frank cases of hyperthyroidism can be diagnosed usually on the basis of the clinical findings and history. A number of clinical aids to diagnosis have been suggested. These consist of:

(1) The tremor test which is performed by having the patient hold the hands outstretched with the fingers spread apart. This tremor is not controlled by counterpressure.

A   B

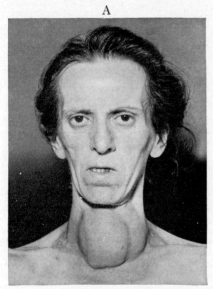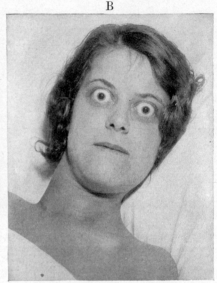

FIG. 164. (A) Toxic goiter. A patient with a large nodular goiter, suffering from severe hyperthyroidism. Note the absence of exophthalmos. (By courtesy of Dr. George Crile, Jr., and the publishers of Surg. Gynec. and Obstet.) (B) Graves' disease. Marked exophthalmos in a patient suffering from severe hyperthyroidism and from whom a large diffuse goiter had been removed. (By courtesy of Dr. George Crile, Jr., and the publishers of Surg. Gynec. and Obstet.)

(2) The duration of voluntary apnea test. Bartlett believed that this is the most useful single aid in the clinical estimation of the severity of thyrotoxicosis.
(3) Reed's formula for estimating the basal metabolic rate on the basis of the pulse rate and pulse pressure.

$$\tfrac{3}{4} \left(\tfrac{3}{4} \text{ PR plus PP}\right) - 72 = \text{BMR}$$

(4) Circulatory response to measured exercise. In thyrotoxicosis there is a prolongation of the acceleration of the pulse rate and a large increase in pulse pressure following measured exercise.

Laboratory Aids to Diagnosis. (1) Basal metabolic rate determinations (BMR) between plus and minus 10% have little significance—those deviating 20% from normal are significant if the test has been performed under basal conditions.

(2) Cholesterol determination. Low blood cholesterol values are a characteristic finding in hyperthyroidism. Some clinicians consider the blood cholesterol finding more significant than the BMR, since they are not modified by nervous or emotional reactions on the part of the patient.

The treatment of hyperthyroidism is both medical and surgical. Cases of recovery are known to have occurred following the elimination of foci of infection, including those of oral origin. The generally accepted form of treatment is a combination of absolute rest, sedation, iodine therapy, surgery and at times roentgen-ray therapy depending on the severity of the individual case. A new drug, thiourea, gives some promise for medical treatment. Spontaneous remissions without any form of treatment are not uncommon.

Oral Aspects. Under oral aspects of hyperthyroidism must be considered (1) the effect of oral infections on diseases of the thyroid, (2) the effect of hyperthyroidism on the development of the teeth, the jaws and the maintenance of the integrity of these structures and (3) the dentist's responsibility in treating the patient with hyperthyroidism.

Focal infection appears to have some injurious effect on the thyroid gland either directly by means of bacteria or their toxins or their influence on iodine metabolism. Billings called attention to cases of thyrotoxicosis due to focal infection. Olsen and Taylor observed a relationship between defective teeth and diseased tonsils in cases where there was no iodine deficiency. Lintz found that 50% of the goiter patients he examined had either infected or extracted teeth while in the control group the incidence was only 17%. Specific cases have been reported where hyperactive thyroids were aggravated by oral infections and were relieved by their elimination. Oral foci of infection may aggravate a hyperthyroid condition or result in exacerbations of symptoms associated with hyperfunction of this gland, but they cannot be considered as playing any direct exciting role.

Infants born of hyperthyroid mothers have been reported to have several teeth erupted at birth. Children with hyperthyroidism exhibit a rapid growth and development of the skeleton, with earlier than normal tooth eruption. The teeth and the jaws are well formed and present no unusual irregularities. The dental development is usually in keeping with the epiphyseal age of these patients, which is also abnormally advanced. Reede called attention to the syndrome of goiter, gingivitis and choreiform movements in children. An exacerbation of the mouth symptoms was frequently associated with thyroid exacerbations.

It has been the experience of the Lahey Clinic that there is a tendency to early and excessive dental decay in hyperthyroid patients and also a co-existent alveolar resorption. Kugelmass noted a high incidence of caries in both hyper- and hypothyroid individuals. Bilanioni also observed rapid alveolar atrophy as well as an increased incidence of caries in hyperthyroidism. Others have reported a marked loss of the alveolar process in hyperthyroid patients or those taking large amounts of desiccated thyroid substance for long periods. The maxillary bones are thin and delicate with an increased radiolucency. Salivary flow is increased. Alveolar absorption due to hyperthyroidism has been produced experimentally in guinea pigs. It was associated with an increased vascularity of the alveolodental periosteum and an increased osteoclastic activity along the *lamina dura*. The increased body metabolism and the increased calcium secretion may account in part for the periodontal findings.

The dentist has an unusual opportunity for detecting signs of thyroid hyperactivity. The objective findings are readily discernible and many of the simpler diagnostic tests are easily performed by the dentist. Unusual nervousness or irritability of the patient may be suggestive of hyperthyroidism. This is particularly true when dental extractions are contemplated. The dentist must differentiate these symptoms from the apprehensiveness which is associated with tooth removal.

Oral operations on hyperthyroid patients are contraindicated. While it is important to eliminate infected foci in the hyperthyroid patient, dental extractions should not be performed until after medical therapy or until the patient's physician sanctions the procedure. Fatalities have resulted from dental extractions on unprepared hyperthyroid patients.

Brams suggested the use of general anesthesia as this lessens the psychic trauma of local anesthesia. Adrenalin is contraindicated. Even the small amount of this drug in the novocaine used for dental anesthesia may produce undesirable reactions in the hyperthyroid patient. At one time the subcutaneous injection of small amounts of adrenalin was the basis of a clinical test for hyperthyroidism (Goetch's test). The serious and fatal reactions which followed its use caused its discontinuance. Even extensive or painful operative procedures are contraindicated on the hyperthyroid patient. If dental treatment is necessary, it should be simple in nature, with short appointments and adequate premedication.

Hypothyroidism

Hypothyroidism results from an insufficiency in the normal function of the thyroid gland. The clinical symptoms which ensue vary, depending on the age at which the deficiency occurs. While marked hypothyroidism produces characteristic clinical findings, mild hypothyroidism is frequently undiagnosed.

The following types of hypothyroidism are recognized: (1) congenital (children born of hypothyroid mothers), (2) childhood form and (3) an adult form of hypothyroidism.

Cretinism is the manifestation of congenital hypothyroidism. Autopsy studies in such cases have shown that there is almost complete lack of thyroid tissue. There is delayed physical and mental development. A lack of normal physical development may be the first indication of the disease. Cretins are physically inactive. These children have a characteristic facial expression. Their head appears too large for the rest of the body. The lips are thickened and the mouth is frequently held in a partially opened position. This may be due in part to the increased size of the tongue. The voice is coarse, hoarse and speech is generally poorly developed. The dental development which is greatly delayed, will be discussed under childhood hypothyroidism.

The early treatment of cretinism with desiccated thyroid will produce marked improvement in the physical development but the mental improvement is less striking. It has no effect on the dental structures which have been previously formed.

Childhood Hypothyroidism. The manifestations of childhood hypothyroidism occur at a later age than those in cretinism. It may be related to iodine deficiency or to unknown damage or insufficiency of the thyroid gland. Physical inactivity, mental dullness, loss of concentration and the inability to carry out instructions may be the first manifestation of hypothyroidism. The symptoms previously enumerated under cretinism are all present. The tissues have a pseudo-edematous appearance and consistency but they do not pit on pressure. The hypothyroid child appears top heavy with the greater length from the *symphysis pubis* upwards. There is a general retardation of osseous development and a marked alteration of the body structure.

ORAL ASPECTS. The oral changes in hypothyroidism, which consist of a retardation of tooth eruption and defective formation of the jaws and facial parts, may give an early clue to diagnosis. The teeth are commonly poorly formed and in some instances appear to be unusually susceptible to dental decay. Large first incisors and small second incisors have been noted. The faulty jaw development is associated with overlapping of the teeth, malocclusion and general facial disharmony. The family dentist or the orthodontist may be the first person to suspect the possibility of mild cases of hypothyroidism.

The dental age of hypothyroid children is many years younger than their chronologic or their epiphyseal age. The dentist can easily estimate the epiphyseal development by taking x-rays of the hands. If there is also delayed epiphyseal development, he is justified in suggesting more elaborate clinical studies.

Adult Hypothyroidism—Myxedema

Adult myxedema will not be seen as frequently by the dentist as the mild forms of thyroid deficiency in children. Adult myxedema develops spontaneously or it is secondary to the surgical removal of too much thyroid tissue in the treatment of hyperthyroidism.

Spontaneous adult hypothyroidism occurs most frequently in women (6:1). It is common at the menopause. The individual is easily fatigued and there is a lack of attention to the surroundings and general mental inactivity. The patient puts on weight in spite of poor appetite. The characteristic nonpitting edema of the subcutaneous tissues occurs. This is particularly evident in the face. The skin gradually becomes dry and scaly. The hair becomes thin and brittle as do the finger nails. The patient may complain of being cold in surroundings that are comfortable for the ordinary individual. The blood pressure is low and the pulse is slow. The basal metabolic rate is significantly lowered and there is usually an increase in the blood cholesterol findings.

The diagnosis of adult myxedema is based on the clinical findings, the basal metabolic rate determinations and blood chemistry studies. Treatment consists of the oral administration of desiccated thyroid substance.

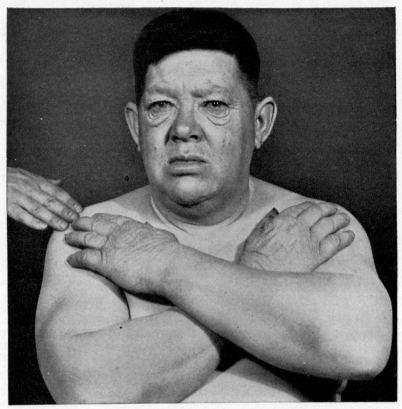

FIG. 165. Myxedema. Note the typical facial expression and shape of the fingers in a man, aged 52, suffering from myxedema. (Grollman, Essentials of Endocrinology, J. B. Lippincott Company.)

ORAL ASPECTS. Abnormally soft dentin and enamel, abnormal root resorption, decalcification of the superior maxilla (and carpal bones) have been reported to be associated with hypothyroidism. Most clinicians agree that there is an increased incidence of caries and probably an increased susceptibility to periodontal diseases in hypothyroidism. Rosenthal reported on the oral findings in 9 adult hypothyroid patients. Marginal gingivitis, lustreless enamel about the necks of the teeth, rampant caries and death of the pulp under shallow fillings and failures in attempts at root canal therapy were common findings.

THYMUS GLAND

The exact function of the thymus gland is not known. This gland is an unpaired structure which is situated in the neck beneath the thyroid gland. It reaches its greatest development between the 8th and 12th years of life after which it regresses in size. An incretion from the thymus gland has not been isolated but animal experiments suggest that this gland may play some minor role in growth.

The thymus gland is of medical and dental interest because it is believed to be associated with sudden death in the young adult, particularly during the administration of a general anesthesia. In these cases the only significant finding at post mortem is a persistent or unusually large thymus gland. Walbott has presented evidence which suggests that "thymic death" may be an anaphylactic reaction. The so-called "thymus type" of an individual is likely to have large adenoids and tonsils. The typical symptoms of thymic death include stridor, dyspnea and shock. If an abnormally large thymus is known to exist it can be reduced in size by roentgen-ray therapy.

THE PARATHYROIDS

The parathyroid glands are 2 to 4 small structures which are posterolateral to the thyroid gland. In rare instances, one or more of the parathyroid glands are located in the thorax beneath the sternum. These thoracic parathyroids assume considerable importance in the surgical treatment of hyperparathyroidism.

The parathyroid glands are concerned with the control of calcium metabolism by means of mobilizing calcium from the bones into the blood stream and maintaining a normal calcium level of 9 to 11.5 mg./100 cc. blood. Parathyroid disturbances affect only those calcified structures which are forming during the period of dysfunction or those which have a readily mobilizable source of calcium.

Hypoparathyroidism

Hypoparathyroidism may result from structural or functional deficiencies occurring usually in early life, or due to disease or accidental removal during thyroidectomy in the adult. The hypocalcemia results in parathyroid tetany. The systemic symptoms of parathyroid tetany demand prompt and active treatment. They overshadow the dental changes which are of secondary origin and importance. Tetany in infancy and childhood is often associated with hypoplasia of the enamel and abnormal dentin formation and calcification. Jaw and facial development is not affected.

Hyperparathyroidism—Osteitis Fibrosa Cystica

Hyperparathyroidism is of more importance to the practicing dentist because of its manifestations in the adult and the common involvement of the oral structures. In hyperparathyroidism there is an excess production of parathormone which is usually the result of hyperplasia or a neoplasm of 1 of the parathyroids. A wide variety of systemic symptoms is associated with this abnormal mobilization of calcium. Renal calculi are likely to develop due to the excess urinary calcium secretion. Secondary infections of the urinary tract are common and serious complications. There are loss of weight and increased thirst. Pain in the extremities, especially the legs, is one of the early and striking symptoms. These painful symptoms are often mistaken for arthritis or neuralgia. Purpuric manifestations are common.

A general demineralization of the skeleton is an early and important finding. Multiple cystic tumors of the bones, including the jaws, give rise to the nomenclature of osteitis fibrosa cystica. Roentgenologic studies often give the first suggestion as to the true nature of the disease. There is a loss of detail of the normal bony trabeculae with a thinning of the cortex. The characteristic multiple bone cysts are seen later in the course of the disease. There is only a slight evidence of new bone formation associated with these changes. Pathologic fractures occur if large cysts develop in weight-bearing bones.

The diagnosis of hyperparathyroidism is made on the basis of the clinical symptoms and the roentgenologic and blood chemistry findings. The serum calcium and the blood phosphatase are markedly elevated while the inorganic phosphorus is low.

The treatment of hyperparathyroidism consists of the removal of the hyperplastic or neoplastic parathyroid glands. This is not easily accomplished, particularly when the involved gland is located in the thorax.

Oral Aspects. This disease should be considered by the dentist whenever unusual areas of decalcification or cysts which are unrelated to the apices of the teeth are observed in the jaws.

The hyperparathyroid patient may consult the dentist because of local oral symptoms which are associated with this disease or in the belief that the loss of weight, the arthritic or neuralgic symptoms are due to oral foci of infection. In many of the reported cases of hyperparathyroidism the patient had an oral tumor or epulis removed a year or more before the systemic disease was recognized. In the case reported by Cohen and Kelly the epulis preceded the generalized symptoms of the disease by 8 years. This emphasizes the importance of having histopathologic studies made of all lesions which are removed from the mouth.

Early loss of teeth is a common finding in persons with hyperparathyroidism and some authors claim that there is an increase in dental decay.

The demineralization of the alveolar process results in extensive alveolar resorption and associated inflammatory changes in the gingiva. In Borke's case portions of the jaw bone were removed when the teeth were extracted. The teeth are not observed to participate in this demineralization. In fact, they appear more dense (radio-opaque) than normal due to the demineralization of the alveolar process. There is extensive diffuse and nodular calcification within the dental pulp.

Following the loss of all the teeth the maxillary and mandibular bone furnishes an unsatisfactory base for artificial dentures because of its poor quality. In hyperparathyroidism, sections of the jaw bones can be removed with ease by means of an ordinary scalpel.

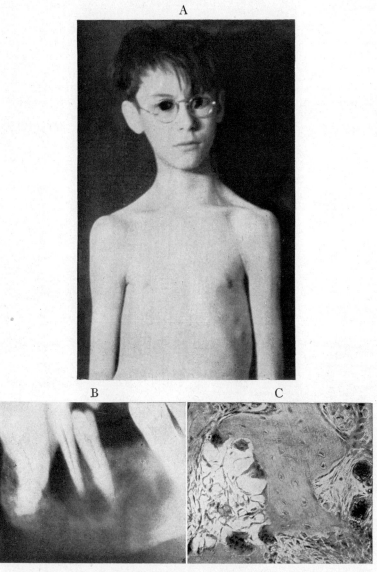

FIG. 166. (A) Generalized osteitis fibrosa (hyperparathyroidism) in a boy aged 15. (B) X-ray of the mandible. (C) Section from the maxilla. (From Thoma's Oral Diagnosis, Ed. 2, W. B. Saunders Company.)

The bone cysts in the jaws or the gingival tumors may be the first evidence of this disease. The finding of these multiple bone cysts in the jaws during a routine roentgenologic examination of these structures is not unusual. These areas consist of large collections of osteoclasts which undergo degeneration or hemorrhage and result in the typical bone cysts. The presence of the multiple radiolucent areas of the jaw bones which are not associated with tooth apices should suggest an oral involvement of some systemic disease, of which hyperparathyroidism is one possibility. The presence of multiple epulides or a recurring epulis should also suggest the possibility of hyperparathyroidism and if bone cysts are also present the diagnosis becomes more probable.

Spingarn and Gerst reported a case of hyperparathyroidism which demonstrated the oral aspects of this disease and emphasized the importance of the dentist ruling out a systemic background for any oral lesion of unusual nature. The patient, a 29-year-old female, was in good health until she experienced severe renal colic which necessitated the removal of an ureteral calculus. Two years later, a mass appeared on the left maxilla which was excised but not studied histologically. A year later the patient experienced a pathologic fracture of the right humerus. Four years later she complained of a painless swelling of the lower jaw. The lower incisors were loose. X-rays of the skeleton now revealed generalized osteitis fibrosa cystica. A surgical exploration for a parathyroid tumor was unsuccessful.

TABLE XVIII

COMPARISON OF THE CLINICAL FEATURES OF HYPERPARATHYROIDISM, PAGET'S DISEASE AND OSTEOMALACIA

	Hyperparathyroidism	Paget's Disease	Osteomalacia
Age	Late childhood to 40 years of age. More common in females.	Usually from 50 to 70 years of age. Males predominate.	Usually 30 to 50 years of age. Occurs in females, particularly those on deficient diet and multiple pregnancies.
Clinical features	Marked systemic symptoms in the GI tract, the urogenital tract and nervous system. Pain marked. Purpuric manifestations. Pain and tenderness on the long bones. Thinning of the bone cortex with loss of detail of bone trabeculae. Bone cysts common, usually in the proximal ends of the long bones. Bone decalcification main feature of disease.	No or few systemic symptoms. Pain a prominent symptom. No purpuric manifestations. Long bones, skull, tibia and spine involved. Cortex of the bone thickened with characteristic "cotton wool" appearance on the x-ray. Bone absorption and bone building with the latter predominating.	Few systemic symptoms. Loss of trabecular detail and generalized demineralization of the skeleton. Pain and tenderness on the long bones. No purpuric manifestations.
Oral changes	Marked loosening of the erupted teeth. No tooth decalcification. Recurrent giant-cell epulides or cysts in the jaws—most common in the mandible.	Loosening and spacing of the teeth. No decalcification of the teeth. Bone cysts do not occur. Marked involvement of the alveolar process common.	Loosening of the teeth. No decalcification of the teeth or increase in dental decay. Bone cysts do not occur. Epulides do not develop.
Blood chemistry	Blood Ca high. Blood phosphatase 2.5 units.	Blood Ca may be normal with normal Ca metabolism. Blood phosphatase may be as high as 40 units.	Blood Ca and P low. Blood phosphatase—little or no change.

The oral findings, particularly those of the jaw bones, must be differentiated from Paget's disease, multiple myeloma, ameloblastoma and osteomalacia. In the former disease the calcium metabolism is normal and bone production exceeds bone destruction. In osteomalacia the blood calcium and phosphorus findings are both low. Ameloblastoma is rarely bilateral and it usually involves the mandible. The roentgenologic findings will permit a differential diagnosis. Biopsy studies may be required to differentiate multiple myeloma. In multiple myeloma the calvarium is commonly involved and the Bence-Jones protein is usually present in the urine.

THE ADRENAL GLANDS

The adrenals or suprarenal glands, 2 in number, are situated on the superior pole of each kidney. The adrenal gland is composed of a medullary portion and a cortical portion. The former is of ectodermal origin and incretes the hormone adrenalin while the latter is of mesodermal origin and incretes cortin. The gland has an important regulatory effect on salt, water and carbohydrate metabolism. Because of the interrelationship between the adrenal cortical hormone and the gonads, gonadal changes are usually associated with diseases of the adrenal cortex. Systemic changes due to hypofunction of the adrenal cortex are best known. Tumors of the adrenal glands result in virilism in women and precocious puberty in children.

ADDISON'S DISEASE

Hypofunction of the adrenal cortex gives rise to the symptoms of Addison's disease. In about half of the cases the hypofunction is due to cortical atrophy. The destruction of the cortical tissue by other diseases, particularly tuberculosis, is another important cause of adrenal hypofunction.

Addison's disease is characterized by progressive weakness, loss of weight, hypotension and pigmentation. The brownish pigmentation of the skin and mucous membranes is one of the prominent symptoms of this disease. The pigmentation is most prominent on those surfaces which are exposed to light or which are subjected to mechanical irritation. The mucosa of the vagina and rectum is not affected. The mechanism of this pigmentation is obscure. It is not influenced by treatment with desoxycorticosterone acetate. Anorexia, vomiting and diarrhea are common in this disease. The patient complains frequently of headache, paresthesias, irritability and loss of memory. Hypotension is one of the most striking symptoms. A systolic pressure as low as 80 to 50 mg. Hg is not unusual, particularly in an adrenal crisis. An acute exacerbation of all symptoms, an adrenal crisis, may follow acute infections or operative procedures on patients with Addison's disease.

The disease is diagnosed on the basis of the clinical symptoms, a low blood pressure and altered blood chemistry findings. There is a decrease in the Na and Cl in the blood plasma with an increase in the secretion of NaCl in the urine. The level of urinary chlorides is one of the laboratory tests utilized in the diagnosis of Addison's disease.

The treatment of Addison's disease is not too successful. The administration of adrenal cortical extract or the synthetic desoxycorticosterone is of definite value. The latter is frequently administered subcutaneously in the form of pellets which are slowly absorbed. Desoxycorticosterone dissolved in propylene glycol has also been administered by the sublingual route. The diet should be high in calories, contain large amounts of NaCl, and be low in K. The above treatment has no effect on the pigmentation.

Oral Aspects

The pigmentation of the oral mucosa may be an early symptom of this disease. At times it is absent in cases of severe Addison's disease. Its presence is of greater diagnostic significance than the dermal pigmentation. It is found on the gums, palate, cheek mucosa and tongue. The cheek is the most common site of involvement. The pigmentation is bluish-black or brownish-gray in color. It appears in the form of streaks or irregular spots or blotches. The oral pigmentation must be differentiated from racial pigmentation, that found in hemochromatosis, that due to heavy metal therapy such as bismuth, and the tattooing of foregin substances such as graphite, charcoal or small particles of amalgam fillings. Loeb never saw the oral mucosal pigmentation disappear under any form of therapy.

Infections or surgical procedures are likely to precipitate an adrenal crisis. Bartels and Jones called attention to the significance and the dangers of dental infection and dental surgery in patients with Addison's disease. They emphasized that these patients should be informed of the seriousness of infection and the need for medical care whenever they are present. From experiences with dental infections in these patients which terminated in fatalities, they have found that whenever extractions are required the administration of a course of sulfathiazole will minimize the dangers to the patient. The sulfathiazole is given 2 days before the extraction and continued for 4 days thereafter. Under this regime local or systemic reactions were not experienced and normal healing took place. When infections were already present the use of penicillin has been advantageous.

17

Diseases of the Bones and Joints

ARTHRITIS	HEREDITARY CRANIOFACIAL DYSOS-
RHEUMATOID ARTHRITIS	TOSIS
OSTEO-ARTHRITIS	ORAL TORI
DISEASES OF THE TEMPOROMAN-	OSTEITIS DEFORMANS—PAGET'S
DIBULAR JOINT	DISEASE
CLEIDOCRANIAL DYSOSTOSIS	OSTEOGENESIS IMPERFECTA
	MULTIPLE MYELOMA

ARTHRITIS

Arthritis is an ancient disease. It is said to be one of the reasons for the extensive baths which the Romans built throughout their empire. "Rheumatism" today affects in one year a greater number of persons than are affected by heart disease and arteriosclerosis combined—and approximately 10 times the tuberculosis prevalence rates (Table No. XIX).

Based on the total cost of medical care for arthritic patients or the number of work days lost, arthritis represents not only a tremendous public health problem but also an increasingly important socio-economic problem.

A satisfactory classification of the various forms of arthritis cannot be achieved until a more complete knowledge of their etiology is known. The following classification will prove convenient and useful.

CLASSIFICATION OF ARTHRITIS *

I. ARTHRITIS DUE TO KNOWN INFECTIOUS AGENTS.
    (a) Tuberculous.
    (b) Gonococcal.
    (c) Pyogenic forms (Streptococcus hemolyticus, staphylococcus, pneumococcus, etc.).
    (d) Luetic arthritis (Charcot's joints).
II. ARTHRITIS PROBABLY DUE TO INFECTIOUS AGENTS, but not proven.
    (a) RHEUMATOID ARTHRITIS (Atrophic arthritis, proliferative arthritis, chronic infectious arthritis).
        1. Known as Still's disease in children.

* Modified from the Classification approved by the Nomenclature Committee of the American Rheumatism Association.

  2. Felty's syndrome when associated with hepatomegaly, splenomegaly and leukopenia.

  3. Marie-Strumpell arthritis—rheumatoid arthritis of the spine. Sex incidence, male:females, 10:1.

 (b) Arthritis associated with rheumatic fever (? arthritis due to hemolytic streptococcus).

III. OSTEO-ARTHRITIS (Hypertrophic arthritis, degenerative arthritis, senile arthritis).

IV. ARTHRITIDES DUE TO DIRECT TRAUMA, INTERNAL OR EXTERNAL PHYS-ICAL INJURIES TO THE JOINT.

 (a) Severe sprains or trauma.

 (b) Arthritis associated with chronic dislocation of a joint—i.e., the shoulder, knee or the temporomandibular joint.

 (c) Hemarthrosis—as in hemophilia.

V. GOUTY ARTHRITIS—actually a disease of metabolism.

TABLE XIX

ESTIMATED PREVALENCE OF SPECIFIED CHRONIC DISEASES IN THE UNITED STATES (1937)

Disease	Number of Cases
Rheumatism	6,850,000
Heart disease	3,700,000
Arteriosclerosis and high blood pressure	3,700,000
Hay fever and asthma	3,450,000
Hernia	2,100,000
Hemorrhoids	2,000,000
Varicose veins	1,750,000
Chronic bronchitis	1,700,000
Nephritis and other kidney diseases	1,550,000
Nervous and mental diseases	1,450,000
Goitre and other thyroid diseases	1,200,000
Sinusitis	1,150,000
Cancer and other tumors	930,000
Diseases of female organs	720,000
Tuberculosis, all forms	680,000
Diabetes mellitus	660,000
Diseases of gallbladder and liver	640,000
Other diseases of the circulatory system	440,000
Chronic tonsillitis and other throat disorders	380,000
Ulcers of stomach and duodenum	330,000
Diseases of bladder and urethra	270,000
Chronic diseases of the skin	270,000
Anemia	240,000
Chronic appendicitis	170,000
Chronic diseases of the eye	150,000
Chronic diseases of the ear	100,000
Chronic pleurisy	90,000
Diseases of the prostate and male genitourinary organs	80,000

From Preliminary Reports, the National Health Survey, Sickness and Medical Care Series Bulletin No. 6, U. S. Public Health Service, Washington, D. C., 1938.
J.A.M.A. Aug. 1, 1942, Vol. 119.

RHEUMATOID ARTHRITIS

Rheumatoid arthritis constitutes the largest single form of arthritis which, along with osteo-arthritis, comprises approxmately ⅔ of all forms of joint disorders. Rheumatoid arthritis is of great economic and social significance as it affects individuals during the height of their productive powers (25 to 50 years).

The cause of rheumatoid arthritis like the common cold remains one of the unsolved problems of medicine. Bacteria, viruses and even protozoa have been suggested as causative agents. Many of the symptoms of rheumatoid arthritis suggest an infectious etiology. In fact the significance of focal infection, including oral foci, in rheumatoid arthritis is based on the premise that the disease is of infectious etiology. While various organisms have been isolated from the fluid of the affected joints, this has not been accomplished by all clinicians. Other theories of etiology include derangements of the carbohydrate, sulphur, cholesterol metabolism and deficiencies of the vitamins, A, B and C.

The articular lesions and the subcutaneous nodules must be considered in the pathosis of rheumatoid arthritis. The early articular lesions are usually associated with an inflammation and proliferative thickening of the synovial lining. At this stage, cartilage changes may be noticed which include a superficial ulceration or a more or less complete involvement by the proliferation of the synovial lining tissue. The articular cartilage may be actually invaded and even completely destroyed, resulting in bony ankylosis.

The subcutaneous nodules represent a proliferative and a degenerative change rather than exudative phenomenon as is seen in rheumatic fever.

Symptoms

The onset of the disease is characteristically insidious, although it may begin as an acute episode. The arthritic symptoms are often preceded by complaints of fatigue, numbness and tingling of the extremities and weight loss. Sometimes the onset of rheumatoid arthritis appears to follow an acute upper respiratory infection, emotional or psychic trauma. During the acute stage of the disease a hyperpyrexia of 99° to 101° F. is common. There is an accompanying tachycardia. Anemia and a leukocytosis of 12,000 to 20,000 leukocytes cu. mm. are usually present.

The joints gradually and progressively become painful and swollen. They exhibit all the characteristics of an acute inflammation. There is usually symmetrical involvement of the joints. The proximal interphalangeal joints are most commonly affected followed by the metacarpal joints, the wrists, the knees, elbows, ankles, shoulders and the hips.

The affected joints have a characteristic fusiform appearance. The swelling results from a thickening and edema of the periarticular tissues. The gradual subsidence of the joint symptoms too often are followed by the painful disabling contractures that have been regarded as characteristic of this disease. Associated muscle atrophy and muscle weakness are common on the hand. The contractures and many of the resulting deformities can be prevented by suitable treatment in the early stages of the disease.

The skin of the affected parts becomes atrophic, smooth, glossy and fine in texture. The subcutaneous nodules are present in 20% of the cases. They are commonly found about the elbows. They may be present during or following the active stages of the disease.

The laboratory aids to diagnosis include roentgenographic studies of the joints. In advanced rheumatoid arthritis, these changes are characteristic with a narrowing of the joint space, resulting from the cartilage destruction. The erythrocyte sedimentation rate is an important diagnostic aid in rheumatoid arthritis. It is usually increased to 20 to 80 mm./hr. It is valuable in differ-

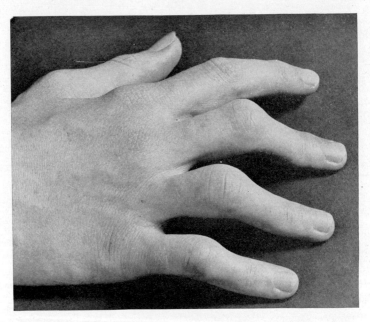

FIG. 167. Rheumatoid arthritis showing swelling and deformities at proximal interphalangeal joints. (Comroe, Arthritis and Allied Conditions, Lea & Febiger.)

entiating rheumatoid arthritis from osteo-arthritis. A positive hemolytic streptococcus agglutination test, when present, is a confirmatory finding.

Diagnosis

Diagnosis is based on the history of onset, the physical and roentgenologic findings, and laboratory tests. A pyogenic arthritis, gonococcal arthritis or rheumatic fever must be considered in the differential diagnosis. On the basis of the symptomatology and various laboratory tests these forms of arthritis can usually be ruled out. The Committee of the American Rheumatic Association calls attention to "a type of arthritis, often indistinguishable from rheumatoid arthritis which seems associated with focal infection as tonsillitis, dental abscesses and sinus infection."

The treatment of rheumatoid arthritis, like many of the other degenerative diseases, taxes the ingenuity, the resourcefulness and the patience of the

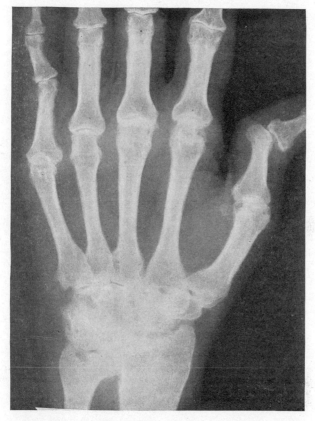

FIG. 168. Rheumatoid arthritis of twelve years'
duration. The changes present are indicative of an
advanced degree of rheumatoid arthritis. Areas of
bony ankylosis are already present. There is subluxation of the distal interphalangeal joints of both
thumbs and partial subluxation of the proximal interphalangeal joint of the left little finger. The most
marked loss of joint cartilage has occurred in the
carpus, where there is evidence of bony ankylosis.
There are numerous scattered juxta-articular cystic
areas and spotty areas of demineralization. (Comroe,
Arthritis and Allied Conditions, Lea & Febiger.)

medical practitioner. Too often the patient "shops" from one physician to
another without ever consenting to adequate diagnostic and clinical studies.
Measures of proven value include proper rest and nutrition, the removal of
infections, the use of drugs (salicylates and barbiturates), and physio-therapy.
In recent years the use of gold salts (chrysotherapy) has assumed a more
prominent place. While good clinical results have been reported, there is con-

siderable danger associated with their use. Dermatitis, fever, stomatitis (see gold stomatitis), purpura, aplastic anemia and even death have been reported.

Oral Aspects. The oral aspects to be considered in rheumatoid arthritis can be divided into (1) temporomandibular joint involvement in this disease and (2) the possible rôle of oral infection as a causative or aggravating factor in this disease.

Temporomandibular Joint Involvement in Rheumatoid Arthritis. The temporomandibular joint can be the initial or the most prominent manifestation of a generalized joint disturbance such as rheumatoid arthritis. When only the temporomandibular joint is involved, local causative factors such as abnormal chewing or sleeping habits or altered occlusal relations resulting from mutilation of the dental arches are looked for rather than a systemic basis for the symptoms.

A consideration of rheumatoid arthritic involvement of the temporomandibular joint has received meagre consideration although a few case reports, notably those by Kazanjian and Riesner called attention to temporomandibular joint involvement in this disease. The observations of Bayles and Russel, a physician and dentist respectively, furnished information about the frequency and the symptomatology of rheumatoid arthritic involvement of the temporomandibular joint and its treatment.

Individuals with temporomandibular joint involvement could be divided into those with (1) transitory, (2) acute and (3) chronic arthritic symptoms. Over 15% of the patients with rheumatoid arthritis had transitory symptoms in the temporomandibular joint. The limitation of motion of this joint and the pain referred to the teeth, maxilla, mandible, ear and muscles of the neck, usually brought the patient to the dentist for diagnosis and treatment. In some patients the jaw opening was limited to 10 mm. for 1 to 3 days.

The acute forms of temporomandibular joint symptoms were noted in approximately 40% of all patients with rheumatoid arthritis. In addition to the symptoms enumerated for the transitory joint involvement, there was definite limitation of motion, local pain, warmth and swelling of the joint. These symptoms persisted from 6 to 10 weeks. The recognition of this form of temporomandibular joint arthritis is important because the ultimate joint function is dependent on proper treatment. Chronic temporomandibular joint symptoms were noted in 45% of all patients with generalized rheumatoid arthritis who entered the hospital for medical or orthopedic care.

The frequency of temporomandibular joint involvement in the transitory, acute and chronic forms of generalized arthritis is given in Table XX.

The recognition of the temporomandibular joint symptoms as a manifestation of rheumatoid arthritis in the absence of other joint symptoms is not easy. The intermittent character of the symptoms with periods of exacerbations and remissions which are associated with swelling and stiffness should arouse suspicion of rheumatoid arthritis. If similar symptoms are present in other joints they will assist in making the diagnosis.

Dingman stressed the importance of the lack of severe constitutional symptoms in the diagnosis of rheumatoid arthritis of the temporomandibular joint.

TABLE XX

ARTHRITIC INVOLVEMENT OF TEMPOROMANDIBULAR JOINT: CLINICAL SUMMARY *

(From Bayles & Russel)

Type of Arthritis	Percentage of Patients with Rheumatoid Arthritis	Degree of Generalized Joint In- volvement	Percentage of Patients with Temporo- mandibular Involvement	Duration	Limitation of Opening of Jaw	Prognosis with Proper Treatment
Transitory......	8	Mild or mod- erate	15.8	1 to 6 days	25 mm. or less	Excellent
Acute..........	20	Moderate to severe	39.2	6 to 10 weeks	Usually 10 mm. or less	Good
Chronic.........	23	Severe	45.0	Over 4 months	25 mm. or less	Fair (good with surgi- cal treat- ment of "burned out" group)
Total........	51					

* On the basis of 100 consecutive admissions for rheumatoid arthritis.

In the patients studied by Bayles and Russel, trauma was a frequent fore-runner of rheumatoid arthritis of the temporomandibular joint. Natural mal-occlusion or that arising from ill-fitting dentures were recognized predispos-ing causes.

The important part of the treatment of acute temporomandibular joint arthritis, whether of traumatic or rheumatic origin, is physiologic rest. The patient may attempt stretching exercises in the fear of ankylosis when com-plete rest is essential. The teeth should be held in a near centric position during talking and eating. In a few days the muscle spasm and pain decrease and controlled use of the joint is advised. Gum-chewing exercises employing first soft and then a harder gum or sponge rubber are recommended. These exercises should not cause pain or fatigue. It may require one or two months to obtain satisfactory joint function.

Patients with temporomandibular joint symptoms which are suspected of being a part of a generalized rheumatoid arthritic process should be referred to a specialist in this field who can make the necessary examinations and laboratory studies to establish or rule out this diagnosis.

Possible Role of Oral Infection as Causative or Aggravating Factor in Rheumatoid Arthritis. Foci of infection, among which oral foci assumed a prominent place, for many years have been considered to play an important role in the causation of rheumatoid arthritis. Many pulpless or "dead" teeth, both those with and without periapical roentgenologic changes suggestive of infection, have been removed in past years in the hope of curing or ameliorating this disease. The dentist has been too frequently "ordered" to remove all the teeth in these patients. The construction of sat-isfactorily functioning artificial dentures has been complicated many times by the unnecessary loss of strategic vital or pulpless teeth. Moreover the den-tist has observed the patient to be still suffering from the joint symptoms after the loss of the teeth, at which time the search for a possible focus of infection has been carried to more remote, inaccessible and less easily re-moved organs.

Within recent years there has developed on the part of both the medical and dental professions a more conservative attitude about the importance of periapical infection. There is little reason to believe that the presence of pulpless teeth in patients with rheumatoid arthritis is of greater hazard than similar teeth in a patient without this disease. While considerable laboratory evidence points to the role of oral foci of infection in the causation of joint symptoms, the conclusions reached in these studies may be questioned because of the technics which were employed or the dosage of the organisms which were used.

The author is of the opinion that periodontal infection is of greater significance than periapical infection (*see* Focal Infection). Numerous studies have emphasized the potential seriousness of periodontal foci of infection, if the joint symptoms are related directly or indirectly to bacterial causation. Cecil, who at one time was impressed with the role of foci of infection and the significance of dental foci in rheumatoid arthritis, has more recently (with Angevine) minimized the significance of foci of infection including those of the oral cavity.

In a small portion of the patients with rheumatoid arthritis, an exacerbation of the joint symptoms, including an elevation of temperature, has followed periodontal treatment or the removal of pulpless teeth. At times severe general reactions follow the superficial scaling of periodontally involved teeth. Under these circumstances, future treatments should be undertaken with great caution and preferably after premedication with one of the sulfonamides. When this type of reaction occurs it is reasonable to believe that the general condition of the patient may benefit from the elimination of the particular focus.

In acute infectious arthritis of short duration the removal of all suspicious teeth may be justified when no other focus can be found. The importance of the teeth as a part of the chewing apparatus should be weighed against their possible role in causing or aggravating the arthritic symptoms.

According to Comroe, the dental care of the patient with rheumatoid arthritis should be undertaken as it would had the patient no arthritis, with the following exceptions:

"(1) No (except emergency) extractions shall be performed during an acute exacerbation of an arthritis, unless the patient is steadily becoming worse or is not improving after a reasonable period of time; *i.e.*, one or two months.

(2) In the case of undernourished, weakened persons, attempts shall be made to build up general resistance and strength before extractions are performed.

(3) Not more than one infected tooth shall be removed at the first sitting, with a rest period of at least three or four days. If a flare-up of arthritic phenomena occurs after extraction, a period of at least a week must be allowed before further extractions are performed. After the first extraction two or three infected teeth may be removed at one sitting, but under no circumstances should more than four infected teeth be removed at any one time."

OSTEO-ARTHRITIS (DEGENERATIVE—SENILE—HYPER-TROPHIC ARTHRITIS)

Osteo-arthritis is a degenerative disease which may be the result of wear and tear of everyday use of the parts. It develops usually after 40 years of

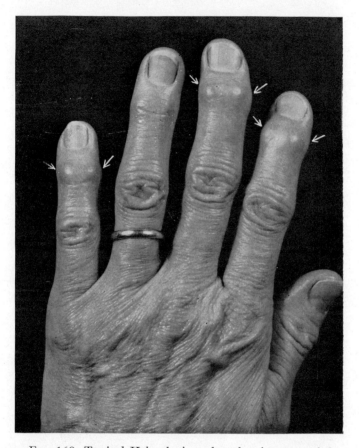

FIG. 169. Typical Heberden's nodes, the signposts of degenerative joint disease (osteo-arthritis). Note their typical characteristic position at the bases of the terminal phalanges, while the proximal phalangeal joints are not usually involved in this process. (Comroe, Arthritis and Allied Conditions, Lea & Febiger.)

age and is common in short heavy individuals. As a rule, the weight-bearing joints are affected, yet one of the most frequent sites of involvement is the terminal phalangeal joints. The enlargement of this joint produces the so-called Heberden's node.

The joint changes in osteo-arthritis consist of a softening and necrosis of the central portion of the interarticular cartilage. The disintegrating cartilage may be worn away with the result that the functioning joint surfaces become

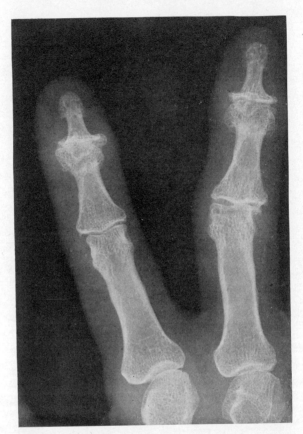

Fig. 170. Degenerative joint disease with formation of Heberden's nodes at terminal phalangeal joints. Note also some involvement of
proximal phalangeal joint (which occurs in a
smaller percentage of cases). Terminal phalangeal
joints are involved characteristically in degenerative joint disease (osteo-arthritis). Note loss of
cartilage in terminal phalangeal joints as evidenced by narrowed or obliterated joint spaces.
Proliferation of bone (hypertrophic changes) are
evident at terminal phalangeal joints. (Comroe,
Arthritis and Allied Conditions, Lea & Febiger.)

composed of dense eburnated bone. About the margins of the joints there is a proliferation of the cartilage and the subchondral and subperiosteal bone. New tissue is also formed which consists of cartilage on the surface and can-cellous bone on the interior. This growth results in the "marginal lipping" of the joints which is a characteristic roentgenologic finding in this form of arthritis. Ankylosis occurs rarely.

Symptoms

Many patients with joint changes characteristic of osteo-arthritis have no painful symptoms. One of the first symptoms may be a slight stiffness of the parts after rest which disappears gradually after use. Pain and discomfort are often present. Slight enlargement of the joints of the toes and the fingers are usually seen. Those of the terminal phalangeal joints are known as Heberden's nodes. Other joints may become involved in time. The general course of the disease is aggravated or accelerated by occupational strain and accidental trauma. Involvement of the spine and the hip joint are particularly painful. While the range of motion of the joints may be restricted by the exostoses about the joint margins, ankylosis is uncommon. These bony exostoses on the spine may cause pressure on the nerve roots.

The early roentgenologic changes consist of a slight sharpening of the joint margins. Later, the "marginal lipping" or exostoses are clearly seen. The changes in the interarticular cartilage result in a narrowing of the joint space. At times in the knees, these exostoses break off and form loose calcified bodies in the joint cavities. Roentgenograms of the hands, which can be easily made by the dentist, are not only easy to interpret but they show the earliest joint changes.

The blood count or the erythrocyte sedimentation rate is not conspicuously altered in osteo-arthritis.

Diagnosis

Important points to consider in the diagnosis of osteo-arthritis are:

(1) Insidious onset of the stiffness and vague joint pains.
(2) The disease occurs usually after the age of 40. In females the onset is frequently at the menopause.
(3) The apparent general well-being of the patient (normal temperature, erythrocyte count and sedimentation rate).
(4) The presence of Heberden's nodes and the frequent involvement of the weight-bearing joints.
(5) "Marginal lipping" or spurs on roentgenographic examination and at times a narrowing of the joint space due to cartilage destruction.

Oral Aspects

Many of the degenerative changes observed in the skeletal joints are also seen in the temporomandibular joints. Abnormal occlusal relations may result in destruction of the interarticular cartilage. Degenerative changes can also be demonstrated in the osseous tissues comprising the temporomandibular joint, although their demonstration in the roentgenogram is more difficult.

Since this form of arthritis is considered to be a degenerative disease which is not even remotely associated with bacterial infection, oral foci of infection are of no direct relation.

DISEASES OF THE TEMPOROMANDIBULAR JOINT

The temporomandibular joint is a complex structure consisting of the condyle of the mandible, the articular meniscus, the glenoid fossa of the temporal bone, the associated capsular and joint ligaments and muscles. The normal functioning of the temporomandibular joint is dependent on (1) the harmonious anatomic relationship of the condyle of the mandible in the glenoid fossa, (2) harmonious muscular function and (3) harmonious dental occlusal relations. Functional disturbances or organic changes which result in disbalance of the above may result in temporomandibular joint disease.

There is a considerable normal variation in the depth and contour of the glenoid fossa and the shape of the condylar head. Vaughn's studies have shown moreover that the temporomandibular joint changes continually throughout life with a constant reduction in the contour of its parts which results in an increase in their working area. Differences in the contour of one glenoid fossa or the shape and size of the condylar head from similar structures on the opposite side of the jaw as seen in the roentgenogram may be due to the roentgenologic technic employed. The x-ray technics employed for examination of this joint must be capable of accurate duplication of results.

The temporomandibular joint is of considerable medical and dental interest because of the diversity of symptoms which occur and the frequent necessity for dental treatment for their elimination or amelioration. Disturbed occlusal relations, whether due to abnormal wear of the teeth, loss of teeth without adequate replacements or prosthetic appliances which have not received periodic servicing are the most common causes of temporomandibular joint disease. While this joint may be affected as a part of a generalized arthritis or as a complication of some systemic disease, most instances of disease of this joint are due to local factors which should be recognized and which are amenable to correction by the dentist.

Associated with Systemic Disease

The frequent involvement of the temporomandibular joint in rheumatoid arthritis has already been discussed. While it may be the initial site of manifestation of this disease, the dentist should first rule out all the common local etiologic causes before assuming that the arthritis is of systemic origin. In doubtful cases it will do no harm to treat the patient as outlined under the oral aspects of rheumatoid arthritis.

This joint may be involved as a part of a generalized septicemia or in association with specific infections such as scarlet fever, diphtheria, typhoid fever, pneumonia, influenza or gonorrhea. Syphilis and tuberculosis rarely involve this joint. The latter results frequently in ankylosis. Infectious processes in the contiguous structures are also important causes of temporomandibular joint arthritis. Joint involvement secondary to furuncles of the external auditory canal or suppurative parotitis have been reported. Shambough observed a case of temporomandibular arthritis secondary to an acute otitis media.

In acute suppurative arthritis of the temporomandibular joint, there are usually swelling and tenderness over the part with a downward and lateral displacement of the jaw which is accompanied by varying degrees of limitation of motion. Fever and leukocytosis are present and the sedimentation rate is increased. X-rays may reveal a widening of the space between the glenoid fossa and the condylar head. An accurate history, which is often difficult to obtain, or the existence of a systemic disease which is known to have joint lesions will assist materially in making the diagnosis. Specific therapy for the systemic disease will result in most cases in an amelioration of the joint symptoms.

Diseases of the temporomandibular joint must be differentiated from lesions which produce swellings and pain in the region of this joint, particularly when the jaw is opened. A furuncle situated on the anterior wall of the external auditory canal produces symptoms similar to those experienced in temporomandibular joint disease. If due to the former cause, intense pain will be experienced when an attempt is made to palpate the condyle through the auditory canal. Pain in the ear while chewing, which is also elicited by pressure applied under the external ear, is suggestive of a furuncle of the external auditory canal. Increased pressure on the temporomandibular joint, without motion, will usually result in painful response in cases of true joint involvement but no pain will be experienced with a furuncle. Enlargement of the small lymph node just anterior to the temporomandibular joint occurs at times in both conditions. Pericementitis of a molar due to overfunction (occlusal trauma) may result in pain which is referred to the region of the temporomandibular joint. The discovery of a tipped, malposed or slightly loosened posterior tooth which is sensitive to percussion, will often permit a correct diagnosis.

Of Local Origin

Temporomandibular joint lesions of local origin of interest to the dentist include: (1) traumatic arthritis, (2) subluxation and/or clicking of the temporomandibular joint, (3) dislocation of the temporomandibular joint, (4) ankylosis of this joint, and (5) an associated group of symptoms known collectively as the temporomandibular joint syndrome or Costen's syndrome.

Traumatic temporomandibular joint disorders in the majority of cases result from (1) a decrease of the intermaxillary space due to premature wear of the teeth or unsatisfactory restoration of lost teeth, (2) naturally occurring malocclusion or (3) abnormal stresses on this joint resulting from muscular imbalance or accidents and (4) abnormal habits. The normal relation of the articulating surfaces is with the mandibular condyle resting in the anterior portion of the glenoid fossa. The posterior teeth (essentially the molars) act as stops to prevent undue pressure on the joint and possible dislocation of the condyle upward and backward.

Thus the relations of the natural teeth or of artificial dentures determine the maxillo-mandibular position when the jaws are closed. The teeth have an important function in maintaining the normal relationship between the condyle and the glenoid fossa. Malalignment of the teeth, abnormal cuspal relations, missing teeth, or artificial appliances that are not properly equilibrated with the remaining natural teeth predispose to temporomandibular reflex disturbances. Sleeping without the dentures in the mouth, usually to be desired, results at times in temporomandibular disturbances with associated reflex phenomenon.

Traumatic forms of arthritis as a rule promptly respond after the elimination of the causative factors.

Subluxation. When the capsular and joint ligaments become stretched or relaxed, abnormal movements of the jaw are often experienced. This results in an abnormal excursion of the meniscus and condylar head forward over the *eminentia articularis*. This dislocation may be spontaneously reducible or require manipulation. The anterior range of motion of the meniscus is not always as great as the anterior range of the mandibular condyle which results in a snapping or clicking sound when the condylar head slips off the meniscus. In other cases there may be an actual wearing through of the meniscus which allows the condylar head to come in contact with the glenoid fossa. This will result in a grating noise when the bony surfaces rub together. These clicking or grating noises are annoying to the patient and to others.

Clicking of the temporomandibular joint is found most frequently in individuals whose joint ligaments have been stretched by frequent subluxation of the joint or in those whose joint has been injured. The clicking will often disappear upon rest of the joint such as by intermaxillary wiring or voluntary rest of the parts. Sinclair believed that the relaxation of the various ligaments was due to a defect of the intercellular substance and collagen in the fibrous connective tissue, secondary to a deficiency of vitamin C. He treated successfully subluxation and clicking of the temporomandibular joint by giving 300 to 500 mg. of ascorbic acid per day.

Severe cases of clicking jaw are treated by the injection of a sclerosing solution, such as sodium psyllate, in the intracapsular space, or the mechanical irritation of this area in the hope of producing scar tissue formation or the more difficult surgical exposure of the parts and removal of the damaged meniscus.

Dislocation. Dislocation of the temporomandibular joint may be in either an anterior or posterior direction. Posterior dislocation is infrequent and it is usually due to trauma such as that received by a blow in which case the glenoid fossa is often fractured. Anterior dislocation of the temporomandibular joint is not uncommon in individuals with relaxed, stretched or otherwise injured capsular ligaments. The condyle overrides anteriorly the *eminentia articularis* and becomes locked in the abnormal forward position with the jaw open. This dislocation may occur when the individual is yawning, laughing, eating or opening the mouth widely for any cause.

Dislocation of the temporomandibular joint at times is experienced during operative dental treatment, during the removal of lower teeth, particularly if the extraction is difficult. In such cases the patient may find it impossible to close the mouth after the rubber dam or mouth prop has been removed.

The reduction of dislocation of the temporomandibular joint a short time after its occurrence is usually not difficult. Dislocations of long duration are more difficult because of the spasm of the muscles of mastication. At times reduction is impossible without the administration of a general anesthesia to furnish adequate muscular relaxation. Every dental practitioner should be familiar with the technic of reducing an anterior dislocation of the temporomandibular joint. The thumbs of the operator's hands should be wrapped with a towel to prevent injury. Standing in front of the patient, the operator should place his thumbs in the molar region parallel to the body of the mandible. The lower border of the mandible should be grasped firmly with the fingers of each hand and with a forceful downward, backward and then upward rotational movement of the jaw the mandible is repositioned. Patients who experience frequent dislocations of the temporomandibular joint can often reposition the jaw without assistance. The treatment of recurring dislocation of the temporomandibular joint is surgical.

Ankylosis of the temporomandibular joint may be true or false. The former occurs within the joint proper where the motion of the parts is limited by osseous or fibrous growths. True ankylosis results usually from an acute infectious arthritis of the joint, or trauma of the involved parts. The author reported a case of true osseous ankylosis of the temporomandibular joint which was present at birth. This deformity was associated with Horner's syndrome.

False ankylosis of this joint results from the limitation of movement of the joint due to osseous or fibrous tissue outside of the joint capsule. The treatment of ankylosis of the temporomandibular joint is usually surgical. It is of historical interest that the first arthroplasty was performed for the relief of an ankylosed temporomandibular joint by Humphrey in 1856.

Costen's Syndrome. Costen, an otolaryngologist, described in 1934 a group of symptoms which were frequently associated with an abnormal functional relationship of the condylar head and the glenoid fossa. Many of the symptoms noted by Costen were similar to those which occur in the head and neck region, due to other causes. The following symptoms were noted:

(1) Mild catarrhal deafness and dizzy spells which were relieved by inflation of the eustachian tubes.

(2) Tinnitus, or at times a snapping noise in the joint which was experienced while chewing. Painful, limited or excessive movement of the affected joint.

(3) Tenderness to palpation over the temporomandibular joint or dull pain in the ears.

(4) Various neuralgic symptoms such as a burning or prickling sensation of the throat, tongue, and side of the nose. Various forms of atypical head pain, particularly that referred to the temporal region or the base of the skull.

(5) Dryness of the mouth due to disturbed salivary gland function.

The early interest in this clinical entity was concerned mainly with the elimination of the "deafness." Later studies made by Costen and others, in which audiometer readings were made, minimized the relationship of catarrhal deafness to abnormalities of the temporomandibular joint, but they emphasized the frequent occurrence of the various reflex neuralgic disturbances. A burning sensation of the tongue, hard palate and pharynx along with tinnitus are commonly experienced. These reflex phenomena are usually found on the side with the abnormal joint relationship.

The temporomandibular joint syndrome is found in patients who present abnormal attrition or wear of the posterior teeth, irregularities or tipping of the teeth, interlocking of steep cusps or occlusal abnormalities resulting from uncompensated anodontia. This produces muscular disbalance and at times actual degenerative changes in the temporomandibular joint. Abnormal cuspal relations occur frequently in patients with a full complement of teeth. Tipped or malposed third molars are frequent offenders. Pain in these cases may arise

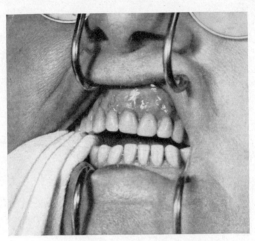

FIG. 171. The use of a folded towel in making a quick test of the effect of increasing the intermaxillary space.

both from the temporomandibular joint and the tooth receiving the abnormal occlusal stress.

Only a small proportion of patients with the abnormalities enumerated develop symptoms referable to the temporomandibular joint. When present, they commonly do not arise until 5 to 8 years after the mutilation of the occlusion or the disturbed occlusal relations. There is some clinical evidence suggesting that the temporomandibular changes and the resulting reflex symptoms are due to tonic contractions of the muscles of mastication which result from subpainful stimuli arising in areas supplied by the mandibular division of the 5th nerve. Many of these patients have premature or abnormal cuspal relations in the third molar region. In the case of tipped third or second molars, abnormal forces are transmitted to the temporomandibular joint.

The diagnosis of the temporomandibular syndrome is not always easy. If the symptoms of this syndrome persist after careful otolaryngologic examination has failed to demonstrate any pathosis, abnormal temporomandibular joint relations should be suspected. The presence of a mutilated occlusion, inadequately serviced dentures and tenderness over the region of the temporomandibular joints lend confirmation to the diagnosis of a temporomandibular syndrome. A simple test which will often indicate the presence of a decreased intermaxillary space, consists of inserting the folded corner of a towel or a tongue depressor in the molar region and having the patient bite firmly. This will frequently afford relief of the painful symptoms. Many times, however, even when this test does not relieve the symptoms the patient will obtain relief following occlusal rehabilitation.

If abnormal cuspal relations are present, occlusal equilibration will often relieve the symptoms. When tipped or malposed teeth are present, their removal and the insertion of an adequate prosthetic appliance are at times necessary to afford relief from the painful stimuli.

More difficult and extensive measures are required in other cases to establish a proper intermaxillary space and satisfactory occlusal relations. In patients with uncompensated anodontia, adequate full or partial dentures may be all that is needed. Other patients will require more elaborate "bite raising" or "repositioning of the mandible" procedures. The rationale of such treatment consists of making the teeth or their substitutes hold the mandible in a position in which joint irritation is eliminated or minimized. The effect of the bite-opening procedures can be evaluated by having the patient wear a temporary appliance for several weeks. This will at times prevent disappointment to both the patient and the dentist after extensive permanent reconstructive measures have been completed. The relief of symptoms is immediate in some cases but in most instances they are gradual. Bite opening or occlusal rehabilitation should not be attempted unless there are definite indications and then only by those experienced in this phase of dentistry. Attempts to open the bite in cases not requiring this form of treatment result in innumerable undesirable and serious complications.

CLEIDOCRANIAL DYSOSTOSIS

Cleidocranial dysostosis is characterized by defective clavicular development and calcification, skull deformities and the frequent occurrence of associated abnormalities in the osseous and dental tissues. This disease occurs spontaneously or as an inherited characteristic, as cases have been reported in which it has been manifested in as many as four generations.

Since cleidocranial dysostosis involves primarily the bones which are formed intramembranously, the cranium and facial structures and the clavicles present the more marked changes. The most characteristic changes are seen in the clavicles which may show all degrees of maldevelopment from their complete absence to faulty calcification of the extremities of this bone. Patients with absent clavicles or those with marked maldevelopment of these bones have an unusual degree of mobility of their shoulders and at times they can be brought forward to meet in the midline. Scoliosis, kyphosis and lordosis of the vertebral column are frequent symptoms. Deformities of the thoracic cage and a contracted and deformed pelvis with lack of ossification of the symphysis and the sacro-iliac articulation are common findings. Cleidocranial dysostosis is not incompatible with life or childbearing.

Cleidocranial dysostosis is diagnosed on the basis of the physical characteristics of the individual, the physical examination and the roentgenologic findings. Other conditions presenting similar clinical findings such as cre-

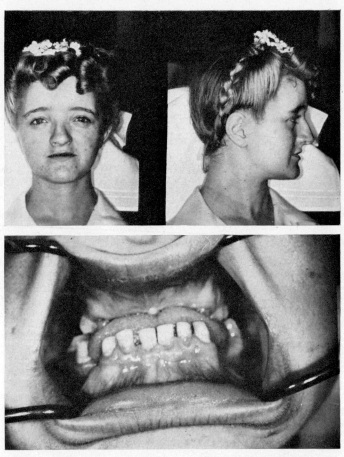

FIG. 172 (*Top*). Cleidocranial dysostosis showing lack of normal facial development in a 19-year-old patient R. S. (*Bottom*) Dental development in patient R. S., age 19 years. Note the unerupted supernumerary teeth in the roentgenograms of the same patient.

tinism, craniofacial dysostosis and osteogenesis imperfecta must be considered in the differential diagnosis.

The dentofacial and cranial changes are prominent because of the intramembranous origin of the bones forming these structures. The skull is shortened (brachycephalic) with an accentuation of the frontal and parietal eminences. The nose is frequently broadened at the base and it has a depressed bridge. The maxillae are underdeveloped and the nasal accessory sinuses are small or absent. The palatal arch is narrow and high and at times a cleft limited to the osseous tissues or comprising both the hard and soft tissues is present. The mandible may be slightly underdeveloped, though not to the same degree as the maxillae.

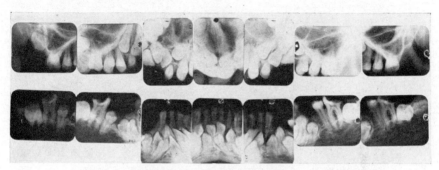

FIG. 173. Dental roentgenograms of R. S. Note the unerupted permanent teeth and the unerupted supernumerary teeth.

Tooth eruption is characteristically delayed and the deciduous teeth are retained abnormally. Many are frequently present in the adult patient. It is not uncommon for most of the permanent teeth to remain unerupted. Supernumerary teeth, also unerupted, are commonly found in the premolar region. The mandibular prognathism, the retention of the deciduous teeth and the

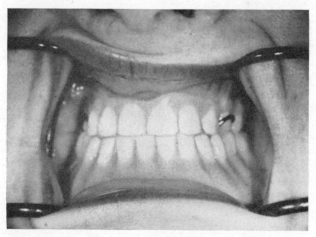

FIG. 174. Patient R. S. following the insertion of
dentures.

failure of the permanent teeth to erupt result in a marked malocclusion and unfortunately one which is frequently not amenable to treatment. The erupted deciduous and permanent teeth are free from enamel hypoplasia although they often present variations in size and shape.

Every effort should be made to restore and maintain all the deciduous and permanent teeth which are erupted. The erupted permanent teeth should receive particular attention because of their importance in partial denture design. Extraction of the deciduous teeth results rarely in eruption of the imbedded permanent members. The removal of the unerupted permanent teeth is difficult because of the crooked and curved roots and it is usually ill-advised even when dentures are to be constructed. Following the stimulation associated with denture wearing or the resorption of the overlying tissues the imbedded teeth may make their appearance in the mouth. They can best be removed at this time.

HEREDITARY CRANIOFACIAL DYSOSTOSIS (CROUZON'S SYNDROME)

This condition is a rare hereditary disease of childhood, which is characterized by marked developmental abnormalities of the skull and upper face. An increased interpupillary width and a slight exophthalmos are early and prominent symptoms.

The frontal eminences are usually prominent. An oxycephalic skull form (tower head) is a striking manifestation of craniofacial dysostosis. When the

TABLE XXI

COMPARISON OF THE CLINICAL FEATURES OF CRANIOFACIAL DYSOSTOSIS AND CLEIDOCRANIAL DYSOSTOSIS

Structures Involved	Craniofacial Dysostosis	Cleidocranial Dysostosis
Skull form	(1) Increased vertical development (oxycephaly) or (2) Increased anterior development (sphenocephaly). (3) Premature suture closure.	(1) Skull usually shortened. (2) Accentuation of frontal and parietal eminences. (3) Delayed suture closure.
Maxillae	(1) Underdeveloped. Narrow and high palatal arch common.	(1) Underdeveloped—particularly the maxillary sinus, cleft of palate at times. (2) Poorly developed infra-orbital ridges.
Mandible	(1) Usually normal in development—apparent prognathism due to hypoplasia of the maxilla.	(1) Slight underdevelopment but not as great as maxilla.
Teeth	(1) No abnormality in eruption or structure. Malocclusion may be present due to lack of development of maxilla.	(1) Persistence of deciduous teeth. Imbedded permanent and supernumerary teeth, especially in premolar area. (2) Enamel not hypoplastic; teeth may show variations in size and shape.
Other structures involved	(1) Skeletal formation normal. (2) Eyes widely spaced—exophthalmos and at times strabismus.	(1) Clavicles may be completely absent or present various degrees of maldevelopment. (2) Pelvic girdle, thoracic cage and long bones may show areas of lack of ossification.

cranial protuberance extends anteriorly it results in a deformity known as sphenocephaly. These cranial abnormalities are the result of increased intracranial pressure in conjunction with an early union of certain of the cranial

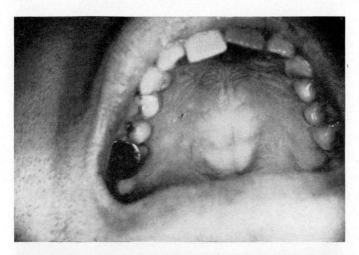

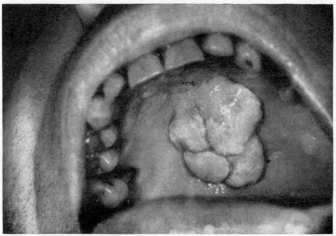

FIG. 175 (*Top*). Small, smooth and symmetrically formed torus palatinus.

FIG. 176 (*Bottom*). Large irregularly shaped torus palatinus with well-developed quadrants. Leukoplakic lesions are present on the mucoperiosteum covering the torus palatinus.

sutures. The facial deformity which results from the lack of development of the maxillae is accentuated by the normally developed mandible. These individuals have frequently a high, narrow palatal arch with a crowding of the upper teeth.

Craniofacial dysostosis must be differentiated from cleidocranial dysostosis.

The retention of the deciduous teeth, the imbedded permanent teeth and the clavicular deficiencies which characterize cleidocranial dysostosis will assist in making a differential diagnosis. The essential features of cleidocranial dysostosis and hereditary craniofacial dysostosis are given in Table XXI.

ORAL TORI

Localized exostoses or tori are found commonly at certain areas of the superior maxilla and on certain areas of the mandible. Tori palatini are found in the midline of the posterior two-thirds of the hard palate. The tori mandibulares are found as a rule lingual to the lower canine or first premolar.

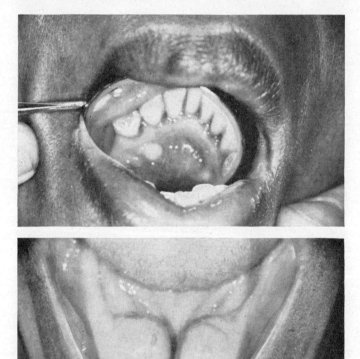

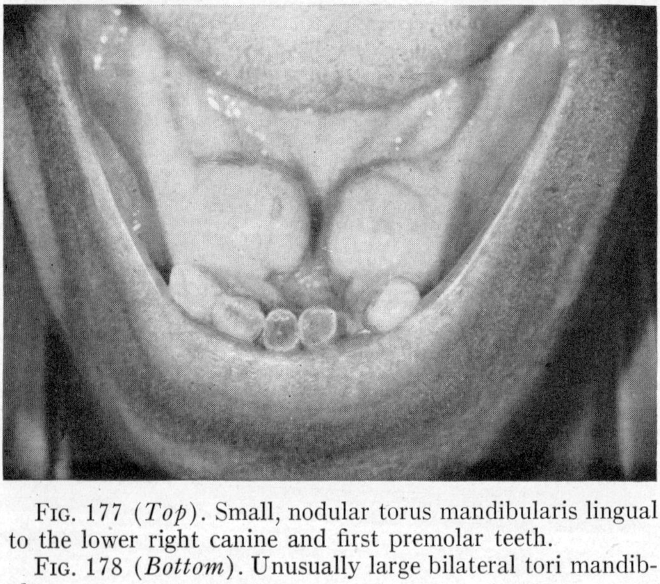

FIG. 177 (Top). Small, nodular torus mandibularis lingual to the lower right canine and first premolar teeth.

FIG. 178 (Bottom). Unusually large bilateral tori mandibulares.

They are usually bilateral but at times they are present only on 1 side. These osseous enlargements are rare in children and adolescents.

Hooton believed that the torus palatinus represents a compensatory adaptation to excessive development of the masticatory apparatus. While this may afford an explanation for the maxillary tori, it is less convincing in explaining the mandibular lesions. Just what stimulates the development of these benign growths is not known.

Miller and Roth carefully studied the tori palatini in over 1,000 patients. They found an incidence of the maxillary tori of approximately 25%. The

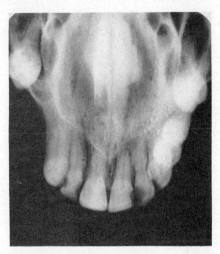

FIG. 179. Roentgenogram of torus palatinus.

careful examination made for these lesions and the inclusion of slight tori in their data account for a higher than usual percentile frequency. They noted the growth twice as frequently in the female as in the male.

Tori do not give rise to symptoms unless there is some irritative lesion of the covering mucosa or they are abnormally large. It is not uncommon for individuals to have a well-developed torus palatinus or mandibularis without being aware of its existence. These lesions show generally slight enlargement from year to year. Miller and Roth noted that the average time required for the lesion to develop from a slight to a marked growth was approximately 15 years. They are commonly recognized first by the dentist. At times, the patient first discovers the growth and he often becomes unduly alarmed before the correct diagnosis is made, occasionally developing cancerphobia. Physicians also are often concerned about finding these growths in their patients' mouths.

There is some evidence of a relationship between these growths and certain systemic conditions. Draper *et al.* found that in 2 large series of breast and uterine carcinomas a torus (palatinus) was observed in 60% of the subjects.

In all their series of carcinoma cases, the percentage incidence of this particular growth was higher than that found in the general population.

These benign growths are of dental importance principally for the complications which they cause in denture construction. Small tori of the maxilla or mandible give rise to no particular problems. If growth be rapid in a denture-wearing patient, poor retention or rocking of the denture may result. The larger tori, especially those with undercuts, offer serious obstacles to satisfactory denture construction and large tori palatini may even interfere with speech.

The mucosa covering a torus palatinus will occasionally become inflamed. Hypertrophy of the palatal glands gives a granular appearance to the overlying mucosa. Hyperkeratosis and even leukoplakia of the mucoperiosteum covering a torus palatinus are seen at times.

Small tori require no treatment. Apprehensive patients should be informed of their benign nature. Large tori or those with undercuts which interfere with proper denture construction, should be removed surgically. Lesions which show a rapid growth and those with leukoplakic involvement of the overlying mucosa should also be removed.

OSTEITIS DEFORMANS—PAGET'S DISEASE

Osteitis deformans is a chronic osseous disturbance of unknown etiology. It is characterized by a hypertrophy and bowing of the long bones and by irregular enlargements and deformities of the flat bones. Paget's description, first given in 1877, is classical.

An etiologic rôle has been ascribed to syphilis, endocrine dysfunction and arteriosclerosis. There is a marked generalized atheromatous condition of the vessels in many of the patients. A hereditary tendency is observed in about 30% of the cases. Malignant growths develop in an unusually large percentage of individuals with osteitis deformans.

The disease usually manifests itself in the 3rd, 4th and 5th decades of life, rarely earlier. There is a slight predominance in the male. The incidence varies in different studies from 1:10,000 to 1:150,000 hospital admissions. If x-rays are taken of all patients evidence of mild osteitis deformans can be found in 1:3,000 patients examined.

The pathologic changes consist of a marked irregularity of the cortex of the bone with hyperemia and increased vascularization of the periosteum. The marrow spaces are filled with fat. The localized areas of osteoporosis and bone-building in the flat bones produce the typical mosaic appearance or "curvilinear markings" which are pathognomonic of this disease. Cysts are rare.

Symptoms

The characteristic symptoms of Paget's disease are objective in nature and they are insidious in onset. There is a thickening and bowing of the long bones, most marked in weight-bearing bones such as the tibia and femur. The bowing of the long bones results in a progressive decrease in height, which may be as much as 6 inches. The feet tend to be everted. The pelvis and sacrum are characteristic sites of involvement.

The skull is commonly involved early in the disease and at times it becomes enormously enlarged. Skull growth may be first evidenced by the necessity for buying larger sizes in hats. In the early course of the disease, and sometimes throughout, the patient experiences pain of a neuralgic nature or vague dull sensations in the involved bones. The pain is usually most severe

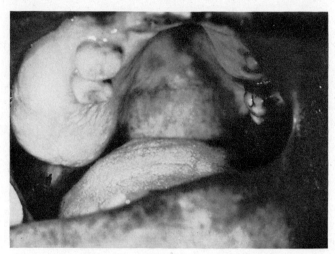

FIG. 180. Enlarged maxillary tuberosity and alveolar process in a case of Paget's disease.

after long standing. Pressure on the affected bones at times causes exquisite pain.

Diagnosis

Diagnosis is based on the presence of the signs or symptoms enumerated in conjunction with x-ray studies of the involved parts, the skull and pelvis. The localized areas of osteoporosis and condensation in the bones are generally pathognomonic. They produce the so-called "cotton-wool" appearance. The pelvis presents striking changes in the generalized form of the disease. Biopsy studies are required for diagnosis of local forms of the disease. Blood studies show approximately normal calcium and phosphorus values while the serum phosphatase is elevated, at times to 40 Bodansky units. The Wassermann reaction is negative unless there is an associated luetic infection.

There is no specific treatment for osteitis deformans. Death is seldom if ever due to the osteitis but rather to diseases of the cardiovascular system, malignant growths or infectious processes. Cases of 20 to 30 years' duration are known.

Oral Aspects

The dentist has an opportunity to see osteitis deformans early in the course of the disease because of the early skull and jaw manifestations which often

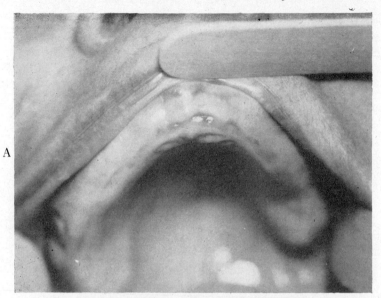

A

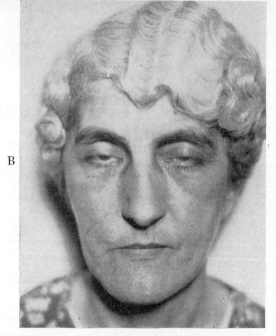

B

Fig. 181. (A) Widening of the edentulous ridges in a patient with Paget's disease. (B) Facial appearance of the same patient. (Novak and Burket, Am. J. Orthodontics and Oral Surg., 30:597-608, 1944.)

precede those in other areas of the body. The most frequent and extensive
changes are observed in the maxilla. In 2 of the patients reported by Novak
and the author, the osseous changes were confined to the maxilla and mandible. Biopsy studies established the diagnosis of osteitis deformans. In the
localized forms of the disease this is necessary to rule out osteitis fibrosa.

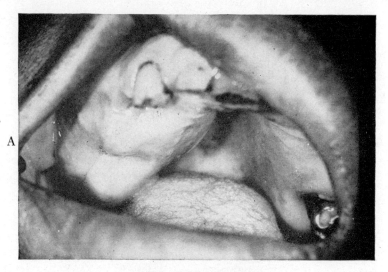

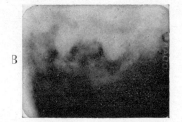

FIG. 182. (A) Showing marked increase in the size of the
alveolar ridges. Craterlike depressions can be seen in the right
premolar region. This was the site of a foul discharge. (B)
Roentgenogram showing loss of trabecular detail in the right
upper premolar region and "cotton wool" appearance of the
bone. (Novak and Burket, Am. J. Orthodontics and Oral
Surg., 30:597-608, 1944.)

There is a marked osteoporosis of the maxilla with localized areas of increased density. These changes result in a loss of the trabecular detail in the
x-rays. With the local areas of increased density the radiolucent areas produce the characteristic "cotton wool" appearance of the bone. There is definite enlargement of the maxilla, particularly around the tuberosity. The size
of the dental arch is increased and spacing of the teeth is common. The
mucosa covering the maxillary bones becomes stretched and numerous fine

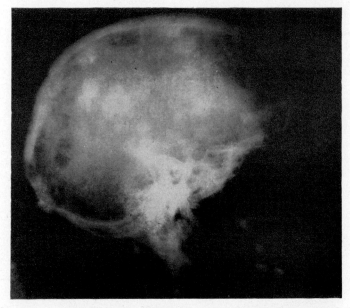

FIG. 183. Skull changes in a patient with generalized Paget's disease. (Novak and Burket, Am. J. Orthodontics and Oral Surg., **30**:597-608, 1944.)

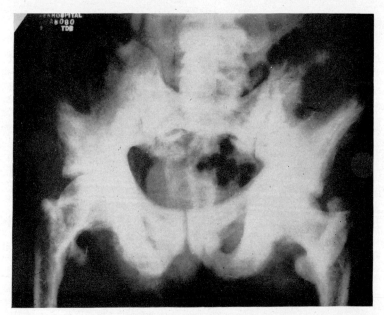

FIG. 184. Pelvic changes in patient with generalized Paget's disease. (Novak and Burket, Am. J. Orthodontics and Oral Surg., **30**:597-608, 1944.)

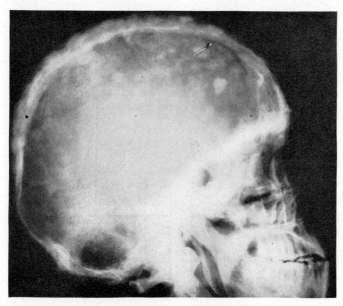

FIG. 185. Typical cotton-wool defects of the skull in a
patient with Paget's disease.

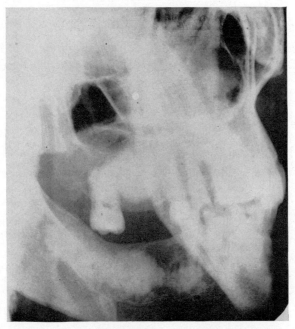

FIG. 186. Left oblique view of the left mandibular
molar region of the patient shown in Fig. 187.

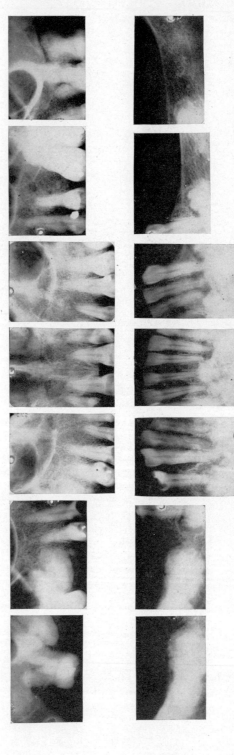

Fig. 187. Dental roentgenograms of patient shown in Fig. 186. These roentgenologic changes in conjunction with the clinical findings suggested the diagnosis of Paget's disease.

capillaries become visible. The disproportionate increase in the size of the maxilla as compared with the mandible produces a facial contour like an inverted triangle. This can be readily differentiated from the ovoid facial contour seen in acromegaly.

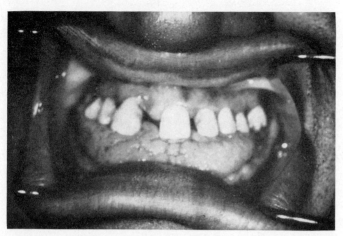

FIG. 188. Fanning of the maxillary anteriors in a case of Paget's disease.

One of the characteristic oral findings consists of the development of osteo-myelitis following dental extractions. These patients often have one or more sinuses which drain a watery yellowish fluid. The oral lesions are at times

TABLE XXII

COMPARISON OF CALCIUM, PHOSPHORUS AND PHOSPHATASE VALUES

	Calcium	Phosphorus	Phosphatase
Normal	9 to 11 mg. Ca/100 cc. blood	2 to 5 mg. P/100 cc. blood	1.4 to 4 units/cc. blood in adult (Bo-dansky)
Rickets	Usually normal except in tetany	Decreased	Increased 20 to 40 × normal
Osteomalacia	Decreased	Decreased	Little if any change
Hyperparathyroidism	Marked increase	Usually decreased	Increased 2 to 50 × normal
Paget's disease	Usually normal	Usually normal	Occasionally elevated
Osteogenesis imperfecta	Usually normal	Usually normal	Usually normal—at times slightly increased
Solitary bone cysts	Normal	Normal	Normal
Metastatic osseous neoplasms	May be elevated	Normal	Normal or may be slightly elevated.
Tetany	7 mg. Ca/100 cc. blood or less	Normal or elevated	Normal

348 DISEASES OF THE BONES AND JOINTS

exquisitely painful. They may require alcoholic injection of one or more divisions of the 5th nerve.

The teeth become loose due to the destruction of the supporting alveolar bone but there is no roentgenologic or histologic evidence of abstraction of calcium from the teeth. X-rays of the teeth show more than normal pulpal calcifications. There is a marked hyperplasia of the cementum histologically and roentgenologically. Fox noted "nobby growths" and irregularity of the roots of all the teeth. The cases studied by the author revealed similar changes throughout both jaws.

Osteitis deformans may be observed in edentulous patients. In such cases frequent denture reconstruction is necessary to obtain satisfactory adaptation of the denture to the continually changing supporting tissues. A progressive and at times irregular hyperplasia of the maxillary tuberosities in a middle-aged patient should sugggest Paget's disease.

OSTEOGENESIS IMPERFECTA (*OSSIUM FRAGILITANS*)

Osteogenesis imperfecta is a rare condition which is characterized by an unusual susceptibility of the bones to fractures, even in intra-uterine life. Bones which are formed intramembranously and those formed from cartilage are affected. The spontaneously occurring fractures and the decreased density of the bones resemble the changes present in rickets but the histopathologic findings are very different. At times osteogenesis imperfecta is associated with an abnormal blue coloring of the sclera and deafness as a hereditary syndrome (Lobstein's disease).

Essentially normal calcium and phosphorus metabolism is present in osteogenesis imperfecta. This condition is not improved by any form of therapy. Hansen *et al.* showed that parathyroid extract and large doses of viosterol resulted in a negative calcium balance and hence their use was contraindicated.

Oral Aspects

In some patients with osteogenesis imperfecta of both the hereditary and nonhereditary types an unusual dental anomaly, hereditary opalescent dentine, is also present. While the enamel may be decreased in amount, the changes represent essentially a mesenchymal dysplasia. This dental hypoplasia is also found in individuals who do not have osteogenesis imperfecta.

Hereditary Opalescent Dentine (*Dentinogenesis Imperfecta*). It is not uncommon to obtain a history of hereditary opalescent dentine in five or more generations. It occurs in both sexes but the patients studied by the author have been predominantly females. The dental changes affect both the root and coronal portion of the permanent dentition, with a disproportion in the size of the crown and the root. The tooth appears on the roentgenogram similar to a member of the deciduous series. A characteristic roentgenologic finding is the early decrease in size of the pulpal chamber and canal by the deposition of adventitious dentine. It is not uncommon to find complete calcification of the pulpal chamber and canal at 15 years of age. This abnormal dentinal deposition contains tubules which run almost at right angles to the

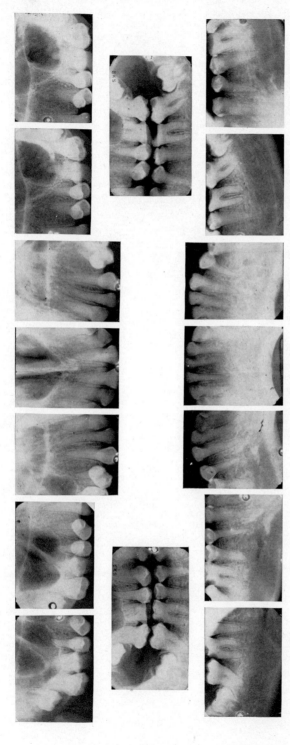

Fig. 189. Dental roentgenologic findings in a 12-year-old girl with hereditary opalescent dentine. Note the disproportion in size of the crowns and roots and the filling-in of the pulp chambers and root canals.

usual course of these tubules. The x-ray absorptive properties of these teeth are low.

When the teeth erupt they present a slight bluish coloration which changes gradually to a purplish opalescent or amber color from which the name of this type of hypoplasia is derived. The structure of the enamel is normal but it is devoid of pigmentation and it has a peculiar refractive phenomenon. The color changes are more marked in the anterior teeth.

Teeth with hereditary opalescent dentine are softer than normal and they fracture easily. Hodge found their hardness to be 70 compared to a normal of 120. In general there is a low caries susceptibility although large masses of the crowns may be fractured and missing. It is common to find several abscessed teeth present in these patients, although their crowns are not extensively involved with dental decay. There is marked enamel and dentine loss through abrasion. Full dentures are usually necessary before 20 years of age, unless jacket crowns are placed before the teeth become too badly destroyed.

MULTIPLE MYELOMA (PLASMOCYTOMA)

Multiple myeloma is a neoplasm of certain cells of the red bone marrow which is of dental interest because of the widespread involvement of the skeletal system including the jaws and the skull. The disease is usually found in late adult life. Pain, which is associated with motion or pressure over the bony nodules or tumor metastases, is an early symptom. Many times the disease is detected during roentgenologic examination for other purposes. A peculiar type of protein, Bence-Jones protein, can be demonstrated in the urine of the majority of the patients with multiple myeloma. The prognosis is poor.

The accidental discovery of lesions in the jaws may be the first evidence of this disease since early symptoms are uncommon. The mandible is more frequently involved because of its greater content of red marrow. Hoepfel found histopathologic evidence of involvement of the jaws in three cases of multiple myeloma which came to necropsy.

Mandibular lesions are most common in the region of the angle of the jaw. In most instances they appear unassociated with the apices of the teeth. In the case reported by Aderes and Boston the teeth were exfoliated. A large elevation of the palate with sloughing of the tissues and a clinical picture resembling carcinoma were present in one of the cases reported by Thoma. Swelling of the right maxilla was the initial symptom in Gross and Waugh's patient.

Gunter and Meloy operated on a 57-year-old woman who had had the first and second molars removed previously because of pain in this area. For a brief period there was freedom from the symptoms when she noticed a circumscribed swelling on the buccal surface of the right jaw. Osteomyelitis was suspected. Roentgenologic examination disclosed a large radiolucent area in the right mandible extending from the premolar area posteriorly to the ramus with a pathologic fracture in the second molar region. Histopathologic studies of the tissue removed at operation revealed a myeloma of the plasma cell type. This diagnosis was readily substantiated when additional roentgenologic studies were made. This case illustrated the desirability of taking x-rays of the skull in all patients with unusual or peculiar osseous lesions.

Multiple myeloma, along with the lipodystrophies, hyperparathyroidism, metastatic carcinoma and syphilis, is a disease which can give rise to oral symptoms or osseous changes which the dentist may be called upon to interpret.

18

Diseases of the Muscles, Nerves, and Nervous System

MUSCLES	NERVES AND NERVOUS SYSTEM

MUSCLES

Trismus

Trismus refers in the strict sense to spasms of the muscles of mastication such as might accompany some irritative lesion of the central nervous system. The term trismus is generally used when referring to an inflammatory or reflex nervous involvement of the muscles of mastication, secondary to disease processes of the teeth and surrounding tissues.

Varying degrees of trismus follow the removal of lower third molars, espe cially unerupted or impacted teeth. This trismus may result in part from a true inflammatory reaction, edema and the trauma incident to the operative procedures. Gingival inflammation about erupting lower third molars, circumcoronitis, is a common cause of trismus. In most instances the fusospirochetal organisms are the etiologic agents. Operative interference in the presence of acute circumcoronitis can result in serious and even fatal infections.

It is a good clinical procedure to make bacterial smears from third molar flaps before operating in this area. This will aid in preventing undesirable postoperative complications, including "dry sockets."

Myositis

Myositis is inflammation of the muscles. Solitary or multiple muscle abscesses or diffuse degenerative changes may occur. The trismus which is so frequently associated with inflammations about lower third molars is not in most cases a true myositis.

An unusual form of myositis is characterized by the formation of calcified material in the affected muscles and their tendons—myositis ossificans. In rare cases this process is generalized throughout the body. Myositis ossificans follows frequently trauma to the affected tissues after which the intramuscular hematoma undergoes ossification. While this ossification process is usually painless, it may seriously interfere with the muscular function.

The muscles of mastication may be involved locally or as a part of a generalized myositis ossificans. In the case observed by Cameron the myositis ossificans was limited to the right masseter muscle. Trauma to this area appeared to be the precipitating factor. Calcification of this muscle and the tendons resulted in ankylosis of the mandible. The calcification of this muscle occurred twice following operative interference.

Myasthenia Gravis

Myasthenia gravis is a rare disease of the muscles whose etiology is not clearly understood. It is believed to be due to a bacterial toxin, although endocrine factors are also considered to be of importance. This disease is characterized by a rapid fatigability of the muscles, particularly those of mastication and facial expression. The individual with myasthenia gravis has a sad and expressionless appearance. It is impossible for him to whistle or to close his eyes completely if the facial muscles are involved. Difficulty in speech and swallowing are frequently encountered. When the muscles of mastication are affected, the maintenance of adequate nourishment may become a serious problem. Sudden fatigability of the muscles of respiration require prompt treatment. After rest, muscular function again returns but it is characterized by a rapidly developing fatigue. The treatment of myasthenia gravis is not successful.

Amylotrophic Lateral Sclerosis

This disease, whose cause is unknown, manifests itself in later life by muscular atrophy, motor weakness and eventual spasticity of the involved parts. Pain is absent and the sensation of the parts is preserved. The disease is usually bilateral, with the initial involvement of the hands.

Disturbed oral function is often a prominent symptom. There is interference with chewing and the normal movements of the lips, tongue and palate. As a result, there may be dysphagia and difficulty in swallowing, with at times regurgitation of fluid through the nose.

Primary Lateral Sclerosis

This is a rare disease of unknown cause, characterized by increasing motor weakness, spasticity and an exaggeration of the tendon reflexes. These changes are not accompanied by pain but the symptoms may persist for many years.

Progressive Bulbar Paralysis (Labio-glosso-pharyngeal Paralysis)

This is a rare disease of unknown cause, which results in degeneration of the motor nuclei of the glossopharyngeal and spinal accessory nerves and at times the motor nucleus of the 5th nerve. These changes are manifested clinically by an atrophy and loss of function of the muscles concerned with chewing, swallowing and speech. At times these symptoms develop following measles or mumps and in these instances a viral etiology is suspected.

The symptoms develop as a rule only in later life. Speech difficulties are encountered, especially those in which the lips play a rôle. The voice may have a "nasal" or cleft palate quality due to paralysis of the muscles of the soft palate. Marked changes in the tongue are common. The extensive muscular atrophy of this organ results in a small flabby structure which shows fibrillary tremors. It may be impossible to protrude the tongue from the mouth. The loss of muscle tone of this organ interferes with the normal partitioning of food, the formation of the food bolus, and its passage into the oropharynx. There are no disturbances of common or special sensation.

True bulbar paralysis must be differentiated from myasthenia gravis. In the latter disease the association of the symptoms with fatigue and the absence of marked muscular atrophy will permit a differential diagnosis. The treatment of true bulbar paralysis is unsatisfactory.

NERVES AND NERVOUS SYSTEM

General Considerations

The terms neuralgia, neuritis and neurosis are often confused or used incorrectly. Neuralgia refers to pain in or along the course of a nerve, irrespective of the nature of the pathologic process which gives rise to the painful stimuli. True neuritis represents an actual inflammation of the nerve. This condition may result in anesthesia or paralysis, depending on the type of nerve involved and at times permanent degeneration of the affected nerve. The term neurosis refers usually to a functional disorder of the nervous system which is not associated with any discoverable lesion. It may be concerned with aberrations in cerebration, which are characterized by the impression that painful stimuli are being received. It is extremely important for the clinician, as well as the patient, to be able to differentiate the true neuralgias and neuritides from the neuroses.

Facial Pain

Pain arising in the orofacial region or pain referred to this area is a common complaint. Because of the frequent association of head pain with the teeth and oral structures these patients will seek frequently dental advice first. It is the responsibility of the dentist to determine whether the pain is associated with some oral lesion, whether it is of referred origin, or whether there exists any pathologic basis for the pain experienced by the patient.

Fay called attention to the fact that little is known about the degeneration of the nerves supplying the deciduous teeth and their redistribution to the permanent teeth. The 5th nerve is unique in this transference of end organs and Fay suggested that disturbances in this complicated process may be a factor in the production of pain in this region.

The extensive peripheral distribution of the 5th nerve, its widely dispersed central connections and its numerous intercommunications with the other cranial and cervical nerves furnish an anatomic basis for the diverse and at times bizarre pain patterns experienced in the head and neck region. Painful stimuli may arise from any of the terminal branches of the 5th nerve, which include the scalp, the eyes, the nose, the ear and the tongue, oral mucosa and the 32 teeth with their high prevalence of pulpal and periodontal disease. Between the sensory receptors of this nerve and its central connections there lie many structures which may also give rise to sensory stimuli. Irritation of the branches of the 2° division of the 5th nerve during their passage along the walls of an infected maxillary sinus results frequently in pain of apparent dental origin. Irritation of a nerve due to any cause during its passage through the various bony canals will also result in pain. Pain which follows the vascular tree is also observed in the head and neck region. There may be a vascular origin for certain of the atypical neuralgias which are characterized by a burning, aching and throbbing pain.

The intensity of the pain stimuli in the head and neck region, particularly those associated with dental lesions, makes its localization by the patient extremely difficult at times. It is a common experience to find the pain referred to the opposite jaw, or the intensity of the stimulus may be sufficient to "overflow" centrally and result in the cerebrated impression of pain arising in some other structure. The typical symptomatology and clinical findings of pain due to acute pulpal and periapical infections are covered in any text book of oral pathology.

Neuritides of Dental Interest

Herpes zoster is an example of neuritis of the 5th nerve or its ganglion. Acute maxillary sinusitis results commonly in neuritis of the maxillary division of the 5th nerve. Pharyngeal infections and periapical abscesses may also produce a true neuritis. Nesbit reported a case in which necropsy studies demonstrated that the infection followed the nerve fibres from the upper teeth into the cranial cavity where a fatal meningitis resulted. Friedman and Olsen described an unusual case of neuritis of the masticatory branches of the 5th nerve which was secondary to arsenic poisoning. Occasionally the pain following the removal of a mandibular third molar represents a true neuritis of the mandibular nerve. Neuritis of the 5th nerve at times follows neuritis of the 7th nerve. Neuritis of the 7th nerve produces the clinical symptomatology of Bell's paralysis or palsy.

The various dietary and nutritional causes of neuritis of the extremities such as pellagra, chronic alcoholism and pernicious anemia do not give rise to symptomatology of this nature in the cephalic region.

Neuralgias of the oral and facial region are classically divided into the Major Neuralgias or Minor Neuralgias.

Trigeminal Neuralgia

Trigeminal neuralgia, or tic douloureux, is the classical example of a major neuralgia. The marked painful symptoms are referred to the areas supplied by the peripheral branches of the 5th nerve, usually the maxillary or mandibular divisions. The facial distortion which is associated with the paroxysms of pain result from a central overflow of stimuli to the nucleus of the 7th nerve.

Trigeminal neuralgia represents a central nerve lesion in which peripheral dental or facial pain serves often as a precipitating factor. The pain does not always arise from the dental structures. Tic douloureux occurs as a rule in middle adult life with a slightly greater frequency in the female. The characteristic feature of tic douloureux is the acute painful spasms which are precipitated by, or related to, pressure on the points of emergence of the peripheral branches of the 5th nerve—such as the infra-orbital or mental nerves. When the attacks can be precipitated by touching a particular area, these areas are called "trigger zones." Washing the face, smiling, shaving or even eating may precipitate a spasm. Because of the severity of the pain, the patients many times will refuse absolutely to allow the examiner to apply pressure over the "trigger points." This is an important diagnostic finding.

The attacks may occur initially at intervals of years, months or weeks. A characteristic feature of this disease is the complete freedom from pain between the spasms. As the disease progresses the attacks occur more often until the patients live in a continual fear of the painful seizures. The distribution of the pain pattern tends to remain the same, although it may involve larger areas.

The pain may seemingly arise from the teeth, the tongue or the lips. Undue attention has been placed in the past on pulpal calcifications as etiologic factors in tic douloureux. These nodular calcific masses in the pulps are an extremely common occurrence, being present in over 85% of all teeth. They are rarely related to the tic douloureux. In suspicious cases a trial nerve block will assist in making the diagnosis and result in the retention of teeth which might otherwise be removed.

The diagnosis of trigeminal neuralgia presents few difficulties, particularly if one of the paroxysms can be witnessed. Tic douloureux must be differentiated from atypical neuralgias in which the acute painful episodes are less intense and in which the pain may persist in mild forms in the interval.

Minor Neuralgias of the Facial Region

The minor neuralgias of the facial region are numerous. They must be differentiated from referred pain. They do not present the acute paroxysms of pain, the typical trigger zones or the pain pattern of tic douloureux. The pain is usually less severe and more likely to be continuous. It may be so severe, however, that it interferes seriously with the patient's routine of living. Neuralgia of the temporomandibular joint and at times the lingual and temporal areas has already been discussed (Costen's syndrome).

A careful clinical and roentgenologic examination is required to determine the cause of minor neuralgias of the facial region. The vitality of all the teeth should be assured either by their reaction to heat or cold or the electric pulp tester. Intra-oral roentgenograms, particularly bite-wing films, are indispensable for detecting small interproximal cavities and secondary decay beneath dental restorations. It should be emphasized that the x-ray is not infallible in the demonstration of small carious lesions or early pathologic changes about the root apex. There is a tendency to place too much emphasis on the results of the x-ray studies and to devote too little time to taking a complete history and making a careful examination of the mouth.

Neuralgia in a clinically edentulous mouth may be due to pathosis in the bone such as unerupted teeth, apical granulomata or cysts, pathosis within the temporomandibular joint or new growths within the jaws.

Pain of apparent dental origin may arise from diseased accessory nasal sinuses. This is particularly true of obscure pain in the upper jaw. Pain referred to the temporomandibular joint may arise from lesions of the external auditory canal, especially furuncles on the anterior wall. Obscure pain in the lower jaw is at times associated with a partially erupted mandibular third molar. Cobb and Mixter observed a patient with lingual spasms which were associated with an atypical facial neuralgia.

A diffuse neuralgia of the temporofacial region is associated commonly with an abnormal occlusal relationship of the molars. The failure to replace an extracted molar may result in tipping and/or extrusion of the remaining teeth, the production of abnormal occlusal stresses on the teeth and an abnormally directed pressure on the temporomandibular joint. The patient is unaware frequently of the origin of the pain although it may be extremely severe. This temporomandibular syndrome is discussed in greater detail in the section devoted to the diseases of the temporomandibular joint.

Psychoneurotic Pain

A considerable number of patients will describe a pain pattern to account for which there is neither any known anatomic pathway nor recognized lesion. These individuals go from one practitioner to another, telling to each their story with ever-increasing detail and vividness. Such patients constitute a real problem in both medical and dental practice.

Psychoneurotic pain is common in highly nervous, anxious individuals, particularly those with a tendency to an inferiority complex. It is found in both sexes. The complexity of the nervous connections in the facial region and the multiplicity of the organs which may give rise to pain in this area account for the frequent complaint of psychoneurotic pain in the head and neck region. Patients with psychoneurotic pain are usually extremely suggestive. Their pain is increased as a rule during periods of relaxation and rest and it will frequently disappear entirely when the mind of the patient is occupied. Psychoneurotic pain may be associated with some benign lesion which the patient considers to be malignant.

One must be cautious about making a diagnosis of psychoneurotic pain. Once the clinician is convinced that no organic lesion is present the patient should be plainly and definitely informed. Temporary relief from pain may follow various forms of therapy including the unnecessary extraction of teeth, but permanent beneficial results are rarely obtained. In general, the practitioner's time, patience and reputation will be protected by refusing treatment, since these individuals will speak freely about practitioners who fail to prescribe effective treatment, but they will comment rarely about those who make a diagnosis of psychoneurosis.

Bell's Palsy—Paralysis of the Facial Nerve

Paralysis of the peripheral portion of the 7th nerve is commonly seen. It occurs usually in adults. It may result from: (1) the exposure to cold or drafts; (2) injury to the nerve due to infection, trauma, or neoplastic growths or (3) in association with numerous systemic diseases.

A history of exposure of the affected region to a draft, cold, or undue chilling is obtained frequently. Paralysis secondary to accidental or operative trauma is not uncommon in this area. One of the possible complications of surgery on the temporomandibular joint, the parotid gland or its duct is injury to the facial nerve. Infections of the parotid gland, face or mouth can give rise directly or indirectly to facial paralysis. In the common variety of facial paralysis which is associated with exposure to cold the paralysis occurs rapidly, often within an hour. The exact pathogenesis is not known but it is believed to result from lymphatic engorgement and pressure on the nerve along its passage through the unyielding facial canal.

Paralysis of the 7th nerve occurs as a manifestation of diphtheria, syphilis, diabetes and multiple neuritis. Syphilis, tuberculosis or intracranial suppurative lesions of the base of the skull may involve the nerve at the base of the skull. Herpes zoster of the geniculate ganglion results occasionally in partial paralysis of the facial nerve. Facial paralysis has been reported following a mandibular injection of a local anesthetic and the removal of an impacted third molar. Instances of partial facial paralysis which develop in association with circumcoronitis of an erupting lower third molar, have also been noted.

The patient is unaware of the paralysis at times until his attention is called to the facial asymmetry. There is a lack of muscular control on the affected side which gives a mask-like expression to half the face. The eyelid on the affected side cannot be closed and it becomes everted so that the conjunctival mucosa is plainly visible. The paralysis of the *orbicularis palpebrarum* gives rise to the characteristic and annoying "tearing" on the paralyzed side. Foreign bodies may become lodged in the eye. The patient is unable to whistle or to blow out the cheeks.

The mouth is pulled towards the sound side while on the paralyzed side the corner drops. The patient's inability to close normally the lips allows the saliva to run from the mouth down over the chin. This constant moisture and folding of the skin results at times in intertrigo or inflammation of the skin folds. Taste sensation on the anterior two-thirds of the tongue is impaired in severe cases.

The diagnosis of facial paralysis is obvious on inspection and examination of the patient. More elaborate studies are required to determine whether the paralysis is central or peripheral in nature. In varying periods of time, depending on the cause and severity of the paralysis, recovery begins to take place in many cases, particularly those associated with exposure to cold. If the paralysis does not disappear by the third month, hope for spontaneous resolution is remote.

In about 20% of the cases recovery is incomplete. About 80% of this group shows the syndrome of "crocodile tears" which consists of lacrimation during eating following apparent recovery from the facial paralysis. Mc-Govern explained this annoying symptom on the basis of the diversion of nerve fibres intended for the submaxillary gland to the lacrimal gland. Blocking the sphenopalatine ganglion relieves the excessive flow of tears.

A   B

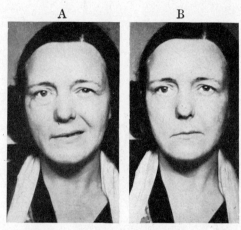

FIG. 190. Typical facial expréssion (A) when smiling and (B) when at rest, in a patient with Bell's palsy on the right side.

There are numerous delicate operations for the surgical treatment of unresolved Bell's paralysis. These vary from actual nerve anastomosis or grafting to facial implants which tend to correct the facial asymmetry and secondary symptoms resulting from the lack of muscle innervation.

Minor Syndromes

Sphenopalatine Neuralgia (Sluder's Syndrome). Neuralgia of the sphenopalatine (nasal) ganglion of the 5th nerve may give rise to a symptom-complex first described by Sluder. This neuralgia is usually unilateral. The symptoms consist of a constant, boring, burning type of pain which seems to rise in the palate, jaw, pharynx and behind the eyeballs on the affected side. At times the pain may be shooting in character. Because of the oral distribution of the pain, the teeth are frequently incriminated and at times removed needlessly in the hope of curing the symptoms. When this pain pattern is noted, the patient should be referred to an otolaryngologist for consultation. Since the pain in sphenopalatine ganglion neuralgia disappears temporarily following cocainization of the sphenopalatine ganglion, this procedure is useful in confirming the diagnosis.

Hunt's Syndrome. In 1907 Hunt described a symptom complex which consisted of a peripheral facial paralysis with herpetic eruption in and around the external auditory meatus, the pillars of the fauces and the anterior two-thirds of the tongue of the same side. The ear pain is usually the first complaint. The vesicles soon make their appearance and the facial paralysis follows in a few days. Spillane called attention recently to the association of Bell's palsy with herpetic eruptions. In the case he reported, there was a temporary loss of taste sensation over the tongue in addition to the other symptoms.

Glossopharyngeal Neuralgia. Coburn & Shafstall described a type of glossopharyngeal neuralgia which is associated with sudden paroxysms of pain in the side of the throat, deep in the base of the tongue or in the ear. The attacks are often precipitated by swallowing. This type of neuralgia can be determined by means of painting the tonsillar area with cocaine. If this prevents the painful spasms when the patient swallows or drinks, it confirms the diagnosis of glossopharyngeal neuralgia. Coburn & Shafstall obtained satisfactory results following the removal of infected teeth and vitamin B therapy. Coleman found that this type of neuralgia cannot be satisfactorily treated by alcoholic nerve injection. It requires intracranial division of the ninth nerve.

Twitching of the Facial Musculature—Facial Tic. Spasmodic twitchings of individual muscles or muscle groups of the facial musculature are not uncommon. These unwanted and unconscious movements are not accompanied by any painful sensations. In some cases the individual is able to control the muscular twitchings through conscious effort. This habit tic develops frequently during childhood. This type of tic can be duplicated by the patient or the examiner. True tics such as described above must be differentiated from rhythmic spasms of the facial musculature which are a manifestation of true Jacksonian epilepsy. The latter are usually unilateral.

Involuntary contractions of unassociated muscle groups of the facial musculature are not unusual after nerve injury or paralysis. The corner of the mouth may be retracted every time the individual blinks his eyes or other dissociated muscular movements may occur. Winking of the eyes with movement of the jaws, the jaw winking or Gunn's phenomenon, is experienced at times in the absence of a history of injury. These phenomena are believed due to the abnormal joining of the nerve fibres during regeneration.

Ehni of the Mayo Clinic observed a form of unilateral facial spasm which is found only in the middle-aged patient. The facial spasms, which have a fibrillary character, occurred only in the muscles supplied by the 7th nerve. These spasms could not be repressed voluntarily and they could not be reproduced at will. Fatigue appeared to aggravate the spasms. This disorder was believed due to some lesion involving the facial nucleus. When indicated, this form of muscular spasm is treated by the sectioning of the facial nerve and joining it to the spinal accessory nerve.

Linguomaxillary Reflex. Blais observed that when the tongue is pinched the lower jaw is dropped. He believed this reflex is particularly important as a measure of the depth of general anesthesia as it disappears gradually in contrast to the corneal or pupillary reflexes. It may also be used to measure the degree of unconsciousness following head injury.

Migraine. Migraine is a syndrome characterized by intense periodic headaches which are preceded at times by certain premonitory symptoms and accompanied by rather severe constitutional reactions. In the female they are experienced frequently at the menstrual period. A family history is obtained in some cases. The exact causative agent is not known. There is considerable evidence that migraine represents a sensitization phenomenon which is analogous to hay fever or urticaria. Nerve strain or the eating of certain foods may give rise to migraine. The disease is most common in middle-aged adults, particularly in middle-aged females.

The severe headache is often preceded by an indefinite feeling of malaise or a variety of sensory impressions which may consist of the sensation of light spots before the eyes, peculiar odors or tastes. At times there are numbness and tingling of the extremities. The patient explains frequently that the headaches are due to some eye strain. The severe intense pain develops rapidly. Any area of the head may be involved but the pain distribution is usually constant in a particular case. The region back of the eyes is a common site. The intense painful symptoms may last for only a few hours or for several days. The patient with migraine experiences as a rule nausea and vomiting after the disappearance of the headache. The occurrence of these headaches at periodic intervals with asymptomatic periods intervening assists in differentiating them from those due to brain tumor.

The treatment of migraine is generally ineffective. A variety of different agents have been used including pituitary preparations, ergotamine tartrate, gynergyn and, in the female, an artificially induced menopause. Therapeutic response is variable and in general unsatisfactory.

Epilepsy

Epilepsy is a disorder of the nervous system which is characterized by attacks of unconsciousness and typical convulsive seizures. There is a strong hereditary background and, while mental deterioration frequently accompanies this disease, many epileptics are mentally brilliant and a few have been considered as geniuses.

In most cases no definite causative factor can be determined. Epilepsy may be the result of intracranial injury occurring at birth or a later date. Brain tumor, hemorrhage, embolism or arteriosclerosis are acquired causes of this disease. Localized cerebral areas of ischemia frequently precede the attack.

Epilepsy is characterized by the epileptic seizures,—convulsions or "fits" or "grand mal" attacks, which are usually followed by periods of coma. Just preceding the convulsion the individual may have a premonition or aura of the impending attack which consists usually of some hallucination of the special senses of sight, smell, or taste. The onset of the convulsion is always sudden. It occurs irrespective of the place, audience or time of day. The epileptic screams commonly at the onset of the attack, the body then becomes rigid, after which the tonic and clonic convulsive movements occur.

The patient is usually completely unconscious during this period and may severely bruise or seriously injure himself. The tongue is frequently bitten or traumatized. During the convulsion the patient often loses control of his sphincters with micturition or defecation. The convulsion terminates spontaneously, leaving the individual tired, stuporous and sleepy.

Less spectacular manifestations of this disease are known as "petit mal" attacks, which may consist of nothing more than momentary spells of unconsciousness or the inability to proceed with the task in hand. This momentary lapse of consciousness passes quickly and the patient himself is frequently totally unaware of any mental lapse.

The diagnosis of epilepsy is usually made on the basis of the history and especially the observation of one of the attacks. Elaborate electrical recordings of brain waves (electro-encephalography) are also used.

It is necessary to determine whether the symptoms are due to acquired causes or whether they exist as an inherent pattern in the individual. In cases of acquired epilepsy, where intracranial lesions are demonstrated, recovery may take place following surgical removal of the lesion.

The general management of the epileptic consists of a thorough search for possible organic causes of the symptoms, the institution of desirable personal hygiene, and a life and environment free from severe emotional disturbances which may predispose to the attacks. Sedative medication is an important part of this treatment in severe cases. The bromides, phenobarbital and particularly dilantin sodium are widely used. Prolonged or injudicious sedation may lead to mental deterioration.

Oral Aspects. The dentist should be on the watch for signs which may suggest an epileptic tendency. Extensive bruises, scarring of the facial areas, the lips and particularly scarring and deformities of the tongue should make one suspect epilepsy. The young patient with tongue scarring should be questioned about the occurrence of "fainting spells." Epileptic patients are particularly prone to grind their teeth during the night (bruxism).

It is important to recognize an epileptic tendency in a patient who is to receive nitrous oxide anesthesia, as the excitement which is often present during induction and the anoxemia which is a frequent accompaniment of this form of anesthesia predispose to seizures. When convulsions occur in a rigidly restrained patient they may result in serious personal injury and considerable damage to the office equipment. Epileptics are usually good patients under local anesthesia if they are not fatigued and if they receive proper premedication.

If a known or an unsuspected epileptic should experience a seizure while in the dental office, prompt measures should be taken to prevent self-inflicted injury. The patient should be removed from the dental chair and placed on the floor where there is little risk of striking the walls, the furniture or office equipment. There is controversy over the advisability of attempting to insert a mouth prop during a convulsion in the hope of preventing tongue injuries. The danger of receiving accidental bites from the epileptic outweighs the danger to the patient of receiving traumatic injuries to the tongue. It is not unusual for teeth to be fractured or dislodged during a seizure. Fixed rather than removable prosthetic appliances should be constructed for the epileptic.

DILANTIN GINGIVAL HYPERPLASIA. Sodium diphenyl hydantoinate (dilantin sodium), which is widely used in the treatment of epilepsy, is frequently

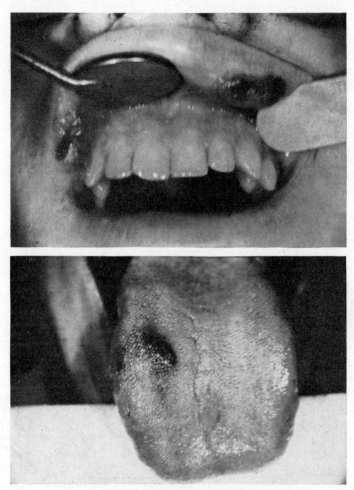

FIG. 191 (*Top*). Bilateral human bites of the upper lip which were received during an epileptic convulsion.

FIG. 192 (*Bottom*). Traumatic injury (bite) to tongue which occurred during an epileptic seizure.

associated with a marked gingival hyperplasia. Kimball first recognized and described these oral findings as a side action of this drug. Various degrees of gingival hyperplasia are observed in from 6 to 50% of the patients receiving this form of sedation. It was believed at first that the hyperplasia was due in part to low levels of blood ascorbic acid and that the changes were more marked in patients with marked deficiencies of vitamin C. Drake and co-workers found in rats that the body supply of vitamin C was gradually decreased by dilantin administration, but others, including the careful studies of Merritt and Foster, could not demonstrate any correlation between vitamin C levels, the administration of dilantin sodium, and the development of the gingival hyperplasia.

The occurrence and the degree of hyperplasia are not directly related to the dosage or the length of administration of the drug, although there is a tendency for the gingival changes to occur in individuals receiving the larger doses of dilantin sodium for some length of time. Sex and age are not predisposing factors although the more marked cases which have been seen by the author occurred in the adolescent patient. Local sources of irritation and poor oral hygiene are important factors in the development of the hyperplasia and its persistence in spite of treatment. Glickman and Lewistun failed to find the hyperplasia in an edentulous area and after the removal of teeth which were surrounded by hyperplastic tissue, normal healing occurred with the disappearance of the gingival enlargement. The exact cause of the hyperplasia is not known. It has been impossible to produce comparable lesions in animals.

The covering epithelium has an unusually thick layer of hornified epithelial cells beneath which there are numerous lymphocytes and plasma cells. Many fibroblasts are observed scattered throughout the fibrous tissue which forms the bulk of the lesion. This histopathologic picture is different from that observed in the hypertrophic gingivitis due to local irritative factors or hormonal disturbances.

These gingival changes are seen first in the interdental papillae, but in advanced cases these proliferations become so large as to cover the tooth almost completely. Frequently only a narrow V of labial enamel surface can be seen. In advanced cases the entire marginal gingiva is involved with the most marked hyperplasia on the buccal or labial surfaces. A well-defined line of demarcation is usually recognized between the normal gum and the hyperplastic tissue.

The patient experiences few if any subjective symptoms. The hyperplastic tissue has a light coral pink color and a slightly more roughened surface than the uninvolved gum. It bleeds rarely. Local inflammatory changes are uncommon because of the thickened keratinized surface. Alveolar resorption occurs less often than in patients with gingival hypertrophy. Dilantin hyperplasia is important because of its undesirable appearance; it makes the maintenance of proper oral hygiene and at times chewing difficult. The gingival lesions, unless severe, do not justify the discontinuance of the drug because of its effectiveness in controlling the "grand mal" type of seizures.

Treatment. Measures directed against the development of the gingival hyperplasia are more effective than the treatment of the frank lesion. Ziskin and Putnam found that rigorous attention to the patient's oral hygiene from the time the drug is first administered is a valuable prophylactic measure. A careful toothbrushing routine and interdental stimulation are important factors in home care. All local predisposing factors should be eliminated by dental treatment. It is frequently difficult to obtain the necessary co-operation from the patient.

When the hyperplasia is confined to the interdental areas and before the tissue has become fibrous, conservative treatment, which consists of interdental stimulation, effective oral hygienic measures and the elimination of

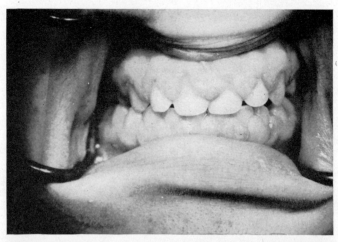

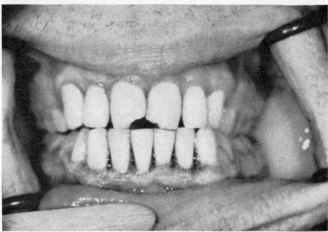

Fig. 193 (*Top*). Dilantin hyperplasia in a 17-year-old girl. The enlarged tissues are light pink in color, fibrous and show no evidence of edema, inflammation or ulceration.

Fig. 194 (*Bottom*). Patient with dilantin hyperplasia following electrocautery of the enlarged gingival tissues. The excess maxillary gingival tissue was removed ten days previously. The excess mandibular gingival tissue was just removed. Fractures of the mesio-incisal angles of the maxillary first incisors occurred during a seizure.

local irritative factors, may result in a disappearance of the hyperplasia or at least prevent its further development.

In extensive dilantin hyperplasia which consists of coral pink fibrous tissue, the surgical removal of the involved tissue is the only satisfactory form of treatment. Stern *et al.* found that the early institution of a rigorous tooth-brushing and interdental stimulation routine are important factors in preventing a recurrence of the lesion. A slight reduction in the dilantin dosage is frequently helpful. Recurrences are common in any form of treatment because the needed patient co-operation can rarely be secured.

Paralysis Agitans (Parkinsonism—Parkinson's Disease)

This is a disease of the central nervous system which is characterized by rhythmical muscular tremors with varying degrees of rigidity. The tremors are usually absent during sleep and they can be controlled for short periods of time by voluntary effort. Individuals with paralysis agitans have slow movements and a bent head and body posture. Paralysis agitans frequently follows encephalitis lethargica but in many cases there is no known previous involvement of the central nervous system.

The patient with paralysis agitans has a staring, fixed, mask-like expression. The typical tremor is commonly present in the muscles of mastication and the tongue may show marked tremor. Speech is as a rule monotonous. Salivation is one of the outstanding symptoms of this disease.

There is no known specific therapy for this disease. Belladonna and its derivatives are used to reduce the muscular rigidity.

Anterior Poliomyelitis (Spinal Meningitis)

Anterior poliomyelitis is an acute infectious disease caused by a filtrable virus. The exact method of transmission of the virus and its portal of entry are not known. Both the nasopharynx and the intestinal tract are possible sites of entry. Aisenberg and Grubb reported the production of poliomyelitis in *Macacus rhesus* monkeys by the inoculation of tooth pulp cavities with the "Creach" strain of virus. Sections of the spinal cord revealed typical poliomyelitis.

Poliomyelitis is characterized by a preparalytic phase with symptoms of irritability, headache, fever and at times diarrhea. When mild, these symptoms are indistinguishable from those of an ordinary upper respiratory infection. The preparalytic stage, when recognized, is followed in 3 or 4 days by the meningitic stage which is characterized by stiffness and rigidity of the neck and back. Paralysis of the various muscle groups may be the initial symptom but it occurs usually within the first 4 days of the meningitic stage. The extent or severity of the paralysis cannot be predicated on the basis of the constitutional symptoms.

Diagnosis is made on the basis of the history, the physical findings and certain characteristic changes in the spinal fluid.

The treatment of the acute disease has been modified in recent years with the more general use of the Sister Kenny method of treatment which consists of hot compresses during the paralytic phase, early passive exercises, and muscle training. This reduces materially the crippling contracture and deformities which result from the muscle spasms. Various prophylactic procedures, such as active and passive immunization and nasal sprays, have not been generally accepted.

Oral Aspects. Cochran believed that atrophy and putrescence of the dental pulp were responsible for poliomyelitis. The only basis for this theory is the experimental studies of Rosenow and coworkers in support of the streptococcal theory of etiology. Thompson observed that poliomyelitis is often found associated with foci of infection—probably as an accompanying finding. Gard reported 2 cases of poliomyelitis which developed within 10 days following dental extractions. It is recognized that tonsillectomy may predispose to the immediate disease. Sabin was unable to demonstrate the poliomyelitis virus in the saliva of the oral secretions of 20 patients.

Poliomyelitis may affect the motor nuclei of the 5th, 7th, 9th and 10th cranial nerves. Sittig and Urban observed a 15-year-old boy with this disease who had permanent bilateral paralysis of the muscles of mastication and weakness of the muscles supplied by the right facial nerve. Cases of permanent facial paralysis following poliomyelitis have been noted.

REFERENCES

THE RESPIRATORY SYSTEM

Brown, J. W., et al.: Epedemic of influenza. Results of prophylactic inoculation of complex influenza. A-distemper vaccine, J. Clin. Investigation, 20:663-69, 1941.

Clayton, M. D., & C. R. Jackson: Foreign body (dental plate) in the esophagus—with erosion of the left primary bronchus, Med. Bull. Vet. Admin., 19:346-7, 1943.

Crawford, J. A.: Pneumococcal stomatitis, Tri-State M. J., 11:2308, 1939.

Finland, M., & J. H. Dingle: Virus pneumonias, New England J. Med., 227:342, 1942.

Grove, R. C., & J. G. Welch: Bacteriologic relationship of dental infection and chronic hyperplastic sinusitis, Laryngoscope, 51:263, 1941.

Harris, L.: The dentist and the recent influenza epidemic, Dental Cosmos, 61:299-301, 1919.

Holinger, Paul H., et al.: Foreign bodies in the air and food passages, Eye, Ear, Nose & Throat Monthly, 22:415, 1943.

Horsfall, F. L., Jr., et al.: Studies on efficacy of complex vaccine against influenza, U. S. Pub. Health Rep., 56:1863-75, 1941.

Kramer, L. R.: Silicosis: A potential hazard in dental laboratories, J. A. D. A., 27:1503, 1940.

Pessin, S. B.: Tularemic pneumonia, pericarditis and ulcerative stomatitis, Arch. Int. Med., 57:1125, 1936.

Pittman, M. A.: Dry ice treatment for hiccough, North Carolina M. J., 1:615, 1940.

Reed, R. R.: A case of persistent singultus ceasing after removal of infected teeth, Am. J. Surg., 34:172, 1928.

Rush, B.: An account of the influenza as it appeared in Philadelphia in the autumn of 1789, in the spring of 1790 and in the winter of 1791, Med. Inq. & Obs., Philadelphia, 2 ed., 2:353-67, 1805.

Shea, J. J.: Infections of the paranasal sinuses of dental origin, Surg., Gynec. & Obst., 66:408, 1938.

Siltzbach, L. E.: The silicosis hazard in mechanical dentistry, J. A. M. A., 113:1116, 1939.

Smith, T. D.: Etiology of primary bronchiectasis, Arch. Surg., 21:1173, 1930.

Stern, Leo: Etiologic factors in the pathogenesis of putrid abscess of the lung, J. Thoracic Surg., 6:202, 1936.

Stern, Leo: Putrid abscess of the lung following dental operations, J. Thoracic Surg., 4:547, 1935.

Tomarkin, E., & W. Loewenthal: Protracted post-influenzal stomatitis with presence of influenza bacillus, Schweiz. med. Wchnschr., 57:770-800, 1927. Abs. J. A. M. A., 89:1463, 1927.

THE CARDIOVASCULAR SYSTEM

Abrahamson, L.: Subacute bacterial endocarditis following removal of septic foci, Brit. M. J., 2:8, 1931.

Ackland, W. R.: Grave cardiac symptoms due to multiple dental abscesses, Bristol Med.-Chir. J., 41:79, 1924.

Barnes, A. R.: A logical approach to the diagnosis of heart disease, Wisconsin M. J., 42:601, 1943.

Bernstein, Mitchell: Subacute bacterial endocarditis, Ann. Int. Med., 5:1138, 1932.

Binkwitz, B.: Blood supply of the tongue—early sign of cardiac decompensation, Med. J. & Rec., 137:426, 1933.

Boisvert, Paul L.: Streptococcosis in children, Am. J. Dis. Child., 64:516, 1942.

Bowers, J. M.: Arteritis of the temporal vessels, Arch. Int. Med., 66:384, 1940.

Boyne, H. N.: The dentist's responsibility to the cardiac patient, J. A. D. A., 23:1451, 1936.

Brown, H. H.: Tooth extraction and chronic infective endocarditis, Brit. M. J., 3:796, 1932.

Capps, J. A.: A consideration of heart disease and syncope in the practice of dentistry, J. A. D. A., 23:1543, 1936.

Carr, J. G., Relationship between dental and cardiovascular disease, J. A. D. A., 24:1979, 1937.

Christian, H. A.: The determinative background of subacute bacterial endocarditis, Am. J. M. Sc., 201:34, 1941.

Clagett, H. Henry: The relation of oral infections to the circulatory system, Mil. Surgeon, 88:662, 1941.

Collins, B. C.: Subacute bacterial endocarditis treated with penicillin, J. A. M. A., 126:233, 1944.

Darlington, C. G.: Death and dentistry, Am. J. Orthodontics & Oral Surg., 27:407, 1941.

Doane, J. C.: Oral sepsis and bacterial endocarditis, Weekly Roster & Med. Dig., Mar. 22, 957, 1941.

Dry, T. J.: Congestive heart failure, J. A. M. A., 118:264, 1943.

Field, Henry, *et al.*: Results of chemotherapy in subacute bacterial endocarditis, Am. J. M. Sc., **202**:798, 1941.

Fleury, J.: Streptococcie maligne lente greffe sur un canal arteriel apres avulsion dentaire, Arch. d. mal du couer, **32**:464, 1939.

Galbreath, W. R., & Edgar Hull: Sulfonamide therapy of bacterial endocarditis, Ann. Int. Med., **18**:201, 1943.

Geiger, A. J.: Relation of fatal subacute bacterial endocarditis to tooth extraction, J. A. D. A., **29**:1023, 1943.

Gilbert, N. C.: Vasomotor changes in coronary arteries and their possible significance, J. A. M. A., **113**:1925, 1939.

Grant, R. T.: After histories for ten years of one thousand men suffering from heart disease: Study in prognosis, Heart, **6**:275, 1933.

Griffith, G. C.: The relationship between dental infections and cardiovascular-renal disease, Dental Cosmos, **77**:167, 1935.

Grollman, A., J. R. Williams, Jr., & T. R. Harrison: Reduction of elevated blood pressure by administration of renal extracts, J. A. M. A., **115**:1169, 1940.

Haden, R. L.: Focal infection as a case of heart disease, Ohio State M. J., **28**:276, 1932.

Holmes, B.: Cardiac disease and the dentist, J. A. D. A., **23**:118, 1936.

Holtz, Edw., & George Friedman: A hemorrhagic eruption of the mouth and throat in the rheumatic state, Am. J. M. Sc., **187**:359, 1943.

Hopkins, J. A.: Bacteremia following extraction of teeth, J. A. D. A., **26**: 2002, 1939.

Horton, B. T., T. B. Magath, & G. E. Brown: Temporal arteritis, Proc. Staff Meetings Mayo Clinic, **12**:548, 1937.

Hoyt, L. H., G. A. Perera, & A. J. Kauvar: Temporal arteritis, New England J. Med., **225**:283, 1941.

Irvine, A. D.: Coarctation of the aorta, Canad. M. A. J., **46**:436, 1942.

Keefer, C. S., *et al.*: Penicillin in the treatment of infections: Statement of the committee on chemotherapeutic and other agents. Division of medical sciences, National Research Council, J. A. M. A., **122**:1217, 1943.

Klestadt, W., & H. Bettinger: Peculiar disease of the tongue and soft palate at onset of periarteritis nordosa, Ztschr. f. laryn. rhin., **30**:2, 1930.

Lathrope, G. H.: Incidence of cardio-vascular renal lesions in oral sepsis, Am. J. Surg. (Anes. Supp.), **38**:40, 1924.

Levy, A. T.: Erythema multiforme bullosum with involvement of the mucous membranes of the mouth, J. A. D. A., **30**:287, 1943.

Lozier, Matthew: Evaluation of anesthetic and surgical risks in dental practice, Dent. Outlook, **29**:15, 1942.

Master, A. M.: Coronary heart disease: angina pectoris acute coronary insufficiency and coronary occlusion, Ann. Int. Med., **20**:661, 1944.

McLean, Jay, *et al.*: Heparin in subacute bacterial endocarditis, J. A. M. A., **117**:1870, 1941.

Montegny, de G.: Question of relation between infected teeth and high blood pressure, Union med. du Canada, **66**:1147, 1937.

Murphy, F. D.: Heart disease and circulatory disturbances in dental practice, J. Wisconsin State Dent. Soc., **17**:163, 1941.

Murray, M., & F. Moosnick: Incidence of bacteremias in patients with dental disease, J. Lab. & Clin. Med., **26**:801, 1941.

Northrop, P. M., & Mary C. Crowley: The dentist's responsibility in the management of the patient with rheumatic heart disease, Am. J. Ortho-dontics & Oral Surg., 30:693, 1944.

Northrop, P. M., & M. C. Crowley: The prophylactic use of sulfathiazole in transient bacteremia following the extraction of teeth, J. Oral Surg., 1:19, 1943.

Okell, C. C., & S. D. Elliott: Bacteremia and oral sepsis with special refer-ence to the etiology of subacute endocarditis, Lancet, 2:869, 1935.

Palmer, B. B., & M. W. Carr: Medico-dental case records: myocarditis, J. Dent. Research, 10:675, 1930.

Palmer, H. D., & B. A. Jempf: Streptococcus viridans following extraction of teeth, J. A. D. A., 26:1788, 1939.

Parkinson, J.: Effort syndrome in soldiers, Brit. M. J., 1:545, 1941.

Parsons-Smith, Basil: The soldier's heart and its treatment, Med. Press & Circular, 2:378, 1940.

Petersen, W. F., & S. J. Nedgel: Dental surgery and endocarditis, J. A. D. A., 25:1462, 1938.

Poston, Mary A., & Edw. S. Orgain: Comparison of the bacteriostatic effect of the sulfonamide drugs upon the growth of 25 strains of streptococcus viridans, Am. J. M. Sc., 203:577, 1942.

Pressman, R. S., & I. B. Bender: Effect of sulfonamide compounds on tran-sient bacteremia following extraction of teeth, Arch. Int. Med., 74:346, 1944.

Raven, R. W.: Recent therapeutic advances in surgery, Post Grad. M. J., 17:190-4, 1941.

Richards, John H.: Bacteremia following irritation of foci of infection, J. A. D. A., 99:1496, 1932.

Rushton, M. A.: Subacute bacterial endocarditis, following extraction of teeth, Guy's Hospital Rep., 80:39, 1930.

Sauer, P. K.: The choice of anesthesia in operative patients with heart dis-ease, Am. J. Surg., 48:532, 1940.

Schwartz, S. P., & I. Salman: The effects of oral surgery on the course of patients with diseases of the heart, Am. J. Orthodontics & Oral Surg., 28:331, 1942.

Smith, C., H. C. Sauls, & C. F. Stone: Subacute bacterial endocarditis due to streptococcus viridans, J. A. D. A., 119:478, 1942.

Smith, Edwin H., Jr., & A. Henry Clagett: Subacute bacterial endocarditis and dental extraction, J. A. D. A., 28:1841, 1941.

Sozzi, E. S.: Dental treatment of patients with rheumatic heart disease, New York J. Dent., 13:342, 1943.

Stevens, R. S.: Present status of treatment of coronary artery disease, Canad. M. A. J., 44:124, 1941.

Stitzel, E. W.: Pediatrist's study of focal infection in children, Pennsyl-vania M. J., 35:395, 1932.

Talbot, W. O.: Unhealthy mouths, public health problem, Texas State J. Med., 26:444, 1930.

Taran, L. M.: Dental care of children with heart disease, J. 2nd Dist. Dent. Soc. State, New York, 28:93-101, 1942.

Tooke, T. B., Jr.: Periarteritis nodosa, Tri-State M. J., 14:2674, 1942.

Volini, I. F., & G. M. Engbring: Coarctation of the aorta, Med. Clinics North Amer., 26:269, 1942.

Weinstein, Joseph: Dental complications in the cardiac patient, Dent. Outlook, 29:258, 1942.
Weiss, Soma: Arteritis: Diseases associated with inflammatory lesions of the peripheral arteries, New England Jour. Med., 225:579, 1941.
Weiss, Harry: Relation of portals of entry to subacute bacterial endocarditis, Arch. Int. Med., 54:710, 1934.
White, P. D.: The soldier's irritable heart, J. A. M. A., 118:270, 1942.

GASTRO-INTESTINAL DISEASES

Achard, P.: Les lesions bucco-dentaires de la fievre typhoide, Abstr. Rev. Odontologique, 57:60, 1934.
Ahlbom, H. E.: Simple achlorhydric anemia. Plummer-Vinson syndrome and carcinoma of the mouth, pharynx and esophagus in women, Brit. M. J., 2:331, 1936.
Albanese, P.: White spot in tooth in the diagnosis of gastric ulcer, Stomatol., 32:224, 1934.
Alvarez, W. C.: What do we really know about the treatment of ulcer?, Atlantic M. J., 31:918, 1928.
Arkwright, J. A.: Foot and mouth disease in man, Lancet, 1:1191, 1928.
Auschultz, Robt. R.: Tularemia with extensive pharyngitis, Am. J. Dis. Child., 62:150, 1941.
Beck, A. L.: Inflammation of the salivary glands, Surg. Gynec. & Obst., 74:604, 1942.
Beebe, E. H.: Gas gangrene following tooth extraction, J. A. D. A., 25:1893, 1938.
Berndt, A. L., R. Buck, & R. von L. Buxton: Pathogenesis of acute suppurative parotitis. Experimental study, Am. J. M. Sc., 182:639, 1931.
Bernstein, A.: Infectious mononucleosis, Medicine, 19:85, 1940.
Black, Donald R.: Nephritic stomatitis, Urol. & Cutan. Rev., 46:75, 1942.
Blackford, R. W.: Recurrent swelling of the parotid and submaxillary glands following bronchoscopy, Ann. Otol. Rhin. & Laryng., 53:54-64, 1944.
Bloomfield, A. L.: Enlargement of superficial lymph nodes in Brucella infection, Am. Rev. Tuberc., 45:741, 1942.
Cahn, Lester R.: The Plummer-Vinson syndrome facies: an oral precancerous sign, Arch. Clin. Oral Path., 2:308, 1938.
Calvin, J. K.: Tetanus, its prevention and treatment, New York State J. Med., 41:1636, 1941.
Castle, W. B., et al.: Etiology and treatment of sprue, Arch. Int. Med., 56:627, 1935.
Chimenti, A.: Osteomielite necrosante del mascellare supiore in rapporte al tifo abdominale, La Stomatologia Gennaio, 33:53, 1935.
Clayton, M. D., & C. R. Jackson: Foreign body (dental plate) in the esophagus, Med. Bull. Vet. Admin., 19:346, 1943.
Clough, P. W.: A case of foot and mouth disease in man, Bull. Johns Hopkins Hosp., 26:351, 1915.
Court, D., & J. K. Halser: Hirschsprung's disease treated by spinal anesthesia, Proc. Roy. Soc. Med., 35:687, 1942.
Crile, G., Jr., & W. R. Manning: Post-operative parotitis, Am. J. Surg., 50:664, 1940.
Crohn, B. B., & R. Drosd: Halitosis, J. A. M. A., 117:2242-5, 1941.

Dockerty, M. B., & C. W. Mayo: Primary malignant tumors of the sub-maxillary gland with special reference to mixed tumors, Proc. Staff Meet. Mayo Clinic, 17:593, 1942.

Egi, S.: Typhoid accompanied by noma, J. Oriental Med., 27:90, 1937.

Enders, J. F., et al.: Immunity in mumps, J. Exper. Med., 81:119-35, 1945.

Figi, F. A., & W. D. Rowland: Primary tumors of Stensen's and Wharton's ducts, Arch. Otolaryng., 41:175, 1944.

Findlay, G. M., & L. P. Clarke: Experimental production of mumps in monkeys, Brit. J. Exper. Path., 15:309-13, 1934.

Ghose, A. K.: Cancrum oris,—complication of bacillary dysentery, Indian M. Gaz., 72:419, 1937.

Goehring, W. O.: A case of toothpick perforation of the intestines, Am. J. Med. Sc., 205:8078, 1943.

Greene, J. A., & R. H. Heeren: Mumps; incidence of palpable splenic enlargement and of "complications" and their relation to salivary gland involvement as evidence that disease is systemic infection, J. Lab. & Clin. Med., 23:129-34, 1937.

Haden, R. L.: Recurrent peptic ulcer from a single focus in presence of multiple foci, M. Clin. North America, 7:1115, 1924.

Halcrow, J. P., et al.: Infectious mononucleosis with an account of an epidemic in an E. M. S. hospital, Brit. M. J., 2:443, 1943.

Holman, W. L.: Focal infection and "elective localization," Arch. Path. & Lab. Med., 5:68, 1928.

Hunter, J. B.: Action of saliva and gastric juice on the clotting of blood, Brit. J. Surg., 16:203, 1928.

Jaenisch, R.: Permanent results in chronic diseases of the gastric-ulcer group after elimination of chronic foci of infection in the mouth, Deut. Med. Wchnschr., 57:2011, 1931.

Jelks, J. L.: Role of focal infection in causation of gastro-intestinal disease, South. M. J., 20:158, 1927.

Johnson, C. D., & E. W. Goodpasture: Investigation of etiology of mumps, J. Exper. Med., 59:1-19, 1934.

Johnson, C. D., & E. W. Goodpasture: Experimental immunity to virus of mumps in monkeys, Am. J. Hyg., 23:329-39, 1936.

Jordon, C. F., et al.: Brucellosis: considerations of its epidemiology, diagnosis and control, Am. J. Pub. Health, 33:773, 1943.

Kilham, L., & A. J. Steigman: Infectious mononucleosis, Lancet, 243:452, 1942.

Kirby, W. M. M., & Charles D. Armstrong: Sarcoidosis with uveoparotid fever, Ann. Int. Med., 21:475, 1944.

Kopeloff, N.: Bacterial content of stomach as influenced by saliva, Proc. Soc. Exper. Biol. & Med., 19:119, 1921-2.

Kutscher, G. W., Jr.: Use of convalescent mumps serum, J. Pediat., 16:166-70, 1940.

Langstroth, L.: The incidence of chronic focal infection in chronic diseases, Am. J. Med. Sc., 155:232, 1918.

Lermann, W. W.: Planned search for foci of infection in chronic disease as means of increasing span of life, with particular reference to gastrointestinal tract, Pennsylvania M. J., 47:699, 1944.

Levy, H., & E. P. Boas: Angina pectoris and the syndrome of peptic ulcer, Arch. Int. Med., 71:307, 1943.

Lintz, W.: Digestive diseases and the teeth, Ann. Int. Med., 4:1188, 1931.

Losch, K. P., & D. Weisberger: High caries susceptibility in diminished salivation, Am. J. Orthodontics & Oral Surg., 26:1102, 1940.

Lourie, R. S.: Rate of secretion of parotid glands in normal children, Am. J. Dis. Child., 65:455, 1943.

Ludden, J. B., J. Flexner, & I. S. Wright: Studies on ascorbic acid deficiency in gastric diseases; incidence, diagnosis and treatment, Am. J. Digest. Dis., 8:249, 1941.

Madding, G. F., & R. E. Fricke: Secondary postoperative parotitis, Surg., 11:45, 1942.

Manson-Bahr, P., & H. Willoughby: Studies on sprue with special reference to treatment; based on the analysis of 200 cases, Quart. J. Med., 23:411, 1930.

Marvell, D. M., & H. J. Parish: Tetanus prophylaxis and circulating antitoxin in men and women, Brit. Med. J., 2:891, 1940.

McKinlay, C. A.: Infectious mononucleosis, J. A. M. A., 105:761, 1935.

Meyer, K. A.: Oral infection in gastro-intestinal disease, J. A. D. A., 27:93-95, 1940.

Miller, J. R., & G. B. Eusterman: Mikulicz's syndrome: report of a case with associated pulmonary and gastric lesions, Proc. Staff Meet. Mayo Clinic, 19:425, 1944.

Moutier, F.: Stomatologie et Gastroenterologie, Revue de stomatol., 33:257-65, 1931.

Mulligan, R. M.: Metastasis of mixed tumors of the salivary glands, Arch. Path., 35:357, 1943.

Newman, N.: Afunctional gingivitis associated with esophageal obstruction, Dent. Survey, 18:1478, 1942.

Nickel, A. C.: The localization in animals of bacteria isolated from foci of infection, J. A. M. A., 87:1117, 1926.

Notti, J. H., H. Ferrer, & A. Grinfeld: Peritonitis por perforcion de la vesicula biliar en el curso de una fiebre tifoideal parotiditis suparada, Arch. argent. pediat., 15:579, 1941.

Orgaz, J.: Buccopharyngeal sepsis preexisting in typhoid, Prensa Medica Argentina, 24:1103, 1937.

Palozzi, S.: White spots on the teeth considered as a sign of gastric ulcer, Stomatol., 32:331, 1934.

Patrick, Adam: Acute diabetes following mumps, Brit. Med. J., 2:802, 1924.

Paul, J. R.: Infectious mononucleosis, Bull. New York Acad. Med., 15:43-55, 1939.

Pelner, Louis: Parotid duct obstruction without calculus, Am. J. Digest. Dis., 9:417, 1942.

Pendergrass, E. P., & P. J. Hodes: Acute post-operative parotitis, Radiology, 38:307, 1942.

Pessin, S. B.: Tularemic pneumonia, pericarditis and ulcerative stomatitis, Arch. Int. Med., 57:1125, 1936.

Pickworth, F. A.: Chronic nasal sinusitis and its relation to mental disorder, London, H. K. Lewis & Co., 1935.

Poe, D. L.: Sarcoidosis of the jaw, Am. J. Orthodontics & Oral Surg., 29:52, 1943.

Poston, M. A., & E. E. Menefee: Acute brucellosis with bacteremia and

oral lesions: treatment with immune human blood, New England J. Med., 219:746-97, 1938.
Price, W. A.: Dental infections and degenerative diseases, clinical researches, Penton Publishing Co., Cleveland, O., 1923.
Queries and Minor Notes: Foot and mouth disease—B. xerosis, J. A. M. A., 104:239, 1935.
Robbins, Guy F.: Tumors of salivary gland origin, Surgery, 14:924, 1943.
Roberts, E. Wendell: Calculi in the parotid region, South. Med. & Surg., 105:373, 1943.
Rosenow, E. C.: Ulcer of the stomach by injection of streptococci, J. A. M. A., 61:1947, 1913.
Rosenow, E. C.: Focal infection and elective localization of bacteria in appendicitis, ulcer of the stomach, cholecystitis and pancreatitis, Surg., Gynec. & Obst., 34:19, 1921.
Rosenow, E. C.: The causation of gastric and duodenal ulcer by streptococci, J. Infect. Dis., 19:333, 1916.
Rowe, S. N.: Mikulicz's syndrome with chronic lymphatic leukemia, New England J. Med., 202:863-5, 1930.
Salivary Calculus or tartar: some notes on case and definition of term "salivary calculus," Brit. Jour. Radiol., 17:31, 1944.
Saphir, W.: Xerostomia successfully treated with nicotinic acid, Am. J. Digest. Dis., 7:298, 1940.
Satterlee, G. R.: The effects of removal of dental infection on chronic gastro-intestinal disorders, Med. J. & Rec., 114:481, 1924.
Schaffer, A. J., & A. W. Jacobsen: Mikulicz's syndrome: a report of ten cases, Am. J. Dis. Child., 34:327, 1927.
Schwindt, L. W.: Specific tongue conditions noted in peptic ulcer cases, M. Times & Long Island M. J., 60:242, 1932.
Simpson, W. M.: New developments in diagnosis and treatment of brucellosis (undulant fever), Minnesota Med., 24:725-38, 1941.
Staggerda, F. R.: Observation on water intake in an adult man with dysfunctioning salivary glands, Am. J. Physiol., 132:517, 1941.
Steigmann, F.: Facial tularemia: diagnostic difficulties of this unusually located primary lesion, Illinois M. J., 67:271, 1935.
Stevens, G. A.: Relationship of dentistry to peptic ulcer and goiter, J. A. D. A., 28:404, 1941.
Sulkin, S. E., & C. G. Harford: Concerning the infectivity of saliva in human rabies, Ann. Int. Med., 19:256, 1943.
Talbot, H. S.: Acute suppurative parotitis; its etiology and pathogenesis and treatment, Am. J. Surg., 25:267, 1934.
Templeton, H. J., & R. T. Sutherland: The exanthem of acute mononucleosis, J. A. M. A., 113:1215, 1939.
Tinney, W. S., H. W. Schmidt, & H. L. Smith: Dysphagia: The result of pressure from a dilated left auricle, Proc. Staff Meet. of Mayo Clinic, 18:476-80, 1943.
Trimble, H. C., et al.: Rate of secretion of saliva and incidence of dental caries, J. Dent. Res., 17:299, 1938.
Upton, C. L.: An unusual case of appendicitis, Boston Med. & Surg. J., 190:623, 1924.
Van Loon, E. L., & Sidney Diamond: Foreign bodies in the gastrointestinal tract, Ann. Otol. Rhinol. & Laryng., 51:1077, 1942.

Vinson, Porter P.: Hysterical Dysphagia, Minnesota Med., **5**:107, 1922.

Walker, V. G.: Treatment of diseases of the salivary glands and ducts, Mil. Surgeon, **89**:656, 1941.

Wardell, W. W., & McL. Birdsong: Tularemia with lesions confined to the tonsils, J. Pediat., **20**:368, 1942.

Warden, E. M.: Epidemic parotitis, Canad. M. A. J., **50**:47, 1944.

Wesselhoeft, C.: Medical progress; mumps, New England J. Med., **226**: 530-34, 1942.

Wilson, G. S., & I. Maier: Treatment with sulphapyridine of guinea pigs infected with brucella abortus, Brit. M. J., **1**:47-50, 1940.

Zaltsberg, I.: Peroral hemorrhage in course of Banti's disease, Klin. med., **16**:118-19, 1938.

THE UROGENITAL SYSTEM

Barr, E. O.: Relation between foci of infection and prostatitis, Urol. & Cutan. Rev., **42**:733, 1938.

Bereston, E. S., & H. Keil: Membranous stomatitis associated with debilitation with uremia, Arch. Dermat. & Syph., **44**:562, 1941.

Bliss, S.: Cause of sore throat in nephritis, J. Biol. Chem., **121**:425-27, 1937.

Brown, R. D.: Sperm fluctuation in health and disease, South. M. J., **36**: 619, 1943.

Fraser, A. D., & J. Menton: Gonococcal stomatitis, Am. Dent. Surg., **51**: 229-32, 1931.

Goldberg, H. A.: Prostatitis and multiple arthritis of dental origin, J. A. D. A., **30**:1378, 1943.

Higgins, C. C., & E. E. Mendenhall: Factors associated with recurrent formation of renal lithiasis, J. Urol., **42**:436, 1939.

Minnich, F. R.: Vulvovaginal mycosis, J. M. A. Georgia, **30**:386-89, 1941.

Oveido, G. F.: Paradental infections as related to prostatic infection: A preliminary report, J. A. D. A. & Dent. Cosmos, **24**:696, 1937.

Rosenow, E. C.: Renal calculi, J. Urol., **44**:19, 1940.

Steiner, W. R., & L. L. Walton: Gonorrheal endocarditis with bilateral parotitis and toxic jaundice as additional complications, Ann. Int. Med., **11**:1464-71, 1938.

Wesson, M. B., R. Albert, & G. Curia: The relationship between dentistry and urology with six case reports, Med. Record., **151**:77-81, 1940.

Whitlow, J. E.: Ulcerative stomatitis and vulvitis, Med. Record., **144**:119, 1936.

Wien, M. S., & M. O. Perlstein: Ulcus vulvae associated with lesions of the mouth, J. A. M. A., **98**:461, 1932.

THE REPRODUCTORY SYSTEM

Agnew, M. C., et al.: Production and prevention of dental caries, J. Pediat., **2**:190, 1933.

d'Alise, C.: Effect of diet during pregnancy and lactation on the teeth of mother and child, Riforma med., **51**:423, 1935.

Beierlein, K. M.: Dental care from the viewpoint of the obstetrician, J. Ind. State Dent. A., **12**:7, 1933.

Birbaum, R., & R. E. Fagnani: The buccal cavity under the influence of menstruation, Boletin Odontologico Mexicano, **21**:209, 1940.

Biro, S.: Untersuchungen über den Einfluss der Graviditat auf die caries der Zähne, Vierteljahr. f. Zahnheilk., 14:371, 1898.

Blum, Theodore: Pregnancy tumors, study of 16 cases, J. A. D. A., 18: 393, 1931.

Bresler, H. E.: Dissertation on gingivitis gravidarum, Dent. Items of Interest, 7:605, 1935.

Brown, R. D.: Sperm fluctuations in health and disease, South. M. J., 36:619, 1943.

Bucher, A.: Prevention of dental caries during pregnancy and lactation, Munchen. med. Woschr., 84:734, 1937.

Burchardt, F.: Gum capillaries in pregnancy, Paradentium, 6:17-22, 1934.

Coles, O.: On the condition of the mouth and teeth during pregnancy, Am. J. Dent. Sc., 8:361, 1874-5.

Costello, M. J.: Eruptions of pregnancy, New York State J. Med., 41:849-55, 1941.

Coven, J. H.: Pregnancy and the teeth, Am. J. Orthodontics & Oral Surg., 29:503, 1943.

Creadick, A. N., & J. M. Gompertz: Preliminary report of the prenatal clinic, J. A. M. A., 12:1236, 1925.

Cross, W. B.: Gum tumors in pregnancy and gingivitis gravidarum, Brit. Dent. J., 75:85, 1943.

Cunningham, R. L.: Relation of dental caries to disease, menstrual experience and physical measurements of young women, J. Dent. Research, 14:439, 1934.

Cunningham, W.: Dental care of the expectant mother, N. Y. Dent. J., 29:157, 1933.

Curtis, A. H.: Streptococcus infection as a cause of spontaneous abortion, J. A. M. A., 84:1262, 1925.

Danforth, W. C.: Care of pregnancy, J. A. M. A., 103:1472, 1934.

Day, B.: Some notes on extraction of teeth during pregnancy, J. Egyptian M. A., 16:214, 1933.

Dayton, A. C.: Cases of metastasis of menstrual secretion from the uterus to mouth, Am. J. Dent. Sc., 10:42-44, 1849-50.

Deakins, M., & J. Looby: The effect of pregnancy on the mineral content of dentin of human teeth, Am. J. Obst. & Gyne., 46:265-7, 1943.

Dudgeon, L. S., & R. C. Jewesbury: Bacteriology of human milk, J. Hyg., 23:64-76, 1924.

Friesell, H. E., & C. C. Vogt: Report concerning the etiology of dental caries, J. A. D. A., 13:748, 1926.

Galloway, C. E.: Focal infection, Am. J. Surg., 14:643, 1931.

Galloway, C. E., & T. D. Paul: Treatment of early abortion, Am. J. Obst. & Gynec., 38:246, 1939.

Gerson, F.: Karies und Schwangerschaft, Zahnärztl. Rundschau., 30:33, 1921.

Gompertz, J. M.: Factors influencing mouth conditions during pregnancy, J. Dent. Research, 6:473, 1924-6.

Graham, W.: Pregnancy and dental health, J. A. D. A., 4:351, 1938.

Greenebaum, J. V., et al.: Studies in rickets; relation of diet during pregnancy to deciduous teeth, J. A. D. A., 17:717, 1930.

Hamann, C. A.: Breast and oral cavity tumors, Proc. Interst. Postgrad. M. A. North America, 5:93, 1930.

Harris, G. B.: Mouth infections and their relation to mother's milk, Dent. Summary, 36:719-22, 1916.

Hunscher, H. A.: Metabolism of women during reproductive cycle; calcium and phosphorus utilization in 2 successive lactation periods, J. Biol. Chem., 86:37-57, 1930.

Jackson, H., Jr., & D. Merril: Agranulocytic angina associated with menstrual cycle, New England J. Med., 210:175-76, 1934.

Jones, M. R.: Studies on inorganic salt metabolism, J. Dent. Research, 10:281, 1930.

Jones, O. V.: Cyclical ulcerative vulvitis and stomatitis, J. Obstet. & Gynec. of Brit. Emp., 47:557-62, 1940.

Kamimura, S.: Pathologic changes in the oral and pharyngeal cavities during menstruation, Oto-rhino-laryng., 9:834, 1936.

Keyes, A. B.: Focal infections and their clinical relations to metastases in the female genitalia, Am. J. Obst. & Gynec., 5:277, 1923.

Klein, A.: Changes in the mouth during menstruation, Zhnarztl. Rundsch., 43:1489 & 1522, 1934.

Klein, H.: The effects of pregnancy on the incidence of the tooth decay, Dental Cosmos, 77:864, 1935.

Lewis, Geo. M.: Herpes gestationis, successful treatment with sulfathiazole, Arch. Dermat. & Syph., 46:841, 1942.

Loomis, F. M.: Possible relation of dental abscesses to toxemia of pregnancy, California State J. Med., 17:399, 1919.

Lozner, E. L., et al.: The so-called "coagulation defect" in menstrual blood, New England J. Med., 226:481, 1942.

Macy, I. G., et al.: Human milk studies, chemical analysis of milk representative of entire first and last halves of nursing period, Am. J. Dis. Child., 42:569-89, 1931.

Mull, J. W., A. H. Bill, & F. M. Kinney: Variation of serum Ca and P during pregnancy effect on occurrence of caries, Am. J. Obst. & Gynec., 27:510, 1934.

Pappworth, M. H.: Cyclical mucosal ulceration, Brit. M. J., 1:271, 1941.

Parma, K.: Gum capillaries in pregnant women, Brit. Dent. J., 68:62, 1940.

Paul, T. D., & C. E. Galloway: Focal infections in pregnancy, Am. J. Obst. & Gynec., 39:694, 1940.

Pierrepont, B. S.: Influence of maternal oral sepsis on the fetus and marasmic children, Lancet, 1:837, 1917.

Racine, W.: Le Syndrome salivaire pre-menstrual, Schweiz. med. Wchnschr., 69:1204, 1939.

Randall, L. M.: Dental hygiene during pregnancy, Brit. J. Dent. Sc., 73:178, 1928.

Raymaker, R. E.: Lecture given before the Greater Philadelphia (Pa.) dental meeting, Feb. 1939.

Reed, C. B.: The mouth in pregnancy, J. A. D. A., 20:1631, 1933.

Schaupp, K. L.: Dental care of the prenatal patient, J. California State Dent. A., 17:143, 1941.

Schour, Isaac: Calcium metabolism of teeth, J. A. M. A., 110:870, 1938.

Shelmire, B.: Pregnancy gingivitis, South. M. J., 21:169, 1928.

Shickele, G.: Anticoagulant factor in uterus secretion, Munchen. med. Wchnschr., 58:123, 1911.

Schour, Isaac: Calcium metabolism, pregnancy and caries, Dent. Outlook, 30:358, 1943.

Sheldon, C. P.: Dental problems associated with pregnancy, New England J. Med., 222:260, 1940.

Solis-Cohen, Myer: The importance of focal infection in obstetrics, Surg., Gynec. & Obstet., 78:44-8, 1944.

Sosada, S.: Catamenia aphthae, Actas dermo-sif., 25:59, 1932.

Starobinsky, I.: Beobachtungen über Zahncaries bei Schwangeren und die Wasserstoffionenkonzentration in ihrem Speichel, Dsche. Monat. f. Zahn., 47:238, 1929.

Storer, H. R.: Submucous injection as cure for the toothache of pregnancy, Am. J. Dent. Sc., 10:138, 1860.

Talbot, J. E.: Focal infection and its relation to toxemia of pregnancy with or without convulsions, Boston M. & Surg. J., 180:469, 1919.

Talbot, J. E.: Chronic sepsis in pregnancy, Surg., Gynec. Obst., 35:42, 1922.

Taylor, E. W.: Cooperation between dentist and physician in diagnosis and treatment of the oral cavity during pregnancy and lactation, J. Tennessee State Dent. A., 14:4, 1934.

Thompson, W. P.: Observations on the possible relation between agranulocytosis and menstruation, with further studies on a case of cyclic neutropenia, New England J. Med., 210:176, 1934.

Waller, H.: Dental disease in nursing women (a note on the association between oral sepsis and deficient lactation), Lancet, 2:785-88, 1916.

Wien, M. S., & M. O. Perlstein: Ulcus vulvae actum associated with lesions of the mouth, J. A. M. A., 98:461, 1932.

Woodward, J.: Catamenia temporarily interrupted in its course by extraction of teeth, Dent. News Letter, 9:252-53, 1855-56.

Zentler, A.: Oral development in the progeny—influenced by the buccal tissues during pregnancy, Dental Cosmos, 54:119, 1912.

Ziserman, A. J.: Ulcerative vulvitis and stomatitis of endocrine origin, J. A. M. A., 104:826, 1935.

Ziskin, D. E.: Incidence of dental caries in pregnant woman, Am. J. Obst. & Gynec., 12:710, 1926.

Ziskin, D. E.: The effect of hormonal treatment on the gums and oral mucosa of women, J. Dent. Res., 16:367-78, 1937.

Ziskin, D. E., S. N. Blackberg, & A. P. Stout: Gingival during pregnancy; experimental study and histopathological interpretation, Surg., Gynec. & Obst., 57:719-26, 1933.

Ziskin, D. E., S. N. Blackberg, & C. A. Slanetz: Effects of subcutaneous injection of estrogenic and gonadotrophic hormones on gums and oral mucosa membranes of normal and castrated rhesus monkey, J. Dent. Research, 15:407-28, 1936.

Ziskin, D. E., & H. Hotelling: Effects of pregnancy, mouth acidity, and age on dental caries, J. Dent. Research, 16:507, 1937.

ENDOCRINES

Austin, L. T.: Basal metabolic rates and dental caries, Am. J. Orthedontics & Oral Surg., 30:50, 1944.

Barr, D. P., & H. A. Bulger: Clinical syndrome of hyperparathyroidism, Am. J. M. Sc., 179:449-76, 1930.

Bartlett, W., Jr.: Diagnosis of diseases of thyroid gland, Am. J. Surg., 56:261, 1942.

Biedl, A.: Successful treatment of paradontosis by means of ovarian preparations, Corresp'blatt f. Zahnaerzte, 55:99, 1931.

Billings, F.: Thyroid intoxications in young girls with focal infection in the tonsils, sinuses and teeth, Focal Infection, N. Y., Appleton, 1918.

Bishop, F. J.: Lingual thyroid, Ann. Otol. Rhinol. & Laryng., 43:294, 1934.

Bohan, P. T.: Ligneous thyroiditis associated with high grade dental infection, M. Clin. N. America, 7:1069, 1924.

Borg, Joseph F.: Hyperparathyroidism, a new consideration for the dentist, J. A. D. A., 22:1683, 1935.

Bram, I.: Role of the dentist in goiter cases: observations on the dental conditions of 6,000 goiter patients, J. A. D. A., 18:1544, 1931.

Buckman, L. T.: Lingual thyroid, Laryngoscope, 46:765, 1936.

Camp, J. D.: Osseous changes in hyperparathyroidism; roentgenologic study, J. A. M. A., 99:1913, 1932.

Goldheizer, Max. A.: The adrenal glands in health and disease, Philadelphia, F. A. Davis Co., 1944.

Goldsmith, Geo. J.: The endocrine factor in periodontia, Dent. Outlook, 31:95, 1944.

Henningsen, M. G.: Caries-free individuals, J. California State Dent. A., 17:1, 1941.

Howard, C. C.: Acromegaloid growth and dwarfism, Internat. J. Orthodontia, 22:992, 1936.

Hutton, J. H.: Relation of endocrine disorder to dental disease, J. A. D. A., 23:227, 1936.

Kerley, C. G.: Subthyroidism with defective dental development, Arch. Pediat., 55:548, 1938.

Keynes, G., & H. Taylor: Case of parathyroid tumour, Brit. J. Surg., 21:20, 1933.

Loeb, Robert F.: Adrenal cortex insufficiency, J. A. M. A., 116:2495, 1941.

Marin, H., & C. L. Graves: Plexiform neurofibroma (von Recklinghausen's disease), invading the oral cavity, Am. J. Orthodontics & Oral Surg., 28:694, 1942.

Markus, M. B.: Facial development in hypopituitary drawfism, Am. J. Orthodontics & Oral Surg., 28:334, 1942.

McCullagh, E. P., & C. A. Resch: Some endocrine factors in dental development and maintenance, J. A. D. A., 28:1436, 1941.

Osborne, O. T.: Relation of mouth infection to thyroid gland, Boston M. & Sc. J., 191:1151, 1924.

Richman, M. J., & A. R. Abarbonel: Effect of estradiol and diethylstilbestrol on atrophic human buccal mucosa with pulmonary report on use of estrogens in management of senile gingivitis, J. Clin. Endocrinology 3:224, 1943.

Rudy, A., & R. Hoffman: Skin disturbances in diabetes mellitus: their relation to vitamin deficiencies, New England J. Med., 227:893, 1943.

Schour, Isaac: Endocrine therapy in dentistry, Bull. Committee on Pharm. & Therapeutics, Jan. 26, No. 14, 1942.

Seligman, Bernard: Reduced dental caries in boys with the transient hereditary adiposogenital syndrome, Urol. & Cutan. Rev., 47:503, 1943.

Shipley, R. A.: Treatment of Addison's disease—pellets of desoxycortico-
sterone acetate, Am. J. M. Sc., 207:19, 1944.
Stevens, G. A.: Relationship of dentistry to peptic ulcer and goiter,
J. A. D. A., 28:404, 1941.
Waldbott, Geo. L.: The allergic theory of so-called thymic death, J. A. M. A.,
105:657, 1935.
Wells, H. G., E. M. Humphreys, & E. G. Work: Significance of the in-
creased frequency of selective cortical necrosis of adrenal, J. A. M. A.,
109:490, 1937.
Wilkins, L., & W. Fleischmann: Diagnosis of hypothyroidism in childhood,
J. A. M. A., 116:2459, 1941.

DISEASES OF THE BONES AND JOINTS

Bayles, T. B., & L. A. Russell: The temporomandibular joint in rheumatoiu
arthritis, J. A. M. A., 116:2842, 1941.
Becks, Hermann: Histologic study of tooth structure in osteogenesis im-
perfecta, Dent. Cosmos, 73:437, 1931.
Block, L. S., & E. Harris: An approach to a rational study and treatment
of temporomandibular joint problems, J. A. D. A., 29:349, 1942.
Bowden, Cornford: A case of Paget's disease with oral symptoms, Am. J.
Surg., 28:11, 1942.
Cecil, Russel L., et al.: Gold salts in the treatment of rheumatoid arthritis,
Ann. Int. Med., 16:811, 1942.
Cook, T. J.: Paget's disease: report of a case with oral manifestations,
J. New York Acad. Dent., 2:147, 1935.
Costen, J. B.: Syndrome of ear and sinus symptoms dependent upon dis-
turbed function of the temporomandibular joint, Ann. Otol., Rhin. &
Laryng., 43:1, 1934.
Costen, J. B.: Reflex effects produced by abnormal movement of the lower
jaw, Arch. Otolaryng., 36:548, 1942.
Dingman, R. O.: Bilateral ankylosis of the temporomandibular joints with
retrusion deformity, J. Oral Surg., 2:71, 1944.
Ellis, R. W. B.: Craniofacial dysostosis, Proc. Roy. Soc. Med., 30:1187,
1937.
Fox, L.: Paget's disease (osteitis deformans) and its effect on maxillary
bones and teeth, J. A. D. A., 20:1823-29, 1933.
Gaing, S., S. Cossy, & O. Giraldes: Gonococcal arthritis in premature new-
born infant; gingival portal of entry, An. Soc. puericult., Buenos Aires,
7:83, 1941.
Galea, M. B., & H. D. Bianchi: Sedimentation speed of erythrocytes in
temporomaxillary arthritis, Semana med., 1:1177-80, 1943.
Gareiso, A., J. E. Viviani, & A. M. Cerdeiro: Craniofacial dysostosis, Am.
J. Dis. Child., 58:857, 1939.
Glickman, Irving, & H. S. Glidden: Paget's disease of the maxillae and
mandible: clinical analysis and case reports, J. A. D. A., 29:2144, 1942.
Goldberg, H. A.: Prostatitis and multiple arthritis of dental origin, J. A.
D. A., 30:1378, 1943.
Hammer, J. L.: Treatment of acute and chronic temporomandibular ar-
thritis, South. Med. & Surg., 105:531, 1943.
Hodge, H. C., et al.: Correlated clinical and structural study of hereditary
opalescent dentine, J. Dent. Research, 15:316, 1936.

Jaffe, H. L., & L. Lichtenstein: Eosinophilic granuloma of bone, Arch. Path., 37:99, 1944.

Kazanjian, V. H.: Ankylosis of the temporomandibular joint, Surg., Gynec. & Obst., 67:333, 1938.

Kennedy, R. L. J., & J. D. Camp: Changes in skull in certain diseases in infants and children, Proc. Staff Meet. Mayo Clinic, 17:365-68, 1942.

Larson, S., & J. A. Lichty: Gargoylism: report of 3 probable cases, Am. J. Roentgenol., 50:61, 1943.

Miller, S. C., & Harry Roth: Torus palatinus: a statistical study, J. A. D. A., 27:1950, 1940.

Nichols, B. H.: Fragilitas osseum. Brittle bones and blue sclera. Hereditary mesenchyme hypoplasia, Cleveland Clin. Quart., 7:58-65, 1940.

Nisenson, A.: An appraisal of the advantage of teeth extraction in arthritis, Med. Bul. Vet. Admin., 18:57, 1941.

Paget, Sir James: Form of chronic inflammation of bones (osteitis deformans), Med.-Chir. Tr., London, 60:37-63, 1877.

Pippin, B. N.: The treatment of temporomandibular joint lesions caused by denture mutilation, Illinois Dent. J., 12:429, 1943.

Rankin, R. M.: Cleidocranial dysostosis, J. Oral Surg., 1:352, 1943.

Rendtorff, H. K.: Paget's disease with special reference to oral manifestations, U. S. Nav. M. Bull., 38:398, 1940.

Repass, F. G.: Cleidocranial dysostosis, Virginia Med. Monthly, 72:121, 1945.

Riesner, S. E.: Temporomandibular joint articulation: its consideration in orthodontic diagnosis, Internat. J. Orthodontia, 22:1, 1936.

Roberts, E., & I. Schour: Hereditary opalescent dentine, Am. J. Orthodontics, 25:267, 1939.

Rosedale, R. B.: Fibrocystic disease of the bones associated with tumor of a parathyroid gland, Am. J. Path., 8:745-51, 1932.

Rushton, M. A.: Studies of the teeth in a late case of osteogenesis imperfecta, J. Path. & Bact., 48:591, 1939.

Russell, L. A., & T. B. Bayles: Temporomandibular joint in rheumatoid arthritis, J. A. D. A., 28:537, 1941.

Salman, I.: Paget's disease (osteitis deformans) with case report involving the maxillary bones, Dental Cosmos, 72:137-40, 1930.

Schultz, L. W., & W. Shriner: Treatment for acute and chronic traumatic temporomandibular arthritis, New York J. Dent., 11:350, 1941.

Shambough, George E.: Involvement of the jaw joint in acute suppurative otitis media, Arch. Otolaryng., 33:975, 1941.

Sheets, C. E., Jr.: The temporomandibular joint, Mil. Surgeon, 88:529, 1941.

Siegel, M.: Osteitis deformans (Paget's disease), Canad. M. A. J., 44:482-84, 1941.

Sinclair, J. A.: Vitamin C deficiency—a factor in subluxation, pain in the temporomandibular area and other dental involvement, Dent. Items of Interest, 63:313, 1941.

Stafne, E. C., & L. T. Austin: Study of dental roentgenograms in cases of Paget's disease (osteitis deformans), osteitis fibrosa cystica and osteoma, J. A. D. A., 25:1202-14, 1938.

Strong, L. V.: Reflex effects of traumatic occlusion, J. Am. Osteopath. A., 42:415, 1942-43.

Thoma, K. H., et al.: An unusual case of hereditary fibrous osteodysplasia (fragilitas ossium) with replacement of dentine by osteocementum, Am. J. Orthodontics & Oral Surg., 29:1-30, 1943.

Thompson, John R.: Constancy of the position of the mandible and its influence on prosthetic restoration, Illinois Dent. J., 12:242, 1943.

Vaughn, H. C.: A study of the temporomandibular joint, Jour. Amer. Dent. Asso., 30:501, 1943.

Vorisek, E. A.: Hereditary craniofacial dysostosis, Amer. Jour. Ophthal., 24:1014, 1941.

Watson, E. M.: Treatment of Paget's disease by cortical preparations, Canad. Med. A. J., 41:561-66, 1939.

Williams, H. L., & E. M. Watson: Hyperphosphatasemia of Paget's disease, J. Lab. Clin. Med., 26:1333-37, 1941.

Willis, L. I.: Temporomandibular joint, U. S. Nav. M. Bull., 41:681, 1943.

Winter, Gordon R.: Dental conditions in cleidocranial dysostosis, Am. J. Orthodontics & Oral Surg., 29:61, 1943.

Wolff, E., & I. E. Nolan: Multiple myeloma first discovered in the mandible, Radiology, 42:76, 1944.

DISEASES OF THE MUSCLES, NERVES, AND NERVOUS SYSTEM

Adams, W. E., & W. Robinson: Trigeminal neuralgia, Lancet, 2:555, 1941.

Aisenberg, M. S., & T. C. Grubb: Poliomyelitis produced by inoculation of tooth pulp cavities, J. Dent. Research, 23:210, 1944.

Blais, J. A., E. Robillard, & H. Laugier: Measure of depth of anesthesia by study of linguo-maxillary reflex, Anesth. & Anal., 22:15, 1943.

Bulleid, A.: Dental sepsis and mental disease, Brit. Dent. J., 22:1211, 1930.

Cahn, L. R.: Traumatic (amputation) neuroma, Am. J. Orthodontics & Oral Surg., 25:190-93, 1939.

Carrea, J. U., & L. Samenico: Epileptiform convulsions considered as reflexes due to lesions of nervous system following faulty eruption of wisdom teeth, Rev. med. latino am., 14:1639-73, 1929.

Cobb, S., & W. J. Mixter: Lingual spasm associated with atypical trigeminal neuralgia, Ann. Surg., 101:49, 1935.

Coburn, D. F., & C. K. Shafstall: Glossopharyngeal neuralgia, Arch. Otolaryng., 33:663, 1941.

Cochran, G. W.: Infantile paralysis of dental origin, Dent. Rev., 30:368, 1916.

Coleman, Claude C.: Neurosurgical procedures for the relief of pain, West Virginia M. J., 39:365, 1943.

Connell, E. S., & B. C. Trowbridge: Cavernous sinus thrombophlebitis, J. Missouri State M. A., 38:320, 1941.

Cooper, M. J.: Associated movements of tongue in epidemic encephalitis controlled by voluntary effort, Arch. Neurol. & Psychiat., 33:148, 1935.

Costen, James B.: Diagnosis of mandibular joint neuralgia and its place in general head pain, Ann. Otolaryng., 53:656, 1944.

Curan, Morven: Cavernous sinus thrombophlebitis, J. Oral Surg., 2:7, 1944.

Douglas, C. M.: The teeth in relation to mental diseases, South. Med. & Surg., 105:531, 1943.

Drake, M. E., C. M. Gruber, & V. G. Haury: The effects of sodium diphenyl hydantinate on vitamin C level in tissues and vitamin excretion in rats, J. Pharm. & Exp. Therapeut., 71:268, 1941.

Ehni, George: Facial twitchings, Proc. Staff Meet. Mayo Clinic, 19:129, 1944.

Esterberg, H. L., & P. H. White: Sodium dilantin gingival hyperplasia, J. A. D. A., 32:16-25, 1945.

Frankel, S. I.: Dilantin sodium in treatment of epilepsy, J. A. M. A., 114: 1320, 1940.

Friedman, A. P., & C. W. Olsen: Paralysis of facial and masticatory nerves following arsenic poisoning, Bull. Los Angeles Neur. Soc., 6:85, 1941.

Glass, R. L.: Focal infection in teeth causing transverse myelitis, J. Mich. M. Soc., 25:187-8, 1926.

Glickman, I., & M. P. Lewitus: Hyperplasia of gingivae associated with dilantin (sodium diphenyl hydantoinate) therapy, J. A. D. A., 28:199, 1941.

Gruhzit, O. M.: Experimental production of gingival hyperplasia with dilantin, Arch. Path., 28:761, 1939.

Gruhzit, O. M.: Sodium diphenyl hydantoinate pharmacologic and histo-pathologic studies, Proc. Am. Soc. Exp. Pathol., Toronto, April 25-29, 1939.

Harris, W.: Trigeminal neuralgia at exceptionally early age; cured by Gasserian alcohol injection, Brit. M. J., 2:39, 1943.

Humphrey, J. H., & M. McClelland: Cranial nerve palsies with herpes following general anesthesia, Brit. M. J., 1:3-5, 1944.

Kimball, O. P.: Treatment of epilepsy with sodium diphenyl hydantoinate, J. A. M. A., 112:1244, 1939.

Klee, F. E.: Atypical neuralgia—the result of impacted teeth, Bull. of U. S. Army Med. Dept., 69:79, 1943.

Livingston, W. K.: Trigeminal neuralgia, treatment by novocain injection of the trigger zones, and a discussion of pain sources, Western J. Surg., 48:205, 1940.

Mallett, S. P., & C. B. Foley: Dilantin in epilepsy, Am. J. Orthodontics & Oral Surg., 27:634-36, 1941.

Martin, H., & G. L. Graves: Plexiform neurofibroma invading the oral cavity, J. A. M. A., 117:1535-39, 1941.

Merrit, H. H., & A. M. Foster: Vitamin C in epilepsy, dilantin sodium not a cause of vitamin C deficiency, Amer. J. M. Sc., 200:541, 1940.

Merwarth, H. R.: The occurrence of peripheral facial paralysis in hypertensive vascular disease, Ann. Int. Med., 17:298, 1942.

Merwarth, H. R.: Facial paralysis, N. Y. State J. Med., 44:1546, 1944.

McGovern, Francis H.: Paroxysmal lacrimation during eating following recovery from facial paralysis, Am. J. Ophth., 23:1388, 1940.

McKaig, C. B., & H. W. Woltman: Neurologic complications of epidemic parotitis; report of parotitic myelitis, Arch. Neurol. & Psychiat., 31:794-808, 1934.

Millhon, J. A., & A. E. Osterberg: Relationship between gingival hyperplasia and ascorbic acid in the blood and urine of epileptic patients undergoing treatment with sodium, 5-diphenyl hydantoinate, J. A. D. A., 29:207, 1942.

Nicol, A. A. McIntosh: A case of bilateral Bell's palsy, Brit. M. J., 1:220, 1942.

Queries and Minor Notes: Permanent facial paralysis following poliomyelitis, J. A. M. A., 107:900, 1936.

Robinson, Leon J.: The gingival changes produced by dilantin sodium, Dis. Nerv. System, 3:88, 1942.

Ross, Grady: Improper nerve impulses resulting from the pressure of impacted teeth, South. Med. & Surg., 105:204, 1943.

Sabin, A. B., & R. Ward: Natural history of human poliomyelitis; elimination of virus, J. Exper. Med., 74:519, 1941.

Shreiber, F.: Brain injuries following multiple extractions of teeth, Internat. J. of Orth. & Oral Surg., 17:183, 1931.

Sittig, O., & J. Urban: Case of poliomyelitis with bilateral paralysis of the masticatory muscles, Lancet, 1:865-6, 1939.

Sperber, I. J.: Dental deformities and mental hygiene, Psychiatric Quart., 4:444-6, 1930.

Spiegel, Leo A.: Syndrome of Garcin—unilateral total involvement of the cranial nerves with report of one case, Ann. Otol. Rhinol. & Laryng., 52:706, 1943.

Stern, Leo, et al.: Analysis of oral reactions to dilantin-sodium, J. Dent. Research, 22:157, 1943.

Sujoy, E., & H. Allemand: Blood groups in acute anterior poliomyelitis, Semana Medica, Buenos Aires, 51:476, 1944.

Thoma, K. H.: Dilantin hyperplasia of the gingivae, Am. J. Orthodontics & Oral Surg., 26:394, 1940.

Thomas, E. A., & J. Peters: Relation of dental disorders to nervous and mental disorders, Am. Dent. Surgeon, 47:711, 1927.

Thompson, R. F.: Focal infection and systemic disease, Southwestern Med., 15:198, 1931.

Tracy, E. A.: Teeth anomalies and epilepsy, Dental Cosmos, 69:410, 1927.

Vallotton, C. F.: Gingival hyperplasia associated with diphenylhydantoin therapy, Virginia M. Monthly, 71:159-61, 1944.

Ziskin, D. E., & E. V. Zegarelli: Dilantin hypertrophy, Arch. Neurol. & Psychiat., 46:897, 1941.

NUTRITIONAL DEFICIENCIES AND DISEASES OF METABOLISM

19

The Vitamins

GENERAL CONSIDERATIONS	VITAMIN D
VITAMIN A	VITAMIN E
VITAMIN B COMPLEX	VITAMIN K
VITAMIN C	VITAMIN P

GENERAL CONSIDERATIONS

The vitamins are one of the five essentials for adequate nutrition and health. As our knowledge increases concerning their chemical composition and physiologic action, their importance to the general body economy becomes better appreciated. Their effect on the activity of the endocrine glands opens up still wider fields.

We may have primary avitaminosis due to an inadequate intake of these substances or a secondary avitaminosis due to increased vitamin requirements (as in certain illnesses), impaired absorption, utilization or retention of these substances. Their administration in cases of known vitamin deficiencies is a potent and valuable therapeutic aid but their indiscriminate use by the public is to be condemned. In certain instances their indiscriminate administration may be even harmful.

Marked deficiencies of any one vitamin, such as C avitaminosis or scurvy, is rare in our nutritional and economic environment but subclinical or mild deficiencies are not uncommon. Due to their frequent occurrence and their less striking symptoms they are often unrecognized and undiagnosed for months or even years. As a group they are more important than the cases of frank deficiencies.

Since the oral cavity is the site where many of these mild nutritional deficiencies are first manifested clinically, the dentist has the unusual opportunity, and responsibility, of making an early diagnosis. This not only aids him in the treatment of the oral lesions which may be present but it also allows the correction of the nutritional deficiency by the physician at a time when less heroic measures may be required.

The rapid advances in the field of nutrition, particularly the vitamins, necessitate constant reference to the professional journals dealing with nutritional developments.

VITAMIN A

Vitamin A is a fat soluble, unsaturated alcohol which is formed in the liver from certain yellow plant pigments called the carotinoids ("provitamin A"). These compounds are fairly stable but when exposed to oxygen at high temperatures or to short wavelength light they undergo decomposition. Vitamin A has the following structural formula:

$$H_3C \quad CH_3$$
$$H_2C \diagdown C \diagup C-CH=CH-\underset{CH_3}{C}=CH-CH=CH-\underset{CH_3}{C}=CH-CH_2OH$$
$$H_2C \quad C$$
$$C$$
$$H_2$$

Vitamin A is necessary for the maintenance of the specialized epithelium of the mucous membranes and glands. In vitamin A deficiency the epithelium of the bladder, ureter and urinary pelves becomes hyperkeratotic while that of the respiratory tract and salivary glands is replaced by a stratified keratinized epithelium. Another function of vitamin A is to influence the structure of growing bone, perhaps through a limitation of the number and the degree of activity of the osteoblasts and osteoclasts. The liver is concerned with the metabolism of vitamin A and the normal blood concentration of this vitamin cannot be maintained unless there is an adequate storage of this substance in the liver. Patients with hypermotility of the small intestine have deficient absorption of this substance. Mineral oil dissolves the carotinoids but is not absorbed itself and when this substance is used regularly as a laxative, deficient A absorption may take place.

Vitamin A is necessary for the synthesis of the visual purple of the retina after exposure to light, the rate of synthesis depending on the vitamin A supply. This fact serves as the basis for a clinical test for A deficiency.

The biophotometer, or more properly the adaptometer, is an instrument which is used clinically to determine the state of A nutrition. This test measures only the efficiency of the visual cycle and more accurate estimates of A nutrition are obtained by determining the amount of this substance in the blood. The normal blood range is 88 to 100 I.U./100 cc. blood.

The average daily adult requirements are estimated to be about 6,000 I.U. Therapeutic doses of over 3,000,000 I.U. have been administered but the usual therapeutic dose is around 40,000 I.U. per day. Intensive therapy is often required for therapeutic results.

Systemic Aspects

Xerophthalmia. Severe deficiencies of this vitamin result in corneal ulceration and necrosis and lack of secretion of the lacrimal glands. This is associated with a conjunctivitis and redness of the eyelids. This clinical picture is recognized as xerophthalmia. Frank A deficiency cases are rare in the U. S. In the case reported by Thorson the patient had bady infected teeth and gums. Several whitish plaques were present on the inner surface of the lower lip. Failure to receive proper treatment in the early stages of the disease may result in permanent loss of sight.

Chronic A Deficiency. Less severe vitamin A deficiencies, arising as a result of insufficient intake or utilization of this vitamin, are more common. Mass nutrition surveys show that about $\frac{2}{3}$ of the people in the lower income groups are not receiving enough vitamin A to assure normal dark adaptation.

Night blindness is one of the earliest and often unrecognized symptoms of chronic A deficiency. This delay in the visual cycle is believed to account in part for the increase in automobile accidents after dark. Itching, burning of the eyes and photophobia are also present.

Characteristic skin and mucosal changes are also observed. The skin becomes dry and rough and at times assumes the appearance of true ichthyosis. Keratosis of the hair follicles is common. The mucosal changes are characterized by an increased keratinization of the epithelium and a metaplasia of highly specialized types of epithelium, such as the ciliated columnar cells lining the respiratory passages, to a transitional form. It has also been suggested that the keratinized epithelium of the urinary tract forms the basis for the increased urinary calculi which are found in cases of vitamin A deficiency.

Vitamin A has received considerable lay publicity as the "anti-infection" vitamin, particularly in respect to the common cold. Careful clinical studies have failed to fulfill the claims of the advertisers. Metaplasia of specialized mucosal tissues may lessen their ability to cope with infectious agents, but in the average population groups studied the supplemental administration of vitamin A did not lessen the incidence or the severity of the common cold.

Oral Aspects

Mellanby and King reported that puppies fed a vitamin A deficient diet developed hyperplasia of the gums, gingivitis and pyorrhea. Abnormalities in calcification of the dentin and enamel were also seen. Arnim showed that experimental A deficiencies in rats result in severe alterations in dental development with a loss of the normal pigmentation of the enamel and the normal strength of the teeth. Severe A deficiencies maintained in rats for long periods of time resulted in tumor-like masses which have many similarities to the human ameloblastoma. The part that infection may play in the production of these growths has not been fully determined.

Vitamin A is important for normal growth and development of children. In hypovitaminosis A enamel formation ceases and the odontoblasts lose their specialized function of forming dentin and they revert to the formation of an osteoid tissue. As a result, striking deformaties are observed in the teeth of the animals who are on the experimental diet. Gordon believed that the lack of adequate vitamin A during this growth period may prove a leading cause of dental difficulties. Bessey and Wolbach went so far as to say that the deficiency of this vitamin during the formative period of the teeth "outranks in the human being all other vitamin deficiencies in importance." Boyle described enamel hypoplasia and disturbed amelogenesis in the human dental structures in vitamin A deficiency.

In the dental tissues of the adult patient there is little evidence that the lack of this vitamin will result in any abnormalities of the teeth or supporting structures. Its importance during the tooth formative period is not denied. Because of the tendency for hyperkeratinization to develop in chronic vitamin A deficiency, it has been suggested that the lack of this vitamin may be an important factor in the causation of leukoplakia. Whatever its importance might be in this respect, the therapeutic use of vitamin A in the treatment of oral leukoplakia has not been encouraging.

Deficiencies of vitamin A are treated by the administration of therapeutic doses of this substance. Extremely high dosage is required at times to effect a therapeutic response.

THE VITAMIN B COMPLEX

The vitamin B complex is composed of at least 12 separate factors; the exact chemical structure and physiologic function of some of these is yet undetermined. The various factors of the B complex are soluble in water, although their degree of solubility varies widely.

The systemic and oral manifestations associated with a deficient intake or utilization of the members of the B complex are varied and symptoms due to a lack of any single factor are uncommon. Thiamin, riboflavin and nicotinic acid are all concerned with cellular respiration and nutrition. They function in part as activators which are being continually regenerated, but they also function as parts of enzyme systems which are used up and require replacement.

In clinical practice it is difficult to identify the lesions which result from a deficiency of only one of the fractions of the B complex, as deficiencies are usually multiple. The generally recognized constituents of the B complex are:

B COMPLEX

	Recommended Daily Intake
Thiamin (B₁)	1.2— 2.3 mg.
Riboflavin (B₂)	2.5— 3.3 mg.
Nicotinic acid (niacin), P-P pellagra preventive factor	15.0—20.0 mg.
Pyridoxine (B₆)	
Pantothenic acid	
Choline	
Folic acid	
Biotin	
Inositol	
Para-aminobenzoic acid	
Other factors	

There is some relation between the development of carcinoma and liver cirrhosis in animals and certain members of the B complex. Certain toxic reactions of the sulfa drugs, including agranulocytosis, probably result from interference with certain components of the B complex.

Thiamin (B₁)

Thiamin has been isolated in crystalline form. The crystalline form and its acid solutions are fairly resistant to oxidation and heat but in neutral or alkaline solutions it is unstable. Thiamin hydrochloride has the following structural formula:

$$
\begin{array}{c}
CH_3 \\
\end{array}
$$

N=C—NH₂·HCl   C====C—CH₂CH₂OH

H₂C—C C—CH₂——N

N—CH   Cl CH——S

Water-soluble
$C_{12}H_{17}N_4OSCl \cdot HCl$ (the hydrochloride)

Thiamin acts as a coenzyme in carbohydrate metabolism, having as its function the oxidation of pyruvic acid. Lack of appreciable gastric acidity and disturbances in intestinal function prevent adequate absorption of thiamin, although sufficient amounts are ingested. Because of its importance in carbohydrate metabolism, it can be readily appreciated that an increased carbohydrate intake will markedly increase the thiamin requirements of an individual.

Unusually rich sources of thiamin include peas, beans, oatmeal, lean pork and peanuts although all the vegetables and fruits contain small amounts of this substance. Breakfast cereals, bread and even candy bars are now "enriched" with thiamin. The daily recommended intake is 1.5 to 2.3 mg., with increasing requirements in fevers, hyperthyroidism or any condition resulting in increased metabolism.

Systemic Aspects. Beri-beri results from a frank deficiency of thiamin. A dry beri-beri in which multiple neuritis is the predominating feature, a wet beri-beri in which there are edema and serous effusion without heart failure, and a cardiac type with circulatory failure have been described. Beri-beri is uncommon in the U. S. The above symptoms respond to intravenous, intramuscular and at times oral administration of thiamin along with other factors of the B complex, if irreversible changes in the involved structures and organs have not taken place. It is not considered good therapy to administer large amounts of any one factor of the B complex without supplying the other factors. Cases of sensitivity to thiamin have been reported.

Chronic thiamin deficiencies result in unco-operative, quarrelsome and even fearful individuals who are easily fatigued. This is why thiamin has been dubbed the "morale vitamin." Other complaints in chronic thiamin deficiency consist of loss of appetite, sensitiveness to noise and pain, headache, backache, painful menses and epigastric burning after meals. Lowered blood pressures (85 to 100 mm. systolic) are common.

Thiamin chloride is useful in stimulating the appetite of invalids and convalescent patients and in preventing certain types of anorexia. Thiamin chloride will lessen the "roentgen sickness" which may follow radiation therapy. It has also been used in the treatment of the vomiting of pregnancy. The neuritis associated with chronic alcoholism and at times pellagra are benefited by thiamin administration. It has been used with success in the treatment of herpes zoster and acrodynia. Varying clinical results have been

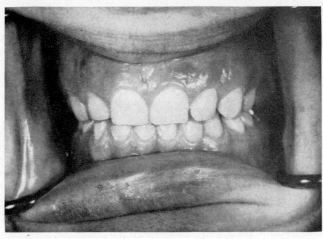

FIG. 195. Gingiva in a patient with thiamin deficiency. The tissues are rose-pink in color, satiny in appearance and they are slightly edematous.

experienced in the treatment of multiple sclerosis, Menière's syndrome and paralysis agitans.

Oral Aspects. Patients with thiamin deficiency will rarely seek dental advice first as the oral lesions and symptoms associated with this deficiency are not sufficiently prominent or serious to require consultation with the dentist. A preliminary study reported by Arvin shows that patients with thiamin deficiency have an increased sensitivity of the teeth and oral mucosa. Simple dental procedures such as scaling and polishing the teeth or taking bite-wing films produced a markedly painful response.

The tongue in thiamin deficiency appears flabby, enlarged and edematous and lacks normal muscle tone. It is not particularly painful. The lateral margins have indentations correponding with the lingual contours of the teeth. The fungiform papillae are enlarged, edematous and hyperemic. Oral mucosal and lingual changes, more clearly associated with other factors of the B complex, are usually present in cases of thiamin deficiency.

The author with Hickman used the B complex, particularly thiamin chloride, in the treatment of herpes simplex, oral aphthae and aphthous stomatitis. In many individuals, recurrent lesions of herpes were controlled by dietary regulation or the supplemental intake of the B complex or thiamin chloride alone. Patients who are prone to develop herpetic lesions following dental treatment were also benefited. (See Herpes Simplex.)

Borsook *et al.* reported the successful use of massive doses of thiamin in the treatment of tic douloureux. There is some doubt whether its use is justified in the treatment of this condition. At times large doses of thiamin chloride (parenterally) will relieve atypical neuralgic pains of the face and jaw region. Whitefield and others claimed that thiamin inserted in the alveolus following the extraction of teeth minimized the chances of dry socket.

Riboflavin (B_2)

Riboflavin has been isolated in crystalline form. Aqueous solutions exhibit the yellow-green fluorescence characteristic of all flavines. This substance is heat stable especially in acid solutions but it is readily decomposed on exposure to light. Riboflavin has the following structural formula:

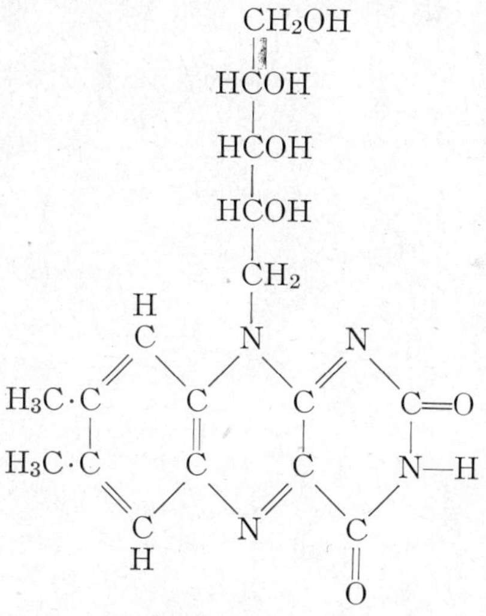

$$CH_2OH$$
$$HCOH$$
$$HCOH$$
$$HCOH$$
$$CH_2$$

$$C_{17}H_{20}N_4O_6$$

Several of the tissue oxidation enzymes are known to contain riboflavin and it is believed to play some rôle in tissue respiration as in experimental deficiencies there is a diminution of the enzymes concerned with cellular respiration.

Milk, liver and vegetables in general are good sources of riboflavin but this substance is widely distributed in animal and plant tissues. The Food and Nutrition Board recommends a daily intake of 2.2 to 3.3 mg. of riboflavin.

Systemic Aspects. The clinical symptoms associated with riboflavin deficiency may be related to the eyes, the skin and the oral structures. Burning and itching of the eyes, ready eye fatigue, diminution in vision and photophobia are important ocular symptoms. Vascularization of the cornea can be seen clinically in advanced cases and slit-lamp examination of the cornea will detect the early corneal changes associated with riboflavin deficiency.

A non-specific dermatitis is frequently present. The earliest dermal changes are noted in the nares, the nasomalar folds, within the helix of the ear and posterior to this structure. They consist of a scaly, greasy desquamation which develops usually on an erythematous base. These dermal changes and the angular cheilosis (see Oral Aspects) may be the first indication of riboflavin deficiency.

Oral Aspects. Angular cheilosis and tongue lesions are early symptoms of ariboflavinosis. Cheilosis was an early and a prominent symptom in the

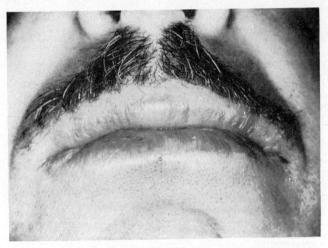

FIG. 196. Desquamation of the vermilion border of the lip and angular cheilosis in a patient with mild vitamin B complex deficiency.

experimental human ariboflavinosis produced by Sebrell and Butler. Ten of the 18 subjects developed these lesions after they had been on a riboflavin deficient diet for 94 to 130 days.

Angular cheilosis and the scaly desquamations are also prominent symptoms of the naturally occurring disease. Cheilosis and inflammation of the borders of the lips were first described by Sebrell and Butler in 1938 as being due to riboflavin deficiency. Machella called attention to the fact that the angular cheilosis may be due to a deficiency of other fractions of the vitamin B complex such as pyridoxine hydrochloride. Such lesions had been known to occur frequently in pellagrins but their etiology had not been determined. The contact area of the lips is intensely reddened, encrusted and bleeds readily when traumatized. In severe cases the entire oral mucosa has a peculiar opalescent sheen.

The characteristic angular cheilosis of hyporiboflavinosis consists of bilateral lesions which extend a few millimeters from the angles of the mouth on the cheek mucosa and laterally on the circumoral skin for 1 to 10 mm.

The base of these lesions or cracks has a moist macerated appearance. In severe cases similar lesions are found on the nasolabial junction. Vertical fissuring of the vermilion border of the lips and the adjacent skin tissues are also observed.

The angular cheilosis associated with hyporiboflavinosis is probably identical with the perlèche lesions which were supposedly due to a specific bac-

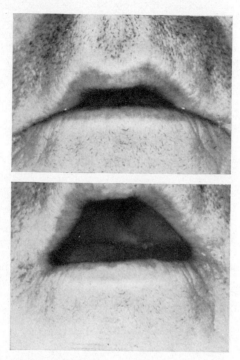

FIG. 197. Pseudocheilosis due to a shortening of the normal intermaxillary space. These lesions do not extend onto the cheek mucosa and they tend to slant downward. (See Color Atlas for angular cheilosis.)

terial infection. Perlèche occurred predominantly in malnourished children and debilitated adults. The angular cheilosis of riboflavin deficiency will show either pure or nearly pure cultures of hemolytic staphylococci in 80% of the cases and beta streptococci in the remaining 20% of the cases. The bacteria represent secondary involvement.

A glossitis is a common symptom of ariboflavinosis. The tongue is a magenta or purplish-red color. The fungiform papillae are prominent, edematous and mushroom-shaped, giving a peculiar granular appearance to the dorsum of the tongue. There may be an accompanying burning sensation or a mild irritation.

Pseudocheilosis. The true angular cheilosis associated with riboflavin deficiency must be differentiated from the "pseudocheilosis" which is related to altered dentofacial relations which result from a decreased intermaxillary space. The angular cheilosis of some patients with ariboflavinosis fails to regress completely until the intermaxillary space is restored by the insertion of artificial dentures. Ellenberg and Pollack reported a group of patients with perlèche-like lesions (angular cheilosis) which had a superficial resemblance to the lesions in riboflavin deficiency who in addition complained of a smooth, burning tongue. The lip lesions were deeply fissured and granulomatous and exhibited spontaneous remissions and exacerbations. Thirty-two of the 34 cases in this study had artificial full dentures.

These lesions were apparently the result of a decreased intermaxillary space, which permitted the upper lip to overlap the lower one, producing a fold at the corners of the mouth. Moisture from retained saliva in this fold in association with bacterial and mechanical irritation gave rise to the lesions. They disappeared when dentures were inserted which restored the intermaxillary space.

Aside from differences in the appearance of the "cheilosis" due to decreased intermaxillary space, which have been described, the author has observed that the lesions resulting from reduced intermaxillary space slant downward as well as outward from the corners of the mouth whereas the angular cheilosis associated with ariboflavinosis is more horizontal.

Treatment. The symptoms of ariboflavinosis are treated by the administration of this substance which should be given in conjunction with the other members of the B complex. Parenteral or intravenous therapy is indicated in severe cases or when there is impaired absorptive function of the small intestine.

Nicotinic Acid

Nicotinic acid has been isolated in the form of white needle-like crystals. The crystalline substance and solutions of nicotinic acid are generally stable. Because of the common and incorrect association of nicotinic acid or its amide with the alkaloid nicotine, the terms niacin and niacinamide have been suggested for lay use instead of nicotinic acid and nicotinamide. These compounds have the following structural formula:

$$C_5H_4NCOOH$$

Nicotinic acid is a component of the tissue enzymes which are concerned with glycogen utilization and cellular respiration. Experimental nicotinic acid deficiencies result in oral lesions of interest to the dentist. As early as 1922

Goldberger stated that canine black tongue (not analogous to human black tongue) was the canine counterpart of human pellagra. Animals on nicotinic

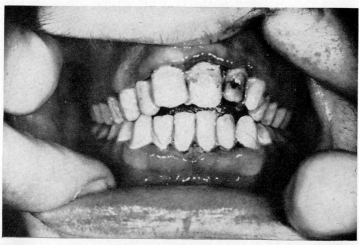

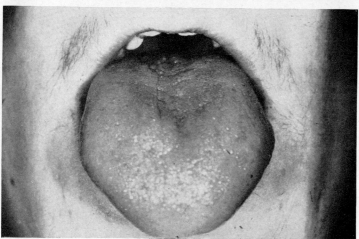

FIG. 198 (*Top*). Fusospirochetal gingivostomatitis secondary to nutritional deficiency (aniacinosis). The gingivostomatitis was unsuccessfully treated by topical medicaments for one month. Response to nicotinamide therapy was prompt and satisfactory.

FIG. 199 (*Bottom*). Early tongue changes in nicotinic acid deficiency. Same patient as in Fig. 198.

acid deficient diets developed frequently gingival and oral mucosal lesions having clinical and bacteriologic similarities to human oral fusospirochetal infection.

Lean meats, liver, potatoes and vegetables are good sources of nicotinic acid. Corn meal and corn products are poor sources of nicotinic acid, which accounts in part for the prevalence of pellagra among the poorer southern population. The Food and Nutrition Board has suggested a daily intake of nicotinic acid (or amide) of 15 to 20 mg.

Systemic Aspects. The pellagrous symptom complex results from a marked deficiency of intake or utilization of nicotinic acid. The typical symptoms include progressive weakness, lassitude, anorexia, diarrhea and the characteristic red, scaly dermatosis of the exposed body parts, particularly the glove and stocking areas. The oral manifestations of pellagra are many

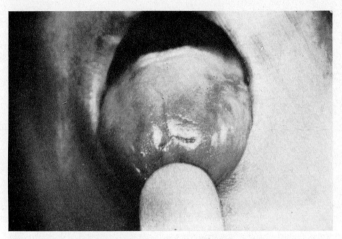

Fig. 200. Atrophic glossitis in a patient with frank nicotinic acid deficiency (pellagra).

times the first and outstanding symptom of the disease. They will be discussed under the oral aspects of nicotinic acid deficiency. One or more of the characteristic pellagrous symptoms may be lacking and in some reported epidemics, a severe glossitis has represented the chief clinical finding.

Pellagra is essentially a disease of the Southern states where it occurs most frequently in individuals subsisting largely on corn products. Milder forms of the disease are being recognized in greater frequency in the Northern states. The best treatment consists of nicotinic acid therapy in conjunction with other factors of the B complex.

The Flushing Reaction. Nicotinic acid has a marked vasodilatory action when taken in sufficient amounts. A sensation of flushing, itching and burning of the skin, particularly of the neck, ears, lips and pharynx, is at times experienced. This reaction does not necessarily indicate that the individual's tissues are saturated with nicotinic acid. The "flushing reaction" is not serious but it may be alarming to the patient. For this reason the amide, which is practically devoid of this side action, is used therapeutically. Because of this vasodilatory effect nicotinic acid has been used in the treatment of anginal attacks with apparent benefit.

Oral Aspects. The early appearance and the severity of the oral manifestations associated with nicotinic acid deficiency may cause these patients to seek dental advice first. It is the dentist's responsibility to recognize the nutri-

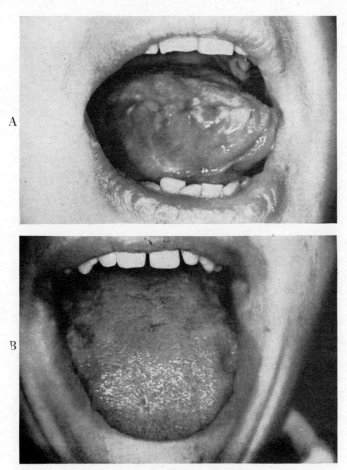

Fig. 201. (A) Tongue and lip changes in a patient with B-complex deficiency of nine years' duration. Note the shallow ulcerated areas on the right lateral margin of the tongue. (B) Same patient three months later following intensive parenteral vitamin therapy and general nutritional support.

tional background of the oral lesions and to see that the patient receives the proper treatment.

The acute glossitis and stomatitis which are associated with nicotinic acid deficiency are intensely painful. They give rise to characteristic changes which are not easily overlooked. The tongue is devoid of papillae, it is painful and it has a fiery red color. Shallow ulcerations on the dorsum and along the margins of this structure, where it is in contact with the teeth, are commonly observed. All stages of developing and healing ulcers can be seen on the tongue and oral mucosa. Pellagrous epidemics in which the lesions have been confined to the tongue have been reported in Palestine and India. The clinical appearance of these shallow ulcerations simulates primary fusospirochetal lesions with the exception that the latter occur rarely on the tongue. The bacteriologic smear findings are typical of a fusospirochetal infection. The ingestion of hot, highly spiced or acid substances is acutely painful.

The lips are inflamed. They have numerous deep encrusted cracks along the vermilion border. Cheilosis is frequently observed in cases of pellagra.

NICOTINIC ACID AND VINCENT'S INFECTION. King reported in 1940 the satisfactory treatment of Vincent's infection in England with the internal administration of nicotinic acid. Attempts to treat fusospirochetal infection in the United States by a similar form of treatment have been discouraging, if not entirely unsatisfactory. Miller et al. found no beneficial results following the administration of 1,000 mg. of nicotinic acid per day. Similar results were experienced by the author from controlled clinical studies where the effectiveness of nicotinic acid 1,000 mg. per day was compared with various topical medicaments in the treatment of acute fusospirochetal stomatitis. Not one of the 15 cases was benefited by the nicotinic acid administration. It is possible that the lesions King and Spies treated and those occurring in Palestine were pellagrous oral mucosal ulcerations which had become secondarily infected with fusospirochetal organisms. Such lesions, due primarily to a nutritional deficiency, would respond promptly to nicotinic acid therapy while those treated by Miller and us were not due primarily to a nutritional deficiency and hence were not benefited by this form of treatment.

Grossman and Schwartzman studied carefully the effectiveness of various topical medicaments as compared with nicotinic acid therapy in the treatment of Vincent's infection in infants and young children. Nicotinic acid was superior to all other forms of treatment. It is difficult to reconcile their results with those observed in adults unless their criteria of Vincent's infection differed from Miller's and ours or unless Vincent's infection in the young child is chiefly secondary to a nutritional deficiency.

More recently Goldberg and Thorp studied the nicotinic acid excretion, a measure of nicotinic acid sufficiency, in a control group of patients and those having acute Vincent's infection. Since no significant differences were found in the nicotinic acid excretion of the 2 groups, it seems unlikely that Vincent's infection is primarily a manifestation of nicotinic acid deficiency.

NICOTINIC ACID AND BLOOD COAGULATION. Calder and Kerby noted the favorable effect of nicotinic acid therapy on blood coagulation when applied topically or administered internally. They found that a 0.6% soluton of nicotinic acid applied to the tooth socket with cotton pledgets produced a firm clot in a few minutes whereas untreated sockets bled for several hours. In other cases, the oral administration of 100 mg. of this substance t.i.d. reduced the clotting time from over 24 hours to 6 minutes. Nicotinic acid acted *in vitro* by neutralizing the antithrombin. Its effectiveness in controlling dental hemorrhage, other than that associated with hemophilia and some of the other blood dyscrasias, has not been sufficiently appreciated by the dentist.

The effect of nicotinic acid on blood coagulation, when used both internally and locally in powdered form, is striking. This combined medication permitted the office treatment of a patient who had required hospitalization on 2 previous occasions for blood transfusions following extractions. The oral administration of 200 mg. nicotinamide a day for 2 days prior to extraction and the packing of equal parts of powdered nicotinic acid and sulfathiazole in the sockets resulted in prompt clot formation with no postoperative bleeding or complications. Repeated extractions were performed on this patient using this treatment with satisfactory results.

Xerostomia, or dry mouth, not due primarily to atrophy of the salivary glands, responds frequently to the administration of 100 mg. of nicotinic acid or its amide per day for several weeks. The restored salivary flow has a soothing effect on the oral mucosa which is usually inflamed. Adams & Robinson found that nicotinic acid gave complete relief in some cases of trigeminal neuralgia and every case receiving this form of treatment improved. Doses up to 75 mg. nicotinic acid 4 times daily were used. This form of therapy for the treatment of trigeminal neuralgia has not been widely used.

Choline

Choline, now considered a member of the B complex, is concerned in some way with the mobilization of fatty acids in the body. In experimental deficiencies, it is associated with fatty degeneration of the liver.

Biotin

Biotin, another member of the B complex, has been assigned the empirical formula of $C_{10}H_{16}O_3N_2S$. Its presence in small quantities is necessary for the growth of micro-organisms. Its significance in nutrition has been appreciated only recently. Its deficiency produces the so-called egg white injury in rats.

Para-aminobenzoic Acid

Para-aminobenzoic acid, also a member of the B complex, exhibits vitamin-like properties. Its exact rôle in human nutrition is not known. Early studies suggest that it may be related to the formation of hair pigment. Another interesting action of this substance is its inhibitory effect on the sulfonamides. Culture media, which are used for making bacteriologic studies on patients receiving sulfonamide therapy, should contain 0.1% para-aminobenzoic acid to neutralize any bacteriostatic effect of the sulfonamides.

Pyridoxine (B₆)

Pyridoxine (B_6) is a white crystalline water-soluble substance. Its exact physiologic properties are not known, but it is probably associated with the tissue enzyme systems. Cereals, especially rice, legumes and milk, are good sources of pyridoxine. The human daily requirement has been estimated to be about 2 mg. Experimental pyridoxine deficiencies have resulted in oral lesions.

A wide variety of clinical conditions such as paralysis agitans, cheilosis and muscular dystrophies have been treated with this substance. The results reported in paralysis agitans have been contradictory, but some of the cases of angular cheilosis which fail to respond satisfactorily to riboflavin administration have been benefited by the addition of this substance. Cantor and Scott found that pyridoxine hydrochloride is effective in the treatment of agranulocytic angina.

Pantothenic Acid

Pantothenic acid is a white crystalline substance whose exact function in human physiology is not known, but experimental and clinical studies suggest that it is related in some manner with changes in hair pigmentation. Pantothenic acid has received considerable publicity in the lay press as the "anti-gray hair vitamin." While it is concerned with hair pigmentation, it does not yet justify this title.

Kniesner, Mann and Spies studied the relationship of dental caries to deficiencies of the B complex in 51 patients. Forty-one patients with clinical deficiency disease averaged 2.1 cavities while 10 patients without clinical symptoms of dietary deficiency averaged 6.1 cavities. Salivary pantothenic acid values varied from 0.012 to 0.19 micrograms per cc. saliva. No significant differences were found in the pantothenic acid content of the saliva from caries-resistant or caries-susceptible patients. No conclusions were reached as to any relationship between dental decay and the salivary pantothenic acid levels.

Folic Acid

Folic acid, one of the fractions of the B complex, has been found to have an important rôle in blood cell production. The lack of this substance in the diet of monkeys results in agranulocytosis. It cured both the anemia and agranulocytosis which were induced in white rats by means of the sulfonamides. Reports of its clinical use have not appeared.

VITAMIN C (ASCORBIC ACID)

For almost 200 years it has been known that certain foodstuffs, such as the citrus fruits, would protect man against scurvy. Scurvy was particularly serious on sailing vessels where fresh foods could not be obtained for long periods. This disease was effectively controlled in the British Navy in 1804 by a regulation which required each sailor to use 1 ounce of lemon juice a day.

The actual vitamin, ascorbic acid, was isolated in 1932 and synthesized a year later. Ascorbic acid is a water-soluble, white, crystalline substance which is a powerful reducing agent. It is fairly heat stable, especially in acid solutions, but it is rapidly destroyed by alkalis, prolonged heating and exposure to light and air.

Ascorbic acid has the following structural formula:

$$O{=}C{\longrightarrow}$$
$$HO{-}C$$
$$HO{-}C \qquad O$$
$$H{-}C{\longrightarrow}$$
$$HO{-}CH$$
$$CH_2OH$$
$$C_6H_8O_6$$

Vitamin C is important in the development of collagen which is the main constituent of connective tissue and the organic matrix of bone. It also plays a rôle in capillary permeability. A diet deficient in vitamin C may lead to failure of the intercellular substance to keep intact the capillary walls or the collagenous fibres enmeshing the endothelium of the capillaries. This vitamin has also been used in animal husbandry where it has been shown that it will restore the fertilizing capacity of bulls.

Fresh vegetables, such as cabbage, cauliflower, tomatoes and citrus fruits, are the best natural sources of this vitamin. The actual vitamin C nutritional value of any food varies considerably, depending on the method of storage, the aging of the food and its manner of preparation for consumption. There is little vitamin C lost in the usual cooking procedures, provided the cooking water is served with the food.

The recommended daily intake for adults is 75 mg. and the usual therapeutic dose for adults is 100 to 300 mg. per day. Large amounts may be given without ill effects, as the excess ascorbic acid is eliminated by the kidneys. This forms the basis of the "saturation test" for vitamin C in the tissues. In spite of our dietary habits the vitamin C intake of our diet is frequently inadequate. The synthetic substance can be administered by the oral, intramuscular or intravenous routes.

Systemic Aspects—Scurvy

Frank vitamin C deficiency results in scurvy or scorbutus. This disease is uncommon in the United States where adequate amounts of C-containing foods are available but it may develop in persons on special diets, those in the lowest economic group and occasionally in artificially fed infants who are not given supplemental vitamin C.

The characteristic symptoms of scurvy include the oral lesions (see Oral Aspect), weakness, easy fatigability, hemorrhages in the skin, muscles, joints and in the oral and intestinal mucosae. When hemorrhages occur in the joints (hemarthrosis), arthritic symptoms are manifested. Large ecchymotic areas are frequently seen on the lower extremities and on the back. Subperiosteal hemorrhages are a characteristic finding and one which can be demonstrated by the roentgenogram even in young children.

All the symptoms of scurvy regress following the administration of vitamin C. In some patients the clinical response to ascorbic acid is less rapid and complete than when natural sources of vitamin C are used.

Differences of opinion exist concerning the clinical entity of subclinical C deficiency and its possible symptoms. Numerous small petechiae which develop about the hair follicles of the lower extremities are one of the earliest signs of C deficiency. Soreness in the legs is frequently experienced.

It is generally agreed that supplemental C is required in many conditions in which it is of definite therapeutic value. Any condition which results in increased metabolism such as hyperthyroidism, pregnancy, and lactation benefits from vitamin C administration. Certain infectious diseases such as tuberculosis, whooping cough, pneumonia, and particularly diphtheria require additional amounts of vitamin C to maintain normal concentrations in the blood and tissues. There is a lowered resistance to infections in general before the clinical onset of scurvy.

Experimental and clinical studies have shown that vitamin C will protect the individual against intolerance to certain drugs such as neo-arsphenamine and mapharsen. Vitamin C will also prevent or lessen the toxic effects of lead poisoning. It is effective in the prevention and treatment of heat cramps and prostration in industrial and military service. Adequate vitamin C is important for normal wound healing. This is particularly true in gastric ulcer patients who may not tolerate foods containing large amounts of vitamin C. Delayed wound healing can be largely prevented by saturation of the blood and tissues with this substance. All surgical patients should receive supplemental vitamin C.

Oral Aspects

The gingival and oral lesions associated with scurvy have been known for many years. They are not manifested before the eruption of the teeth. The gums are hypertrophied, spongy and bluish-red in color. They are sore and bleed on the slightest pressure. The connective tissue fibres of the alveolo-dental periosteum are also affected. The teeth become loose and in severe cases they are exfoliated. Secondary infection of the gums with fusospirochetal organisms develops commonly. This, with the gingival hemorrhage, gives rise to a particularly foul mouth odor. Submucosal hemorrhages may be a conspicuous finding.

In subclinical vitamin C deficiency such striking oral changes are not seen. Hirschfeld called attention to an old rose color of the gums as the first oral symptom. A chronic gingivitis or bleeding gums which does not respond to prophylactic treatment and proper oral hygiene at home should suggest the possibility of subclinical vitamin C deficiency or some other nutritional deficiency. Kent found that the lack of an accompanying cervical adenitis in early cases of gingivitis was an important diagnostic finding in hypovitaminosis C.

There is experimental evidence demonstrating the importance of this vitamin during odontogenesis and for the maintenance of the attachment apparatus after tooth eruption. The exact importance of vitamin C to dental health in man is still not fully understood. Many of the experimental animal studies have not been corroborated by clinical experience. The problem is further complicated by the fact that natural sources of vitamin C were used in some of the studies and ascorbic acid in others.

The changes in the dental tissues of guinea pigs were of considerable biologic significance during the early studies on vitamin C. Structural and functional defects of the odontoblasts with the production of an osteoid tissue instead of tubular dentin furnished one of the better methods for the bioassay of this vitamin. Pulpal hemorrhages in the region of the odontoblasts were also a common finding. In severe deficiencies, the ameloblasts became functionally impaired or disappeared. These changes gave rise to enamel defects in the erupted teeth of the experimental animals. Boyle produced lesions in the attachment apparatus and gums of guinea pigs by means of a chronic C deficient diet which were comparable to those seen in certain forms of periodontal disease in man. The author noted changes in the dental pulps of specimens obtained from human necropsies which were similar to those observed in the teeth of scorbutic guinea pigs. The pulpal hemorrhages were marked at the base of the odontoblastic layer. An analysis of these case histories revealed that in every instance the individuals had succumbed to lobar pneumonia.

Clinical studies have been inconclusive, if not contradictory, as to the rôle of vitamin C on the teeth and supporting structures (except in scurvy). Crandon *et al.* were the subjects for the first experimental studies on scurvy in humans. Their teeth and gums did not show any significant changes until long after general symptoms of scurvy appeared and extremely low levels of blood ascorbic acid had been reached. At the end of the 6th month of the experiment, when clinical scurvy had been present for 3 months, the gums were only slightly boggy on pressure. A gingival biopsy taken at this time failed to show any of the changes which are associated with vitamin C deficiency. The dental roentgenograms showed occasional discontinuities of the *lamina dura*. From these studies they concluded, contrary to past opinion, that oral symptoms develop late in scurvy. The good oral hygiene of these experimenters may account for the delay in the development of the dental symptoms and for their mild nature.

Hanke *et al.* studied 500 private patients and 340 institutionalized children to determine the protective effect of vitamin C (as found in orange and lemon juice) on the dental structures. Eight ounces of orange juice and the juice of ½ lemon were prescribed once or twice daily. Certain types of gingivitis often disappeared after 30 to 90 days of this regime. They concluded that "orange and lemon juice contain something antagonistic to gingivitis, that this something might be vitamin C. . . . We have never proved that the active agent is vitamin C, and we do not claim it is." Familiarity with Hanke's conclusions would have eliminated much of the criticism of his studies.

Mead later called attention to the beneficial effect of the citrus fruits on the health of the periodontal tissues. Kruse's biomicroscopic studies demonstrated that the health of the gums formed a satisfactory basis for determining the vitamin C status of an individual although at any given time the blood ascorbic acid levels and the gingival findings may not be in agreement. Slobody observed a close correlation between the subcutaneous vitamin C test perfected by him, the degree of vitamin C saturation of the tissues and the condition of the gums. He also called attention to the discrepancy between the blood plasma ascorbic acid level and the condition of the gums as determined by the subcutaneous vitamin C test, biomicroscopic and clinical examinations.

Other studies have minimized the importance of vitamin C other than that required for good nutrition, for the health of the gingival and periodontal diseases. Radusch found that a vitamin C intake above the daily recommended requirement was not associated with any diminution in the amount or degree of periodontal disease. Burrill accounted for the frequent finding of a suboptimal level of vitamin C in patients with periodontal disease, by suggesting that the factors which might contribute to periodontal disease were similar to those which might also contribute to a faulty diet.

The findings of Howe, Radusch, Burrill and others are not actually contradictory to those reported by Hanke and coworkers. Most of the more recent reports have been concerned with the importance of vitamin C as ascorbic acid, while Hanke studied the effect of the citrus fruit juices in the treatment of gingival and periodontal lesions. It is now known that the natural fruit juices contain other factors beside vitamin C, such as citrin, which might have an important action on the periodontal tissues.

The final judgment as to the therapeutic value of an intake of vitamin C, above the normal optimum, in the treatment of the common oral lesions, cannot be made at this time. An increased vitamin C intake will produce a desirable therapeutic response if the patient has some absorptive defect which did not permit adequate tissue utilization on a normal intake. In such a case the increased vitamin C intake compensated for faulty absorptive function. It has not been shown that vitamin C administration above that which is required for tissue saturation, produces any beneficial action on the gums or periodontal tissues.

VITAMIN D (THE ANTIRACHITIC VITAMIN)

At least 10 different sterol derivatives exhibit the properties of vitamin D, but ergosterol (D_2) and 9-dehydrocholesterol are the most important. D_1, D_2, D_3, and D_4 have been assigned chemical formulae. Such substances acquire antirachitic properties when exposed to ultraviolet light. The structural formula of ergosterol (D_2) is shown on page 405.

Vitamin D is concerned primarily with the absorption of Ca and P from the intestinal tract and the formation and maintenance of the skeletal system and the teeth. The main function of vitamin D is the regulation of the Ca and P absorption so that they exist in normal amounts and ratios within wide dietary variations.

Fish liver oils, such as those derived from the halibut or the cod, are extremely rich in vitamin D. It is also found in smaller quantities in eggs, milk and all dairy products. Today many staple foodstuffs such as milk, bread, breakfast cereals and even candy bars are irradiated to increase their vitamin D content.

$$CH_3$$

$$CH-CH=CH$$

$$C_{28}H_{43}OH$$

Vitamin D as present in viosterol (irradiated ergosterol)

The daily requirements of vitamin D have been set at 625 U.S.P. vitamin D units. The requirements are increased during lactation and pregnancy. Massive doses of vitamin D, over 100,000 U.S.P. units, have been given for the treatment of arthritis. Symptoms of overdosage in the human being are rare.

Rickets

Frank deficiency of vitamin D in the infant produces the clinical symptoms of tetany (spasmophilia) or rickets. Childhood rickets and tetany are uncommon with the present-day prenatal and pediatric care and the irradiation of the milk unless the infant is on a very restricted diet or some gastrointestinal disturbance prevents proper absorption of the ingested food.

Rickets is usually manifested during the first 2 years of life, being commonest between the 6th and 18th months. It is seen chiefly in the temperate zones, where it is particularly common in the winter months. Unusual irritability, restlessness and sweating of the head and neck region may call attention to the disease but the chief manifestations of rickets are seen in the bones. Craniotabes, the development of soft parchment-like spots in the skull, is frequently the first evidence of the disease. The rachitic child has large, prominent frontal bones which give an enlarged, square appearance to the head.

The characteristic bowing of the legs and the enlargement of the wrists and ankles are common symptoms of clinical rickets. Small bony and cartilaginous nodules develop where the ribs join the sternum, giving rise to the "rachitic rosary." Other chest deformities are also common in rickets.

The typical roentgenologic changes are seen best in the lower ends of the radius and ulna. The normal distinct transverse convex line of the metaphyses appears widened, irregular and at times indefinite. Partial or complete fractures are seen occasionally.

The diagnosis of rickets is based on the clinical, roentgenologic and blood chemistry findings. The roentgenologic changes in rickets constitute one of the most important diagnostic criterion. The blood calcium or phosphorus is decreased and there is a disturbance in the normal Ca:P ratio.

Osteomalacia (Adult Rickets)

Osteomalacia is a manifestation of vitamin D deficiency in the adult. Osteomalacia is rare in the United States, but it is observed commonly in China and the Punjab (India). It may develop: (1) whenever the general diet is deficient in calcium or vitamin D or (2) when there is an abnormal calcium drain on the body. In the areas mentioned, vitamin D deficiency may be due to the absence of foods in the diet containing this substance or the lack of exposure to sunlight. Gastro-intestinal disturbances which interfere with the normal fat digestion and absorption can result in vitamin D deficiency.

In osteomalacia there is an irregular increase in the thickness of both the cortex and the trabeculae of the bones. These tissues are poorly calcified and contain fibrous bone marrow and islands of osteoid tissue.

Oral Aspects

It would be expected that any substance which plays such an important rôle in skeletal formation and calcium and phosphorus utilization would have a marked influence on the teeth and jaws. The effect of vitamin D deficiency on the dental tissues during (1) the tooth formative period and (2) in the posteruptive period will be discussed separately.

Deficiency During the Tooth Formative Period

Day studied the teeth and jaws of a group of children born of osteo-malaciac mothers in the Punjab. The dental structure of the developing fetus did not seem to be adversely affected. Severe enamel hypoplasia of the teeth was noted but the quality of the tissues seemed good as the teeth of the children studied were remarkably free from cavities. The author has seen extensive enamel hypoplasia of the deciduous dentition in a child born of a mother with osteomalacia.

Enamel hypoplasia of the permanent incisors and the first molars is a common manifestation of childhood rickets. While these teeth are obviously imperfectly calcified they are not abnormally susceptible to dental caries. Although numerous other diseases will result in enamel hypoplasia, few will produce the extensive involvement which is associated with rickets.

The hypoplasia in the molars is limited essentially to the enamel and the general morphologic features of the crown and roots are not involved as in prenatal syphilis. Other factors besides the lack of vitamin D are concerned in the production of this enamel hypoplasia. In fact, Taylor & Day concluded that vitamin D deficiency alone does not cause enamel hypoplasia. A delayed dentition has been noted in rickets.

Deficiency in the Posteruptive Period

While vitamin D is particularly important during the formative period of the teeth, it also exerts a beneficial influence when it is given late in the formative period and to a lesser extent after the teeth have erupted. In view of the relatively slight metabolic exchange in the erupted tooth, it is more difficult to explain the mechanism for this protective effect on the erupted tooth. It has been estimated that the replacement of 1% of the phosphorus in the tooth by dietary phosphorus requires approximately 250 days.

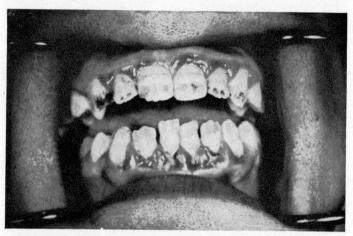

FIG. 202. Enamel hypoplasia and an open bite malocclusion which were associated with childhood rickets. Note the hypertrophic gingivitis and poor oral hygiene.

Research workers are not all agreed that vitamin D above the generally accepted requirements exerts any beneficial effect on tooth decay in the erupted tooth. There is considerable evidence however which points to a caries-protective effect of vitamin D. No satisfactory explanation, based on known dental anatomic and physiologic facts, has been advanced for this apparent caries-protective effect which is obtained from a high vitamin D intake.

When vitamin D is added to the diet of institutionalized children there is observed a decrease in the caries incidence as compared with the control group. McBeath found that the results were equally effective when vitamin D, milk or cod liver oil were used. The relation between dental caries and sunshine has been studied extensively. East found an inverse correlation between the amount of sunlight and the incidence of new cavities. These findings were based on the caries attack rates in 24 states as compared to the number of hours of sunshine recorded by the U. S. Weather Bureau. The number of hours' sunshine and the number of hours' exposure to sunlight are obviously different as local environmental conditions such as smoke, dust, buildings and shade will all effect the amount of effective radiation. In regions where over 3,000 sunshine hours per year were experienced the caries attack rate was 290.5 cavities per 100 white boys of 12 to 14 years of age. In areas where there was less than 2,200 hours, the attack rate was 485.75 per 100 boys.

Brodsky *et al.* presented evidence which indicates that a single massive dose of vitamin D (305,000 U.S.P. units) and vitamin A (2,455,000 U.S.P. units) significantly reduced the number of new cavities in the experimental groups. No toxic effects were noted. Fosdick and Hatton demonstrated that the administration of both vitamin A (12,000 U.S.P. units) and vitamin D (900 U.S.P. units) per day resulted in a remarkable decrease in caries susceptibility as determined by the rate of acid production of the saliva.

Relatively few toxic symptoms due to high vitamin D administration have been observed in man. The effect of vitamin D overdosage on the dental and periodontal structures in dogs has been studied by Becks. He noted an overgrowth of the cementum, an irregular laminated dentin, malformations and malocclusions of the teeth and delayed dental development. There was generalized osteosclerosis of the jaw bones and the periodontal structures. The dosage of vitamin D employed was not comparable with that which has been used in man.

The effect of increased vitamin D intake on the caries attack rates in adults has not been so clearly demonstrated. Robinson called attention to the lack of a satisfactory physiologic mechanism whereby vitamin D or the supplemental administration of calcium or phosphorus could affect the enamel of the erupted tooth. Recent studies utilizing the radio-isotopes have demonstrated a slight metabolic exchange in the dentin, but that in the enamel was almost infinitesimal. Most of the experimental evidence supports the view that the fully erupted tooth of the adult cannot be significantly modified by the addition of calcium, phosphorus or vitamin D. Even in severe demineralizing diseases such as hyperparathyroidism and osteomalacia no roentgenologic or chemical changes can be demonstrated in the teeth. Taylor & Day found an average of only 1.54 cavities in the 22 women with osteomalacia which they examined. Of equal interest was the fact that only 2 cavities were found in the 144 teeth of 7 rachitic children of these osteomalaciac mothers.

In summary it can be said that there is general agreement as to the importance of vitamin D during the period of tooth formation. There is considerable clinical evidence to show that an increased vitamin D intake may have a caries-protective effect during childhood, although other factors such as the type of the diet are also extremely important. The evidence of a beneficial effect of an increased vitamin D intake on the erupted teeth of adults is less definite. Most of the studies indicate that erupted teeth are relatively unaffected by calcium, phosphorus or vitamin D. This does not hold, however, for the alveolar process which may be seriously involved in any metabolic disturbance which affects the general skeletal system. The indiscriminate administration of dicalcium phosphate in the hope of arresting caries in the adult has no scientific basis and in fact it may be harmful.

VITAMIN E (TOCOPHEROL)

Vitamin E has been called the fertility vitamin. It is fat soluble and it occurs widespread in nature. Grains, vegetable oils and green vegetables are good sources of vitamin E. The daily requirements for man have not been determined. Manifestations of toxicity have not been reported.

Most of the knowledge about this vitamin has been obtained from experimental animal studies where a deficiency of this substance in the female is known to result in abortion or degenerative changes in the developing embryo. In the male, a deficiency of this vitamin results in a loss of sperm, of fertilizing power, and a loss of sex interest. Some animals on a vitamin E deficient diet develop muscular dystrophy and paralysis.

The chief clinical use of vitamin E has been in the treatment of habitual abortion or threatened abortion. There is some evidence that adequate vitamin E intake during pregnancy may aid in preventing developmental anomalies.

No dental or oral changes have been reported associated with a deficiency of this vitamin.

VITAMIN K (MENADIONE)

Vitamin K is a water insoluble, heat stable substance which is found in green leaves, notably alfalfa, spinach and putrid fish meal. Numerous synthetic compounds including K_5 have been isolated. Phthiocol (2-methyl-1,4-napthoquinone) or its derivatives has largely replaced the natural sources of this substance. It has the following structural formula:

$$H_3C-CH-(CH_2)_3-CH-(CH_2)_3-CH-(CH_2)_3-CH$$

(structural formula with naphthoquinone ring bearing H, O, CH₃ substituents and side chain)

$$C_{31}H_{46}O_2$$

Vitamin K is necessary for the formation of prothrombin. Dietary deficiencies of vitamin K are rare in adults but its inadequate utilization because of liver dysfunction, obstructive jaundice, lack of bile salts or impaired small intestine absorptive function are associated with hemorrhagic phenomena related to prothrombin deficiency.

The determination of prothrombin time and the vitamin K level of the blood plasma are valuable diagnostic aids in suspected cases of vitamin K deficiency. Normal values for prothrombin time vary depending with the method used.

The daily requirements of vitamin K are not known. The customary daily dose of synthetic vitamin K is 2 mg. No toxic reactions have been reported following its administration.

Systemic Aspects

The most important use of vitamin K is in curing or preventing the bleeding associated with obstructive jaundice and primary hepatic disease. Patients with obstructive jaundice or primary hepatic disease should receive vitamin K before any surgery is attempted. Vitamin K can be administered by mouth, but bile salts are necessary for its absorption from the intestinal tract.

This vitamin has also been used successfully in the treatment of hemorrhagic disease of the newborn. It is often given to the mother prior to delivery. Vitamin K is not effective in the treatment of hemophilia and thrombocytopenic purpura.

Oral Aspects

Quick showed experimentally that chicks on a low vitamin K diet have a tendency for spontaneous mucosal hemorrhages. Graham stated that vitamin K is valuable in controlling certain forms of postoperative dental hemorrhage—the author did not make more specific statements. If oral surgery must be performed on a jaundiced patient, vitamin K would be a desirable pre-operative treatment.

Fosdick reported that the presence of vitamin K in the oral cavity reduced markedly the number of lactobacilli and yeasts which could be cultured from the saliva. It was suggested that this vitamin might be used in some manner as a prophylactic agent against dental caries. Additional studies are being conducted to determine the practicability of this procedure.

VITAMIN P (CITRIN—HESPERIDIN)

As early as 1936, Szent-Györgyi suggested that another vitamin, tentatively called vitamin P because of its effect on capillary permeabililty and fragility, existed in lemon peel. The chemical structure of this substance was determined in 1942 by Waura and Webb. It is a flavone glucoside, hesperidin.

The exact function of hesperidin and its derivatives is not known, but this substance has a beneficial effect on capillary health and probably plays a rôle in tissue respiration. The lack of a suitable experimental animal is one of the chief deterents to studies on vitamin P. The daily requirements have not been determined. Exact laboratory procedures for determining the vitamin P nutrition have not been devised. The capillary fragility test (tourniquet test) may give suggestive information.

Systemic Aspects

The hemorrhagic phenomena believed to be associated with vitamin P deficiency consist of small hemorrhages which are found most commonly in the skin. Easy fatigue, lassitude and pain in the eyes and shoulders have been described by Scarborough. The capillary resistance of the subjects studied by him was not benefited by the administration of vitamins A, B_1, C, or D.

Hesperidin has been used effectively in the treatment of thrombocytopenic purpura as well as nutritional, allergic and infectious forms of purpura. Purpura resulting from arsenical and bismuth therapy has responded favorably to the administration of this vitamin. Raunert even reported that after all other methods had failed the daily administration of citrin and calcium stopped the bleeding in patients with hemophilia, gastric hemorrhage and hematuria. The therapeutic use of citrin is still in the experimental stage. No toxic effects have been reported.

Oral Aspects

Kreshover and the author determined the blood ascorbic level and the capillary fragility findings (petechial count) in patients with periodontal disease and suitable controls. When a standardized positive pressure technic was used for determining the capillary fragility it was found that a high percentage of the patients with periodontal disease had an abnormally high petechial count as compared to a low percentage in the control group of the same age range.

There was no correlation between the petechial count and the blood ascorbic acid levels before and after saturation of the patient with ascorbic acid, although the blood ascorbic acid level could be correlated with the administration of vitamin C. The capillary fragility findings were not altered by this treatment. In a few patients who have been subsequently studied, the petechial count dropped following the administration of large amounts of orange juice.

The author believes that abnormal capillary fragility findings may be an indication, among other things, of a deficiency of vitamin P. Since the patients with periodontal disease had a consistently high petechial count it is possible that the altered capillary permeability in these patients was a factor contributing to the periodontal disease. The administration of citrin, when available, may have a beneficial effect on both the capillary permeability and the periodontal disturbances. The vitamin P content of the natural citrus fruit juices may be responsible for their beneficial effect in some forms of periodontal disease.

20

Diseases of Metabolism

DIABETES MELLITUS	GOUT—GOUTY ARTHRITIS
PERNICIOUS ANEMIA	THE XANTHOMATOSES
SPRUE	

DIABETES MELLITUS

Diabetes is a metabolic disease associated with insufficient insulin production in the pancreas or increased demands for this substance. This metabolic derangement affects primarily carbohydrate utilization and formation but the normal utilization of fats and proteins is also affected.

It is estimated that there are approximately 660,000 diabetics in the United States and the number is increasing. Part of this increase is due to the greater life expectancy of the juvenile diabetic which results from modern methods of treatment. This disease ranked in 9th place in 1938 as primary cause of death. Diabetes is essentially a disease of middle adult life, the 4th and 5th decades, although juvenile diabetes is not uncommon. It has predilection for the Jewish race and exhibits a hereditary predisposition in all races.

An analysis of diabetics according to their occupation reveals a high incidence in the professional groups and those who lead a sedentary life. Physical exercise and moderation in the diet appear to have a protective effect. Diabetes is also related to the *per capita* income, being greater in those with larger incomes although the belief that the increased consumption of carbohydrates predisposes to the disease is not necessarily true.

While diabetes is believed to be related to insufficient insulin production for the immediate body needs, it does not follow that the insular tissues of the pancreas are always at fault. The activity of this gland, because of the interrelationship of all the endocrines, may be considerably modified by disturbances in other glands of internal secretion such as the pituitary. There may be increased insulin demands. It is not always possible to correlate histopathologic changes in the insular tissue with the severity of the diabetes.

Symptoms

The early recognition of diabetes is not always easy. It is estimated that 12% of the people with this disease present no clinical symptoms whatsoever.

TABLE XXIII

Diabetes and Occupation, Occupations in Order of Rank of Mortality from Diabetes.* Metropolitan Life Insurance Company, Industrial Department, 1922-1924

(After Joslin, Dublin and Marks)

	Occupation	Standardized Relative Index, Ages 15 to 64
High diabetes mortality (index 115 or over)	Merchants and storekeepers.............	204
	Tailors and other clothing workers........	185
	Saloonkeepers and bartenders............	157
	Railway enginemen and trainmen.........	154
	Electricians.............................	140
	Store clerks and salesmen................	137
	Watchmen and guards...................	125
	Clerks, bookkeepers and office assistants...	121
	Stationary engineers and firemen.........	118
Average diabetes mortality (index 86 to 114)	Machinists.............................	107
	Iron and steel-mill workers..............	107
	All occupations (excluding retired)........	100
	Railway track and yard workers..........	97
	Plumbers, gasfitters, and steamfitters......	96
	Textile (except cordage, hemp, dyeing and finishing) millworkers.................	91
Low diabetes mortality (index 85 or less)	Teamsters and drivers...................	84
	Furniture and other woodworkers........	81
	Farmers and farm laborers..............	77
	Laborers...............................	68
	Janitors and building employees..........	68
	Painters, paperhangers, and varnishers....	61
	Carpenters.............................	59
	Coalminers (underground)..............	51

* Occupations with less than 15 deaths excluded except where the mortality is very high or low.

For explanation of this term the reader is referred to Dublin, L. I., and Vane, R. J., Jr., Causes of Death by Occupation, Bull. U. S. Bureau of Labor Statistics, No. 507.

Courtesy of W. B. Saunders Company, Duncan's "Diseases of Metabolism," 1942.

The initiating symptoms are frequently so gradual and diverse that their true significance and nature is not realized until one of the varied complications of the disease ensues. Many cases are detected during routine urinary examinations for other purposes, *i.e.*, life insurance examinations. If this procedure were more routine with the physician, more cases might be diagnosed in the early stages.

General weakness, the loss of weight accompanied by an increase in appetite, and the frequent desire for food (polyphagia), pruritus, the consumption of large amounts of water (polydypsia) and the passage of large amounts of urine (polyuria) are common symptoms. A lowered resistance to pyogenic infections as manifest by frequent boils, carbuncles, styes, paronychiae, parietal root abscesses or marked periodontal disease are diabetic complications which may first call attention to the underlying disease. The early recognition of diabetes by the physician or dentist is a real contribution to the health of the patient as all too frequently diabetics do not seek professional attention until the complications associated with the disease develop.

The clinical signs and symptoms mentioned above may suggest diabetes

but the final diagnosis rests on the results of the appropriate laboratory findings, glycosuria and altered sugar tolerance curves. Glycosuria suggests a
diagnosis of diabetes and a repeatedly elevated blood sugar is diagnostic.

Treatment

The treatment of diabetes is in the province of the physician. It is also his
duty to inform the patient that should dental extractions be necessary the

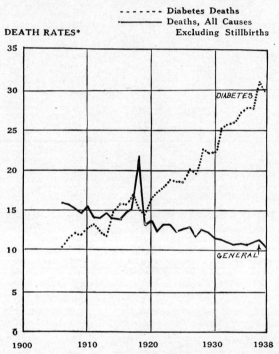

FIG. 203. Comparison of death rates due to
diabetes and those due to other causes. General
death rates are per 1,000 population. Diabetes
death rates are per 100,000 population. (Duncan,
Diseases of Metabolism, W. B. Saunders Company.)

patient should inform the dentist of his diabetic condition. It is important
for the physician to stress the necessity for more frequent dental attention
in the diabetic, not only from the diabetic standpoint but to prevent possible
oral complications.

The physician aims to keep the diabetic patient with the urine almost
sugar-free and to avoid the 2 chief complications of this disease—diabetic
coma and insulin reactions. The first results from hyperglycemia and acidosis
and the latter from too low a blood sugar level which may follow acciden-

tally taking more insulin than is required or failure to take sufficient nourishment at the proper time. The dentist should be familiar with both these complications.

Diabetic Coma

In diabetic coma the patient exhibits symptoms of air hunger. They are dehydrated, the skin and mucosae being dry. The breath may have the char-

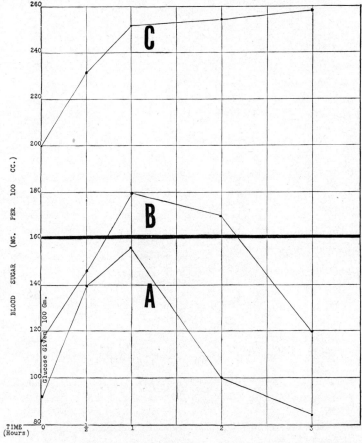

FIG. 204. Three glucose tolerance curves. A depicts the normal glycemic response to the oral administration of 100 Gm. of glucose. The rise in blood sugar level is rapid, but a normal value is restored in two hours. In B the glycemic response is slower and normal values are not restored until the third hour as is found in mild diabetes. C depicts the fasting hyperglycemic and the continued increase in the blood sugar level even at the third hour as seen in severe diabetes. Glycosuria usually occurs when the blood sugar level is maintained (for several hours) about 160 mg. per 100 cc. as depicted by the heavy black line. (Duncan, Diseases of Metabolism, W. B. Saunders Company.)

acteristic acetone odor. The blood pressure is low, the pulse is rapid and the extremities are usually cold to touch. Complete unconsciousness usually comes on gradually.

Insulin Reactions (Insulin Shock—Hypoglycemic Reactions)

These patients complain of nervousness, weakness, headache and at times numbness of the extremities. They are often hungry. The skin surface may be moist or clammy and the individuals appear slightly dazed. They are unable to concentrate on any particular object or subject. Paresthesias of the tongue or mucosa and lips are frequent symptoms. Muscular twitching, actual convulsions, mental confusion and frank unconsciousness may be present. The pupils are usually dilated.

In cases of doubt as to whether the patient is in diabetic coma or hypoglycemia, a lump of sugar should be placed between the cheeks and the teeth, or if the patient is conscious enough to take nourishment, he should be given some orange juice.

Oral Aspects

Because of the common occurrence of this disease every dentist should be familiar with its oral manifestations and the dental aspects of diabetes mellitus. For convenience of discussion the oral changes associated with diabetes can be divided into:

(1) The effect of diabetes on the periodontal structures and the oral mucosa.
(2) The effect of diabetes on the incidence of dental caries and odontalgia.
(3) The effect of oral foci of infection on diabetes mellitus.
(4) Precautions for performing dental surgery on diabetic patients.

(1) **Effect on the Periodontal Structures and Oral Mucosa.** The association of diabetes and periodontal disease was first noted by Seiffert in 1862. Magitot believed that the oral cavity presented constant symptoms in this disease. The exact incidence of periodontal involvement in diabetes is difficult to determine because adult diabetes occurs most frequently in the age range in which periodontal disease is also most prevalent.

The effect of diabetes on the periodontal structures can be studied in juvenile diabetics where the occurrence of periodontal disease is less likely to be a complicating factor. Rutledge studied the periodontal structures in 29 children between the ages of 8 and 19 who were under treatment for diabetes. In 80% of the cases gingival lesions with marginal and vertical atrophy of the alveolar bone and marginal widening of the periodontal membrane space could be found alone or together. Individuals 14 to 18 years of age may be wearing full dentures. The oral manifestations in juvenile diabetes constituted an important symptom of the disease and marked periodontal involvement in the adolescent should always suggest juvenile diabetes.

Some form of periodontal disease is present in approximately 75% of all diabetics. This will vary in extent and clinical manifestations depending on the severity of the diabetes, the duration of the disease before treatment is

instituted and the general hygienic habits of the patient and local predisposing factors. The high incidence of periodontal disease in uncontrolled adult
diabetes is probably due to the diabetic state, although many clinicians do
not agree with this view. The periodontal lesions in juvenile and adult diabetes are similar, being modified only by changes in the dental structures at
the different age periods.

The gums in the uncontrolled diabetic are usually deep red in color, slightly
hypertrophied and extremely dry. Proliferating masses of granulation tissue
which protrude from beneath the marginal gingiva, are characteristic findings

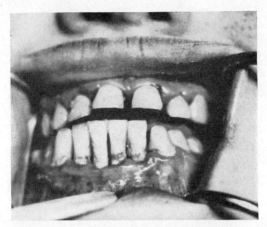

FIG. 205. Marked periodontal disease in an
18-year-old patient with unsuspected diabetes. One year previously this patient was
a professional model for dentifrice advertisements.

in uncontrolled diabetics. Generalized suppuration of the marginal gum, including the interdental papillae, is another common finding. This extensive
suppuration aids in differentiating diabetic periodontosis from the functional
forms of the disease. Pain is often present in diabetic periodontosis and the
teeth are sensitive to percussion. Extensive alveolar atrophy with loosening
of the teeth may develop within a short time. The reduced alkaline reserve
in uncontrolled diabetes favors the removal of calcium salts from the alveolar
process. There is evidence that diabetes depresses the activity of some of the
vitamins, especially C. This weakens still further the supporting mechanism
of the tooth. Calcareous deposits form rapidly and are usually abundant. The
subgingival accretions are extremely hard. The extent of the alveolar resorption and the calcareous deposits are clearly shown by the x-ray. Recurrent
periodontal or parietal root abscesses should suggest the possibility of underlying diabetes.

The author has seen several cases of extensive alveolar destruction involving 1 or 2 teeth which could not be explained by local factors. Within a year
or 2 these individuals developed symptoms of diabetes. This emphasizes the

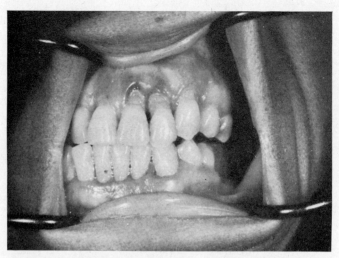

FIG. 206. Periodontal disease in an uncontrolled diabetic patient.

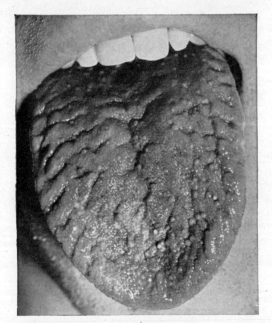

FIG. 207. Xanthomatous nodules on the tongue in a patient with diabetes. (Duncan, Diseases of Metabolism, W. B. Saunders Company.)

importance of routine urine examinations in all cases of periodontal disease.

Dryness and burning of the tongue may be an early symptom in diabetes. The fissures of the tongue are more pronounced and the fungiform papillae are frequently enlarged and hyperemic. The musculature is flabby and the indentation markings of the teeth are commonly observed on the edges of this organ.

In controlled diabetics there are no characteristic gingival or periodontal lesions. If the oral hygiene is poor, the gums may be slightly cyanotic and

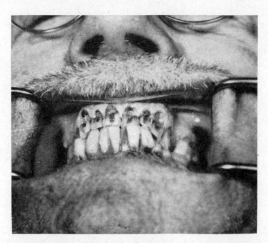

Fig. 208. Marked abrasion (erosion?) of the labial surfaces of the teeth in a diabetic patient 52 years of age. No symptoms were experienced due to this abnormal loss of tooth substance.

appear flabby. Even in controlled diabetics there is lessened tissue resistance and slight irritating agents of any kind may elicit a marked tissue response.

Effect on Dental Caries and Odontalgia. A study of the incidence of caries in controlled and uncontrolled diabetics presents some interesting findings. A sudden onset of caries or its active progression is often associated with clinical diabetes. Zilz noted an increased incidence of dental decay in uncontrolled diabetes. The decreased salivary flow may also be a predisposing factor.

Kirk and Simon also contended that there is an increased fermentable content in the saliva of the diabetic which furnishes a suitable medium for acid production. The presence of sugar in the saliva of diabetics is not a constant finding, although cases of glucosialorrhea have been reported. The presence of glucose in the saliva is more dependent on the glucose threshold of the salivary gland than the severity of the diabetes. Salivary glands have normally a higher glucose threshold than the kidneys. In general, salivary studies made on diabetics have failed to reveal the temporal relationship between the collection of the saliva and insulin administration or the time of day. Gore believed that the susceptibility to caries is largely dependent on the amount of insulin in the salivary glands. The mechanism responsible for the increase in dental caries in the uncontrolled diabetic is not clearly understood but there is ample evidence of its occurrence.

There is no indication that dental caries is increased in controlled diabetes. In fact, diabetic children fed a diet low in refined carbohydrates are relatively immune to dental caries. Adult diabetic patients who are on a well-balanced dietary regime or those who take insulin regularly are also relatively free from dental caries.

Odontalgia or pulpitis occurs occasionally in diabetics unassociated with clinical dental lesions. This is due to a diabetic arteritis of the dental pulp. This diabetic arteritis may result in death of the pulp even in the absence of caries. The tooth becomes dark in color and pain is increasingly severe. The author has observed the pulp of an extracted intact lower incisor that presented the typical histologic picture of diabetic arteritis. Prinz described an increased sensitivity in and about the necks of the teeth in diabetics.

Relation to Oral Foci of Infection

Periapical or periodontal foci of infection are of particular significance in the diabetic as they may transform a less serious case of diabetes into a grave or even fatal one. Any source of infection reduces the body's ability to metabolize carbohydrates. An abscessed tooth or an acute periodontal infection is sufficient to produce glycosuria in a diabetic patient or, in rare instances, diabetic coma. Joslin observed diabetes to grow worse in the presence of inflammatory conditions of the teeth and gums.

The question often arises whether all pulpless teeth should be removed in diabetics. Most certainly teeth with large suppurating areas should be eliminated. On the other hand, if the root canals have been properly treated, there is no reason why a pulpless tooth presents any undue hazard.

Periodontal infection is of greater significance to the diabetic. Here the areas for septic absorption are larger and the tissues are constantly being traumatized during chewing. Such a condition may aggravate the diabetic state. Teeth remaining loose after the control of diabetes and appropriate local treatment should be removed. The necessity for conservatism in the treatment of periodontal disease in the diabetic must be emphasized. Caustics and strong iodine-containing preparations should not be used.

The diabetic requires frequent and regular dental care. The oral cavity should be maintained in the best hygienic state possible. All foci of infection must be removed or eliminated by suitable and satisfactory treatment. With the elimination of oral sepsis it is not unusual to note a decreased insulin requirement.

Dental Surgery in Diabetic Patients

Dental surgery in the diabetic requires a consideration of (1) steps that may be taken to prevent an elevation in blood sugar, (2) the choice of the anesthetic and (3) steps that may be taken to prevent postoperative complications. A routine medical history will acquaint the dentist with known cases of diabetes, or elicit symptoms suggestive of the disease. Dental extractions should not be performed in cases of uncontrolled diabetes unless the co-operating physician wishes to assume all responsibility.

Steps Taken to Prevent an Elevation in Blood Sugar

A calm, confident, assuring attitude on the part of the dentist is most important. Adequate premedication prior to dental surgery is important. The nervous and emotional excitement associated with even minor operations causes an elevated blood sugar level, due to increased adrenalin output.

The best time for dental surgery is during the descending portion of the blood sugar curve. This will vary, depending on the type of insulin, the time insulin is taken and the time relationship of the extraction to meals. Extractions under local anesthesia are best performed 1½ to 3 hours following breakfast and the administration of insulin. Provided suitable precautions are taken, teeth can be removed when the blood sugar level is elevated without undue complications, but in any case only a few teeth should be removed at a sitting. The chance of inducing shock is increased as the number of teeth removed increases. Baker at the Mayo Clinic reported 2 cases of diabetic coma following dental extractions. Others have been recorded.

Local anesthesia without adrenalin is preferred. The use of adrenalin increases the blood sugar level and the marked ischemia resulting from its use predisposes to tissue slough and postoperative infection. Adrenalin is also contraindicated in coronary artery disease which is common in the diabetic. Adequate local anesthesia can be obtained with a plain 2% procaine or ¾% monocaine hydrochloride solution. Blaustein found that monocaine (¾%) produced the smallest average milligram change in higher blood sugar levels. If a vasoconstrictor is required, cobefrin does not have the sympathetic stimulatory effect of adrenalin, although it produces a marked and prolonged elevation in blood pressure.

Since all general anesthetics cause a marked rise in blood sugar, their use requires close co-operation with the patient's physician. The glycogen reserves of the individual should be built up prior to the operation and a careful watch kept to detect early signs of acidosis. While ether is the general anesthetic of choice, it is impractical for the usual dental operation. Satisfactory results, with nitrous oxide in diabetics, were reported by Blaustein.

He found that nitrous oxide was best given to the diabetic on a fasting stomach. The patients were instructed to take ¼ to ½ of the regular morning insulin dosage at the regular time. No food was eaten and surgery was performed approximately 3 hours after the insulin was taken. Ten minutes after the patient returned to consciousness the remainder of the insulin was administered and the patient was given the regular caloric food intake. Good results were obtained. If special preparation is not convenient, the surgery should be performed about 3½ hours following insulin and breakfast. Vomiting may cause additional complications. Diabetic patients requiring general anesthesia should be hospitalized so facilities and personnel are readily available to care for any complications.

All surgical procedures in diabetics should be as atraumatic as possible. Marginal necrosis of the tissues about extraction sockets is common. Extensive necrosis or gangrene following dental surgery may be the first evidence of diabetes. Unlike diabetic gangrene of the extremities, age plays little rôle in oral diabetic gangrene. Millet observed oral diabetic gangrene in children as well as the aged. It is stated that the mechanism producing gangrene of the face is different from that in the extremities where an obliterative arteritis is the exciting cause. When one considers the high bacterial population in the oral cavity, it is remarkable that oral gangrene does not occur more often. Although there may be extensive loss of tissue, the prognosis in oral diabetic gangrene is not unfavorable.

The so-called "dry socket" occurs more frequently in diabetics, even when under control, than in the normal patient. The incidence of "dry socket" and local periostitis can be lessened by the elimination of the periodontal disease and the administration of adequate amounts of vitamin C before extraction in conjunction with the local use of sulfanilamide or sulfathiazole in the tooth socket.

There is an impression that the tendency for hemorrhage is greater in the diabetic patient. There is no significant variation in the bleeding or clotting time for the different blood sugar levels in diabetic patients. The occasional tendency to hemorrhage may be associated with a vitamin deficiency or secondary infection of the blood clot.

Summary

Dental treatment in a diabetic requires a fundamental understanding of the nature of the disease by the dentist. Trauma should be avoided during periodontal treatment or tooth extractions. Caustic drugs should not be used in the mouth of a diabetic. The patient should be instructed in the proper tooth-brushing technic to prevent unnecessary irritation of the soft tissues.

All foci of infection should be removed or eliminated, including teeth remaining loose after adequate periodontal treatment in controlled diabetics. There is no reason why adequately treated pulpless teeth should be extracted.

Dental surgery in diabetic patients should be performed during the descending portion of the blood sugar curve; that is approximately 1½ to 3 hours after insulin and breakfast. Local anesthesia, preferably without adrenalin, is the anesthetic of choice and monocaine hydrochloride (¾%) causes the smallest elevation of the blood sugar. Adequate pre-operative medication is advised for both local and general anesthesia. All surgery should be as atraumatic as possible. The use of one of the sulfonamides in the tooth socket and the pre-operative administration of adequate vitamin C and B complex will reduce secondary infection and promote ready wound healing.

PERNICIOUS ANEMIA (ADDISON'S ANEMIA—BERMIER'S ANEMIA)

Pernicious anemia is a chronic disease which results from a deficiency of the "intrinsic factor" produced in the gastric mucosa, a deficiency of the "extrinsic principle" of the consumed food, deficiencies of absorption or a combination of the above.

Pernicious anemia is a disease of late adult life, with about equal incidence in both sexes. There is some suggestion of a hereditary background. Gastric achlorhydria predisposes to the disease.

The onset of pernicious anemia is insidious and the initial symptoms may be referable to many organ systems, including the oral cavity. Gastrointestinal symptoms, which are common and prominent in this disease, include anorexia and alternating diarrhea. In severe cases nausea and vomiting are experienced. Patients often complain of breathlessness, dizziness, faintness and palpitation. The skin has a peculiar yellowish pallor which is characteristic.

Symptoms referable to the nervous system may be the first evidence of the disease. Numbness and tingling of the extremities are common early symptoms. Short, stabbing pains may be experienced and in advanced stages of the disease, when degeneration of the cord has occurred, there is loss of both deep and superficial reflexes and loss of function of the extremities. The neuritic changes are believed to be associated with B complex deficiencies.

Diagnosis

The diagnosis of pernicious anemia is made on the basis of the history, the hematologic and gastric findings. The blood count is diagnostic. In addition to the marked decrease in the number of the erythrocytes, at times less than 1,000,000 per cu. mm., there is a marked variation in the size (anisocytosis) and shape (poikilocytosis) of the cells. The hemoglobin is not decreased in proportion to the red cell count which results in a color index (C.I.) greater than 1. Immature red cells and reticulocytes are common. The average diameter of the red cells is greater than normal. There is also a decreased white cell count.

Gastric achlorhydria, even after histamine stimulation, is a characteristic finding. The gastric achylia in some cases is known to precede the pernicious anemia.

The treatment of pernicious anemia is in the province of the physician. Today the prognosis of the pernicious anemia patient is much more hopeful than in past years due to the availability and the extensive use of liver preparations of high potency. The neuritic symptoms may not respond to treatment. In this disease treatment does not result in a permanent cure but it just supplies the deficiency.

Oral Aspects

In 1877 Moeller described certain atrophic lingual changes which were believed to be a clinical entity. In 1909 Hunter first called attention to the relationship between oral sepsis and pernicious anemia. He believed that the swallowed purulent material gave rise to some hemolytic substance which resulted in the marked anemia. In all probability, the atrophic lesions described by Moeller and Hunter are a single clinical entity and the atrophic lingual changes which develop in certain parasitic infections are similar in appearance. Waldenstrom's hypothesis of the mechanism of the atrophic lingual changes explains the similarity of the clinical lesions which might result from a variety of causes.

The tongue symptoms and changes are prominent in pernicious anemia. A painful glossitis and glossopyrosis may be an early symptom of this disease and one which causes the patient to seek dental advice. The glossitis associated with pernicious anemia is characterized by its fiery red color and its usual distribution to the tip and margins of the tongue with papillary atrophy

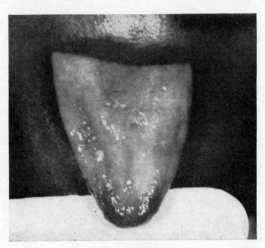

FIG. 209. Fiery red glossitis involving the lateral margins and tip of the tongue in a patient with pernicious anemia. The initial symptom in this patient was the inability to wear full dentures because of the painful tongue and denture-supporting areas. Typical hematologic and gastric findings were present.

of the affected areas. In advanced cases there is a diminution of the papillary anatomy of the entire tongue with a loss of the normal muscle tone. The tongue becomes smooth and has a stiff feel to the patient. In severe cases degeneration and atrophy of the cheek mucosa occur.

Schneider and Carey believed that the *Streptococcus viridans* is responsible for the inflammatory appearance of the oral lesions. Middleton considered an erythematous and swollen tongue an important diagnostic aid in this disease. The oral mucosa also presents the greenish-yellow color noted on the skin. This is best seen at the junction of the hard and soft palates when daylight is used for illumination.

The dental practitioner must differentiate between the glossitis associated with pernicious anemia from simple mechanical irritative lesions, the atrophic glossitis of syphilis, glossopyrosis, glossodynia and possible allergic lesions. Important points in the differential diagnosis include the fiery red appearance of the tongue, the areas involved and the fact that spontaneous remissions and exacerbations are experienced which are usually associated with more disseminated symptoms. A hemogram will usually establish the diagnosis. It should be requested in all cases where local causes cannot be found for persisting tongue lesions.

Local treatment, other than the removal of mechanical causes of irritation, will give little relief for the tongue lesions. Topical application of medicaments may lessen the bacterial flora but it does not relieve the painful symptoms.

SPRUE

Sprue is a symptom complex which develops in individuals who live for long periods of time on diets consisting mainly of carbohydrates and fats. It is common in tropical countries and certain of the southern states of the United States.

Systemic Aspects

The onset of this disease is insidious with slowly developing weakness, mental irritability and loss of weight. The passage of numerous bulky, frothy, fatty, foul-smelling stools is usually the symptom which attracts the most attention. These stools contain large amounts of fat. A brownish pigmentation of the skin may develop. There is an associated macrocytic anemia which is indistinguishable from that found in pernicious anemia.

The treatment of sprue consists of the oral or intramuscular administration of liver extract and general dietary regulation.

Oral Aspects

The oral lesions in sprue are prominent and some clinicians consider their presence necessary for the diagnosis of this disease. The oral manifestations appear usually after the diarrhea. The patients complain of a burning sensation of the oral mucosa and tongue. Numerous minute herpetic vesicles form and soon rupture, leaving painful superficial erosions. The tongue becomes swollen and the fungiform papillae become enlarged and prominent. At times superficial cracks or aphthous-like lesions develop. These lingual symptoms have given rise to the term "sprue tongue." Angular cheilosis is common. In general the oral mucosal lesions associated with sprue are similar to those observed in B complex deficiency.

The oral lesions respond to the general therapy of the disease and the institution of satisfactory oral hygienic measures.

GOUT—GOUTY ARTHRITIS

Gout is a form of recurring arthritis which is associated with disturbed purine metabolism. The exact etiology is unknown.

About 5% of all "arthritis patients" have gout and approximately 95% of those afflicted with this disease are males. It is uncommon before 35 years of age. Patients who have gout are usually overweight. Many but not all consume abnormally large amounts of alcohol, meats and purine-containing foods. Some give a history of a hereditary tendency.

The typical attack of gout is characterized by severe pain which is characteristically localized in the big toe but the ankle, wrist or finger may be affected. The patient is awakened from sleep by the pain or he notices it early in the morning. The involved joint soon becomes swollen, red and exquisitely tender. Fever may or may not be present.

The acute attack lasts a week or 10 days at which time all the symptoms may disappear. With repeated attacks, which may be precipitated by excessive physical exertion, the use of certain medicines or dietary indiscretions, the joints fail to recover completely and some pain, stiffness and deformity persist. Later in the disease the characteristic gouty tophi develop. Tophi are hard nodular swellings composed of sodium urate crystals. They are found most often about the margins of the ears, over the olecranon region and occasionally about the joints. Large tophi at times ulcerate through the overlying soft tissues.

Laboratory aids to the diagnosis of gout include x-ray examinations and blood chemistry findings. During the acute stage of the disease, the x-ray findings are negative but after repeated attacks osseous tophi can be demonstrated as punched out areas in the bones of the fingers and the toes. A blood uric acid level of over 1 mg. per 100 cc. of whole blood in a patient with symptoms of gout confirms the clinical impression. In chronic gout the blood uric acid may reach 8 to 10 mg. per 100 cc.

Diagnosis is made on the basis of the history, the physical and laboratory findings. In doubtful cases a therapeutic test with colchicine may be used. This drug spectacularly relieves the pain of acute gout but it is ineffective in other forms of arthritis with which gout may be confused. Gout is treated in the acute state by rest of the affected part and the administration of colchicine or salicylic acid. During the chronic stage a low purine diet and a moderate regime of living are advised.

There is no known relationship between gout and focal infection or gout and diseases of the oral tissues.

THE XANTHOMATOSES—DISEASES OF LIPOID METABOLISM

The xanthomatoses are of dental interest, as oral symptoms and lesions are often the first evidence of the disease. The xanthomatoses are due to a constitutional defect in lipoid metabolism which results in lipoids overflowing into the blood stream. The elimination of these lipoid substances however is more difficult than the hyperglycemia in diabetes. Since the lipoids are normally handled by the reticulo-endothelial cells, we find that the organs comprised of large numbers of these cells, such as the liver and spleen, show the most marked changes. These granulomatous masses of lipoid cells produce pressure symptoms, result in dysfunction of the involved organs and produce at times osteoporotic areas in the bones.

Schüller-Christian's disease, Gaucher's disease and Nieman-Picks disease will be discussed. They are associated with faulty cholesterol, kerasin and phospholecithin metabolism respectfully.

Schüller-Christian's Disease

Schüller-Christian's disease may be regarded as a chronic osseous form of xanthomatosis, with a predilection for Jewish males. It occurs usually in young individuals, although all ages may be affected.

The diagnostic triad for Schüller-Christian's disease consists of: (1) exophthalmos—due to lipoid-containing cells in the circumorbital tissues, (2) diabetes insipidus—due to derangement of the function of the posterior

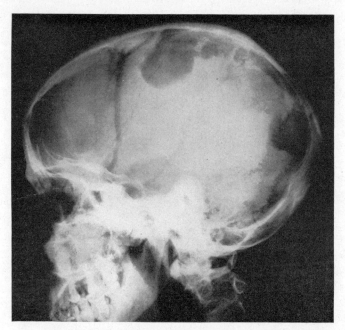

Fig. 210. Skull of a patient with Schüller-Christian's disease. No dental changes were noted in this case.

pituitary and (3) defects in the membranous bones. Like Hutchinson's triad, all these symptoms are rarely observed in a particular case.

The characteristic lesions of the skull consist of a moth-eaten appearance of the bone with sharply defined borders and a complete loss of trabecular structure in the area of the lesions. Subperiosteal swellings are also observed.

Oral Aspects. The oral manifestations many times develop early in the course of the disease, causing the individual to seek dental advice. A gingivostomatitis which is often mistaken for a fusospirochetosis is commonly present. The gums become increasingly spongy and swollen but ulceration is not an outstanding symptom. There are progressive loosening and exfoliation of the teeth resulting from the replacement of the bony supporting tissues by the xanthomatous granuloma. The "pus" seen in advanced cases is high in cholesterol and this crystalline substance can be readily identified.

In cases of obscure, persistent jaw pain without apparent clinical cause, dental x-rays may reveal areas of bone rarefaction apart from the tooth apexes. When the granulomatous areas are more closely associated with the teeth, they have been mistaken for cysts. The contents of these lesions have a fatty appearance and consistency which permit ready differentiation from the common dental granuloma. Histologic examination of the tissue will prove valuable in doubtful cases. Tooth vitality tests are as a rule within the normal range of values.

Diagnosis is made on the basis of the clinical findings, the x-ray and biopsy studies. When unusual radiolucent areas are noted in the jaws which are associated with vital teeth, or which are apart from the apex of the tooth, the possibility of a xanthomatous granuloma should be considered. The granulomatous masses in the jaws offer favorable sites to obtain material for biopsy studies. This condition must be differentiated from Paget's disease, multiple myeloma, osteitis fibrosa cystica, malignant growths and ameloblastomas.

Loose teeth should be removed and good oral hygiene established by conservative means in patients with Schüller-Christian's disease before deep x-ray therapy is administered. The general prognosis as far as life is concerned is good.

Gaucher's Disease

Gaucher's disease occurs next in frequency to Schüller-Christian's disease. It occurs predominantly in the Jewish race and shows a 2:1 predominance for females. The general symptoms consist of splenomegaly and hepatomegaly and a brown discoloration of the skin. During the later stages of the disease, there is a leukopenia, anemia and thrombocytopenia. Gross skeletal bone involvement and pain are rare. Bleeding from the nose and oral cavity is a common symptom. It is due to the secondary thrombocytopenia. The diagnosis is made on the basis of the physical findings, the x-ray and biopsy studies. Good oral hygiene should be established. When hemorrhagic phenomena are absent, teeth may be extracted without danger. While there is no specific treatment for Gaucher's disease the prognosis is fair.

Oral Aspects. Bender described the dental changes in Gaucher's disease and has since confirmed his original observations by additional case reports. There is a general porosity of the jaw bones. Large rarefactions having a cyst-like appearance in the mandible (molar, premolar and rarely the mental region) and in the maxilla (premolar area) are characteristic findings. Areas of abnormal bone porosity apart from the tooth apexes or those associated with vital teeth are also common. Biopsy studies of these areas have revealed the presence of the typical Gaucher's cells. In the x-rays the long bones appear less opaque, coarse grained and "worm eaten."

Niemann-Pick's Disease

Niemann-Pick's disease, which is associated with disturbances of phospholecithin metabolism, occurs usually in infants. It runs an acute and fatal course. No dental changes have been reported.

REFERENCES

THE VITAMINS

Barker, L. F.: Diagnosis and treatment of vitamin deficiencies, J. Iowa Med. Soc., 30:1-8, 1940.

Black, A.: Recent work in vitamin therapy, South. Med. & Surg., 102: 609, 1940.

Boyle, P. E.: Effect of various dietary deficiencies on the periodontal tissues of the guinea pig and man, J. A. D. A., 28:1788, 1941.

Cayer, D., et al.: Clinical significance of glossitis and cheilosis •in deficiencies, South. M. J., 38:11, 1945.

Fancher, O. E., J. C. Calandra, & L. S. Fosdick: The effect of vitamins on acid formation in saliva, J. Dent. Research, 23:23, 1944.

Faust, Homer E.: Effects of vitamins A, C, and D on teeth, J. Dent. for Children, 10:87, 1943.

Fosdick, L. S., & E. H. Hatton: Effect of vitamins on susceptibility to caries, Illinois Dent. J., 7:302, 1938.

Goldman, H. M.: Report of histopathologic study of jaws of diet-deficiency in monkeys, and its relation to Vincent's infection, Am. J. Orthodontics (Oral Surg. Sect.), 29:480-8, 1943.

Jeghers, Harold: Nutrition: The appearance of the tongue as an index of nutritional deficiency, New England J. Med., 227:221, 1942.

Kaufman, W. H., & D. C. Smith: Cutaneous changes in the sprue syndrome, J. A. M. A., 121:168, 1943.

Kelly, Herbert T.: Appraise vitamin formulas and not titles, Pennsylvania M. J., 46:961, 1943.

Lapira, E.: Ulcerative stomatitis associated with avitaminosis in Malta, Brit. Dent. J., 74:257, 1943.

Spies, T. D., A. P. Swain, & J. M. Grant: Clinically associated deficiency diseases, Am. J. M. Sc., 200:536, 1940.

Thompson, D. L.: Twelve principles of nutrition, New York J. Dent., 13:225-31, 1943.

Tomlinson, T. H.: Oral pathology in monkeys in various experimental dietary deficiencies, Pub. Health Rep., 54:431, 1939.

Topping, N. H., & H. F. Fraser: Mouth lesions associated with dietary deficiencies in monkeys, Pub. Health Rep., 54:416, 1939.

Youmans, J. B.: Nutritional Deficiencies, Philadelphia, J. B. Lippincott Co., 1941.

Vitamin A

Burn, C. G.: Changes in the structure of the developing tooth in rats maintained on a diet deficient in vitamin A, Yale J. Biol. & Med., 13:817, 1941.

Council on Dental Therapeutics: J. A. D. A., 27:1986, 1940.

Mellanby, H.: Effect of maternal dietary deficiency of vitamin A on dental tissues in rats, J. Dent. Research, 20:489, 1941.

Orten, A. N., C. G. Burn, & A. H. Smith: Vitamin A deficiency and the enamel organ, Proc. Exp. Soc. Biol. & Med., 36:82, 1937.

Schour, I., M. M. Hoffman, & M. C. Smith: Changes in the incisor teeth of albino rats with vitamin A deficiency and the effects of replacement therapy, Am. J. Path., 17:529, 1941.

Steffens, Lincoln: Dark adaptation and dietary deficiency in vitamin A, Am. J. Ophth., 23:1325, 1940.
Swift, B. H.: Relation of vitamin A to leukoplakia, J. Obst. & Gynec. Brit. Emp., 43:1053, 1936.
Thorson, J. A.: Nutritional xerophthalmia, J. A. M. A., 103:1438, 1934.

Vitamin B

Adams, W. E., & W. Robinson: Trigeminal neuralgia, Lancet, 2:555, 1941.
Borsook, H., M. Y. Kremers, & C. G. Wiggins: The relief of symptoms of major trigeminal neuralgia (tic douloureux), J. A. M. A., 114:1421, 1940.
Calder, R. M., & G. P. Kerby: The effect of nicotinic acid on blood coagulation, Am. J. M. Sc., 200:590, 1940.
Cantor, M. M., & John W. Scott: Effect of vitamin B_6 (pyridoxine) in the treatment of leukopenia and granulocytopenia of toxic origin in humans. Preliminary report, Science, 100:545, 1944.
Clarke, A. G., & F. Prescott: Studies in vitamin B deficiency, Brit. M. J., 2:503, 1943.
Damianovich, J., & R. Ravizzoli: Nicotinic acid and aphthous stomatitis, Arch. Dermat. & Syph., 48:66, 1943.
Ellenburg, M., & H. Pollack: Pseudoariboflavinosis, J. A. M. A., 119:790, 1942.
Elvehjem, C. A.: The water soluble vitamins, J. A. M. A., 120:1388, 1942.
Finnerud, Clark W.: Perlèche: Its nosologic status, J. A. M. A., 126:737, 1944.
Goldberg, L., & J. M. Thorp: Nicotinic acid excretion in normal men and in cases of Vincent's gingivitis, South African J. M. Sc., 7:85, 1942.
Jolliffe, N.: Newer knowledge of the vitamin B complex, Bull. New York Acad. Med., 17:195-204, 1941.
Jones, H. E., T. G. Armstrong, H. F. Green, & V. Chadwick: Stomatitis due to riboflavin deficiency, Lancet, 1:720, 1944.
Katzenellenbogen, I.: Nicotinic acid in the treatment of endemic glossitis, Dent. Rec., 60:34, 1940.
King, J. D.: Vincent's disease treated with nicotinic acid, Lancet, 2:32, 1940.
Kniesner, A. H., A. W. Mann, & T. D. Spies: Relationship of dental caries to deficiencies of the vitamin B group, J. Dent. Research, 21:259-62, 1942.
Mann, Arvin W.: Nutrition as it affects the teeth, M. Clin. North America, 27:545, 1943.
Martin, H., & C. E. Koop: Precancerous mouth lesions of avitaminosis B; their etiology, response to therapy and relationship to intra-oral cancer, Am. J. Surg., 57:195, 1942.
Najjar, V. A., & L. E. Holt: Studies in thiamine excretion, Bull. Johns Hopkins Hosp., 67:107, 1940.
Nippert, P. H., *et al.*: Riboflavin deficiency versus Perlèche: differential diagnosis of fissuring of labial commissures, Georgia M. A. J., 32:295, 1943.
Riddle, J. W., T. D. Spies, & N. P. Hudson: Unpublished observations— cited by Spies, T. D., *et al.* Endemic riboflavin deficiency, Am. J. M. Sc., 200:697, 1940.

Rose, A. S., & B. M. Jacobson: Treatment of trigeminal neuralgia with vitamin B_1, Arch. Neurol. & Psychiat., **44**:1307, 1941.

Sebrell, William H.: The clinical symptoms and signs of vitamin B complex deficiency, Ann. Int. Med., **15**:953, 1941.

Sebrell, W. H., & R. E. Butler: Riboflavin deficiency in man, Pub. Health Rep., **53**:2282, 1938.

Sebrell, W. H., et al.: Human riboflavin requirements estimated by urinary excretion of subjects on a controlled intake, Pub. Health Rep., **56**:570, 1941.

Shields, Wm. P.: Riboflavin deficiency, New England J. Med., **223**:215, 1940.

Sinclair, J. A.: Vitamin A and B deficiency in Vincent's infection, J. A. D. A., **26**:1611, 1939.

Smith, S. F.: Regional injection of thiamine chloride in herpes zoster, J. M. Soc. New Jersey, **38**:396, 1941.

Spies, Tom D., et al.: Endemic riboflavin deficiency in infants and children, Am. J. M. Sc., **200**:697, 1940.

Spies, T. D., C. Cooper, & M. A. Blankenhorn: The use of nicotinic acid in the treatment of pellagra, J. A. M. A., **110**:622, 1938.

Stannus, H. S.: Some problems in riboflavin and allied deficiencies, Brit. M. J., **29**:140, 1944.

Sydenstricker, V. P., et al.: Riboflavin deficiency in human subjects, J. A. M. A., **113**:1697-1700, 1939.

Sydenstricker, V. P.: Nicotinic acid and riboflavin deficiency, Ann. Int. Med., **14**:1499, 1941.

Vitamin C

Bromer, R. S.: A critical analysis of the roentgen signs of infantile scurvy, Am. J. Roentgenol., **49**:575, 1943.

Burril, D. Y.: Relationship of blood plasma vitamin C level to gingival and periodontal disease, J. Dent. Research, **21**:353, 1942.

Campbell, H. G., & R. P. Cook: Incidence and treatment of "gingivitis" at the Dundee Dental Hospital, Brit. Dent. J., **72**:213, 1942.

Conwit, M. I.: Scurvy—scorbutus, Dent. Outlook, **29**:450-3, 1942.

Crandon, T. H., et al.: Experimental human scurvy, New England J. Med., **223**:353, 1940.

Day, C. D. M.: A consideration of latent scurvy and its relation to dental defects, Dental Cosmos, **76**:291, 1934.

Fish, E. W., & L. J. Harris: Vitamin C deficiency effects on tooth structure in guinea pigs, Brit. Dent. J., **58**:3, 1935.

Hanke, M. T.: Diet and Dental Health, Univ. of Chicago Press, Chicago, 1933.

Hanke, M. T., et al.: Nutritional studies on children. The effect upon gingivitis of adding orange and lemon juice to the diet, Dental Cosmos, **75**:570, 1933.

Hanke, M. T., et al.: Relation of diet to general health and particularly to inflammation of the oral tissues and dental caries, J. A. D. A., **17**:957, 1930.

Hirschfeld, I.: Scurvy; report on 3 cases in adults, J. A. D. A., **16**:796, 1929.

Hojer, A.: Tooth changes in scurvy, Acta. Pediat., **2**:8, 1942.

Hunt, A. L.: The role of vitamin C in wound healing, Brit. J. Surg., 28: 436, 1941.

King, J. D., & A. B. Francklyn: Gingival disease in Gibraltar evacuee children, Lancet, 1:495, 1944.

Kruse, H. D.: The gingival manifestations of avitaminosis C, with especial consideration of the detection of early changes by biomicroscopy, Milbank Memorial Fund Quart., 20:290, 1942.

Levcowich, T., & E. L. Batchelder: Ascorbic acid excretion at known levels of intake as related to capillary resistance, dietary estimates and human requirements, J. Nutrition, 23:399-408, 1942.

McMillan, R. B.: Scurvy: A survey of fifty-three cases, Brit. M. J., 1:234, 1944.

Pijoan, M., & E. L. Lozner: The physiologic significance of vitamin C in man, New England J. Med., 231:14, 1944.

Radusch, Dorothy F.: Vitamin C in periodontal disease, J. A. D. A., 29: 1652, 1942.

Radusch, D. F.: Relation between periodontal condition and certain dietary factors, J. Dent. Research, 18:305, 1939.

Restarski, J. S., & M. Pijoan: Gingivitis and vitamin C, J. A. D. A., 31:1323, 1944.

Ruskin, S. L.: The influence of vitamin C on Wassermann fastness in syphilis, Am. J. Digest. Dis., 10:170, 1943.

Stuhl, Frederick: Vitamin-C subnutrition in gingivostomatitis, Lancet, 1:640, 1943.

Wohlback, S. B., & P. E. Howe: Intercellular substances in experimental scorbutus, Arch. Path. & Lab. Med., 1:1, 1926.

Vitamin D

Anderson, B. G.: Developmental enamel defects, Am. J. Dis. Child., 63:154, 1942.

Anderson, B. G., & V. O. Hurme: Malocclusion in a group of postrachitic adolescent children, Am. J. Orthodontics & Oral Surg., 26:119, 1940.

Becks, H.: Dangerous effects of vitamin D overdosage on dental and paradental structures, J. A. D. A., 29:1947, 1942.

Brodsky, R. H., B. Schick, & H. Vollmer: Prevention of dental caries by massive doses of Vitamin D, Am. J. Dis. Child., 62:1183-87, 1941.

East, B. R.: Sunshine and incidence of dental caries, Am. J. Pub. Health, 29:777, 1939.

Eliot, Martha M., et al.: A study of the teeth of a group of school children previously examined for rickets, Am. J. Dis. Child., 48:713, 1934.

Hatfield, H. K.: A preliminary study of the effect of rickets on the jaws, Internat. J. Orthodontia, 5:367, 1919.

Henningsen, M. G.: Caries free individuals, J. California State Dent. Assn., 17:1, 1941.

McBeath, E. C.: Experiments on dietary control of dental caries in children, J. Dent. Research, 12:723-47, 1932.

McBeath, E. C., & W. A. Verlin: Further studies on the role of vitamin D in the nutritional control of dental caries in children, J. A. D. A., 29:1393, 1942.

McCauley, H. B.: Significance of radioactive isotopes in dental research, J. A. D. A., 29:1219, 1942.

Robinson, H. B. G.: Dental caries and metabolism of calcium, J. A. D. A., 30:357, 1943.

Schour, Isaac: Vitamin D, and calcium and phosphorous compounds in dental therapy, Univ. of Ill. Committee on Pharm. & Therap. Bull. No. 13, 1942.

Taylor, G. F., & C. D. M. Day: Relation of vitamin D and mineral deficiencies to dental caries, Brit. M. J., 1:919-21, 1939.

Taylor, G. F., & C. D. M. Day: Osteomalacia and dental caries, Brit. M. J., 2:221, 1940.

Volker, J. F.: Tooth metabolism as indicated by studies with radio-active phosphorus, Dentistry, 4:224, 1943.

Vitamins K and P

Calandra, J. C., O. E. Fancher, & L. S. Fosdick: The effect of synthetic vitamin K and related compounds on the rate of acid formation in saliva, J. Dent. Research, 23:31-39, 1944.

Editorial: Vitamin P, Am. J. Orthodontics & Oral Surg., 29:239-40, 1943.

Elmby, A., & E. Warburg: The inadequacy of synthetic vitamin C as an antiscorbutic agent, Lancet, 2:1353, 1937.

Graham, J. W.: Oral manifestations of vitamin deficiency, J. Canad. Dent. A., 7:7, 1941.

Higby, R. H.: Chemical nature of hesperidin and its experimental medical use as source of vitamin P—review, J. Am. Pharm. A., 30:629-35, 1941 (Scient. Ed.).

Jersild, T.: Therapeutic effect of vitamin P in Schonlein-Henoch's purpura, Lancet, 1:1445, 1938.

Kugelmass, I. N.: Vitamin P in vascular purpura, J. A. M. A., 115:519-20, 1940.

Mead, S. V.: Studies of the effect of ingestion of citrus fruit upon gingival hemorrhage, J. Dent. Research, 23:73-78, 1944.

Rapaport, H. G.: Vitamin P and capillary fragility, J. Pediat., 18:321-7, 1941.

Raunert, M.: Die blutstillende Wirkung des citrins (P-vitamins), Ztschr. f. Urol., 32:630-3, 1938.

Scarborough, H.: Deficiency of vitamin C and vitamin P in man, Lancet, 2:644-7, 1940.

Scarborough, H., & C. P. Stewart: Effect of hesperidin (vitamin P) on capillary fragility, Lancet, 2:610, 1938.

Scarborough, H.: Vitamin P, Biochem. J., 33:1400-07, 1939.

Waddell, W. W., & DuPont Guerry: Effect of vitamin K on the clotting time of the prothrombin and the blood, J. A. M. A., 112:2259, 1939.

Wawra, C. Z., & J. L. Webb: The isolation of a new oxidation-reduction enzyme from lemon peel (vitamin P), Science, 96:302, 1942.

Weir, James F., H. R. Butt, & A. M. Snell: Further observations on clinical use of vitamin K, Am. J. Digest. Dis., 7:485, 1940.

DISEASES OF METABOLISM
Diabetes

Aiguier, J. E.: The dental care of the diabetic patient, J. New York Acad. Dent., 2:99, 1935.

Aleman, I., & I. Uleia: New ideas on the oral lesions of diabetes, Rev. de stomatol., 37:595, 1935.

Baker, T. W.: A clinical survey of 108 consecutive cases of diabetic coma, Arch. Int. Med., 58:373, 1936.

Beardwood, J. T., Jr.: Modern diabetic care, Pennsylvania M. J., 44:1022, 1941.

Blaustein, S.: Observations of anesthesia and exodontia for the diabetic, J. Second District Dent. Soc., New York, 25:413, 1940.

Blaustein, S.: New nitrous oxide technic for dental surgery in diabetes mellitus, Anesth. & Analg., 19:345, 1940.

Blaustein, S., & E. Ferguson: Dental cooperation in diabetes mellitus, J. Lab. & Clin. Med., 25:47, 1939.

Brizi, C.: Rapporti tra il diabetec il cavo orale, Stomatol. ital., 2:409, 1940.

Brucker, M.: The endocrine glands and the teeth, Dent. Items of Interest, 55:186-90, 1933.

Duncan, G. G.: Diabetic coma, Pennsylvania M. J., 44:725, 1941.

Dysart, B. R.: Diabetic gangrene involving the sinuses, Arch. Otolaryng., 41:143, 1945.

Gore, J. T.: Saliva and enamel decalcification, J. Dent. Research, 20:107-15, 1941.

Greene, J. A., et al.: Control of diabetes mellitus, relation to healing of clean and infected wounds and to incidence of infection in clean wounds, J. A. M. A., 115:1518, 1940.

Gundersen, E.: Is diabetes of infectious origin?, J. Infect. Dis., 41:197-202, 1927.

Hector, G. A., & D. G. Evans: Dental agenesis in the presence of diabetes mellitus, Dent. Cosmos, 74:986, 1932.

Hirschfeld, I.: Periodontal symptoms associated with diabetes, J. Periodontology, 5:37-47, 1934.

Holcomb, B.: Influence of focal infections in diabetes as shown by alterations of blood sugar curve, J. Lab. & Clin. Med., 11:874-78, 1926.

Kent, H. A.: Dental service for diabetics, New York State J. Med., 33:1083, 1933.

Millett, Joseph: Diabetic gangrene of the face, J. A. D. A., 112:1143, 1939.

N. Y. Institute of Clinical Oral Pathology: Osteomyelitis associated with diabetes. Case report, Arch. Clin. Oral Path., 1:223, 1937.

Niles, J. G.: Early recognition of diabetes mellitus through interstitial alveolar resorption, Dental Cosmos, 74:161-64, 1932.

Osborne, O. T.: Question of diabetes caused by oral infection, New York State M. J., 2:20, 1918.

Ralli, E. P.: Teeth in diabetes—problem in nutrition, Ann. Dent., 4:129, 1938.

Rathery, F., & L. Binet: Saliva in diabetics, Presse méd., 28:363, 1920.

Rosenthal, L. S.: The gums in diabetes, Dent. Record, 49:489, 1929.

Rudy, A., & M. M. Cohen: The oral aspects of diabetes mellitus, New England J. Med., 219:503, 1938.

Rudy, A., & R. Hoffman: Skin disturbances in diabetes mellitus, New England J. Med., **227**:893, 1942.
Rutledge, C. E.: Oral and roentgenographic aspects of the teeth and jaws of juvenile diabetics, J. A. D. A., **27**:1740, 1940.
Simon, F. J.: The glucose content of human saliva, Dental Cosmos, **68**:622, 1926.
Vaccari, A.: Buccodental changes in diabetes, Stomatol., **36**:398, 1938.
Williams, J. B.: Diabetic periodontovlasia, J. A. D. A., **15**:523, 1928.
Zilz, J.: Statistical observations on diabetes and pyorrhea alveolaris, Dent. Cosmos, **57**:102-03, 1915.
Ziskin, D. E., *et al.:* Diabetes in relation to certain oral and systemic problems, J. Dent. Research, **23**:317, 1944.

Other Diseases of Metabolism

Bender, I. B.: Dental observations in Gaucher's disease, J. Dent. Res., **17**: 359, 1938.
Cecil, R. L.: Diagnosis and treatment of gout, Northwest Med., **40**:411-14, 1941.
Isaacs, R., C. C. Sturgis, & M. Smith: Treatment of pernicious anemia, J. A. M. A., **91**:1687, 1928.
Kaufman, W. H., & Dudley C. Smith: Cutaneous changes in the sprue syndrome, J. A. M. A., **121**:168, 1943.
Levine, S., & L. Solis-Cohen: Gaucher's disease, Am. J. Roentgenol. & Rad. Therapy, **50**:765, 1943.
Schüller, A.: Diagnosis of Schüller-Christian's disease, Brit. J. Radiology, **12**:225, 1939.
Tassman, G. C., & I. B. Bender: Report of a case of Gaucher's disease, J. A. D. A., **27**:1268, 1940.
Tucker, John: Hand-Schüller-Christian disease, Cleveland Clinic Quart., **10**:55, 1943.
Versiani, O., J. M. Figueiro, & M. A. Junqueira: Hand-Schüller-Christian's syndrome and "eosinophilic or solitary granuloma of bone," Am. J. Med. Sc., **207**:161, 1944.

DISEASES OF THE BLOOD AND BLOOD-FORMING ORGANS

21

The Blood Dyscrasias

GENERAL CONSIDERATIONS	HEREDITARY HEMORRHAGIC TELAN-
MALIGNANT NEUTROPENIA	GIECTASIA
THE LEUKEMIAS	THE PURPURAS
HEMOPHILIA	POLYCYTHEMIA
PSEUDOHEMOPHILIA	PRIMARY ERYTHROBLASTIC ANEMIA

GENERAL CONSIDERATIONS

In spite of the rarity of the blood dyscrasias they are of considerable dental importance since the dentist is frequently consulted first for the treatment of the gingival hypertrophy, the bleeding gums or the ulcerative lesions. The early diagnosis of certain of these diseases, such as the leukemias, is only of academic interest at present as effective curative treatment is not known. Dental operations on these patients are ill-advised and they result often in a fulminating spread of the painful ulcerative lesions. While the dentist may not be blamed directly for this unfavorable turn of events, at best he may be criticized for not realizing the true nature of the oral lesion.

On the other hand, an early diagnosis of malignant neutropenia (agranulocytosis) may be life saving. The dangers of extracting teeth in hemophiliacs are well known, but a history of being a "bleeder" is often discounted by the dentist because of the rarity of this disease.

The dentist should always be on the alert for lesions which might be due to one of these diseases. From the practicing dentist's viewpoint the incidence of oral lesions in the blood dyscrasias is high. They deserve serious consideration in any patient who has a persistent gingival hypertrophy, ulcerogangrenous lesions or persistent bleeding from the gums or tooth extraction wounds. A determination of the bleeding and clotting times or a complete blood count are simple procedures which can be performed in the dentist's office. They will usually establish the diagnosis or will give the dentist more confidence in the local treatment of obscure ulcerative lesions of the oral mucosa and the gingival tissues.

MALIGNANT NEUTROPENIA (AGRANULOCYTOSIS—AGRANULOCYTIC ANGINA)

Malignant neutropenia or agranulocytosis is a syndrome characterized by ulcerative lesions of the oral and pharyngeal mucosa accompanied frequently by malaise, fever and splenomegaly. It was first described in 1922 by Schultz. The circulating granulocytes are always markedly reduced in number.

The attention of the dental profession was first called to this disease by Appleton. The initial lesions are commonly found in the mouth and as a consequence the patient seeks dental treatment first. The extraction of teeth in a patient with malignant neutropenia may result in a fatality. It is important for the dentist to differentiate the lesions of agranulocytosis from those of oral fusospirochetal infection before instituting treatment.

Accurate figures on the incidence of malignant neutropenia are not available but in a three-year period ending in 1934 the number of deaths due to this disease in the United States was over 1,500. The incidence would be undoubtedly higher if there was accurate reporting of all deaths.

The disease is most common in women over 30 years of age. It occurs rarely in the colored race and when present it is usually related to arsphenamine administration. Givan and Shapiro reported 29 cases of agranulocytosis occurring in children, most of which followed an acute infectious disease.

Malignant neutropenia is peculiar in that it is more prevalent in the well-to-do. It is uncommon in the municipal clinics and charity hospitals. It is about 8 times more common among the so-called professional group of physicians, dentists, interns, nurses and technicians. Kracke suggests that this may be the result of "oversampling of samples." The geographic distribution of the disease is closely related to the consumption of synthetic drugs.

Etiology

There are four general etiologic theories for this syndrome, namely: (1) bacterial, (2) dietary deficiency, (3) hormonal dysfunction and (4) chemical or drug allergy or idiosyncrasy.

While it is well known that certain infectious diseases such as typhoid fever and influenza will produce a leukopenia, all attempts to substantiate this theory by means of animal inoculations with bacteria or bacterial toxins have been unsuccessful. Ulcerative stomatitis has been produced in dogs fed a nicotinic acid-free diet, but the hematologic findings in these animals were characteristic for aplastic anemia and they failed to develop an absolute drop in the granulocyte count.

Leukopenia is associated commonly with hormonal disturbances such as adrenal cortical deficiency. The onset of malignant neutropenia is related to menstruation and in some individuals a regular cyclic agranulopenia is observed at each menstrual period. This cyclic agranulocytosis was so severe in one case observed by the author that x-ray sterilization was performed in a 30-year-old patient. Thompson has reported 18 cases of agranulocytic angina in young women in which the subjective symptoms occurred within a day or two of the onset of the menstrual flow and all the patients were menstruating at the time of admission. The patients in this group were in the habit of taking drugs at this time which may have been a factor in causing the low granulocyte count.

The first case of agranulocytosis related to drug administration (acetphenetidin) was reported in 1930. Numerous cases of agranulocytic angina following the administration of a wide variety of drugs were observed thereafter. Amidopyrine, or proprietary products containing this drug, were responsible for the majority of the cases. Madison and Squier gave a small dose of amidopyrine to two patients who had recovered from agranulocytosis associated previously with the use of this drug. There was a marked drop in the leukocyte count and a recurrence of the typical agranulocytic attack. Plum gave 3 grs. of amidopyrine to a recovered patient and in $1\frac{1}{2}$ hours the leukocyte count dropped from 9,000 to 1,900 leukocytes per cu. mm. and remained at this level for 24 hours.

Attempts to produce malignant neutropenia in animals by the administration of this drug have been discouraging. Later studies have shown that the oxidation products of amidopyrine which are produced in the human intestinal tract, catechol and quinone, will produce a marked drop in the granulocytes when administered to animals.

Agranulocytosis follows occasionally the administration of gold salts or arsenic preparations. With the recent extensive use of the sulfonamides, there have appeared numerous instances of agranulocytosis following the administration of sulfanilamide, sulfathiazole, sulfamerazine, sulfapyridine and sulfadiazine. Malignant neutropenia develops usually after considerable amounts of the sulfonamides have been taken, as a rule over 60 Gm. While the complication is infrequent, it must be considered whenever these compounds are administered. Jones and Miller reported an attack of agranulocytosis following sulfanilamide therapy in a patient who had experienced previously the same reaction with amidopyrine. Agranulocytosis secondary to the administration of quinine which was used in the treatment of therapeutically induced malaria was reported by Franks and Davis.

The lack of folic acid, a component of the vitamin B complex, results in agranulocytosis in monkeys. It cures sulfonamide-induced agranulocytosis in white rats.

A careful study of the pathosis was made by Fitz-Hugh who found that the red blood cells, the platelets or coagulating factors of the blood are not involved. The essential lesion consisted of an arrest in maturation of the myeloid series at about the myeloblastic level. In some cases, there was an accompanying arrest or non-migration of the other leukocytes into the blood stream. The ulcerative lesions which are observed clinically are the result of invasion by opportunist bacteria into tissues without adequate cellular defense.

Symptoms

In the first cases described by Schultz the syndrome was characterized by a severe gangrenous stomatitis, a changed blood picture and systemic symptoms of fever, malaise and splenomegaly. The onset of clinical symptoms may be sudden or gradual. The patient complains on many occasions of a gradually increasing weakness which is complicated later by the more acute ulcerative lesions of the mouth and throat. Fever, malaise, and headache are common.

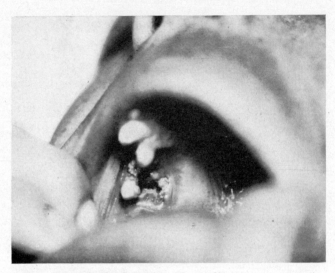

Fig. 211. Oral ulcerations in malignant neutropenia. The patient requested the removal of the retained roots in the ulcerated area. W.B.C. 1,750 cu. mm. with polymorphonuclear neutrophiles 2%. Case responded satisfactorily to liver therapy and pentnucleotides. (More modern treatment pyridoxine HCl and penicillin.)

The general symptoms often are passed off as "grippe" or "flu." The systemic symptoms are usually out of all proportion to the extent of the oral lesions.

In a series of cases studied by the author, over 80% of the patients gave a history of boils or carbuncles during the weeks prior to the clinical onset of the disease. In the female, the clinical onset was frequently coincident with or aggravated by the menstrual period.

The typical oral lesions consist of irregular-shaped necrotic areas which may or may not be contiguous with the gingival tissues. The ulcers have a dirty gray or even black appearance which aids in differentiating them from those commonly seen in fusospirochetal stomatitis. There is little inflammatory reaction about the margins of the lesions due to the lack of granulocytes in the circulating blood. Hemorrhage from the gingival tissues is common and herpetic lesions are occasionally present on the lips or cheeks. The odor from the mouth in cases with extensive oral lesions is characteristic of decomposing tissue. Ptyalism is common. Local adenopathy of varying degrees may be present.

The patient believes in many instances that the oral ulcerations are the result of retained root fragments or carious teeth and they will request their extraction. The peculiar appearance of the ulcers, the lack of inflammatory reaction about their margins and the accompanying systemic manifestations should suggest the true nature of the condition. To extract teeth in a patient with malignant neutropenia is to court serious consequences.

It is possible to have the typical hematologic findings of malignant neutropenia without the development of oral lesions. The oral lesions are the result, not the cause, of the hematologic findings.

Diagnosis

Diagnosis can be made on the basis of the clinical history, the appearance of the lesions, and the differential blood count which shows an absolute or relative decrease in granulocytes. The red cell count and hemoglobin are usually within normal range of values.

Laboratory Aids to Diagnosis

A positive diagnosis cannot be made, regardless of the typical clinical symptoms, without a complete blood count. All surgery should be postponed until this has been done. The characteristic hematologic findings include an absence of young granulocytes, a decrease in the number of the granulocytes and at times their complete disappearance. The red cell count and the hemoglobin, which are usually within the normal range of values, aid in differentiating this disease from an aleukemic phase of leukemia. Appleton observed that cases which terminated fatally also had a decreased lymphocyte count.

The bacteriologic smear is of little diagnostic significance. Fusospirochetal organisms are found less frequently than one would expect from the clinical picture, but at times the smear may be typical for a fusospirochetal infection. Anaerobic bacteriologic studies in malignant neutropenia have been incomplete.

Differential Diagnosis. The differential diagnosis should include a consideration of acute follicular tonsillitis with ulceration, fusospirochetal angina, noma, infectious mononucleosis, diphtheria and diabetic gangrene.

Treatment

Malignant neutropenia requires prompt and energetic treatment. All drugs which might cause this disease, with the possible exception of the sulfonamides, should be stopped immediately. Dameshek and Wolfson made a preliminary report in 1942 on the successful treatment of this disease with sulfathiazole. Heilig and Visveswar treated the disease successfully with sulfapyridine and more recently Eckert et al. reported several cases of agranulocytosis in which the successful outcome was believed to be due to the administration of large amounts of sulfadiazine. Eckert et al. believed that the bone marrow depression associated with "sulfa" drug administration is temporary and that, if the infectious processes are held in check during this temporary depression, the chances of recovery are greater. Several of their patients had already received from 52 to 72 Gm. of sulfadiazine, yet a blood level of 10-20 mg./100 cc. blood was maintained during the time of the temporary bone marrow depression until the normal protective mechanisms were again functioning.

Transfusions are given frequently to tide the patient over until measures directed at stimulating granulocyte maturation or production again become operative. The intramuscular injection of sodium pentnucleotide 40 cc. per day plus injections of liver extract are believed to be beneficial. Ruskin reported adenylic acid to be the factor in the pentnucleotides which produces the clinical improvement. He advised the use of adenylic acid for the treatment of malignant neutropenia.

Keefer *et al.* and Smith *et al.* reported the successful treatment of three cases of agranulocytosis with penicillin. The penicillin controlled the secondary infection and allowed spontaneous leukocyte regeneration to occur. In one case, the agranulocytosis was associated with sulfonamide therapy and in the other two with mapharsen treatment.

Cantor and Scott treated three cases of agranulocytic angina with intravenously administered pyridoxine hydrochloride (B_6). The precipitating factor in one case was sulfathiazole, in the second it was thiouracil and in the third case there was no medication other than aspirin.

Pyridoxine hydrochloride was administered in doses of from 125 to 200 mg. daily. In each case, the temperature fell to normal limits and the symptoms disappeared within 48 hours. There was an increase in the leukocyte count and the reappearance of granulocytes. The authors suggested that pyridoxine acted by direct stimulation of the myelocytic elements of the bone marrow.

A combination of penicillin and pyridoxine may prove to be an effective treatment for this disease.

Oral treatment should be conservative. All surgical procedures, extractions or dental prophylaxis or the use of caustic drugs are contraindicated. The outcome of the oral lesions is dependent more on the general response of the patient than any local treatment. A mild alkaline mouth wash is indicated and the local lesions can be painted with crystal violet or proflavin to keep the secondary bacterial infection to a minimum. Zinc peroxide paste is effective.

Prognosis

The prognosis depends on the duration of the disease before therapy is instituted and the individual response of the patient. Jackson and Tighe reported a mortality of 35% under the most favorable conditions. If the initial reports of the successful treatment of agranulocytosis by penicillin and pyridoxine hydrochloride are borne out by additional studies, the prognosis of this disease will be more favorable. Since early diagnosis contributes materially to a favorable prognosis, the dentist can play an important rôle.

THE LEUKEMIAS

The leukemias are characterized by a marked increase in the number of the white blood cells in the circulating blood and in the tissues. Depending on which cell types are increased in number we have myelogenous, lymphatic or monocytic leukemia. The oral lesions and systemic symptoms of all types of acute leukemia are so similar that they can be advantageously considered together. In the chronic forms of the disease there is considerable variation in the duration of the different types of leukemia and in the severity of the oral lesions.

Hippocrates in 460 B.C. described a disease which may have been leukemia. "In many who have enlargement of the spleen the gums may become detached from the teeth." In 1845 the disease was recognized by John Hughes Bennet and shortly thereafter it was described independently by Virchow who called it leukemia.

The actual prevalence of leukemia is hard to determine. There are approximately 2 cases of leukemia in every 1,000 hospital admittances. The incidence is apparently increasing due largely to more accurate diagnoses. The percentage distribution of the various forms of leukemia and the frequency of oral lesions are given in Table XXIV.

TABLE XXIV

The Percentage Distribution of the Various Forms of Leukemia and Associated Oral Lesions

(Based on 455 cases)

	Age Average	Percentage Distribution	Percentage with Oral Lesions
Acute myelogenous	20	29 ⎫ 63	40
Chronic myelogenous	35	34 ⎭	
Acute lymphatic	50	7 ⎫ 27	23
Chronic lymphatic	69	20 ⎭	
Monocytic	Adolescents	3.2	87

The exact cause of leukemia in man is not known. A comparable disease in fowls has been shown to be due to a virus but human leukemia is not known to be infectious or contagious. Transfusions have been made accidentally from patients with leukemia without the disease resulting in the recipient. There is some evidence that the disease may exist as a familial trait. Six cases have been reported in one family, five being verified by necropsy studies.

The pathogenesis of all types of leukemia is essentially similar. The exact site of the abnormal (malignant?) cellular activity varies naturally in the different forms of the disease. In myelogenous leukemia, the neutrophile is usually the cell type involved, although eosinophilic and basophilic types of leukemia have been reported. The marked hyperactivity of the myeloblasts may occur without a great increase in the number of circulating leukocytes (aleukemic phase of leukemia). However, in spite of the near-normal leukocyte count there is usually an increased percentage of immature cells. In such cases bone marrow smears will reveal evidence of hyperactivity.

The Acute Leukemias (Myelogenous, Monocytic and Lymphatic Leukemia)

The symptoms of acute leukemia, particularly the myelogenous and monocytic varieties, resemble an acute infection. There are profound exhaustion,

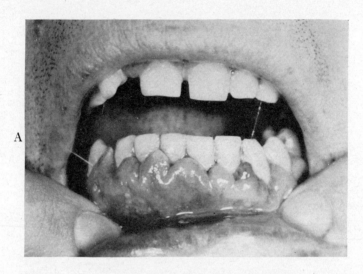

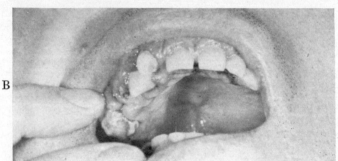

Fig. 212. (A) Gingival hypertrophy associated with myelogenous leukemia. Patient sought dental treatment for hypertrophied gums. W.B.C. 180,000 cu. m. with 92% polymorphonuclear leukocytes. (B) Gingival hypertrophy and necrosis about retained molar roots in the same patient.

fever (102° to 104° F.), diarrhea, headache and body pains. Generalized lymphadenopathy and splenomegaly may be present. Anemia is not a prominent finding in acute leukemia. At times gingival hypertrophy or ulceration, acute tonsillitis or a tonsillar abscess ushers in the disease. Purpuric manifestations in the skin, nasal and oral mucosae are observed frequently. The oral lesions may be the most serious from the patient's point of view.

Diagnosis. The diagnosis of acute leukemia is based on the suggestive clinical findings and the hemogram or bone marrow smears. A positive diagnosis cannot be made on clinical findings alone.

Oral Aspects. Patients with oral lesions associated with the acute leukemias may seek dental advice and treatment first. It is the responsibility

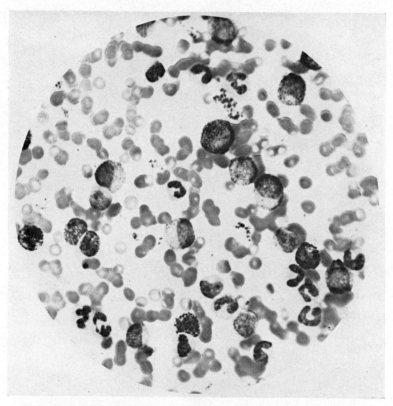

Fig. 212 (C) Blood smear. (Photograph by Wardlaw M. Hammond, Research Associate in Microscopy, School of Dentistry, University of Pennsylvania.)

of the dentist to recognize the systemic basis for the oral lesions so that he will plan his local treatment accordingly as well as refer the patient to the physician for positive diagnosis and general care. While the frequency of oral symptoms is not high when all cases of leukemia are considered, from the practicing dentist's standpoint the incidence of the oral lesions is large.

Gingival and Oral Mocosal Lesions. The oral lesions of all forms of acute leukemia are similar. They consist of a marked hypertrophy and ulceration of considerable areas of the gums. The earliest mouth lesions are seen usually in the maxillary molar region and in the lower anterior region,

446 THE BLOOD DYSCRASIAS

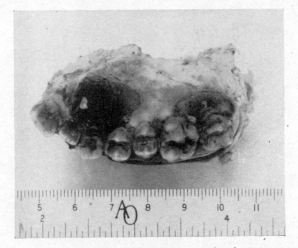

FIG. 213. Gross specimen, palatal aspect. (Burket, Am. J. Orthodontics and Oral Surg., 30:516, 1944.)

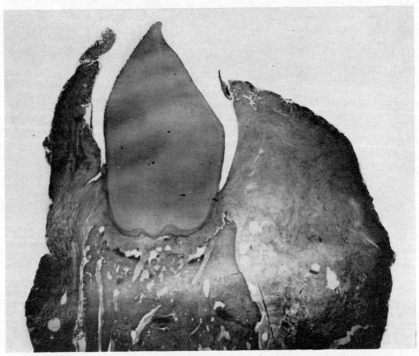

FIG. 214. Marked hypertrophy and necrosis of the gingival tissues in the canine region ($\times 2\frac{1}{2}$). (Burket, Am. J. Orthodontics and Oral Surg., 30:516, 1944.)

although they may be present in any area of the mouth. The tongue is rarely involved. The marked hypertrophy of the gums is accounted for in part by the necrosis and edema of these tissues and the marked extravascular accumulation of the abnormal leukocytes. The extensive tissue necrosis develops as the result of multiple thrombi forming in the smaller blood vessels. The hypertrophied tissue reaches frequently the occlusal surfaces of the teeth.

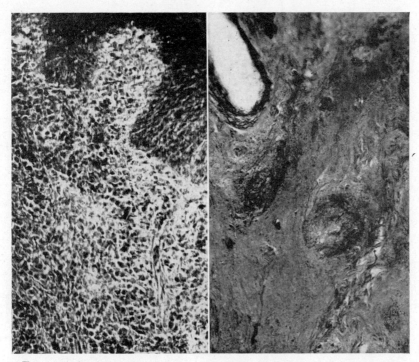

Fig. 215 (*Left*). Mononuclear infiltration in the gingival tissues.
Fig. 216 (*Right*). Thrombosed vessels and necrosis in the gingival tissues with more marked lesions ($\times$ 35). (Burket, Am. J. Orthodontics and Oral Surg., **30**:516, 1944.)

Pulpal Lesions. All the other soft dental tissues may become involved. Pulpal "abscesses" or areas of liquification necrosis are frequently observed in noncarious teeth. These patients complain at times of a severe odontalgia without apparent clinical cause. The large numbers of extravascular immature leukocytes that can be demonstrated in the pulp furnish a pathologic explanation for the clinical symptoms. The dental periosteum is likewise involved causing rapid loosening of the teeth. The architecture and function of this tissue is destroyed.

The treatment of the oral lesions in leukemia should be directed towards maintaining the best possible oral hygiene, relieving pain and refraining from aggravating the local necrotic process. Oral surgery of any kind is contraindicated. It may result in massive necrosis, severe hemorrhage and rapid death. Following oral surgery the "asymptomatic" leukemia patient may exhibit suddenly an acute and rapidly fatal form of the disease.

Irritant and caustic drugs are contraindicated. Oral hygiene can be maintained by the use of 1½% hydrogen peroxide mouth wash or better yet a

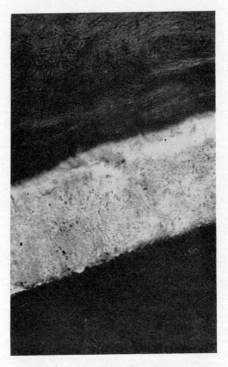

Fig. 217. Necrosis of the dental periosteum (× 35). (Burket, Am. J. Orthodontics and Oral Surg., 30:516, 1944.)

sodium bicarbonate mouth wash. A thick aqueous paste of zinc peroxide is excellent for controlling the secondary infection in the necrotic lesions as well as the accompanying extremely foul odor. Appleton has suggested the use of a urea mouth wash. Toothbrushing is usually out of the question.

The diet should be liquid or semisolid in nature. Anesthetic troches can be administered prior to eating in cases of severe pain. Extractions should be postponed during the acute stage of the disease. If the leukocyte count drops following therapy or during a remission of the disease to near normal limits, dental extractions can be performed without undue danger of hemorrhage or necrosis.

Acute Monocytic Leukemia, Post-Mortem Oral Pathologic Findings

Case Report: The patient, a 12-year-old boy, was admitted to the New Haven Hospital complaining of toothache and pain in the lower jaw, decreased appetite, a sallow color and intermittent pains in the abdomen for 2 weeks. The day before admission the patient was taken to the dentist, who extracted a lower left first molar. There was an acute reaction following the removal of this tooth and the next morning there was a

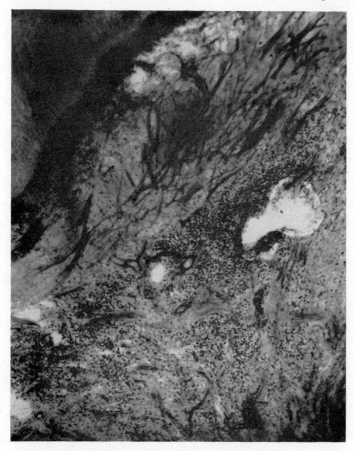

FIG. 218. Fibrosis and mononuclear infiltration of the dental pulp (× 35). (Burket, Am. J. Orthodontics and Oral Surg., 30:516, 1944.)

marked increase in swelling on the left side of the neck and the patient had a temperature of 102° F. He was hospitalized for observation and diagnosis.

The patient was a pale, ill-looking boy who was breathing through his mouth. There was a foul, putrid odor to his breath. The lips were pale and dry and the tongue was heavily coated. The gums were swollen, red and tender. Many carious teeth were present. The gingival hypertrophy and the ulceration were especially marked in the region of the recent extraction.

The cervical lymph nodes were large, discrete, non-fluctuant and freely movable. In the left side of the abdomen, a mass was palpable which was thought to be the spleen. No petechiae were noted anywhere on the body. The other findings were essentially negative.

The dental consultant thought that the gingivitis and adenitis were secondary to some blood dyscrasia. The swelling of the face, lips and gingivae increased in size as did that of the spleen. The necrosis of the gums became more extensive. Pain and a foul putrid odor were outstanding symptoms.

The patient died 3 weeks after he first began to tire easily, 2 weeks after the onset of the jaw and abdominal symptoms and 8 days following the removal of the lower left molar.

The blood counts on various occasions were as follows:

	R.B.C. c. mm.	Hg. %	W.B.C. c. mm.	PMN. %	LYM. %	MONOS. %
7/29/34	1,870,000	40	6,100	27	53	10
7/30/34	2,610,000	46	13,700	13	74	11
8/1/34	2,100,000	44	28,000	5	7	86
8/3/34	1,890,000	40	40,600	0	15	85
8/5/34	850,000	30	78,800	2	23	75
8/3/34	Bleeding time: 3 minutes.					

Clotting time: Capillary tube, 4 minutes; large tube, 1 minute.

Clinical Diagnosis: Monocytic leukemia.
Anatomical Diagnosis: Generalized lymph node enlargement; hyperplasia of the bone marrow; splenomegaly; multiple petechiae in the skin, conjunctivae, sclerae, pleurae, liver and kidneys; necrotizing gingivitis. Clinically—monocytic leukemia.

Oral Pathologic Findings. The specimen obtained for oral pathologic studies consisted of that portion of the right maxillae containing the teeth from the first incisor to the third molar. The gums were reddish purple in color and hypertrophied throughout. The interdental papillae were markedly enlarged and ulcerated. Extensive areas of necrosis were observed buccally and lingually in the region of the second incisor, canine and first premolar teeth and on the lingual in the region of the second molar.

GINGIVA. There is a marked hypertrophy of both the marginal and alveolar gingivae. The epithelium is missing over the marginal gingivae. Where the structural elements are still distinguishable, the usual architecture of the gingival tissues is almost entirely replaced by a dense accumulation of large mononuclear cells. In other regions, the *tunica propria* is markedly widened and stains poorly indicating beginning necrosis. The necrosis of the gums is most marked about the thrombosed vessels in the marginal and alveolar gingivae.

DENTAL PERIOSTEUM. The usual structural architecture of the dental periosteum is well preserved in the apical region of the teeth. In the middle third of the dental periosteum next to the alveolar bone, there are numerous localized areas where there is a loss of the usual structural elements and staining qualities of the tissues which are suggestive of beginning necrosis. In the dental periosteum adjacent to these areas, many extravascular large mononucleated cells are seen. Small thrombosed blood vessels could be observed in these regions. Few cellular elements could be distinguished in the gingival third of the dental periosteum of the most extensively involved teeth. There was diffuse necrosis of the tissue elements in this region with only an occasional "ghost" mononuclear cell scattered throughout the amorphous faintly staining tissue.

ALVEOLAR BONE. The adipose tissue which occupies normally the alveolar marrow spaces of the upper jaw was infiltrated by a large number of mononuclear cells which gave a highly cellular appearance to this tissue.

DENTAL PULP. There was a diffuse fibrosis of the pulpal tissues. Many of the small blood vessels were completely filled with closely packed monocytic cells. Large numbers of similarly appearing cells were scattered throughout the dental pulp. These extravascular mononuclear cells were particularly prominent in the subodontoblastic layer.

Chronic Lymphatic Leukemia

The onset of lymphatic leukemia is insidious and an unexplained lymphadenopathy is frequently the first evidence of the disease. Weakness, dyspnea, anemia and a peculiar yellow pallor develop gradually. Spontaneous hemorrhages are common. The anemia appears earlier in chronic lymphatic leukemia than in chronic myelogenous leukemia. Oral lesions are less common than in chronic myelogenous leukemia and when present they may represent

THE LEUKEMIAS 451

any combination of those mentioned under acute leukemia. The lymph nodes do not tend to mat together—which aids in differentiating this disease from lymphosarcoma. The nodes do not break down as in tuberculosis. Splenomegaly is not as characteristic a symptom as in myelogenous leukemia.

The diagnosis of chronic leukemia is also made on the hematologic findings. The leukocyte count is usually from 60,000 to 100,000 white blood cells c. mm., but it may be even higher. The immature and adult lymphocytes total frequently 95 to 98% of the total leukocytes. The young cell forms contain less cytoplasm than normal. A secondary anemia is a characteristic finding and the lowered blood platelets account for the purpuric symptoms.

Myelogenous and Monocytic Leukemia

Chronic myelogenous leukemia is also insidious in its onset. Wintrobe and Basenbach have shown that a persistent unexplained leukocytosis may be present several years before clinical symptoms appear. Splenomegaly and secondary hepatic enlargement are also common. These patients complain frequently of gastro-intestinal disturbances, vertigo, palpitation and asthenia. They also have a peculiar greenish yellow color. Fever and spontaneous hemorrhages are common in the advanced disease. Lymphadenopathy is variable.

Local gangrenous lesions are common in the later stages of the disease. If the teeth are removed accidentally before the patient develops the more characteristic general symptoms, an acute and perhaps fatal exacerbation may occur.

In monocytic leukemia peculiar blue-red raised areas are frequently seen in the skin. They consist of infiltrations of the monocytic cells. These lesions may be confused with moniliasis and other diseases. Oral lesions are common in monocytic leukemia.

The diagnosis of chronic myelogenous and monocytic leukemia is based on the hematologic findings. In the former, total counts of 100,000 to 500,000 leukocytes c. mm. are not uncommon. With such high counts the blood has a sticky feel and a milky appearance. The relative percentage of myelocytes and the large number of young forms are significant findings. In monocytic leukemia the total and differential counts are lower but the relative percentage of monocytes is markedly elevated. A severe anemia is a characteristic of chronic leukemia.

Diagnosis. Certain diseases which give rise to a marked lymphocytosis such as influenza, whooping cough, or infectious mononucleosis may be mistaken for leukemia. The age of the patient and the physical findings will aid in the diagnosis. The differential diagnosis of infectious mononucleosis and monocytic leukemia may offer some difficulties. The sheep cell antigen test (Paul-Bunnel) is of assistance.

Bacterial smears of the gums are of little diagnostic significance. They may show only a few fusospirochetal organisms or they may be typically positive for a fusospirochetal infection.

Treatment. The treatment of leukemia is at best but palliative. Unsuccessful attempts have been made to reduce the leukocytes by chemical, physiologic and biologic means. X-ray radiation of the long bones is useful, especially in chronic myelogenous leukemia. This form of treatment requires extreme caution. The symptomatic improvement and the reduction in the peripheral blood counts and the effective duration of the remissions becomes less after each series of radiations until the patient receives no further benefit. Blood transfusions are used in the acute stage of the disease to combat the anemia.

The radio-isotopes of phosphorus, made by bombarding phosphorus salts in the cyclotron, have been used in the treatment of leukemia. This form of therapy has prolonged life but no cures have been reported.

Prognosis. The prognosis in leukemia is very unfavorable. Kracke believes that the life expectancy of a patient with leukemia is roughly proportional to the stage of maturity of the circulating leukocytes.

HEMOPHILIA

Hemophilia is a hereditary disease which is manifested clinically in the male. The disease is transmitted by the female who presents no clinical symptoms. It is characterized by a prolongation of the clotting time of the blood. The hemophilic tendency is a recessive sex-linked characteristic which appears in approximately $\frac{2}{3}$ of the offspring of the female transmitters.*

Hemophilia is a rare disease but, since dental extractions are commonly the first evidence of the condition or the cause of serious hemorrhage, it is of considerable importance to dentists. It is most common in the Teutonic race and it has affected several royal families.

The etiology of the disease is not known. It was once believed to be due to a qualitative defect of the blood platelets which resulted in an increased resistance to disintegration. The more recent studies indicate that the defect is not in the platelets but that it is related to the plasma globulin fraction of blood plasma. Szent-Gyorgi has been reported to have isolated an unknown property of human blood called plasma chinin which plays a decisive part in the process of blood coagulation. The lack of this material is said to cause hereditary hemophilia. All the hemophiliacs studied by Kubanyi belonged to the same blood group (Group A Landsteiner—II Moss or Jansky). This observation has not been substantiated by the studies of Tinney and Watkins or the author.

Symptoms

The disease is manifested rarely in infancy. It is recognized usually in early childhood by the development of extensive subcutaneous hemorrhages following the slightest trauma. Unfortunately for the dentist, the first evidence of the disease may be manifest during the eruption of a tooth or following a dental extraction.

The joints are a common site of involvement. Hemorrhage into the joints produces an acute hemarthrosis as well as a chronic form of arthritis with

* It is possible theoretically to have true hemophilia in the female and cases have been reported occurring in females which fulfill the diagnostic criteria of hemophilia. They are extremely rare.

permanent joint damage. Severe spontaneous nosebleeds are often experienced. Because of the seriousness of the slightest cut or injury the normal life habits of a hemophiliac are definitely curtailed. It is not possible for them to engage in active sports or to go far from places where treatment is readily available.

Bleeding episodes in hemophiliacs often develop spontaneously with a localized infection or a few days later. A marked gingival hemorrhage may be associated with an abscessed tooth. The extraction of a tooth in a hemophiliac is a major surgical operation.

Diagnosis

The patient (male) is often aware of his inherited trait. All patients, both male and female, who give a history of prolonged bleeding following slight injury should have a bleeding and clotting time performed prior to extraction or other surgical procedures. Not all individuals who are said to be "bleeders" are hemophiliacs but the seriousness of performing operations on true hemophiliacs does not justify the dentist taking the slightest chance. It is imperative that a bleeding and clotting time be performed on all patients, giving a history of prolonged bleeding following past dental extractions or following slight cuts.

Laboratory Findings

The laboratory findings in hemophilia are characteristic. The clotting time is prolonged, whereas the bleeding time is not affected. Once the clot is formed, however, it retracts in a normal manner. Bleeding does not occur from pin or needle pricks such as for blood counts or myringotomy wounds as sufficient thromboplastic substance is eliminated from the wound edges to start the clotting process. The other cellular elements of the blood are unchanged, unless there is a secondary anemia as a result of frequent or prolonged hemorrhage.

Differential Diagnosis

The condition most likely to be confused with hemophilia is thrombocytopenic purpura. (See Table XXV.) The bleeding and clotting values and the Rumpel-Leeds test will permit a differential diagnosis. Rarer entities such as pseudohemophilia, familial epistaxis, hereditary familial telangiectasia and hereditary hemoptysis need not be considered as a rule.

Treatment

The treatment of hemophilia resolves itself into procedures which should be instituted before surgery is undertaken and measures which may be effective in controlling hemorrhage once it has occurred.

General prophylactic measures include the use of blood transfusions and more recently the use intravenously of lyophile human plasma. Johnson found that solutions of dried human plasma administered intravenously were particularly effective in eliminating the fear of tooth extraction. An infusion of 150 cc. of the restored blood plasma reduced the blood coagulation time to normal in most cases after which 2 or 3 teeth were extracted. Dried plasma was also packed into the tooth sockets. Sufficient plasma was administered for a few days, following tooth extraction to keep the coagulation time under 20 minutes. The use of dried human plasma eliminates the need for cross matching of blood and storage does not destroy its thromboplastic activity.

Fibrin foam, which is a preparation made from human fibrinogen and thrombin, is an excellent hemostatic. This substance is a porous mass of fibrillar fibrin which contains numerous air spaces. When this material is moistened with a solution of human thrombin and applied to the bleeding area excellent hemostasis is obtained. This material can be held in contact with the oral tissues by means of a shellac base plate.

Countless other preparations such as female sex hormones, placental extract, oxalic acid preparations and 1:3,000 Russl Viper Venom have been used. In general they have not been universally effective.

Birch successfully used small orthodontic rubber bands for exfoliating teeth in hemophiliacs. No special general or local treatment is needed with this method other than placing the small rubber band over the tooth. The dental periosteal fibres are separated gradually from the cementum, closing the vascular channels without bleeding during this procedure. At times it was necessary to separate the roots of multirooted teeth. Exfoliation took place within 4 to 30 days during which time the patient did not experience undue pain. In view of Birch's experience in hemophilia, and his successful use of this method, it is worthy of trial. It is the only method that should be attempted in ambulatory patients.

Oral Aspects

Hemorrhage following dental extractions can be controlled effectively by pressure plus the use of some hemostatic substance—however, repeated oozing of blood and bleeding are generally the rule. If several teeth are removed, it is desirable to make a modelling compound or shellac base plate impression of the socket area at the time of operation. If postoperative bleeding occurs in spite of general treatment it can be controlled by placing several layers of gauze moistened with thromboplastin or cephalin (Kaomagin) in the impression and holding this gently but firmly in place for 10 to 15 minutes. While bleeding can be readily controlled by this method, it does not prevent recurrence. The use of fresh human or animal (pigeon) muscles sutured over the socket is of value.

Atraumatic surgery is imperative in these patients. Particular attention should be paid to an aseptic technic and the careful trimming of all rough alveolar margins. The extraction of teeth in the hemophiliac is a major surgical procedure which should be performed in a hospital where professional assistance and facilities are available to cope with any emergencies that may arise.

Prognosis

The general prognosis of the hemophiliac is not good. Of the 152 boys studied by Grandidier one-half died before the 7th year. The extraction of teeth can usually be performed in hemophiliacs without serious consequences.

Birch's conservative technic with rubber bands deserves serious consideration in cases of elective extraction and the use of dried plasma affords an effective and practical form of general therapy prior to dental extraction by the usual technic.

TABLE XXV

COMPARISON OF THE CLINICAL AND LABORATORY FINDINGS IN HEMOPHILIA, PSEUDOHEMO-
PHILIA AND THROMBOCYTOPENIC PURPURA

	Hemophilia	*Pseudohemophilia*	*Thrombocytopenic Purpura*
Sex	Males only (with rare exceptions).	Occurs in both sexes.	Occurs usually in the female.
Hereditary aspects	Transmitted by the female who shows no symptoms of the disease. Associated with x-chromosomes, a recessive characteristic.	Transmitted directly by the affected individual to members of the next generation. Associated with autochromosomes, a dominant characteristic.	No known hereditary aspect.
Bleeding time	Normal.	Increased.	Increased.
Clotting time	Increased	Normal.	Normal.
Clot retraction	Normal.	Normal.	Poor clot retraction.
Platelets	May be slightly increased.		Marked reduction in the number of platelets.

PSEUDOHEMOPHILIA

Pseudohemophilia is an entirely different disease from true hemophilia. Pseudohemophilia occurs in both sexes and is transmitted by either the male or the female to the next generation. This disease resembles purpura in that the coagulation time is normal but the bleeding time is prolonged. There is apparently an insufficient agglutination of the blood platelets resulting in faulty clot formation.

The symptoms of pseudohemophilia are similar to those of true hemophilia, although they are usually less severe. Persistent bleeding following dental extractions is encountered frequently. In males the determination of the bleeding and clotting time will differentiate this condition from true hemophilia. In the female a platelet count will differentiate the disease from thrombocytopenic purpura. A familial history is necessary in both cases to establish the diagnosis.

HEREDITARY HEMORRHAGIC TELANGIECTASIA

Hereditary hemorrhagic telangiectasia was first completely described by Osler. It is a rare vascular anomaly which is characterized by numerous localized telangiectases or angiomata on the skin and mucous membranes. This disease occurs in equal frequency in both sexes and it is not associated with any derangement of the bleeding time, the clotting time, clot retraction or the platelet count.

This condition is of some dental interest because the lesions occur most frequently on the nasal and oral mucosa. These bleeding angiomata may occur in any part of the gastro-intestinal tract. Severe and at times fatal hemorrhages are an outstanding symptom. The angiomatous lesions appear clinically similar to those commonly seen on the skin or oral mucosa, but histologic study reveals an abnormal thinness of the vessel walls in this condition.

The nasal mucosa is the most common site of the lesions, followed next by the tongue, lips and face. The dorsum and tip of the tongue are commonly involved. The author saw a case which was characterized by profuse oral hemorrhage arising from a small lesion of the lingual alveolar gingiva of a lower third molar.

This disease is diagnosed on the basis of the familial history and the presence of multiple angiomata of the skin and mucosa which have a tendency to profuse recurrent hemorrhages. The hemorrhage can usually be controlled by pressure if it occurs at a site where this can be applied. Coagulation

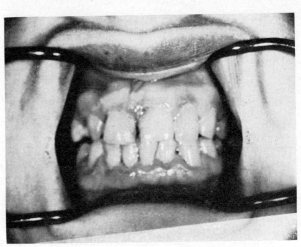

FIG. 219. Gums of a patient with Osler's disease—
hereditary familial telangiectasis.

by means of chemical agents such as 50% trichloracetic acid or electro-coagulation is usually effective for the oral lesions. Figi and Watkins found that electrocoagulation was particularly effective for the control of oral hemorrhages.

THE PURPURAS

The purpuras comprise a group of diseases which are characterized by the extravasation of blood beneath or from the skin and mucous membranes. They can be classified as follows:

(A) Thrombocytopenic purpuras (in which there is an actual numerical deficiency in blood platelets).
    (1) Primary or essential form—etiology unknown.
    (2) Secondary forms—due to infections, tumors or drugs that affect platelet formation in the bone marrow.
(B) Vascular purpuras—due to damage or change in capillary walls rather than platelet deficiency.
    (1) Purpura simplex
    (2) Henoch's purpura ⎱ Allergic purpura?
    (3) Schonlein's purpura ⎰

(4) Secondary or symptomatic purpuras—due to infections, malnutrition, liver diseases, poisons, drugs, etc.

Essential Thrombocytopenic Purpura

Essential thrombocytopenic purpura is characterized by a marked reduction in the number of blood platelets, an increased bleeding time and a failure of normal clot retraction. This form of purpura is most common in early life—before the age of 15. There is a slightly higher incidence in females. Frequent remissions are not unusual in young individuals and many times there are repeated hospitalizations for periodic transfusions.

The etiology of this form of purpura is unknown, but it is perhaps related to some abnormal splenic activity. Familial tendencies for low platelet counts are also known. There are 3 general hypotheses for the low platelet count: (1) Some abnormal splenic function, (2) a scarcity of megakaryocytes in the bone marrow and (3) a defect or deficiency in the maturation of the platelets.

Symptoms. The sudden appearance of large purpuric spots beneath the skin or mucosa is a characteristic finding. Hemorrhage may also occur in any of the internal organs producing symptoms referable to the particular structure involved. Nosebleed is a common and at times distressing symptom. In typical cases of thrombocytopenic purpura the physical examination reveals an enlarged spleen. A mild fever and a leukocytosis are present during an acute attack.

Diagnosis. Diagnosis of thrombocytopenic purpura is made on the basis of the history, the physical examination and the characteristic hematologic findings. These include (1) an increased bleeding time, (2) a marked reduction in the number of blood platelets, (3) a normal clotting time, (4) the formation of a non-retractile clot and (5) a positive Rumpel-Leeds test.

General treatment is the responsibility of the pediatrician or the physician. Transfusions will tide the patient over an acute episode. Vitamin C as well as vitamin P have been of value in some cases. Snake venom results at times in symptomatic improvement of the capillary oozing but it does not improve the platelet count. Splenectomy results in a rapid and marked increase in the platelet count.

Oral Aspects of Purpura (All Forms)

The first evidence of purpura is frequently severe gingival hemorrhage. This gingival bleeding may be localized to areas of previous inflammation or trauma or it may be generalized. Capillary oozing from the entire marginal gingivae is not an unusual finding. The decomposing blood about the gums and in the interdental areas produces a fetid odor and forms a favorable medium for bacterial growth.

Small reddish purple spots may appear beneath the oral mucosa, particularly prominent near the junction of the hard and soft palates. These reddish areas do not blanch on pressure. This aids in differentiating petechiae or purpuric spots from vascular anomalies in which the blood is still intravascular.

Spontaneous pulpal hemorrhage has also been observed, particularly in the symptomatic varieties of the disease.

The gingival hemorrhages can be controlled usually by the local use of hemostatics of the non-caustic type such as thromboplastin or clotting globulin. At times a 1½% strength hydrogen peroxide mouthwash will stop the gingival oozing and at other times all measures are ineffective in controlling the gingival bleeding.

No operative procedures should be attempted when purpuric symptoms are present. The diet should be soft or semisolid in order to minimize the trauma to the gums. It should contain large amounts of vitamin C and P for the possible beneficial effects of these substances. As the platelet count increases, due to more general therapeutic measures, the local oral lesions will be improved correspondingly.

Secondary Thrombocytopenic Purpura

This form of purpura results from chemical poisons, infections or the crowding of the megakaryocytes from the bone marrow such as that due to neoplastic growths. Secondary forms of thrombocytopenic purpura occur usually in adults and there is rarely a previous history of purpura.

Frequent causes of secondary thrombocytopenic purpura are:

(1) Tumors of the bone marrow such as multiple myeloma or metastatic carcinoma.
(2) Diseases of the blood such as aplastic anemia, leukemia (myelogenous), pernicious anemia and rarely malignant neutropenia.
(3) Severe infections.
(4) Radio-active substances.
(5) Drug idiosyncrasies or allergies to arsphenamine, benzene, quinine, phenobarbital, aniline, colloidal silver, sedoramid and numerous other proprietary drugs.

Symptoms. The symptoms of secondary purpura are similar to those described previously. The oral manifestations will be modified by existing disease processes which might also produce lesions of the oral mucosa such as those associated with aplastic anemia or leukemia.

Diagnosis. Diagnosis is made on the basis of the medical history, the history of drug administration in conjunction with the usual hematologic studies.

Treatment. In the case of purpuric reactions to drugs, prompt response follows usually the discontinuance of the medication. In most cases the purpuric symptoms are secondary to those of the general disease. Moccasin snake venom 0.4 cc. to 1 cc. of a 1:3,000 solution administered subcutaneously at various time intervals has been effective in all types of purpura other than the thrombocytopenic variety. Nicotinic acid should also be tried. (See Vitamins.)

Vascular Purpuras

Purpura simplex occurs usually in children. Its etiology is unknown. It lasts 2 to 4 weeks and may recur. Oral manifestations are observed rarely.

Henoch's purpura is found usually in young adults (males) and it is characterized by gastro-intestinal symptoms, abdominal pain which often simulates appendicitis, urticaria and edema. It is thought that this form of purpura may be related to some food allergy. Recovery is usually spontaneous.

Schoenlein's purpura is often called "rheumatic purpura" because of the frequent joint involvement which is present in addition to the gastro-intestinal and abdominal symptoms enumerated under Henoch's purpura. While the etiology is as yet unknown, allergy is believed to play a role in the causation of the disease.

POLYCYTHEMIA

Polycythemia refers to an increased number of circulating erythrocytes, usually above 6,000,000 cells per c. mm. Polycythemia may be primary in nature, that resulting from an actual proliferation of the erythropoietic tissues (polycythemia rubra vera, Vaquez's disease) or it may be symptomatic. Symptomatic or secondary polycythemia is observed commonly in individuals living at high altitudes, in patients with congenital heart disease, in patients with sclerosis of the pulmonary arteries (Ayerza's disease), pulmonary emphysema, marked dehydration, acidosis and following the ingestion of certain drugs such as acetanilid. In symptomatic polycythemia the oral and systemic symptoms, which are characteristic of primary polycythemia, are observed rarely.

Primary Polycythemia (Polycythemia Rubra Vera, Vaquez's Disease)

Primary polycythemia is uncommon. The disease is known to show a familial tendency and a predisposition for Russian and Polish Jews. Males are usually affected. The etiology of this disease is unknown, but it can be considered as an erythropoietic analogue of leukemia.

Primary polycythemia is characterized by a marked purplish-red coloration which gives the afflicted individual the appearance of extreme anger. The superficial veins are dark and distended. The patients complain of nervousness, headache, tinnitus and neuralgias. Paresthesias are common, particularly those involving the cranial nerves. They result from localized areas of cerebral anemia due to the increased viscosity of the blood, hemorrhage or thrombosis. The arms are congested when lowered and anemic when raised—indicating capillary congestion. Hypertension is a common but not a universal finding. An enlarged, hard, non-tender spleen is common.

Oral Findings. The purplish-red discoloration of the ears, oral mucosa, gums and tongue is one of the outstanding symptoms of the disease. The tongue may appear as if it had been painted with gentian violet. The gums are markedly swollen, they frequently bleed spontaneously but they show no tendency to ulcerate. Petechiae of the mucosa and skin are common.

Laboratory Findings. The red blood cells are usually 8,000,000 per c. mm. or higher. Counts of 16,000,000 erythrocytes per c. mm. have been reported but on theoretical grounds counts above 12 to 13,000,000 red blood cells per c. mm. are incompatible with life because of spontaneous clotting of the blood. The hemoglobin is elevated with a color index of approximately 0.8. The leukocyte count is also elevated. Nucleated red blood cells and considerable variation in the size and the shape of the cells are noted on the blood smears. Diagnosis of polycythemia is made on the characteristic clinical findings, the history of the disease and the laboratory findings. Possible causes of secondary polycythemia must be considered. A study of the erythrocyte cell mass and the blood volume will permit differentiation. Argyrosis and congestive heart failure must be distinguished on clinical grounds.

Treatment. Venisection or oxygen inhalation may be employed to avert a circulatory or respiratory crisis. X-ray radiation is of little value as it also

A   B

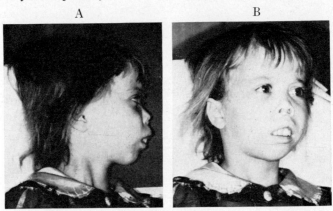

FIG. 220. (A) Profile and (B) front views of a 9-year-old girl with Cooley's anemia. (Courtesy of Novak, Philadelphia, Pa.)

tends to depress the white blood cell production. Phenylhydrazine or the less toxic acetylphenylhydrazine has a destructive action (hemolytic) on the red blood cells and will control the disease for long periods of time. Patients with primary polycythemia should lead a moderate life, avoid purine-containing foods and those stimulating erythoblastic activity.

Oral treatment consists of maintaining good oral hygiene during the acute stage (markedly elevated erythrocyte count) of the disease. Operative procedures can be carried out usually in mild cases without danger, although severe hemorrhages have been experienced following extractions during periods when the red cell count was high. A moderate hemorrhage in these patients is of no great consequence.

PRIMARY ERYTHROBLASTIC ANEMIA—COOLEY'S ANEMIA

Cooley's anemia is a manifestation of some congenital defect in the erythroblastic tissues. It is found chiefly in both the male and female children of Greeks, Italians and Syrians, although it has been observed occasionally in other racial groups such as the English and Chinese. Not all members of the family are affected.

The disease usually becomes manifest before the second year of life. The extreme pallor and yellowish tint to the skin is often the first clinical manifestation of the disease. The icteric color results from an excess of bile pigments which are produced by the hemolysis of the abnormal erythrocytes. There is a marked enlargement of the spleen which results in a protruding abdomen. The liver may also be enlarged and vague gastro-intestinal disturbances are common. Individuals with Cooley's anemia complain usually of

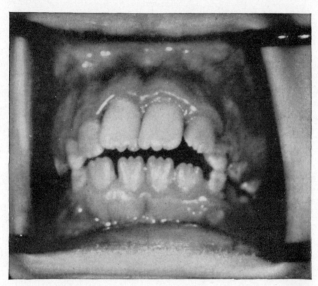

FIG. 221. Open bite and prominent enamel tubercles on the incisal edges of the teeth in a patient with Cooley's anemia. Same patient as shown in Fig. 220. (Novak, Am. J. Orthodontics and Oral Surg., 30:542-6, 1944.)

weakness. They are lethargic and appear mentally sluggish for their age. The disease is slowly progressive with periods of remissions and exacerbations. Infections result commonly in an accentuation of the hemolytic symptoms. They are the usual cause of death.

Roentgenologic examination of the long bones shows osteoporosis with a widening of the medullary space at the expense of the cortex. Bony spicules are frequently observed radiating from the cortex. The skull changes are discussed under the Oral Aspects of this disease. The hematologic findings are characteristic. The color index is low with a great variation in the size and shape of the erythrocytes. Many immature red blood cells are observed in the peripheral circulation. There is a slight increase in the number of leukocytes.

This disease is diagnosed by the characteristic clinical findings of splenomegaly, the facial changes to be described and the typical hematologic and roentgenologic changes. Cooley's anemia must be differentiated from mongolism, sickle cell anemia, cleidocranial dysostosis and congenital syphilis.

A differential diagnosis can easily be made when the x-ray and hematologic findings are available.

The treatment of this disease is unsatisfactory and the ultimate prognosis of the individual is poor, although an occasional patient will survive to adult life. Splenectomy results in a temporary improvement but the only treatment of value is repeated transfusions.

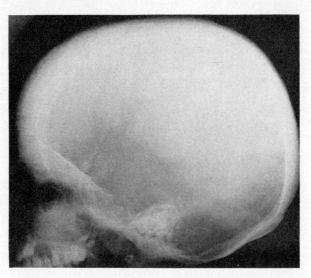

FIG. 222. Skull changes in Cooley's anemia. Note the marked thickening of the cortex and a radial arrangement of the bone trabeculae. Same patient as shown in Figs. 220-221. (Novak, A. J., Am. J. Orthodontics and Oral Surg., 30:542-6, 1944.)

Oral Aspects. The craniofacial and dental changes in Cooley's anemia are striking. By the second year of life the afflicted child begins to develop a characteristic mongoloid appearance with prominent frontal and parietal bosses, a marked overdevelopment of the maxillae and malar bones, which is associated with a short nose with a depressed bridge. The overdevelopment of the maxillae results frequently in malocclusion, an open bite and spacing of the teeth of the maxillary arch. Ziskin reported a retarded development of the permanent teeth and a progressively increasing space between the premolar and molar teeth.

The oral mucosa is extremely pale and has a lemon yellow tint which is best seen just posterior to the termination of the hard palate. Unusual bleeding following dental extractions in these patients has not been reported.

The x-ray changes of the skull represent one of the most striking findings in this disease. They are usually present in long-standing cases. They consist of a marked thickening and rarefaction of the cranium. The trabeculae which join the inner and outer tables of the skull, appear on the x-ray as radially

TABLE XXVI

TABULATION OF THE HEMATOLOGIC FINDINGS IN SOME OF THE DISEASES IN WHICH HEMOGRAMS ARE OF IMPORTANCE IN DIAGNOSIS

Disease	R.B.C. c. mm.	Hg. Gm./100 cc.	C.I.	W.B.C. c. mm.	Neutrophils %	Lymphocytes %	Monocytes %	Primitive Cell Forms %	Platelets c. mm.	Remarks
Normal	5,000,000	15.6	1.0	6,000-9,000	64	33	2	..	350,000	
Pernicious anemia	1,000,000	5.8	1.5	3,900	49	50	..	..	40,000	Anisocytosis and poikilocytosis on smears
Secondary hypochromic anemia	3,000,000	6.0	.5	9,000	65	30	3	..	500,000	Hypochromia-microcytosis
Aplastic anemia	1,000,000	3.0	1.0	1,650	8	92	..	..	10,000	
Polycythemia	8,500,000	17.0	0.9	20,000	60	25	..	15	500,000	
Malignant neutropenia	4,500,000	15.0	1.0	900	3	97	..	..	250,000	
Acute lymphatic leukemia	2,000,000	6.0	1.0	70,000	2	98	..	Many lymphoblasts	50,000	
Acute myeloplastic leukemia	2,000,000	6.0	1.0	150,000-250,000	98	2	..	Many myeloblasts	100,000	
Acute monocytic leukemia	3,500,000	11.4	1.0	50,000	20	20	60	Many monoblasts	150,000	
Infectious mononucleosis	5,000,000	15.6	1.0	30,000	25	63	12	Atypical lymphocyte	300,000	Heterophilic antibody test positive

arranged calcified spicules which appear to extend beyond the outer table. On the x-ray they give the appearance of calcified hairs standing on end. Roentgenograms of the maxillae reveal a marked increase in size of these bones with a decreased density and loss of trabecular detail.

REFERENCES

BLOOD DYSCRASIAS

Malignant Neutropenia

Anday, G. J., & R. L. Ferguson: Changes in the white cell count following tooth extraction in albino rats and rabbits, J. Dent. Research, 24:17-30, 1945.

Appleton, J. L. T.: Agranulocytosis, Dental Cosmos, 74:267-76, 1932.

Barlow, H. C.: Case of agranulocytosis in infant: with recovery, Brit. M. J., 1:669-70, 1941.

Bromberg, L., & P. Murphy: Agranulocytic angina following prophylactic typhoid vaccination, J. A. M. A., 92:1266-67, 1929.

Cantor, M. M., & John W. Scott: Effect of vitamin B6 (pyridoxine) in the treatment of leucopenia and granulocytopenia of toxic origin in humans. Preliminary report, Science, 100:545, 1944.

Copley, E. L.: Agranulocytic angina—a drug hazard, Virginia M. Monthly, 71:416, 1944.

Daft, F. S., & W. H. Sebrell: The successful treatment of granulocytopenia and leukopenia in rats with crystalline folic acid, Pub. Health Rep., 58:1542, 1943.

Dameshek, Wm., & L. E. Wolfson: A preliminary report on the treatment of agranulocytosis with sulfathiazole, Am. J. M. Sc., 203:819, 1942.

Eckert, J. F., et al.: The treatment of agranulocytosis with sulfadiazine, Am. J. M. Sc., 206:713, 1943.

Favorite, G. O., L. Reiner, & R. London: Acute agranulocytosis during sulfamerazine therapy, J. Lab. & Clin. Med., 29:899, 1944.

Fitz-Hugh, T.: Etiology and pathology of agranulocytic angina; present-day findings and hypotheses, Am. J. Clin. Path., 7:524-30, 1937.

Fitz-Hugh, T., Jr.: Sensitivity reactions of blood and bone marrow to certain drugs, J. A. M. A., 111:1643-47, 1938.

Franks, A. G., & M. I. J. Davis: Agranulocytosis—complication following quinine in a case of malaria therapy, Am. J. Syph. Gonorr. & Ven. Dis., 27:314, 1943.

Gordon, W. H.: Etiology of malignant neutropenia, J. Oklahoma M. A., 36:376, 1943.

Hanzlik, P. J.: Agranulocytosis, a critical review of causes and treatment, J. A. D. A., 22:487, 1935.

Heilig, R., & S. K. Visveswar: Malignant leukopenia successfully treated with sulfapyridine, J. A. M. A., 122:591, 1943.

Ives, R. F.: Hemolytic streptococci angina with agranulocytosis treated with prontosil and sulphanilamide, Ann. Int. Med., 12:882-87, 1938.

Jackson, H., Jr., & D. Merril: Agranulocytic angina associated with menstrual cycle, New England J. Med., 210:175-76, 1934.

Jackson, H., Jr., & T. J. G. Tighe: Analysis of treatment and mortality of

390 cases of acute agranulocytic angina, New England J. Med., 220:729-33, 1939.

Johnson, S. A. M.: Acute agranulocytosis due to administration of succinyl-sulfathiazole, J. A. M. A., 122:668, 1943.

Kopp, Israel: Chronic leucopenia with fatal termination due to agranulocytic angina, Am. J. Orthodontics & Oral Surg., 27:245, 1941.

Kopp, I.: Chronic leukopenia with fatal termination due to agranulocytic angina; case report, Ann. Int. Med., 13:2347-54, 1940.

Kracke, R. R., & F. P. Parker: Relationship of drug therapy to agranulocytosis, J. A. M. A., 105:1047, 1935.

Lawrence, J. S.: Leukopenia: discussion of the various modes of production, J. A. M. A., 116:478-84, 1941.

Madison, F. W., & T. L. Squier: Etiology of primary granulocytopenia (agranulocytic angina), J. A. M. A., 102:755-59, 1934.

Meyer, A. H.: Agranulocytosis: Report of case caused by sulfadiazine, California & West. Med. J., 60:277, 1944.

Meyer, A. H.: Granulocytopenia: A case caused by thiouracil, California & West. Med., 61:54, 1944.

McCarthy, F. P., & R. Wilson: Blood dyscrasias following arsphenamine, J. A. M. A., 99:1557, 1932.

Muether, R. O., L. T. Moore, J. W. Stewart, & G. O. Broun: Chronic granulocytopenia caused by excessive splenic lysis of granulocytes; report of case, J. A. M. A., 116:2255-57, 1941.

Newcomb, P. B., & E. W. Deane: Thiourea causing granulopenia and thrombopenia, Lancet, 1:179, 1944.

Plafker, M.: Agranulocytosis following anti-luetic treatment; report of a case, Dental Cosmos, 78:181-84, 1936.

Ruskin, S. L.: Adenylic acid in the treatment of agranulocytic angina and mucous membrane lesions, Am. J. Digest. Dis., 10:81, 1943.

Shecket, H. A., & A. E. Price: Fatal granulocytopenia following administration of sulfanilamide, J. A. M. A., 112:823-28, 1939.

Smith, L. B., F. Cohen, & R. G. Nichols: Agranulocytosis treated with penicillin, J. A. M. A., 126:1027, 1944.

Stealy, C. L.: Chronic granulocytopenia of 5 years' duration with recurrent acute attacks; case report, Am. J. M. Sc., 189:633-38, 1935.

Thompson, W. P.: Observations on possible relation between agranulocytosis and menstruation with further studies on case of cyclic neutropenia, New England J. Med., 210:176-78, 1934.

Weinberg, H. B.: Agranulocytosis following sulfadiazine administration, J. Iowa M. Soc., 34:63, 1944.

Leukemia

Amidon, E. L.: Reaction of leukemic patients to sulfonamides, J. Lab. & Clin. Med., 28:1691, 1943.

Aseltine, Lyle F.: Monocytic leukemia with oral manifestations: report of case, J. Oral Surg., 2:266, 1944.

Bethel, Frank H.: Leukemia: The relative incidence of its various forms, and their response to radiation therapy, Ann. Int. Med., 18:757, 1943.

Brunner, Hans: Changes of the temporal bone in luekemia and osteitis fibrosa, Arch. Otolaryng., 39:1, 1944.

Burket, L. W.: A histopathologic explanation for the oral lesions in the acute leukemias, Am. J. Orthodontics & Oral Surg., 30:516, 1944.

Clough, P. W.: Monocytic leukemia, Bull. Johns Hopkins Hosp., 51:148, 1932.

Craver, L. F.: Treatment of leukemia by radioactive phosphorus, Bull. New York Acad. Med., 18:254, 1942.

Cross, Frank S.: Congenital leucemia, J. Pediat., 24:191, 1944.

Dameshek, W.: Acute monocytic leukemia, Arch. Int. Med., 46:718, 1930.

Forkner, C. E.: Clinical and pathologic differentiation of acute leukemias with special references to acute monocytic leukemia, Arch. Int. Med., 53:1, 1934.

Friedman, M., et al.: Eosinophil leukemia, Am. J. Med. Sc., 208:333, 1944.

Garvey, P. H., & J. S. Lawrence: Facial diplegia in lymphatic leukemia, J. A. M. A., 101:1941-4, 1933.

Hansen-Pruss, O. C., & E. G. Goodman: Acute leukemia as terminal event in polycythemia vera; report of 2 cases with autopsies, North Carolina M. J., 4:254-58, 1943.

Henshaw, P. S., & J. W. Hawkins: Incidence of leukemia in physicians, J. Nat. Cancer Inst., 4:339, 1944.

Hill, J. M., & C. N. Duncan: Leukemoid reactions, Am. J. M. Sc., 201:847, 1941.

Kracke, R. R., & H. E. Garver: Differential diagnosis of the leukemic states with particular reference to immature cell types, J. A. M. A., 104:697-702, 1935.

Krumbharr, E. B.: Leukemoid blood pictures in various clinical conditions, Am. J. M. Sc., 172:519, 1926.

Legal intelligence: Negligence alleged against doctor and dentist, Brit. M. J., 1:283, 1935.

Love, A. A.: Manifestations of leukemia encountered in otolaryngologic and stomatologic practice, Arch. Otolaryng., 23:173, 1936.

Lucia, S. P.: Leukemia: evaluation of the therapy, California & West. Med., 55:119, 1941.

Mason, H.: Gingival hypertrophy due to myelogenous leucemia, Am. J. Orthodontics & Oral Surg., 28:738, 1942.

Morrison, M. J., F. Feldman, & A. A. Samwick: Carcinoma and leukemia, Ann. Int. Med., 20:75, 1944.

Neger, M.: An unusual manifestation of leukemia, Am. J. Orthodontics & Oral Surg., 25:481, 1939.

Paul, J. T., W. O. Brown, & L. R. Limarzi: The effect of colchicine on chronic myeloid leukemia, Am. J. Clin. Path., 2:210, 1941.

Resch, C. A.: Oral manifestations of leukemia, Am. J. Orthodontics & Oral Surg., 26:701, 1940.

Rosenthal, N., & W. Harris: Leukemia—its diagnosis and treatment, J. A. M. A., 104:702, 1935.

Saghirian, L. M., & Chas. A. Jones: Acute monocytic leukemia, Am. J. Orthodontics & Oral Surg., 28:561, 1942.

Shapiro, B. B.: The oral lesions and blood picture of pernicious anemia, leukemia and agranulocytosis, Dent. Items of Interest, 62:113-26, 1940.

Walmesley, W. C. D.: Excessive hemorrhage after tooth extraction, due to acute leukemia, Brit. M. J., 1:1159-90, 1929.

Hemophilia

Baird, K. H., & M. S. Fox: Severe sublingual and paratracheal hemorrhage in hemophilia with recovery following tracheotomy, J. Pediat., 32:90, 1943.

Birch, C. L.: Hemophilia, J. A. M. A., 99:1566-72, 1932.

Birch, C. L., & F. F. Snider: Tooth extraction in hemophilia, J. A. D. A., 26:1933-42, 1939.

Cambrook, J. D.: Some observations on the extraction of teeth in cases of haemophilia, Proc. Roy. Soc. Med., 26:962, 1933.

Copley, A. L.: The influence of blood transfusion and injections of bursa pastoris (Shepherd's Purse) extract on the clot resistance in two hemophiliacs, Am. J. M. Sc., 204:665, 1942.

Creveld, S. van, & R. Hamber: Coagulation-globulin in hemorrhages after extraction of teeth, especially in hemophilic patients, Amer. Jour. Orthodontics & Oral Surg., 29:6-28, 1943.

Dalitsch, W. W.: Dental extractions in hemophilia, J. A. D. A., 21:1804-11, 1934.

Dalitsch, W. W.: Removal of teeth by exfoliation with elastic ligatures, Dent. Digest, 45:310-14, 1939.

Eley, R. C.: Hemophilia, Internat. Clin., 2:202-22, 1936.

Foulis, M. A., & J. W. Crawford: Female "bleeders," Brit. M. J., 2:594, 1934.

Johnson, J. B.: Management of hemophilia with lyophile human plasma intravenously injected, J. A. M. A., 118:799-802, 1942.

Kubanyi, A.: Blood groups in hemophilic family, Klin. Wchnschr., 5:321-22, 1926.

Lozner, E. L., et al.: The use of rabbit thrombin as a local hemostatic, Am. J. Med. Sc., 202:593, 1941.

Macklin, M. T.: Sex ratios in families with hemophilia, Am. J. Dis. Child., 58:1215-27, 1939.

Munro, F. L., & Harold W. Jones: The detrimental effect of frequent transfusions in hemophilia, Am. J. M. Sc., 206:710, 1943.

Paliard, F., et al.: Un cas d'hémophilie chez une jeune fille de 17 ans, Lyon med., 162:208-12, 1938.

Parfentjev, I. A., M. A. Goodline, & F. L. Clapp: Preparation and properties of a dry powdered mixture of sulfanilamide and hemostatic globulin, J. Lab. & Clin. Med., 28:1465, 1943.

Peck, S. M., & N. Rosenthal: Effect of moccasin snake venom in hemorrhagic conditions, J. A. M. A., 104:1066, 1935.

Peiper, A.: Sporadische Haemophilie bei einem Mädchen, Med. Welt., 11:1492-93, 1937.

Quick, A. J.: Diagnosis of hemophilia, Am. J. M. Sc., 201:469-74, 1941.

Reed, C. P. B.: Dental hemorrhage arrested by egg-white derivative, Dental Digest, 49:75, 1943; Brit. Dent. Jour., 73:111, 1943.

The Purpuras and Other Blood Dyscrasias

Cappon, D.: Hereditary haemorrhagic telangiectasia, Brit. M. J., 1:440, 1945.

Cook, T. J.: Blood dyscrasias from dental point of view, Am. J. Orthodontics, 24:467, 1938.

Cooley, T. B., & O. P. Lee: Erythroblastic anemia: additional comments, Am. J. Dis. Child., 43:705-08, 1932.

Corcoran, M. J.: Erythroblastic anemia, Radiology, 43:373, 1944.

Dameshek, W.: Hematology, New England J. Med., 228:157, 188, 1943.

Davis, E.: Hereditary familial purpura simplex, Lancet, 2:1110-14, 1939.

Erf, Lowell A.: Radio-phosphorus—an agent for the satisfactory treatment of polycythemia and its associated manifestations, Ann. Int. Med., 19:587, 1943.

Evans, H., & K. M. A. Perry: Thrombocytopenic purpura, Lancet, 2:410, 1943.

Falconer, E. H., & I. C. Schumacher: Purpura haemorrhagica due to ingestion of sedormid (allylisopropylacetylcarbamide); experimental observations and report of case, Arch. Int. Med., 65:122-37, 1940.

Figi, F. A., & C. H. Watkins: Hereditary hemorrhagic telangiectasia, Ann. Otol., Rhin. & Laryng., 52:330, 1943.

Flynn, J. M.: Erythroblastic anemia with review of the literature, Brit. J. Radiol., 16:157, 1943.

Herrman, J. B.: Schonlein-Henoch's purpura simulating acute surgical abdomen, Connecticut M. J., 4:202-07, 1940.

Houser, K. M.: Hereditary hemorrhagic telangectasia, Tr. Am. Laryng. A., 56:86, 1934.

Jersild, T.: Therapeutic effect of vitamin P in Schonlein-Henoch's purpura, Lancet, 1:1445-47, 1938.

Larrabee, R. C., & D. Littman: Hereditary hemorrhagic telangiectasis, New England J. Med., 207:1177, 1932.

Limarzi, L. R.: Hemorrhagic diseases, Dent. Outlook, 31:142, 1944.

Newerla, G. J.: Erythroblastosis fetalis: report of a case, New England J. Med., 229:533, 1943.

Osler, William: On a family form of recurring epistaxis, associated with multiple telangiectases of the skin and mucous membranes, Bull. Johns Hopkins Hosp., 12:333, 1901.

Peck, S. M., & N. Rosenthal: Effect of moccasin snake (Ancistrodon piscivorus) in hemorrhagic conditions, J. A. M. A., 104:1066-70, 1935.

Rosenfeld, S., & F. Feldman: Thrombopenic purpura due to sulfathiazole, J. A. M. A., 118:974-5, 1942.

Rucks, L. W., & J. J. Hobson: Purpura fulminans (Waterhouse-Friderichsen syndrome), J. Pediat., 22:226, 1943.

Schamp, H. M., & C. M. Giddings: Effects of certain sulpha and other drugs on blood clotting, J. California State Dent. A., 20:1, 1944.

Steiner, W. R.: Hereditary hemorrhagic telangiectasia: with report of three families and a review of those previously recorded, Arch. Int. Med., 19:194, 1917.

Thoma, Kurt, et al.: Erythroblastic anemia, Am. J. Orthodontics & Oral Surg., 30:643, 1944.

White, James W.: Thrombocytopenic purpura and tooth extraction, Brit. M. J., 2:341, 1944.

Whitehouse, F. R., & C. H. Watkins: Acute thrombocytopenic purpura following sulfadiazine therapy, Proc. Staff Meet., Mayo Clinic, 17:140-3, 1942.

THE SPECIFIC INFECTIOUS GRANULOMATA

22

Syphilis

GENERAL CONSIDERATIONS

The specific infectious granulomata include tuberculosis, actinomycosis, blastomycosis, leprosy, syphilis (tertiary), Hodgkin's disease, lymphogranuloma venereum and other rarer diseases. The etiologic agents for this group of diseases include viruses, bacteria and fungi.

The oral lesions of the specific infectious granulomata have many characteristics in common and from the standpoint of oral medicine and oral diagnosis it is well to consider these diseases as a group. The lesions of the infectious granulomata are characterized by a marked proliferation of connective tissue rather than a marked vascular and exudative change. This connective tissue proliferation, with the accompanying growth of capillaries (granulation tissue), furnishes the basis for the term granulomata.

Most of these diseases are characterized by a marked chronicity. Acute fulminating symptoms are uncommon unless blood stream invasion occurs. The exact time of onset is difficult to determine. Since these diseases present infrequently oral lesions they are usually incorrectly diagnosed. The oral mucosal lesions of many of these diseases are characterized by the appearance of recurrent small "pimples" or small abscesses, which rupture, forming shallow ulcers along whose margins new miliary lesions develop. While the appearance of the individual lesions differ somewhat for the various diseases, they all have the same general characteristics of chronicity, the production of granulation tissue and frequently the history of miliary lesions forming about the periphery of the ulcer.

The importance of syphilis from the medical and public health point of view has been brought to the attention of the public through educational programs sponsored by the Surgeon General's Office, professional groups, the press and radio. The medical and public health aspects of the disease must assume greater importance than the associated moral issues. This does not imply that promiscuity should be sanctioned, or that moral issues are not involved but the public must consider syphilis first as a disease that requires prompt professional attention and then determine the moral issues.

Osler called syphilis "the great imitator" because of its protean manifestations. It is said that, if one knows syphilis in all of its manifestations, one will know all of medicine. To a lesser degree this is true of the oral mucosal lesions encountered in this disease. The clinical manifestations of the oral lesions are varied and they present peculiarities of their own. The dentist should be familiar with the oral findings in the various stages of the disease for his personal protection, for the welfare of his patient and the safety of society. Since oral lesions may be present in all stages of the disease and since they are second in frequency to the genital lesions, the dentist has an unusual opportunity for diagnosing unsuspected syphilis.

The prevalence of syphilis is variable depending on the geographic locality and the relative proportion of the colored race in the population group. Vonderlehr and Usilton summarized the serologic findings of 1,895,778 selectees between the ages of 21 and 35. The prevalence of syphilis was 47.7 per thousand. Based on these findings the estimated rate for the entire male Negro population aged 21 to 35 is 272 per thousand, for the entire male white population of the same age group 23.5 per thousand. The highest prevalence rates for whites and Negroes are found in the southeastern states. Marriage laws have been enacted in many of the states which require proof of non-infectious syphilis in both partners to the marriage prior to the granting of the license. Data from such sources indicate a prevalence of from 50 to 325 per thousand.

The most common mode of infection is through sexual intercourse with an infected partner. If syphilis were transmitted through some prosaic medium like the drinking water, the disease would have long since been controlled. Extragenital lesions and modes of transmission are also well known but they constitute less than 5% of the total cases. They will be discussed in greater detail under the oral lesions of syphilis.

Syphilis may also be contracted by the dentist, the physician and their assistants during the course of their professional duties. Vonderlehr stated that extragenital lesions are more common among dentists than any other group of professional men. (See Occupational Diseases of Dental Practice.) After a course of intensive antiluetic therapy or in the chronic stages of the disease the chances of infection are minimal. It is the patient with undiagnosed syphilis, not the patient with known syphilis, who is dangerous.

The classical and time-honored division of syphilis into the primary, secondary and tertiary stages is being supplanted by the terms acute and chronic syphilis. The primary chancre, the macular or papular eruption and the mucous patches are grouped as manifestations of acute syphilis, while the gummatous lesions, the osseous and central nervous system involvements are considered manifestations of chronic syphilis. From the standpoint of infectiousness, treatment and prognosis, this grouping of luetic manifestations into acute and chronic syphilis is desirable.

ACUTE AND CHRONIC SYPHILIS

The syphilitic chancre develops usually within 14 to 21 days at the site of inoculation with the *Treponema pallidum*. The typical, brown, encrusted, painless, indurated lesion associated with regional lymphadenopathy does not always develop. If secondary infection occurs the usual appearance may be altered considerably.

Genital lesions are rarely observed in the female. Because of the anatomy of the parts, they are more commonly observed in the male. It is not unusual for the general macular eruption to be the first manifestation of the disease in either sex. Constitutional symptoms are mild or entirely absent when the chancre is present. After periods varying from 3 weeks to 2 months, the primary lesion regresses spontaneously.

The location and appearance of the lesion usually suggest the correct diagnosis. Darkfield examination is the most valuable diagnostic aid in the first 2 to 3 weeks of the lesion. After this time the various blood serologic reactions become positive, until by the end of the 6th week all the blood serologic reactions are usually strongly positive.

Following the disappearance of the chancre, there is usually a period during which there is no clinical evidence of the disease except for the positive serologic findings.

The generalized manifestations of the syphilitic infection (secondary stage) develop usually about 6 weeks after the appearance of the primary lesion but they may appear years later. They consist of the generalized skin eruption, the mucous patches on the mucous membranes, pharyngitis and mild to moderate constitutional symptoms. The typical skin eruption consists of a generalized macular or papular coppery-red or ham-colored spots which are most prominent on the face, hands, feet and genitalia. Pain and itching are rare symptoms. A generalized adenopathy commonly accompanies the eruption. Constitutional symptoms of malaise, anorexia, headaches, bone pains and a mild elevation of temperature frequently accompany these cutaneous manifestations. The appearance of the eruption varies and it may simulate a variety of dermatologic conditions.

An acute pharyngitis—syphilitic angina—is often a manifestation of acute (secondary) syphilis. The involved tissues appear swollen, dry and have a beefy red color. The patient may complain of a recently developed hoarseness. Biederman observed a dark, dusky-red band 6 to 10 mm. wide on the anterior pillars of the fauces beginning at their base and extending upwards from 0.5 to 2.5 cm. in approximately 70% of the luetics examined. He considered this sign a useful diagnostic aid.

The diagnosis of acute syphilis is made on the history of exposure (when obtained), the history of a primary lesion or positive blood serologic reactions which are strongly positive in later stages of acute syphilis. Darkfield examination of material obtained from the mucous patches is also strongly positive. The *Treponema pallidum* and the oral *Treponema microdentium* have many common morphologic features which make the interpretation of darkfield examination of material from suspected oral syphilitic lesions difficult for even the experienced syphilologist.

The manifestations of chronic syphilis are so varied and widespread that they may simulate almost any disease entity and the clinician should always consider syphilis as a possibility in the diagnosis of any unusual symptom complex. The syphilitic gumma, an infectious granuloma, may involve any structure of the body. It seems to have a predilection for bones which are formed intramembranously such as the bones of the face (especially the palatal and nasal bones) and certain of the solid viscera such as the liver and spleen. Luetic involvement of the liver results in jaundice.

Syphilitic involvement of the cardiovascular system is particularly important. Syphilis affects primarily the aortic valves and the ascending portion of the aorta. This involvement of the aortic valves and the base of the aorta results in aortic insufficiency and a whole train of associated cardiac changes of a serious nature. The syphilitic aortitis, affecting primarily the media, is characterized by a loss of the elastic tissue and a weakening of the muscular layer of the aorta, which results in insufficiency of the aortic valves and at times aneuryms and fatal rupture of the aorta.

Short, shooting, knife-like pains are frequently experienced in the abdominal region in the "tabetic crises." They result from involvement of the posterior root ganglia. These sporadic pains are frequently mistaken for symptoms of organic disease in the organs supplied by these nerves and at times operations have been performed before the true cause of the pains has been determined.

Nervous system involvement in chronic syphilis produces a wide variety of symptoms, depending on the location and the extent of the lesion. A single cerebral gumma may produce symptoms suggestive of a brain tumor. Involvement of the cranial nerves results in pupils which react to accommodation but not to light—the Argyl-Robertson pupils. Involvement of the spinal cord—tabes dorsalis—is a common late manifestation. A patient with tabes dorsalis soon loses the position sense of this extremity and walks with a characteristic slapping step. This change of gait may be accompanied by burning or prickly sensations of the extremities, parethesias or actual anesthesia of the parts. Such an individual is unable to stand erect unaided with his eyes closed—a positive Romberg's sign.

PRENATAL SYPHILIS

Systemic Aspects

The term prenatal syphilis is preferable to congenital or hereditary syphilis, as the fetus actually "acquires" the infection *in utero*.

The incidence of prenatal syphilis is dropping significantly as a result of the more general acceptance of prenatal clinics in which tests for maternal syphilis are a routine procedure. Luetic pregnant women will usually give birth to nonsyphilitic children if appropriate antiluetic therapy is begun by the 5th month of gestation.

A primary lesion is not observed in prenatal luetics. The characteristic macular eruption, the snuffles, the loss of weight, the cracking and scaling of the reddened soles of the feet and palms are a manifestation of acute or secondary syphilis. The cracking and scaling of the skin gives a weazened-old-man-appearance to the infant. The head has frequently a squarish configuration with prominent frontal lobes. Later in life such individuals have

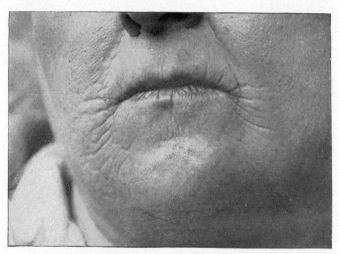

FIG. 223. Rhagades forming permanent scars radiating from the lips. (Thoma, Oral Pathology, C. V. Mosby Co.)

as a rule coarse, dry hair and a pasty complexion. Symptoms of tertiary or chronic syphilis may develop at an early age and children of 10 or 12 years of age may show the typical "saddle-nose" deformity due to gummatous destruction of the nasal bones or perforation of the palate.

Oral Aspects

The oral changes associated with prenatal syphilis represent at times the only visual symptoms of the infection and since these changes persist or are manifest years after the acute infection, the dentist may be the first to suspect this disease. The patient is seldom infectious after the acute stage of the disease. The oral aspects of prenatal syphilis include: (1) the post rhagadic scarring about the mouth, (2) the changes in the teeth and (3) other dentofacial abnormalities.

Postrhagadic Scarring—Syphilitic Rhagades. Postrhagadic scars are linear markings that are found about the oral or anal orifices. They are the result of a diffuse luetic involvement of the skin of these parts which develop usually between the 3rd to 7th week of life. The acute lesion appears as a red or coppery-colored linear area covered with a necrotic crust. Strakosh stated that the rhagades are seen more frequently on the lower lip because of the thinness of the epithelium covering this structure and its greater mobility.

The healed syphilitic rhagades appear clinically as ordinary cicatrices but histologic study reveals specific pathologic changes. The linear scars are

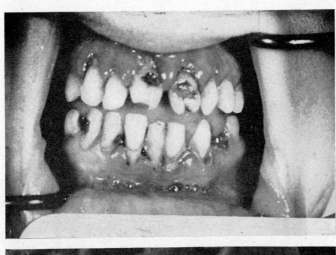

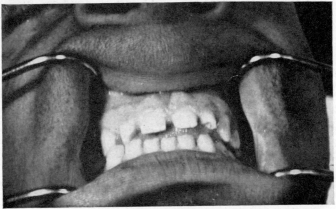

FIG. 224 (*Top*). Notched incisors and peg-shaped teeth present in a patient with prenatal syphilis.

FIG. 225 (*Bottom*). Screwdriver incisors, the spacing of the maxillary teeth and the open bite deformity are commonly found in individuals having prenatal lues.

radially arranged, perpendicular to the mucocutaneous junction, and they are most prominent on the lower lip near the angles of the mouth. Frequently there is a diminished coloring of the lip and a lack of distinctness of the mucocutaneous border.

Hutchinson's Triad. The deciduous dentition is rarely affected since any fetal luetic infection which occurs during the formation of the crowns of these teeth, results usually in abortion. Abnormalities in color, size and shape of the deciduous teeth have been described and the author has demonstrated histologic changes confined to the dentin of these teeth. A retarded root absorption of the deciduous dentition is frequently noted in prenatal luetics.

Sir Jonathon Hutchinson described in 1856 the typical defects of the permanent incisors associated with prenatal syphilis and in 1859 before the London Pathological Society he proposed the diagnostic triad for prenatal

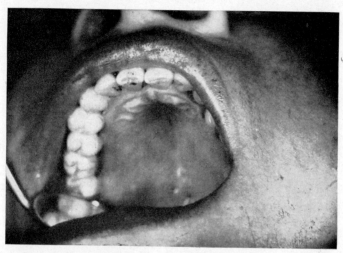

FIG. 226. Mulberry maxillary first molar in a patient with prenatal syphilis. Observe how the cusps of the first molar are more centrally placed than those of the premolars.

syphilis which now bears his name. The Hutchinson's Triad includes: (1) the characteristic defects (hypoplasia) of the permanent incisors and molar teeth, (2) eighth nerve deafness and (3) interstitial keratitis. Clinical experience has shown that the entire triad is seldom present and that the effects of this disease on the dentofacial structures are more profound than those originally described by Hutchinson.

The dental hypoplasias associated with prenatal syphilis affect primarily the permanent incisors, the cuspids and the first molars since these teeth are being formed during the period of the luetic infection. Hutchinson described the characteristic notching of the edges of the permanent incisors. However, the morphology of the entire tooth is characteristically altered. There is a general constriction of the crown towards the incisal edge which gives rise to the common "screwdriver" and "peg-shaped" incisors frequently associated with this disease. There is also a rounding of the mesial and distal marginal ridges which gives to the erupted tooth a characteristic clinical appearance. The tip of the cuspid is frequently involved and a spacing between the incisors and this tooth is a common observation.

The molar lesions are characterized by a marked constriction of the cusps toward the central portion of the crown, giving the tooth a bud-shaped or shrunken appearance on the occlusal surface. The enamel covering the cusps may be intact, although marked defects are present in the grooves and fissures of the tooth. A prominent Carabelli's cusp (accessory bucco-lingual cusp of the upper molars) was once believed to be indicative of prenatal lues. Campbell has presented clinical evidence of altered permanent tooth form occurring in the children of prenatal luetics which appears as peg-shaped or missing incisors, usually the second.

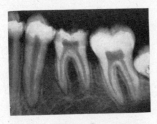

FIG. 227. Roentgenogram of mandibular molar area in a patient with prenatal syphilis, demonstrating the dwarfing of both the crown and the root of the first permanent molar.

There is considerable speculation whether these dental deformities are the direct result of the *T. pallidum* in the enamel organ or whether they represent a general interference with the function of highly specialized cells (ameloblasts) resulting from endocrine or nutritional disturbances secondary to the *T. pallidum*. Luetic infections are certainly the most common cause of such dental deformities. Bauer, Hill and Gottlieb have demonstrated the *T. pallidum* in the enamel organ of developing teeth, but other investigators have not been so fortunate. Kreshover has shown experimentally that enamel hypoplasias produced by numerous different causes have essentially the same histologic findings and he suggests that the *T. pallidum per se* has no specific effect in the dental hypoplasias commonly associated with prenatal syphilis.

These dental changes associated with prenatal syphilis must be distinguished from those associated with rachitis or the exanthematous fevers. The general contour of the tooth is usually unaltered in the enamel hypoplasias associated with these conditions, and the defects are confined to linear or zonal areas on the labial or cuspal surfaces. While there may be marked local areas of hypoplasia of the enamel and dentin, a constriction of the crowns of the teeth or the cusps is rarely seen unless a prenatal luetic infection is also present.

Dental X-ray Findings. The characteristic notching of the permanent incisors may be demonstrated by means of a roentgenogram before the eruption of this tooth if prenatal syphilis is

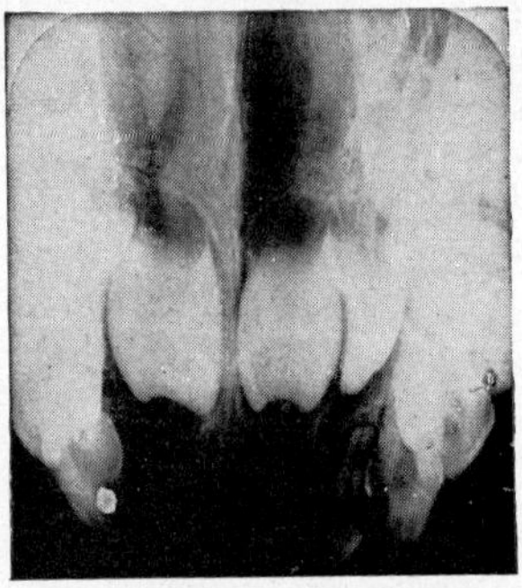

FIG. 228. Demonstration of Hutchinsonian incisors prior to their eruption by means of the dental roentgenogram. (Stokes, Beerman and Ingraham, Clinical Syphililology, W. B. Saunders Company.)

suspected. This has been done by Stokes and also Schour. While this finding is highly suggestive if the typical notched incisor is present, the other variations of the incisors will not produce as conclusive a picture. An equally characteristic but less universally appreciated roentgenographic finding is the altered general morphology of the mandibular first permanent molar. Not only the clinical crown but also the root of this tooth is dwarfed.

Johnston *et al*. have demonstrated that the mesiodistal diameter of this tooth and the general size of the tooth are usually smaller in prenatal luetics than the adjacent second molar; the reverse of the condition is seen usually in normal individuals. While the crown of the first mandibular molar may be markedly affected in the enamel hypoplasias associated with rickets, the root of the tooth is not involved.

Dentofacial Changes. Malocclusion is frequently observed in prenatal luetics. Klauder considered the "open bite" which may be found in these patients to be of the same diagnostic value as the Hutchinsonian tooth. Johnston *et al*. noted an "open bite" deformity in approximately one-third of the children studied. This deformity results apparently from a lack of development of the premaxilla. While the open bite is not diagnostic when taken alone, when associated with any of the other stigmata of prenatal syphilis it is more significant. Stathers does not consider that any particular type of malocclusion occurs sufficiently frequently to be considered characteristic of prenatal syphilis. Stathers & Skidmore found that many times the dental changes were asymmetric in distribution.

TABLE XXVII *

DISTRIBUTION OF EXTRAGENITAL CHANCRES BY SITE, RACE, AND SEX

	Males		Females	
Site	White	Negro	White	Negro
Lip.	5	3	3	2
Tonsil.	..	..	1	1
Tongue.	1	..	..	..
Mouth.	..	..	1	..
Nose.	..	..	1	..
Breast.	..	..	1	..
Wrist.	..	..	1	..
Finger.	..	1	1	..
Abdomen.	2	..	..	..
Groin.	..	1	..	..
Totals.	8	5	9	3

* Rudolph H. Kampmeier, M.D. "Essentials of Syphilology," J. B. Lippincott Co.

SYPHILITIC CHANCRE

General Features

The oral cavity is the most frequent site of extragenital syphilitic lesions and their recognition by the dentist is of particular importance as the clinical appearance and symptomatology of these lesions differ considerably from those found on the genitalia. Since the lesions of acute syphilis (primary and secondary) are highly contagious, they represent a serious public health problem and a potential source of infection of the dentist in the performance

of his professional duties. The lesions of chronic syphilis are equally important but they do not offer such a hazard to the dentist or society.

Chancres of Orofacial Region

Location. Chancres are found on the lips, oral mucosa, tongue, soft palate,
tonsillar and pharyngeal region and the gums. The lip alone accounted for
57% of the extragenital chancres studied by Wile and Holman. The lesions are
found more frequently on the lower lip in the male. No unusual histories were

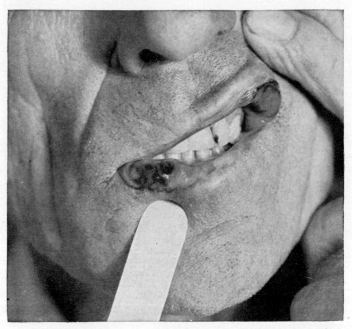

Fig. 229. Primary syphilis—multiple chancres. (Kampmeier,
Essentials of Syphilology, J. B. Lippincott Company.)

obtained regarding the acquisition of the lesions. A history of a bruise, a
cigaret burn, razor trauma or a "cold sore" were common. Many of the
lesions were not contracted through sexual relations.

Chancres of the gum are uncommon.* An interesting case of chancre developing following dental extraction was observed recently.

A 25-year-old male was referred to the clinic by his dentist for the diagnosis and treatment of a shallow spreading ulcer which developed following the removal of an upper
right third molar. Normal healing of the alveolus occurred for the first 2 weeks, at which
time a shallow, slightly painful "ulceration" developed at the alveolus and spread gradually onto the palate. This lesion was treated as a fusospirochetal infection and then by
the repeated application of a mild caustic without response.

When the patient was first seen in the clinic, the lesion in question did not present the
clinical characteristics of either a fusospirochetal ulceration or a chancre. It was shallow
and grayish-white and not particularly painful on palpation. It appeared as an erosion

* Epstein & Zeisler, Straith, Sadusk & Anderson reported chancres on the gingiva.

rather than an ulcer. There was no induration or surrounding area of erythema. A blood Wassermann and darkfield examination of the superficial lesion were both negative. Nothing out of the ordinary was seen in a smear, stained in the usual way. A blood Wassermann and darkfield examination of material aspirated from the alveolus 1 week later

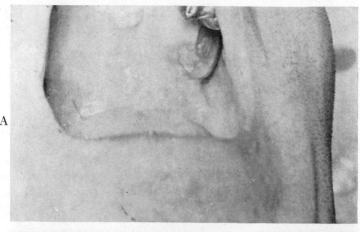

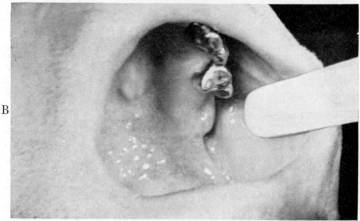

Fig. 230. (A) Primary syphilitic chancre which developed at the site of a healing socket. Adenopathy was present at the left angle of the mandible. (B) Same patient following ten days of antiluetic treatment showing marked regression of the local lesion.

were strongly positive. A history of buccogenital contact 10 days following the removal of the tooth was then obtained from the patient. The granulation tissue of the healing socket formed a satisfactory site for the implantation of the *T. pallidum*.

Appearance. As this case history illustrates, chancres of the oral cavity do not present the typical painless, brown, crusted, indurated lesion found on the genitalia because of the moisture, the trauma and bacterial flora present in the mouth. Oral chancres are usually slightly painful and they are covered with a grayish-white film or slough. Extra-oral portions of lip chancres may have a brown, crusted appearance while the intra-oral portion of the same lesions will have the grayish-white surface. Induration of the underlying tissues is not as prominent a symptom as on other body surfaces. Smears, made from such lesions and stained by the usual aniline dyes, show usually few bacterial forms and *T. pallidum* is refractory to the usual aniline stains. Occasionally the bacterial smear may show a picture simulating a mild fuso-spirochetal infection.

Exposure to infection, if known or admitted, is an important aid in making a tentative diagnosis. Enlargement of the lymph nodes draining the area of

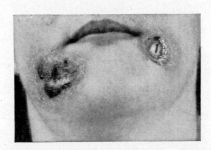

FIG. 231. Appearance of two chancres located on the chin. (Lever, New Eng. J. Med., 10: 231, 1944.)

the lesion is one of the most significant and valuable diagnostic aids. The lymphadenopathy is usually hard and slightly painful. Thurmon did not feel that the clinical appearance of the lesion or even the darkfield examination is specifically diagnostic for lesions well within the oral cavity as there are other organisms inhabiting this region (*T. microdentium*) which are difficult to differentiate from *T. pallidum.*

Herpetic lesions of the lip offer a problem in diagnosis. The superficial crusting which occurs following the rupture of a large vesicle or a group of small vesicles simulates a chancre. However, the encrusted surface of a herpetic lesion is usually yellow in contrast with the brownish-black of the chancre. The history of onset of the herpetic lesion is usually characteristic. It is more painful, it is of shorter duration and it is frequently associated with an upper respiratory infection. Lymphadenopathy is uncommon. A "herpetic lesion" which requires more than 2 weeks for involution, especially if accompanied by unilateral adenopathy, should be suspected of being of luetic origin.

Diagnosis of a syphilitic oral chancre is based on the history, darkfield examination made by a competent observer and, in the later stages of the lesion, blood serologic reactions.

SYPHILITIC MUCOUS PATCHES

General Features

Syphilitic mucous patches represent the mucous membrane analogue of the papular or macular skin eruption. They are found on the genital mucosa, the oral mucosa, the tongue, the tonsillar and pharyngeal region and on the lips. Their development on the gums is uncommon. The oral commissure is a fre-

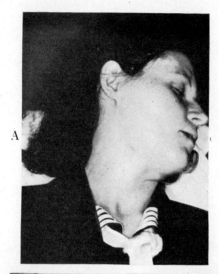

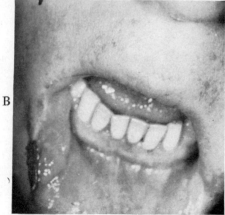

FIG. 232. (A) Syphilitic chancre of the lip and incision below the right angle of the jaw. The adenopathy was considered to be secondary to a diseased lower molar. (B) Syphilitic chancre of the lip in the same patient.

quent site, and, in this location, the lesions present a split or folded appearance caused by the folding of the tissue.

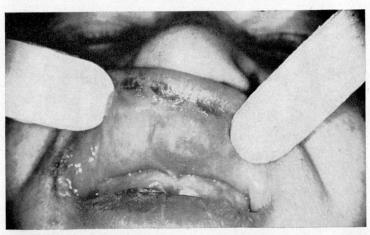

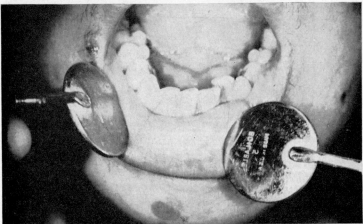

FIG. 233 (*Top*). Mucous patch of the upper lip and syphilitic lesions of the vermilion borders of the lips and oral commissures. Note the oval shape of the mucous patch and its translucent surface.

FIG. 234 (*Bottom*). Patient with generalized lesions of acute syphilis. A split papula is present at the right oral commissure, a mucous patch on the lip and a papular skin lesion on the chin. (Also see color plates.)

The mucous patches are the most infectious lesion of acute syphilis. They appear as slightly raised, grayish-white lesions which are surrounded by an erythematous base. They are moderately painful when they develop on movable tissues. Trauma to the surface of the lesion results in a raw bleeding surface. Mucous patches are frequently observed on the tongue. The partial loss of the lingual papillae over the lesions clearly demarcates them from the uninvolved tissue.

Oral Mucous Patches

Oral mucous patches may be mistaken for fusospirochetal ulcerations, healing herpetic or traumatic lesions. A history of an associated dermal eruption is useful in making the diagnosis. Fusospirochetal ulcerations are more acutely painful and they are usually asociated with the typical gingival lesions. Aniline-dye stained bacterial smears are of no diagnostic value and, while dark-field examination is almost always positive for *T. pallidum,* it presents the

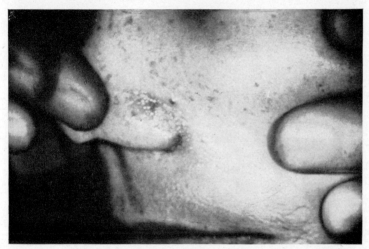

Fig. 235. Moist syphilitic lesions at the nasolabial fold.

same difficulties discussed under the diagnosis of oral chancres. The blood serologic tests for syphilis are positive at this stage of the disease and they furnish the best means of diagnosis.

SYPHILITIC GUMMATA

Location

The lesions of chronic (tertiary) syphilis which are most frequently found in the mouth are confined to the palate and the tongue. Gummatous destruction of the palatal bones is the most frequent cause of pathologic palatal defects. Gummata may involve the salivary glands and the jaw bones.

Of Palate and Tongue

Gummatous involvement of the tongue is not unusual in late untreated syphilis. Single gummas are usually found on the dorsum of this organ and their differential diagnosis when ulcerated presents a problem as malignant growths and tuberculous lesions must be considered. Since the blood serology may be negative in this stage of the disease biopsy is indicated. Numerous small gummata may form in the tongue. In the healing process which follows, a series of nodules, scars and sulci are formed on the dorsum of the tongue which give it an upholstered appearance—the typical luetic interstitial glos-

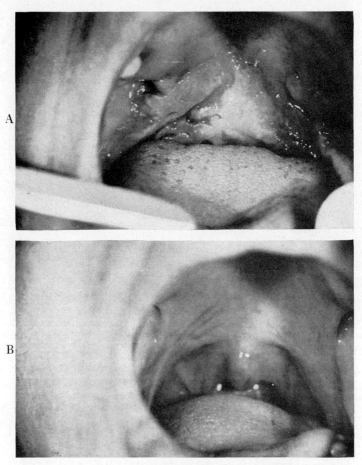

A

B

FIG. 236. (A) Extensive mucous patches of the soft palate. (B) Same patient following antiluetic treatment with penicillin.

sitis. Such a tongue with its distorted appearance, fibrous texture, and loss of covering papillae is also called a luetic bald tongue.

Leukoplakia is frequently associated with the various forms of luetic glossitis but the exact nature of the relationship has not been established. (See Leukoplakia.) Syphilis may be one of the many conditions predisposing to leukoplakia. Malignant degeneration of these leukoplakic areas occurs frequently, probably because of the advanced state of the condition before diagnosis is made and treatment is instigated.

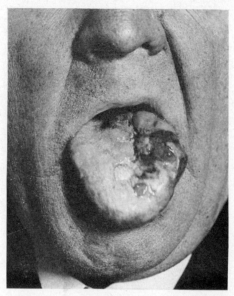

FIG. 237. Syphilitic interstitial glossitis, smooth atrophy of tongue, leukoplakia, and squamous carcinoma. (Courtesy of Dr. George M. MacKee.) (From Sutton and Sutton, Diseases of the Skin, C. V. Mosby Co.)

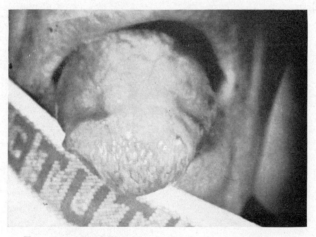

FIG. 238. Syphilitic interstitial glossitis with associated leukoplakic changes and squamous cell carcinoma of the tip of the tongue.

SYPHILIS OF THE NERVOUS SYSTEM

Certain strains of the *Treponema pallidum* have a predilection for nervous tissue. Paresis, syphilitic involvement of the cerebral tissue and tabes dorsalis,

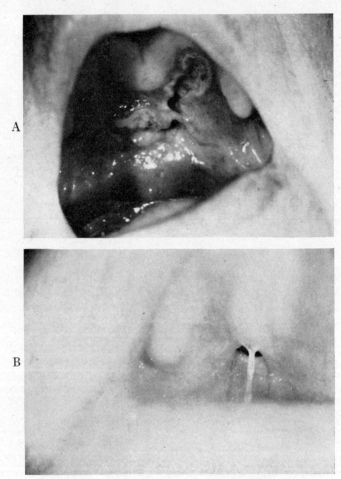

FIG. 239. (A) Active gumma of the palate. The marginal bluish purple coloration is typical. Perforation of the palate was not complete at this time. (B) Perforation of the palate which developed following treatment. Mucus is dropping from the nasal cavity into the mouth.

syphilitic involvement of the posterior root ganglia, are the common forms of neurosyphilis.

Paresis and Tabes Dorsalis

Paretic neurosyphilis develops in approximately 3% of the patients with syphilis with a marked predominance in males. The symptoms of paresis are extremely varied and they may mimic almost any disease. Personality changes are often the first manifestation of neurosyphilis. Increased irritability, fatigability, mental sluggishness, or carelessness in personal habits are other early symptoms. There is a loss of fine muscular co-ordination, as indicated by the inability to enunciate clearly or to perform delicate tests with the hands. In the classical case of paresis, the patient develops ideas of grandeur,

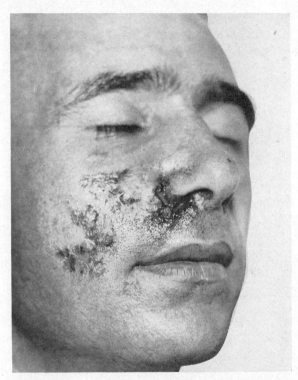

FIG. 240. Syphilitic osteomyelitis associated with an impacted supernumerary tooth in the upper incisor region. Note the numerous fistulous openings.

wealth and ability far beyond his station in life. Occasionally these euphoric symptoms first suggest the diagnosis. Eventually the affected individual loses his memory, his ability to reason and to perform the acts of speech and writing, and he becomes more or less a vegetable. Paretic neurosyphilis is treated with artificial fever, therapeutic infection with malarial parasites and the arsenical tryparsamide.

Tabes dorsalis is a late manifestation of untreated or inadequately treated syphilis which occurs in approximately 2 to 3% of all luetics. Symptoms develop usually 10 to 20 years following the initial infection. The patient often experiences abnormal sensations of warmth and coldness. Pain of an agonizing, burning or gnawing variety may be experienced. Sharp, stabbing, knife-like pains, the tabetic crises, which appear to be localized to certain definite areas, or which dart from place to place, are an early and fairly constant symptom in tabes dorsalis. They are commonly more severe at night. The recurrent paroxysms of abdominal pain which are often accompanied by nausea and vomiting (gastric crises) are at times mistaken for organic disease processes of the affected organ. Following the acute painful episode, the individual feels well and has no gastro-intestinal symptoms.

Some of the more important diagnostic signs of tabes dorsalis, such as the Argyll-Robertson pupil and the ataxic gait, may be detected by the dentist. The Argyll-Robertson pupil is one which fails to react to light (pupillary con-

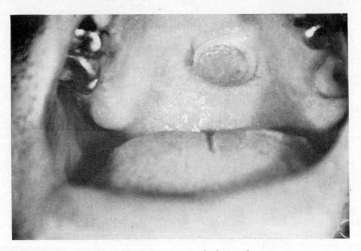

FIG. 241. Gumma of the palate.

striction) but which still reacts to accommodation. The pupils may be unequal as to size or maintain a somewhat contracted state.

In the well-developed case of tabes dorsalis, the characteristic unsteady, staggering, slap-footed gait of the patient is a striking and conspicuous symptom. The muscle and position sense of the extremities are impaired and the affected individual has great difficulty in maintaining a steady posture when standing with the eyes closed and the feet together (Romberg's sign). Lack of muscular co-ordination and position sense are manifested by the inability to touch the tip of the nose with a finger. Trophic changes consist of deep perforating ulcers and painless destruction of the larger joints (Charcot joint).

The diagnosis of tabes dorsalis is made on the history of a past luetic infection, the subjective symptoms and the presence of some of the clinical signs of the infection in conjunction with certain laboratory studies. The blood Wassermann may or may not be positive, but the spinal Wassermann and the colloidal gold reaction are usually positive.

Oral Aspects. Severe neuralgic pains of the head and neck may be present in tabes dorsalis. They must be differentiated from neuralgic pains due to dental or pharyngeal foci which would have a similar distribution. Winkelman reported several cases of trigeminal neuralgia due entirely to syphilis and stated that it is not unusual in tabes dorsalis to have degeneration of the sensory portion of the 5th cranial nerve with complete integrity of the motor root. This condition is analogous to that commonly observed in the spinal nerves. Strauss called attention to tenderness of the masseter and temporal muscles in trigeminal neuritis of syphilitic origin.

A   B

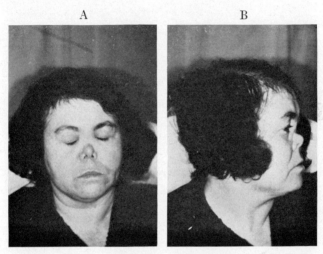

FIG. 242. (A) Front and (B) profile views of the saddle-nose facial deformity resulting from gummatous destruction of the nasal bones in a patient with prenatal syphilis.

Loss of taste and spontaneous necrosis of the alveolar process without any observable cause have been described in tabetic patients. Paresthesias are common in all parts of the body, including the lips, tongue and cheeks. More or less painless ulcerations of the palate and nasal septum are often seen. Kron and Pentz reported the extraction of teeth without anesthesia. Spontaneous death of the dental pulp in the absence of recognizable precipitating factors has been observed in both tabetic and paretic patients.

Penz observed that the vital reaction of the dental pulp to induced currents is considerably modified in tabetic and paretic patients. Abnormal variations ranging from hyperesthesia to anesthesia were found in 94% of the cases. The amount of current necessary to reach the "irritation point" in these patients varied, but it tended toward a decreased irritability or partial anesthesia of this tissue. The thresholds of sensitivity were found to be erratic and irregular in contrast with the more definite and regular curve obtained in the control subjects. Histologic studies of the dental pulps of these patients revealed changes similar to those observed in other nerve tissue in neurosyphilis. Syphilitic degeneration of the Gasserian ganglion was also demonstrated.

23

Tuberculosis

GENERAL CONSIDERATIONS

Tuberculosis is a widespread infectious disease affecting not only man but the lower animals. It is important from the medical, social and economic standpoints. While marked advances have been made in the diagnosis and treatment of tuberculosis many cases are still diagnosed too late for effective treatment and for the protection of society.

A tuberculous infection is frequently referred to as an "acid-fast infection" because of the staining properties of the tubercle bacillus. The term "acid-fast infection" furnishes a satisfactory manner of referring to this disease in the presence of the patient.

Human or bovine strains of *Mycobacterium tuberculosis* are responsible for the disease in man. The population morbidity is high, estimated at around 95 to 98%. Tuberculosis is still responsible for 7 to 9% of all deaths. The American Indian and Negro and the Irish race are particularly susceptible. When tuberculosis has been introduced to primitive peoples, it runs an acute form with a high mortality.

Tuberculosis is more common in the female. Most deaths occur between the ages of 25 and 45 years. Individuals with a family history of tuberculosis are more susceptible than others. Inadequate nutrition, physical exertion, general debilitating diseases, overcrowding, and other respiratory disease such as silicosis are important predisposing factors in the clinical onset of the infection.

SYSTEMIC ASPECTS

The initial symptoms of chronic ulcerative or fibroid pulmonary tuberculosis may be subtle and unrecognized. Undue fatigability, loss of weight and anorexia, a rapid pulse, pallor and amenorrhea in the female are common initial symptoms. A regular elevation of temperature of 0.5 to 2° F. is a common finding in early infections. A persistent cough, particularly when productive of blood-stained sputum, should make one suspicious of tuberculosis. Hemoptysis is said to occur at some time in about 60% of all cases and, while this symptom is alarming, it is rarely fatal. At times hemoptysis is an initial symptom and one which often permits an early diagnosis of tuberculosis.

Forms

Tuberculosis may develop as an acute pulmonary infection with rapid, and usually fatal, spread throughout the body by means of the blood or lymphatic systems. Such patients present usually the symptoms of an acute pulmonary infection which persists unduly and which is usually accompanied by a rapid general deterioration of the patient. This form of the disease is known as acute miliary tuberculosis.

The usual form of the disease consists of a chronic process which is characterized by fibrotic or ulcerative lesions, cavitation, or a combination of these lesions. This form of tuberculosis, the chronic ulcerative or fibroid type, is responsible for by far the greater number of deaths.

A glandular form of the disease occurred frequently in children in past years. This was characterized by lesions in the intestinal tract and a marked enlargement of the cervical lymph nodes with caseation and often break down of the glands. These infections were usually due to the consumption of raw milk from tuberculous cows. Tuberculous involvement of the cervical nodes is called scrofula. Tuberculous caries of the spine, usually a disease of childhood, is known as Pott's disease.

Other body structures may be the primary tuberculous focus or they may be secondarily involved from pulmonary lesions. Involvement of the cervical glands in scrofula and the intestinal tract in childhood tuberculosis have already been mentioned. Tuberculosis of the spine, long bones and joints results in marked deformity and loss of function. Cerebral involvement, in the form of a single large abscess, a tuberculoma, may give symptoms indistinguishable from brain tumor. Tuberculous meningitis is generally fatal. Tuberculosis of the adrenal cortex is a common cause of Addison's disease.

Tuberculous abscesses may form in any organ or structure of the body. The chronicity of a tuberculous abscess and its lack of marked painful or inflammatory symptoms has resulted in the title of "cold abscess" as distinct from the usual pyogenic abscess.

Diagnosis

The diagnosis of pulmonary tuberculosis is based on the family history, the presence of one or more of the common symptoms of the disease, the physical findings, fluoroscopic or roentgenologic findings in the chest and certain laboratory studies. Symptoms of the disease may be present long before physical signs can be picked up in the chest even when the examination is done carefully and painstakingly by an expert. Repeated sputum examinations or gastric washings will reveal usually the presence of the tubercle bacillus. Sputum examinations, however, may remain negative even in the presence of pulmonary lesions which are readily demonstrable by the x-ray.

Fluoroscopy and stereoroentgenograms of the chest are the best methods of detecting early tubercular lesions and for estimating the extent of involvement in the more advanced stages of the disease. A regular chest x-ray survey of the adult population would go far to control this disease.

Laboratory Aids

Laboratory aids to diagnosis include the microscopic examination of Ziehl-Neelson stained sputum, exudate or scrapings, the tuberculin test, the erythrocyte sedimentation rate and guinea pig inoculations of suspected tuberculous material and biopsy studies. The technic for sputum examination and guinea pig inoculations have been discussed in the Chapter on Laboratory Procedures.

Tuberculin testing is more useful in the younger age groups. A "positive" reaction indicates sensitization of the tested tissues to the tubercle bacillus but it does not establish the temporal relation of the infection nor does it indicate whether the process is "active."

The erythrocyte sedimentation rate is usually elevated in tuberculous infections. It furnishes a rough estimate of the activity of the process but of course is not specific for tuberculous infections alone.

Treatment

The treatment of tuberculosis still consists mainly of mental and physical rest of the individual and the affected parts, an optimum diet, sunlight in certain forms of the disease, and measures which are taken to prevent the development of complications or the extension of the disease. Purely medical treatment of the tuberculous patient is most effective in the treatment of early lesions.

Recent developments in treatment have consisted mainly of new methods of applying long-known principles. These have consisted of measures taken to immobilize the involved portions of the lung by phrenectomy, phrenicotomy, collapse of the lung by means of air introduced in the intrapleural space—pneumothorax—or more radical procedures such as resection of the ribs and collapse of the lung—thoracoplasty.

Tuberculosis is one of the important diseases for which no satisfactory therapeutic serum, vaccine or chemotherapeutic agent has been found. Experimental studies have suggested that promin, a derivative of the sulfonamides, might be a useful therapeutic agent. The meagre human studies reported in which this drug have been used are not encouraging.

ORAL ASPECTS

Regular and complete dental care is of utmost importance in the successful management of the tuberculous patient. The maintenance of a healthy mouth and an adequate masticatory apparatus is a requisite for successful treatment of the active disease and the prevention of certain complications.

The oral aspects of the tuberculous patient can be grouped as follows:

(1) Healthy teeth and periodontal tissues are necessary for optimal general body resistance. Oral infections may represent a serious load on the general resistance of the patient.
(2) Good oral hygiene and healthy periodontal tissues are important factors in minimizing secondary pyogenic involvement of tuberculous cavities and the development of tuberculous lesions of the oral mucosa and tongue.
(3) Oral mucosal tuberculous lesions, an explanation of their infrequency, location on the oral mucosa, tongue, in the periapical tissues, the salivary glands and the bones.
(4) Dental lesions said to be associated with tuberculosis such as:
    (a) Vincent's infection.
    (b) Periodontal disease.
    (c) Increased dental caries—particularly the Class V cavity.
(5) The treatment of the oral mucosal lesions.

Optimal nutrition is paramount in the tuberculous patient and this cannot be achieved without an adequate number of serviceable teeth or replacements, which are surrounded by healthy supporting tissues. Suppurative periodontal lesions are particularly undesirable in the tuberculous patient. In addition to their effect on lowering the resistance of the patient, the swallowed exudate may interfere with normal digestive function. The transient bacteremias which occur frequently while chewing may give rise to metastatic pyogenic lesions in the lungs or other body areas which would have an unfavorable influence on the general course of the disease. The tuberculous patient requires frequent periodic dental care of a comprehensive nature.

Permanent restorative work is essential for establishing and maintaining a satisfactory nutritional state and in addition it promotes a desirable psychologic attitude on the part of the patient. The treatment of tuberculosis is measured in terms of years rather than weeks or months and the dental treatment of the tuberculous patient should be planned accordingly.

Oral Mucosal Lesions

Involvement of the oral cavity in tuberculosis is comparatively rare. The incidence of mouth lesions vary from 0.35 to 3.65% in all types of tubercular infections. Bryant observed only 17 cases in over 7,000 patients with advanced tuberculosis. Farber *et al.* observed 9 cases of tuberculous ulcers of the tongue in 9,000 cases he reviewed.

Several explanations have been offered for the infrequent occurrence of the oral lesions considering the number of patients with positive sputum. The resistance of the oral tissues may be unusually high for this type of infection. The mechanical cleansing action of the saliva and food may play an important rôle in hindering the development of the lesions. Preliminary studies made by Appleton, Kanter & Dietz have shown that the saliva exerted a bacteriostatic effect on the tubercle bacillus but it does not alter the virulence. The constituent of the saliva responsible for this effect has not been determined.

Oral tuberculous lesions are more common in the male probably because of their generally poor oral hygiene. The tongue is the most frequent site of the lesions, but the cheeks, gums and lips and palate are often involved. Tuberculous involvement of the salivary glands, particularly the parotid, tuberculous osteomyelitis and tuberculous apical dental granulomata occur less frequently.

The method of inoculation of the oral lesions is still undetermined. Some believe that the inoculation occurs as a result of infected sputum passing over

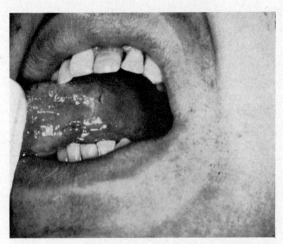

FIG. 243. Tuberculous ulcer of the lateral margin of the tongue. The lesion developed where the tongue margin was irritated by a broken-down tooth.

these tissues, while others assert that the organisms are carried to these tissues by the blood or lymphatic systems. The lingual lesions develop frequently at the site of previous traumatic lesions. Darlington and Salman reported 12 cases of tuberculous apical dental granulomata. Looseness of the teeth was the outstanding clinical symptom. In view of their experience with tuberculous apical dental granulomata, these authors believed that the organisms were distributed to these areas by the blood stream and not the sputum.

Tongue Lesions

Oral lesions of the tongue favor the theory of sputum inoculation. The lingual lesions develop frequently at the site of previous traumatic injuries. The anachoretic effect in the periapical tissues or in other regions of the mouth which are the site of chronic irritation lend support to the hematogenous route of inoculation.

Oral tuberculous lesions represent usually secondary manifestations of far advanced pulmonary disease which has an unfavorable prognosis. In a few instances, as for example the case reported by Collins and Cook, the oral lesions were believed to be primary. Proof of the primary nature of a lesion is difficult to establish.

The oral tuberculous lesions, particularly those of the lips, develop frequently as small "pimples" which break down to form ulcers. About the margins of the ulcer new "pimples" form and go through the same cycle. These small "pimples" represent miliary tubercles. This chronic process is repeated until marked tissue destruction occurs. The lesions are usually multiple.

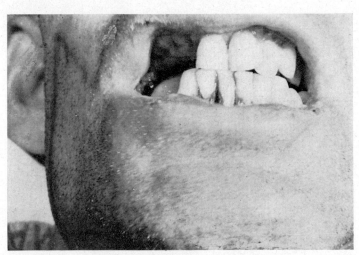

FIG. 244. Tuberculous ulcerations of the oral commissures and cheeks. A small tubercle is visible just to the right of the mandibular right canine. Direct smears from the lesions were positive for tubercle bacilli.

The initial site of oral tuberculous ulcers is frequently at the corners of the mouth but they may appear at any location. In some instances lesions develop on areas of the lip and cheek which were traumatized or which were the site of nonspecific irritations. The tuberculous ulcer is characterized by an irregular, undermined "mouse-eaten" border. The base of the ulcer is usually covered with a yellowish exudate or mucus. A less common oral manifestation consists of a productive granulomatous type of lesion.

Tongue lesions develop commonly at the site where this organ rests against rough, sharp or broken-down teeth, or at the sites of other trauma. The tip and lateral margins of the tongue are consequently the areas most commonly involved but deep ulcerated median fissures of the dorsum of the tongue are not uncommon. Ferber *et al.* described a case where the patient bit the left side of the tongue following the insertion of a dental bridge. The indolent ulcer which developed at this site was tuberculous in nature.

Oral mucosal tuberculous lesions are characterized by severe, unremitting and progressive pain which interferes seriously with the proper nutrition of the patient. Marked sialorrhea is common. These patients give often a history of repeated treatments for "Vincent's" infection without benefit. The oral tuberculous lesions are usually aggravated by intravenous therapy with arsphenamine or mapharsen.

Diagnosis. The diagnosis of oral tuberculous lesions may be difficult in cases where tuberculosis is not suspected. Chancre, gumma, carcinoma, traumatic and infectious ulcers of other causes must be considered. Ziehl-Neelson stained smears will occasionally demonstrate the causative organisms. While biopsy studies or animal inoculation studies are useful in diagnosing the oral

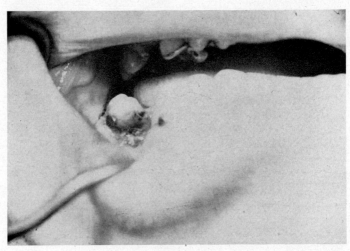

Fig. 245. Tuberculous lesion mesial to the lower right second molar. Direct smears were negative for tubercle bacilli. Repeated biopsy studies and animal inoculations were positive for tuberculosis.

lesions, any patient with suspicious oral lesions should be referred to a competent physician for thorough chest x-ray studies and physical examination. Morrow and Miller advised the complete removal of the lesion for biopsy study as they felt that, if only a part of it is removed, a marked reaction may occur.

Treatment. The treatment of oral tuberculous lesions is only an adjunct to the general management of the patient. Banyai found that the local application of cod liver oil is beneficial. Brodsky secured excellent results with Grenz ray radiation of oral lesions, even in some cases where osseous involvement has occurred. The actual cautery, CO_2 snow and ultraviolet radiation are used at times. The correction or removal of irritating teeth, broken dentures or appliances should precede any form of local treatment.

The prognosis of patients with oral tuberculous lesions is generally poor as the development of oral lesions indicates usually an unfavorable response of the body to the infection.

Oral Lesions Related to Tuberculosis

Numerous dental changes have been associated with tuberculosis. These changes include: (1) an increased incidence of periodontal diseases and (2) an increased incidence of dental decay, particularly the cervical or Class V cavity. Recent carefully controlled studies have not substantiated these earlier clinical impressions.

Tanchester and Sorrin did not find a higher incidence of periodontal disease in the tuberculous patient. Dental decay was not unusually high and the "typical cervical caries of the tubercular patient" was not found. The unusual cervical caries that was observed by some clinicians may be due in part to the habit of holding medicated lozenges or fruit-flavored drops containing large amounts of refined carbohydrates in the oral vestibule.

Gruber studied a group of tuberculous individuals in all stages of the disease who had experienced the infection for varying periods of time. These patients did not show an increased incidence of periodontal disease as determined by clinical and roentgenologic studies. The caries experience of these patients, in terms of DMF values, was slightly less than the generally accepted average. In this group, infection with tuberculosis did not have any deleterious effect on the teeth or the periodontal tissues.

Any disease which lowers markedly general body resistance may have a detrimental influence on the periodontal tissues. The excellent nutrition and the special attention which is paid to oral hygiene and dental care in these patients may be important factors in maintaining the integrity of the oral tissues.

Cruickshank found that the zinc content of the teeth in patients with tuberculosis was consistently higher than in normal individuals. The mechanism of the increased zinc content of the teeth or the significance of this observation was not explained.

During pneumothorax therapy, air may be accidentally injected into the blood stream. The gas embolism which follows the refilling of the pleural space produces a marked pallor of the tongue. This is known as Liebermeister's syndrome. This oral symptom may be the first indication of a fatal air embolism.

24

Miscellaneous Infectious Granulomata

ACTINOMYCOSIS	GRANULOMA INGUINALE
BLASTOMYCOSIS	LYMPHOPATHIA VENEREUM
MONILIASIS	HODGKIN'S DISEASE
HISTOPLASMOSIS	VIRUS DISEASES
LEPROSY	PARASITIC INFECTIONS
GLANDERS	GONORRHEA
LEISHMANIASIS	

ACTINOMYCOSIS

Actinomycosis is a chronic infectious granuloma which occurs frequently in cattle and less often in man. It is characterized by multiple abscesses and fistula formation. In cattle the bone is more often involved (Lumpy Jaw) than the soft tissues, while in man the reverse is true.

The disease is widespread and its distribution in man follows that in animals. It is most prevalent in the plains country such as the Mississippi Valley. While the majority of the cases of cervicofacial actinomycosis occurs in male agricultural workers, it is believed that this is due to a greater exposure to infection rather than an occupational or sexual predisposition. The disease is usually found in middle life.

The Actinomycetes are normally found in the soil, on grasses and grains and in the mouth. Aerobic forms are isolated from the soil while those from the mouth are micro-aerophilic or anerobic in type. Typical actinomycotic lesions have been produced in guinea pigs by the intraperitoneal inoculation of material removed from carious teeth. Naeslund demonstrated the pathogenic anaerobic type just as often in the dental film of healthy teeth as in carious teeth.

A previous history of a cut, abrasion of the oral mucosa, or the extraction of a tooth precedes frequently the clinical development of the disease. At one time it was believed that the organism was implanted in the oral tissues by chewing splinters, blades of grass or timothy stalks. These habits probably furnished a favorable implantation site for the organisms already present in the mouth. The infection is now believed to be chiefly endogenous.

The *Actinomyces bovis* is generally stated to be the etiologic agent responsible for the clinical disease; however, organisms morphologically indistinguishable from the pathogenic forms have been isolated from the oral cavity. This organism consists of filaments and clubs. The filaments stain characteristically Gram positive and the clubs Gram negative. The clubbing may represent a reaction of the organism to the culture media or body tissue.

Actinomyces bovis grows in a typical ray-like arrangement which appears clinically as a small yellowish granule—the "sulphur granule." These "sulphur granules" are important clinical diagnostic signs.

Symptoms

The gastro-intestinal and thoracic forms of actinomycosis will produce symptoms related to chronic infectious processes in these systems. Diagnosis may be difficult without the demonstration of the causative organism.

Oral Aspects

Approximately 60% of all cases of actinomycosis are of the cervicofacial type and 15 to 20% seem to follow the extraction of teeth. The cervicofacial form of the disease is so common that it is considered as characteristic. The submaxillary region is the most frequent site of involvement in cervicofacial actinomycosis. The process spreads usually by direct tissue invasion and rarely by way of the lymphatics or the blood stream. The cheeks, the masseter region and the parotid gland may be involved. Extension has occurred to the skull and meninges.

One of the characteristics of actinomycosis is the lack of immediate tissue reaction following implantation of the infection. An actinomycotic infection and a carious or pulpless tooth will produce similar swellings in the submaxillary region. In actinomycosis, the swelling and trismus persist after the removal of the tooth. Several hard, circumscribed tumor-like swellings may develop which break down eventually and discharge a yellowish fluid containing the characteristic "sulphur granules." There are usually several discharging sinuses which alone are almost pathognomonic of the disease. The involved area has a hard doughy consistency rather than being fluctuant. The skin surrounding the discharging fistulae has a purplish color and may present small areas of hypertrophic granulation tissue.

It takes as a rule 6 weeks or longer for an actinomycotic swelling to break down. Acute pain is usually absent. These are important diagnostic signs. Many times the true nature of the process is not appreciated until the persistent multiple sinuses develop.

The tongue is frequently the primary site of the disease. It is involved in approximately 3.7% of all cases. Primary actinomycosis of the tongue must be differentiated from primary neoplasms, tuberculous ulceration and syphilitic gumma. In actinomycosis of the tongue a small deep-seated nodule is usually found which is painless at first and causes no discomfort. The lesion increases gradually in size and the overlying tissues soften and rupture. There may be temporary healing and then the process is repeated with a more extensive lesion resulting. Dysphagia is a prominent symptom in cases of extensive involvement.

Diagnosis

Any indolent inflammatory process with induration and persistently drain-ing multiple fistulae is suggestive of actinomycosis. A purplish or dark-red discoloration of the skin surrounding the sinuses is additional confirmatory

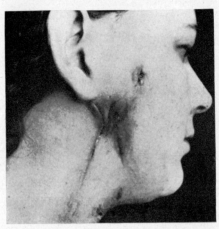

FIG. 246. Multiple fistulae in a patient with actinomycosis of the cervicofacial region. (Courtesy of Dr. Robert H. Ivy, Philadelphia, Pa.)

evidence. The discharge should be examined grossly for the sulphur granules and cultured for the causative organism.

Actinomycosis of the cervicofacial region is frequently confused with osteo-myelitis of the mandible. In osteomyelitis, pain is more severe, there is greater destruction of bone and the suppuration occurs usually more quickly. X-ray studies will aid in the diagnosis. Tuberculous adenitis must be considered if the individual is young. In this disease, multiple sinuses may also be present but the tissues do not have the board-like induration seen in actinomycosis and the examination of the exudate for acid-fast organisms will aid in estab-lishing a diagnosis.* Multiple fistula formation is not the rule in blastomy-cosis. Cervical forms of lymphopathia venereum present considerable diffi-culty in diagnosis. Biopsy studies are frequently required to make or to verify the diagnosis.

Treatment

The treatment of actinomycosis is in the province of the oral surgeon and the physician. The establishment of free drainage, radium or roentgen ray

---

* Some non-pathogenic forms of Actinomyces are also acid-fast.

therapy plus KI to the limit of tolerance are accepted forms of treatment. Extensive scarring usually results. Excellent results have been obtained recently in all forms of actinomycosis by the use of penicillin and the sulfonamides.

The prognosis is good in the cervicofacial form of the disease, less favorable in the thoracic and abdominal forms. Recovery may take many months.

BLASTOMYCOSIS

Blastomycosis is an uncommon chronic infectious disease caused by a yeast-like fungus Blastomycetes. This disease may involve all the organs of the body, especially the lungs, the cutaneous surfaces and occasionally the oral mucosa.

The clinical symptoms are similar to those observed in actinomycosis, except that the suppuration and the epithelial hyperplasia about the margins of the lesions are less marked. Both the cutaneous and the systemic form of blastomycosis may affect the oral cavity. The palate and the tongue are often involved. Aubrey reported a case of blastomycotic infection of the gums and mandible. This case also illustrates the importance of a careful study of all "loose teeth," as they may be the first manifestation of some systemic disease or malignancy.

In Aubrey's case the lower left first incisor of a 56-year-old male was removed by the patient's physician because of "infection." Ten days later a marked hyperplasia of the epithelial tissues developed about the alveolus and a large ulcer appeared on the buccal alveolar gum. The ulcer was painless, fiery red in color and it had a small contracted opening in the center which extended to the socket of the recently extracted tooth. The swelling was soft and granulomatous. The regional lymph nodes were swollen and hard. A careful history revealed symptoms of respiratory infection, night sweats, cough, blood-stained sputum and mild fever several months prior to the extraction. X-rays of the chest revealed an infiltrative lesion at the left apex.

Three small elevated yellowish nodules were noticed in the gum about 1 cm. from the center of the lesion. A tiny bead of pus could be expelled from each nodule. Histopathologic study of this tissue and additional laboratory procedures established the diagnosis of blastomycosis. A week later numerous small dull red nodular swellings appeared on the legs.

Diagnosis is based on the clinical appearance of the lesion, biopsy studies and the culture of the causative organism. There is no specific treatment for the systemic or oral lesions.

MONILIASIS (THRUSH)

Moniliasis is a specific infection caused by the yeast-like fungus, *Monilia albicans*. Monilial infections are known to involve the gastro-intestinal and respiratory tracts, the vagina and rarely the blood stream. When the oral cavity is involved the condition is known as thrush.

Thrush is usually found in infants, young children or the aged. In adults it is rare except when it is associated with a protracted wasting disease such as colitis, carcinoma, dysentery or tuberculosis. Monilial infections are said to occur frequently in the mouths of diabetics because of the high carbohydrate concentration of all the body secretions. The disease is common in institutions where infants are crowded together and where mouth hygiene and the cleanliness of nursing bottles and nipples are neglected. It is practically impossible for thrush to develop on a healthy mucous membrane. The incidence of the disease is clearly related to hygienic standards and economic groups.

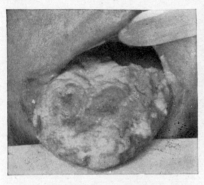 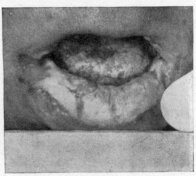

Fig. 247 (*Left*). Thrush (Kent). (From Thoma's Oral Diagnosis, W. B. Saunders Company.)
Fig. 248 (*Right*). Thrush affecting the lip (Kent). (From Thoma's Oral Diagnosis, W. B. Saunders Company.)

Epidemics of thrush have been traced to accumulations of dust. The disease is known to be transmitted by means of infected rubber nipples, clothes used for cleaning infants' mouths and by the nipples of nurses or mothers. Waters and Cartwright found no relation between vaginal moniliasis and the incidence of thrush in the newborn. Woodruff and Hesseltine's study indicated on the other hand that babies born of mothers with vaginal moniliasis had 35 times the chance of developing thrush as babies born of non-infected mothers.

In the United States a 1% incidence of thrush has been reported from one of our large maternity hospitals. In a recent study of neonatal thrush made by Ludlam and Henderson in England an incidence of 6.4% was reported. There was no evidence in this careful study that local trauma, debility or prematurity predisposed to the infection, nor was there any relationship observed between vaginal moniliasis and the incidence of neonatal thrush. Airborne infection was of little importance. Monilial organisms were found in a high proportion of the samples of pooled human milk. The incidence of thrush declined following the boiling of the milk. An important source of infection was shown to be the throats and fingers of the nursing staff.

Moniliasis is due to a vegetable parasite, *Monilia albicans*, which is characterized by the presence of branching hyphae or pseudomycelium and blastospores. The structure of the monilial forms can be readily seen in smears that have been treated with 10% KOH.

Symptoms

There are few systemic symptoms in thrush. The oral lesions appear first on the edges of the tongue, the buccal and labial mucosal surfaces and the palate. The entire oral cavity and larynx may be involved. The mouth is dry and a peculiar acid-sweet odor may be present. The lesions appear as irregular, small, whitish flakes resembling bits of coagulated milk. These spots are firmly adherent to the underlying tissues and when forcibly removed they leave raw bleeding surfaces. These spots are composed of epithelial cells and the branching monilial hyphae.

Diagnosis

Diagnosis is usually made on the appearance of the lesions and the absence of constitutional symptoms. Bacteriologic smears, treated with 10% KOH, will aid in verifying the diagnosis. Monilial forms may be cultured, and also observed occasionally in smears obtained from mouths without clinical manifestations of the disease.

The differential diagnosis must rule out diphtheria (severe constitutional symptoms), lichen planus (rare in infants and children and usually associated with dermal lesions), mucous patches (Wassermann) and a fusospirochetal infection (smear).

Gastro-intestinal and respiratory forms of the disease are resistant to treatment. Oral moniliasis is easily treated and controlled. As much of the milk-white lesions should be removed as is possible without producing bleeding. Freshly prepared 1% aqueous crystal violet should be applied topically 3 times a day (after feeding) for several days or until there is no further evidence of the disease. Silver picrate preparations are equally effective and do not have the undesirable staining properties of the aniline dyes. Boric acid solutions are worthless. The fungus will survive for over a week in a saturated solution of boric acid.

Oral moniliasis is rarely fatal. In poorly nourished infants noma has been known to follow thrush. Prognosis of systemic moniliasis is not so favorable.

HISTOPLASMOSIS

Histoplasmosis is essentially a disease of the semi-tropical regions, which is being recognized clinically with increasing frequency in the United States. This disease is due to a yeast-like organism, the *Histoplasma capsulatum*. Splenomegaly and hepatomegaly are common symptoms, as is lymph node involvement, which at times simulates that seen in leukemia. The disease often runs a febrile course with pulmonary symptoms. Anemia and leukopenia are common hematologic findings. Ulcerative skin and mucosal lesions are present occasionally.

Oral Aspects

Oral lesions may be present. Palmer *et al.* described the oral mucosal manifestations which they observed in a 45-year-old male. The patient complained of hoarseness, dysphagia and ulceration of the upper lip of 4 months' duration. Ulcers also developed on the penis and around the anus. The lip ulcer had a punched-out crusted appearance and involved over half this structure.

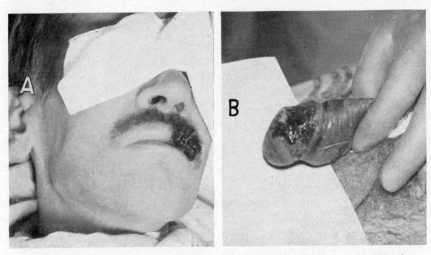

FIG. 249. Lesions of histoplasmosis of (A) the lip and (B) the penis. (Palmer, Amolsch and Shaffer, Arch. Dermat. and Syph., **45**: 912, 1943.)

There were numerous superficial ulcerations of the mucosa of the tongue and palate. The lesions were not indurated. Diagnosis was made by means of biopsy study.

LEPROSY

Leprosy is a slightly contagious infectious granuloma caused by the *Mycobacterium leprae* (Hansen's bacillus). It is characterized by destruction of all the body tissues by the granulomatous infiltration which results in marked deformity, ulceration and local anesthesia of the affected parts.

This disease occurs chiefly in tropical climates but sufficient cases are found in the U. S. to justify a National Leprosarium at Carville, La., and one on the island of Molokai in Hawaii. Most of the cases in the states come from New York, California, Texas, Florida and Louisiana. Diagnosis can be made on the appearance of the lesions, the demonstration of the organisms in the lesions and biopsy studies. Leprous patients are isolated not so much for contagious reasons as because of the marked deformity and destruction which occur in leprosy. The disease is characterized by acute exacerbations and spontaneous remissions. Each episode results in further destruction, scarring or deformity of the parts. Pain is not a prominent symptom.

Oral Aspects

The oral lesions of nodular leprosy are characterized by small tumor masses, lepromas, which break down frequently and ulcerate, due to trauma or secondary infection. The hard palate, the lips, and the tongue are common sites for the lesions. A frequent area of involvement is the tissue palatal to the upper incisors. When the lesions are present in the gum margins, the irritant action of calculus and that of chewing results in marked hypertrophy of

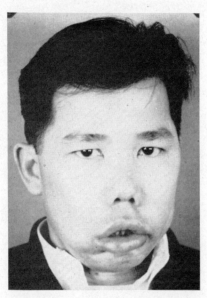

FIG. 250. Facial deformities resulting from scar formation associated with leprosy. (Prejean, Dental Survey, 119:1152, 1943.)

the tissue. The teeth become loosened and partially buried in the hypertrophied tissue. The lesions bleed easily. The saliva is extremely viscid. Perforation of the palate is extremely rare compared with that associated with luetic infections. Increased bone absorption has been reported occurring beneath dentures in the leprous patient. Marked scarring in the region of the orbicularis oris results in a "button-hole" mouth which may require surgical intervention in order to obtain sufficient space to insert dentures or perform needed dental work.

Del Rio found lingual involvement in 20% of the cases. The tongue presents a deep folded appearance due to the lepromas and later deformity as cicatrix formation occurs. The lingual leprous lesions are frequently associated with leukoplakia at the same area and ulcerated broken-down nodules are common. The tongue lesions are not particularly painful. The 5th and 7th cranial nerves are commonly involved in the anesthetic form of the disease.

Prejean has observed that facial paralysis in leprosy is usually bilateral. The muscles of the face, lips and soft palate are frequently affected but the muscles of mastication are not involved.

The usual prophylactic measures and the use of mild antiseptics are of value in the treatment of the ulcers.

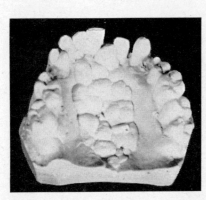 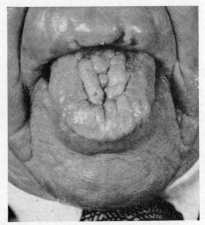

Fig. 251 (*Left*). Leprous lesions involving the hard palate. (Prejean, Dental Survey, 119:1152, 1943.)

Fig. 252 (*Right*). Tongue lesions in nodular leprosy. (Prejean, Dental Survey, 119:1152, 1943.)

GLANDERS (FARCY)

Glanders is an infectious granuloma of horses and asses which rarely affects men who come in contact with infected animals. The human infection may occur in (1) an acute form which terminates within a short time with pulmonary symptoms or (2) a chronic form which remains frequently undiagnosed for some time. The disease is characterized by periods of quiescence and recrudescence. Glanders is diagnosed on the basis of the history of contact with infected animals, agglutination tests and the actual demonstration of the *Malleomyces mallei* in the lesions.

Oral Aspects

The oral and nasal mucosae are the usual sites of the chronic lesions. They appear as sluggish ulcers which simulate those seen in tuberculosis.

LEISHMANIASIS (KALA-AZAR)

Leishmaniasis, or kala-azar, is an infectious disease characterized by splenic enlargement, anemia and leukopenia. It is caused by a protozoön, *Leishmania donovani*. This disease is rare in the United States, but occurs commonly along the Mediterranean, in China and India.

It is usually insidious in onset. At times a high continuous temperature with a rapid pulse will usher in the disease. Soon the characteristic double remittent (Pel-Ebstein) type of fever develops. Ascites, edema of the feet and splenomegaly develop early in the course of the disease. A marked anemia, thrombocytopenia and a granulopenia are consistent hematologic findings.

Hemorrhages from the nose and gums are common in kala-azar. Cancrum oris is the most frequent and serious complication of the disease. It commences usually as a small ulceration on the buccal mucosa or the palate which spreads rapidly and results frequently in death.

GRANULOMA INGUINALE (LYMPHOGRANULOMA INGUINALE)

Granuloma inguinale is an infectious granuloma which is usually found in the inguinal and the genito-anal regions. Within recent years it has been recognized that this disease is more common in the United States than was formerly believed, especially among the Negro population in the southern states. It is not of proven venereal origin. Granuloma inguinale is believed to represent a protozoön parasitic infection—possibly a form of leishmaniasis. The characteristic cytologic feature of this disease, the Donovan bodies, can nearly always be demonstrated in the mononuclear cells of the biopsy specimen and at times in the exudate.

The lesion begins as a small papule which ulcerates, increases slowly in size and gives rise eventually to the granulomatous spreading ulcerating lesions of the inguinal and genito-anal regions. Constitutional symptoms, pain or suppuration are uncommon. Granuloma inguinale is diagnosed on the clinical appearance and distribution of the lesion and the demonstration of Donovan bodies in the smear or biopsy preparations from the lesion. Intravenous potassium antimony tartrate and fuadin are effective therapeutic agents.

Oral Aspects

Fox stated that about 6% of the lesions of granuloma inguinale are found on areas other than the inguinal and genito-anal regions. Donovan described the first oral, extragenital lesion in 1905. It had the typical granulomatous appearance and intranuclear Donovan bodies were demonstrated in scrapings from the lesion. Hales studied an extragenital lip lesion which was characterized by extensive superficial ulceration with a well-defined elevated granulomatous margin. Hunter reported a case of granuloma inguinale with severe oral and laryngeal lesions which were associated with complete destruction of the mouth, dysphagia and "bilateral ankylosis of the jaws." Numerous other cases have been reported in the literature.

An interesting lesion of granuloma inguinale which was confined to the gums of the lower jaw was observed by the author in a 25-year-old Negro. The patient came to the clinic because of "bleeding and a feeling of fullness of the lower gums." A small granular area was noted on the lower gum near the left canine about 5 months previously. During the intervening time the previously normal gums increased markedly in size, bled easily, and turned a bluish-red color. The patient's past medical history was negative aside from a hemorrhoidectomy which was performed 5 years previously. There was said to be a slight recurrence of this latter complaint.

The essential findings on clinical examination were confined to the lower gums and teeth. The general mouth hygiene was poor. The labiobuccal and lingual alveolar gums were composed of a mass of bluish-purple tissue which bled on the slightest trauma. The tissues could be readily separated from the teeth and the alveolar process. There were no visible areas of necrosis or ulceration. The lower teeth presented a grade 2 mobility. Roentgenologic examination of the teeth and jaws revealed a moderate degree of alveolar resorption which was most marked in the lower jaw, where there was diffuse widening of the dental periosteal space.

The clinical appearance of the lesion suggested some infectious granulomata such as lues, tuberculosis, blastomycosis or moniliasis. Bacterial smears using appropriate stain-

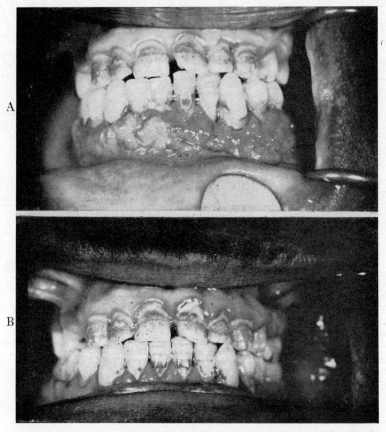

FIG. 253. (A) Granulomatous lesions of granuloma inguinale affecting the mandibular gums. The oral lesions resulted from self-inoculation of the gums from the anal lesions. (B) Improvement in clinical appearance of the gums after systemic treatment with potassium antimony tartrate. X-rays of this patient shown in Fig. 258.

ing methods were of no assistance in making the diagnosis. The blood Wassermann was repeatedly negative. The Frei test was negative with several different antigens. A biopsy study of the involved gum revealed the presence of cellular inclusion bodies suggestive of Donovan bodies.

A complete physical examination revealed a shallow ulceration with a granulomatous margin extending on the right buttock from the anal region. Biopsy study of this lesion presented a histopathologic picture similar to the gingival biopsy. It was suggestive of the diagnosis of granuloma inguinale.

The anal and the gingival lesions responded rapidy to intravenous potassium antimony tartrate injections. The friable granulation tissue covering the mandibular alveolar gums was replaced by more normal-appearing gum tissue. The teeth became firmer, but no new bone formation was observed in check-up roentgenograms. This case of suspected extragenital granuloma inguinale which involved the mandibular gingivae was probably auto-inoculated from the anal lesion by the patient's fingers.

LYMPHOPATHIA VENEREUM (LYMPHOGRANULOMA INGUINALE)

Lymphopathia venereum is a venereal disease caused by a filtrable virus. The initial lesion (vesicle) which develops on the site of inoculation is followed in 2 to 3 weeks by painful regional adenopathy and general symptoms of malaise, chilliness and a mild febrile reaction. The original adenopathy increases, with eventual breakdown of the nodes and the discharge of yellow pus. Marked scarring occurs, particularly in the female, which gives rise to marked deformity of the affected parts, abscesses and fistulae.

The intradermal Frei test and biopsy studies are used to confirm the clinical diagnosis. Lymphopathia venereum has been treated by sulfonamide therapy, Frei antigen and in selected cases surgical excision of the involved nodes.

Oral Aspects

Extragenital oral lesions of lymphopathia venereum are uncommon as judged by the cases reported in the dental literature. When one considers the increasing prevalence of this disease and the fact that extragenital lesions are not rare, it is evident that a wider knowledge of the oral manifestations is desirable.

The oral lesions result from *coitus buccalis,* kissing and auto-inoculation. Coutts *et al.* observed a frequent symptomatic triad consisting of (1) iritis, (2) aphthoid lesions of the mouth and penis and (3) a positive Frei test. Many of these patients present ulcerative tonsillar lesions simulating Vincent's infection. Coutts said that "judging from the confirmed cases and mentioned coincidences we may think that many up to the present undetermined or wrongly attributed cases of gingivitis, stomatitis, etc., may be caused by the virus of lymphogranuloma inguinale."

The tongue is a common site of oral involvement, particularly in prostitutes. The usual tongue lesions consist of small, slightly painful, superficial ulcerations with nonindurated borders which appear on the extreme tip of this organ. In long-standing cases, there are zones of cicatricial retraction, limited areas of a dark red color with loss of the superficial epithelium and opaque lichenoid papules of a grayish color. Dysphagia, a red soft palate and small red granulomatous lesions accompanied by regional lymphadenopathy are common associated symptoms. In most of the cases presenting primary oral lesions, the true nature of the process has not been determined until incision, secondary infection or considerable secondary change has occurred.

Cervical adenopathy is a prominent symptom when the infection enters through the mouth. This disease may be difficult to differentiate clinically from tuberculous adenitis if only the cervical nodes are involved. The skin covering the swollen nodes is violaceous in color, indurated and it presents usually one or more sinuses. Slaughter reported an interesting case of pre-cervical lymphopathia venereum in a patient who also presented anogenital lesions. Pressure over the enlarged cervical nodes caused a thick, yellow, purulent material to escape into the mouth from around the lower left first molar. There was considerable bone destruction.

Lymphopathia venereum infections of the cervical region must be differentiated from actinomycosis, tuberculous adenitis and blastomycosis. The tongue lesions must be differentiated from syphilitic gumma, actinomycosis, tuberculosis and lichen planus.

The diagnosis of the oral lesions can be made on the basis of a suggestive history, particularly when anogenital lesions are present, a positive Frei test and biopsy studies. The local lesions will disappear under general systemic therapy, but they should be treated symptomatically to reduce the secondary infection. At times, surgical intervention is indicated.

HODGKIN'S DISEASE

Hodgkin's disease is a chronic disease which is characterized by painless and progressive enlargement of the lymph nodes and the organs of the reticuloendothelial system, fever, anemia and general wasting. The disease is found more commonly in adults where it shows a predilection for the male sex. The causative agent is not known. Tuberculosis is an accompanying finding at times.

The onset of the disease is usually gradual. An alveolodental abscess, an acute exanthematous fever or an acute upper respiratory infection may precede the increasing weakness, pallor and fever which is constant or remittent in nature. Itching of the skin is an important symptom in Hodgkin's disease, preceding at times the adenopathy. The enlargement of the lymph nodes and their associated pressure phenomena are early and prominent symptoms in 60 to 75% of all the cases. The cervical, supraclavicular, axillary and the inguinal nodes are especially involved. The lymph nodes are soft to firm in consistency depending on the stage of the disease. They remain discrete and show no tendency to break down. The adenopathy in the early stages of the disease is commonly unilateral which aids in the clinical differentiation from lymphosarcoma and leukemia where it is usually bilateral.

The pressure exerted by the enlargement of the lymph nodes and the organs of the reticuloendothelial system on the adjacent structures gives rise to varied symptoms. Hoarseness is a common finding due to pressure on the recurrent laryngeal nerves and many patients also complain of difficulty in swallowing.

There are no characteristic hematologic findings in Hodgkin's disease. An eosinophilia is frequently present and in the later stages of the disease there is a leukocytosis. Hodgkin's disease is diagnosed on the basis of the history of onset, the clinical and x-ray findings and biopsy studies of one of the affected lymph nodes. There is no effective therapy for this disease but irradiation of the enlarged lymph nodes relieves temporarily the pressure symptoms. Fowler's solution is believed to be beneficial. The prognosis is very unfavorable.

The child or adolescent patient with Hodgkin's disease may be seen first by the dentist in the belief that the cervical adenopathy is secondary to dental infection. Gingival hypertrophy, gingival hemorrhage and secondary infection with the fusospirochetal organisms are not uncommon in patients with Hodgkin's disease.

VIRUS DISEASES

Viruses are highly specialized intracellular parasites which show special adaptations to the kind of cells that they invade. Some have a tendency to involve nervous tissue (neurotropic), others skin (dermotropic), etc. Viruses at times are also host specific and the virus producing the oral papillomatosis in dogs will only produce the disease in this animal. Viruses are known to affect plants, insects, and animals as well as man. They cause such serious diseases as smallpox, yellow fever and anterior poliomyelitis. Less serious but more common virus diseases are measles, chicken pox, mumps, possibly epidemic influenza, herpes zoster and simplex, possibly the common cold and the lowly wart.

Viruses are protein in nature. Because of their small size they have the ability to pass through mineral earth filters which are impermeable to bacteria. Viruses are submicroscopic (optical microscope) in size, varying from 10 to 275 millimicrons.

The first scientifically established virus disease was the tobacco mosaic virus (1892) and this same virus was the first to be "seen" by means of the electron microscope, in 1939.

A characteristic of many viruses is the production of intranuclear inclusion bodies in certain cells of the host. While these structures are not present in all virus diseases, they are not found in other than virus diseases. Another characteristic of many virus diseases is the immunity which follows infection. In smallpox, chicken pox and anterior poliomyelitis this immunity is relatively permanent but in herpes simplex it is of short duration. They have a variable susceptibility to heat, drying and ultraviolet radiation.

Foot and Mouth Disease—Epizoötic Stomatitis

Epizoötic stomatitis is an acute contagious disease characterized by fever, chills, malaise and the formation of vesicles on the fingers, toes, oral mucosa and the lips.

Epizoötic stomatitis is caused by the smallest known virus, the one which was first demonstrated to produce disease in man. It retains its infectiousness in extremely high dilutions ($1:10^7$). The disease is rare in this country. Dairymen, farmers and butchers are relatively often infected. Direct contamination from infected animal secretions such as raw milk is the common method of transmission. The hedgehog has been found to be naturally infected and it is believed by some to be an animal vector. Guinea pigs are susceptible to the disease and it has been produced experimentally in man with the development of the classical symptoms.

After an incubation period of 3 to 4 days the patient complains of headache, lassitude, chills or fever. Pains in the neck muscles, dysphagia or a burning sensation of the palmar surfaces of the hands are common.

The primary vesicles appear at the point of entry of the virus, most often on the lips, the oral mucosa, or the fingers. The feet are rarely involved in man. The exanthem consists of various-sized vesicles which develop rapidly, break and heal usually without leaving any trace of their existence. There is a marked increase in salivation and mandibular adenopathy. The disease usually reaches a crisis about the 10th day but it requires 3 to 4 weeks before the eruptions cease forming and heal.

The diagnosis of foot-and-mouth disease is made on the basis of the constitutional symptoms, the characteristic location and appearance of the vesicular eruption in conjunction with a history of possible contact with the virus. It can be corroborated by animal inoculations.*

In the differential diagnosis pemphigus, herpetic infections, varicella, allergic conditions and, more rarely, erythema multiforme must be considered.

The treatment of the oral lesions is largely symptomatic. The topical application of 1% aqueous proflavin, and the use of a mild alkaline mouth wash is all that is required. The prognosis is good in adults but in children the outcome is dependent on the maintenance of adequate nutrition in the presence of the painful mouth lesions.

PARASITIC INFECTIONS

The parasites inhabiting the oral cavity have received comparatively little study because of the infrequency with which they give rise to clinical symptoms and lesions. Parasites may gain entrance to the oral cavity by means of infected food or articles which are placed in the mouth. In addition, parasites which are present in the blood stream during some stage of their life cycle may become lodged in the oral tissues. The most detailed study of the parasitic flora of the mouth has been made by Kofoid et al.

Entamoeba Gingivalis

As early as 1849, Gros described the common oral ameba. It was the first parasitic ameba to be found in man. This oral protozoön received little attention until 1914-15 when Barret & Smith and Bass & Jones called attention independently to its common occurrence in the mouths of individuals with pyorrhea. They suggested that it might be of etiologic significance. These observations formed the basis for the use of amebocides, such as emetin hydrochloride, in the treatment of periodontal diseases. It was soon determined, however, that the E. gingivalis was a common habitant in any mouth with poor oral hygiene and it was frequently found in patients with good oral hygiene. Its prevalence bore little relationship to the presence or absence of periodontal disease.

* Permission to inoculate animals with suspected material is not granted to anyone other than State and Federal veterinarians who are charged with the responsibility of making diagnoses in cases where foot-and-mouth disease is suspected (Sutton & Sutton).

In experimental animals, monkeys, a temporary increase in the number of *E. gingivalis* was noted just prior to and during the loss of the deciduous teeth. This observation has not been noted in man.

These parasites should be regarded as a normal member of the micro-organisms of the oral cavity. *E. gingivalis* can be readily demonstrated in smears made from the gingival crevice or periodontal pocket, which are stained and examined in the usual manner. Subjective symptoms or patho-logic changes of the oral tissues associated with the presence of these para-sites have not been observed.

Trichomonads

This group of parasites represents a slightly higher stage of unicellular development than the amebae. Trichomonads are found in the bronchi, intes-

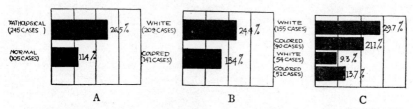

FIG. 254. Percentage distribution of *T. buccalis* (350 cases). (A) According to condition of mouths. (B) According to color of patients. (C) According to condition of mouths and color of patients—*upper pair:* morbid mouths; *lower pair:* normal mouths. (Beatman, Jour. Dent. Res., **13**:339, 1933.)

tinal tract, oral cavity and the vagina. They are characterized by the pres-ence of flagella and an undulating membrane which aid in locomotion. The best-known member of this group is the *Trichomonas vaginalis* which gives rise to a vulvovaginitis.

Bland and Rakoff studied the incidence of *Trichomonas vaginalis, T. tenax* (*buccalis*) and *T. hominis* (*intestinalis*) in 200 patients attending a gyneco-logic clinic. They found an incidence of 23.5%, 16.5% and 1.5% from the vagina, mouth and intestinal tract respectively. Vaginal auto-infestation with *T. tenax* has been emphasized by Lynch but the study of Bland & Rakoff does not substantiate this view.

The *T. tenax* is a frequent inhabitant of the oral cavity but it cannot be readily demonstrated in the smears which are prepared and stained in the usual manner. A warm stage technic using specially stained wet specimens is required to demonstrate satisfactorily this parasite. *T. tenax* was found in approximately 90% of the San Quentin prisoners with pyorrhea who were examined by Hinshaw. In a younger group and in those individuals with little clinical pathosis these parasites were uncommon. Cobe found the *T. buccalis* in 36% of the cases of periodontal disease which he studied from a bacteriologic standpoint. These parasites were found more frequently in mouths containing large calcareous deposits. Beatman concluded that the incidence of *T. buccalis* was roughly related to the state of oral hygiene of the individual. He found that the *T. buccalis* was associated with disease-producing organisms and that unsanitary oral conditions favored its growth.

There is little evidence that the *T. buccalis* is pathogenic although Glaubach & Guller reported a case of pneumonia which was apparently caused by it.

Trichinae

Trichiniasis or infection with the *Trichinella spiralis* is more common than is generally realized. Mild infections go unrecognized. Trichiniasis is commonly acquired through the consumption of infected meat such as improperly cooked pork products. Generalized muscle aches and pains which are accompanied by a moderate elevation of temperature are the characteristic constitutional symptoms of this disease. Edema of the eyelids, photophobia, rose spots on the skin and at times "splinter" hemorrhages beneath the nails are also present. Eosinophilia is a common finding. This disease is diagnosed on the basis of the history, the clinical findings and a fairly reliable specific skin test.

The trichinae have a predilection for muscle tissue and their lodgement in the muscles in and about the mouth have been reported. According to Prinz they have a predilection for the muscles of the tongue where their presence may give rise to small hemorrhages. Edema of the soft palate, pharynx and the muscles of mastication is common. Cook found encysted trichinae in tissue removed from the third molar region of a patient who had previously experienced this disease.

Other Oral Parasites

Oral lesions associated with many other parasitic forms have been recognized. Shira reported a case of oral myiasis (fly or maggot infection) due to the screwworm fly. An acute inflammatory reaction which extended from the gingival margin to the mucobuccal fold was present in the region of the upper incisors. A small sinus was noted about 5 mm. above the gingival margin. Six white, active larvae, approximately 6 mm. in length, were removed from beneath the gum in this area. Healing was uneventful. Myiasis of the tongue has also been reported.

Various members of the genus *Gongylonema* have been recovered from the mouths of humans where they have been observed to cause a swelling and hyperemia of the lower lip. These parasites are common in the pig. Simpson reported a case of mite infection of the genus *Tyroglyphus* in a carcinomatous growth which was invading the mandible in a 54-year-old woman. Some of the mites were living in the lesions and eggs were present. An echinococcal infection of the tongue was reported by Fernandez, and Schilling observed a patient with an allergic glossitis due to a dead tape worm.

GONORRHEA (GLEET—CLAP)

Gonorrhea is an acute venereal disease caused by the *Neisseria gonorrhoeae,* a Gram-negative diplococcus. The initial lesion is usually in the genital tract.

Manifestations in other parts of the body result from spread to adjacent structures by the regional lymphatics or to more distant structures by way of the blood stream. Gonorrhea is known professionally as a "Neisserian infection."

The prevalence of gonorrhea varies widely in the different racial groups and geographic areas. Possibly 5% of the population is, or has been, infected. The prevalence of the disease in adults parallels roughly the prevalence of sexual promiscuity. Sexual intercourse is the main means of transmission.

Males are more commonly infected than females. Infection can be transmitted by means of contaminated fingers, clothing, instruments and possibly toilet seats. Gonococcal vaginitis in children arises as a result of contamination from infected nurses, relatives or articles of clothing. Passage through an infected birth canal is responsible for gonococcal ophthalmia and stomatitis.

The gonococcus is a kidney-bean-shaped, Gram-negative diplococcus which is found characteristically within the polymorphonuclear leukocyte. Its cultivation is difficult. Predisposing causes for reactivation of infection in the female are pregnancy, menstruation, abortion or pelvic surgery. Marked physical exertion, traumatism, alcoholism and excessive sexual stimulation are important predisposing causes in both sexes.

Symptoms

Gonorrhea has an acute and a chronic stage with many complications. The acute symptoms develop within 3 to 7 days following exposure. Malaise, anorexia, grippe-like aches and pains are common general symptoms. The characteristic local symptom is an acute anterior urethritis. At first there is itching, burning or stinging of the urethral meatus but later severe pain is experienced. The penis is acutely inflamed and a copious, thick, yellowish discharge appears. These acute symptoms subside usually in a week or 2 except for a scant discharge which is only observed in the morning, the characteristic "morning drop."

The complications of gonorrhea are important. Most significant and common in the male is the development of urethral strictures many years after the acute infection. Involvement of the pelvic structures in the female such as the uterine cervix, the Fallopian tubes (sterility) and the pelvic peritoneum are common. These complications occur most frequently in untreated or inadequately treated cases.

Less common complications consist of gonococcal septicemia, endocarditis and arthritis. Gonococcal septicemia and endocarditis present the usual symptoms of septicemia and endocarditis with embolic phenomenon. Solitary joint involvement is not unusual.

Diagnosis

Acute gonorrhea can be diagnosed tentatively on the basis of the symptomatology and an accurate clinical history. Gram-stained smears of any discharge will assist materially. Positive diagnosis in doubtful cases rests with the cultivation of the gonococcus from the discharge, or lesion. The complement fixation test affords valuable information in the so-called closed forms of the disease where distant structures are involved.

Rigid measures should be taken to prevent spread of the disease. Rest is desirable and coffee, tea, alcohol and highly spiced foods are contraindicated. Antiseptic urethral instillations of potassium permanganate, acriflavine or silver solutions are older forms of treatment. The sulfonamides are particularly useful when administered internally. Penicillin has produced spectacular results in the treatment of both acute as well as chronic gonococcal infections. It is effective in the so-called sulfonamide-resistant cases. Theelin is used in children (vaginitis) as this stimulates a rapid transition of the infantile vaginal mucosa to the adult type.

Oral Aspects

Gonococcal arthritis of the temporomandibular joint and gonococcal stomatitis are the 2 main dental aspects of this disease. Specific joint complications in gonorrhea are uncommon but in such cases the temporomandibular joint is involved frequently. A 23-year-old ward maid was seen recently who complained of severe pain in 1 temporomandibular joint. Local causes such as trauma, disturbed occlusal relations, altered vertical dimension and possible rheumatic involvement, were ruled out. A careful history, physical examination and laboratory studies revealed an acute gonococcal infection of several weeks' duration. With proper treatment of the general infection the arthritic symptoms disappeared.

Neisserian stomatitis is essentially a surface infection of the oral mucosa. It occurs: (1) in infants who become infected during birth; (2) in children who have gonococcal vaginitis; (3) in adults through auto-inoculation of the oral mucosa by means of contaminated fingers and (4) in sexual perverts through orogenital contact. It is rare.

Gonococcal stomatitis in infants is characterized by the formation of yellowish plaques on the tongue and hard palate. A whitish creamy exudate may cover the oral mucosa in more advanced cases. The acute symptoms last rarely more than a week.

The adult patient complains of dryness and an intense burning or itching of the mouth. The oral mucosa is fiery red and a thick yellowish green exudate can be seen in localized areas or throughout the mucosa. New epithelium covers the eroded areas and healing takes place without scar formation. There is an abundance of thick ropy saliva. The salivary glands are not infected.

The diagnosis of Neisserian stomatitis follows the procedures discussed previously. A history of concurrent urethral or vaginal discharge is significant. Do not be misled by the social position of the patient. With modern methods of isolation, the isolation of the organism from the mouth should be required before a positive diagnosis would be justified.

Local treatment consists of mouth irrigations with boric acid, half-strength hydrogen peroxide or 1:200 Metaphen. The eyes of the operator should be protected well to prevent accidental infection. Eroded areas can be painted with 10% protargol solution. The topical and parenteral use of penicillin should prove almost a specific in this type of stomatitis.

The patient, or the parents, should be told of the contagious nature of the infection.

REFERENCES

SYPHILIS

Anderson, B. G.: Dental defects in congenital syphilis, Am. J. Dis. Child., 57:52, 1939.

Assinder, E. W.: Oral manifestations of venereal diseases, Proc. Roy. Soc. Med., 29:503, 1936.

Astrachan, G. D.: Unsuspected syphilis, Dental Outlook, 29:348, 1942.

Barnes, C. M.: Bilateral and complete trigeminal paralysis without involvement of other cranial nerves, Bull. Johns Hopkins Hosp., 27:138, 1916.

Barnett, C. W., & G. V. Kulchar: The infectivity of saliva in early syphilis, J. Invest. Dermat., 2:327, 1939.

Bauer, W. H.: Tooth buds and jaws in patients with congenital syphilis, Am. J. Path., 20:297-310, 1944.

Bauer, W.: Observations on tooth pulp and maxillary bone in congenital syphilis, Wien. Klin. Wchnschr., 44:879, 1931.

Biederman, J. B.: Preliminary report of another diagnostic sign in syphilis, Am. J. Syph. & Neurol., 18:306, 1934.

Brauer, J. C., & C. H. Blackston: Dental aspects of congenital syphilis, J. A. D. A., 28:1633-39, 1941.

Buschke, A., & A. Joseph: Can syphilis be transmitted by lipsticks?, Med. Welt., 2:1417, 1928.

Cannon, A. B.: A study of two hundred cases of congenital syphilis, J. A. M. A., 89:666, 1927.

Casilli, A. R.: Luetic glossitis, Urol. & Cutan. Rev., 44:744, 1940.

Cavallaro, J.: Syphilis in its relation to dentition, Dental Cosmos, 50:1151 and 61; 1325, 1908.

Combes, F. C., & S. M. Bleufarb: Annular papular syphilis of the tongue, Arch. Dermat. & Syph., 43:383, 1941.

DeWilde, Herman: Stigmata of congenital syphilis in the deciduous dentition, Am. J. Orthodontics & Oral Surg., 29:368, 1943.

Downing, J. G.: Incidence of extragenital chancres, Arch. Dermat. & Syph., 39:50, 1939.

Editorial: The responsibility of the dentist in diagnosing syphilis, J. A. D. A., 28:298, 1941.

Eliseht, F. C., & A. Agüero: Chancre of tonsils, Revista de la Assoc. Méd., Buenos Aires, 53:221, 1939.

Epstein, C. M., & E. P. Zeisler: Chancre of the gingiva, J. A. D. A., 20:2228, 1933.

Felici, M.: Bilateral lingual atrophy in tabes, Riv. sper. freniat., 30:315, 1937.

Fournier, A.: Syphilitic teeth, Dental Cosmos, 26:12, 1884.

Goodman, Herman: Oral syphilis, Dental Cosmos, 62:59, 1920.

Greenbaum, S.: The modern diagnosis of contagious buccal syphilis, Dental Cosmos, 71:271, 1929.

Hill, T. J.: An investigation on spirochetosis of the dental anlage in congenital syphilis, Am. J. Path., 7:515-17, 1931.

Hollander, S., & B. A. Goldman: Syphilis of the oral mucosa, Dent. Digest, 40:90-94, 103-105, 1934.

Houston, Trim: Syphilis as the dentist sees it, J. A. D. A., 26:1362, 1939.

Hudson, E. H.: The childhood syphilis of the Bedouins, J. A. D. A., 24: 219, 1937.

Hutchinson, Jonathan: Report on the effects of infantile syphilis in marring the development of the teeth, Trans. Pathological Soc. London, 9:449, 1858.

Hutchinson, Jonathan: Hutchinson's triad, Trans. Pathological Soc. London, 10:287, 1859.

Hutchinson, Jonathan: Syphilis—diagnosis in the late periods—the teeth, Trans. Pathological Soc. London, 38:85, 1887.

Hutchinson, Jonathan: On the influence of hereditary syphilis on the teeth, Lancet, 9:449 and 10:187, 1856.

Hutchinson, Jonathan: Heredito-syphilitic struma and on the teeth as a means of diagnosis, Brit. M. J., 1:515, 1861.

Johnston, W. D., B. G. Anderson, & P. F. McAlenney: Effects of congenital syphilis on the teeth and associated structures in children, Am. J. Orthodontics & Oral Surg., 27:667, 1941.

Karnosh, L. J.: Histo-pathology of syphilitic hypoplasia of the teeth, Arch. Dermat. & Syph., 13:25, 1926.

LaPage, C. P.: Congenital syphilis with obscure initial signs, Lancet, 2:503, 1944.

Leifer, William: Accidental syphilitic infection of dentists: report of two cases, J. A. D. A., 29:435, 1942.

Leonard, P.: Syphilis, chancre of the cheek, Ann. d. mal. vén., 35:65, 1940.

Lever, Walter F.: Multiple extragenital giant chancres, New England J. Med., 231:227, 1944.

Lewis, G. R.: Gumma of the tongue, J. Missouri State Dent. A., 23:185, 1943.

Moody, E.: Congenital syphilis and the eruption of the first teeth, J. Missouri M. A., 19:295-6, 1922.

Norman, T.: Oral syphilis, Internat. Clin., 3:93, 1937.

O'Leary, Paul A.: Significance of syphilis to the dentist, J. A. D. A., 23: 1523, 1936.

Parounagian, M. B., & H. Goodman: Chancre of the lip, Am. J. Syphilis, 7:563-8, 1923.

Pentz, Wm. R.: Vital reactions of the pulp of teeth in syphilis produced by induced currents, Arch. Dermat. & Syph., 28:163, 1933.

Pentz, W. R., & M. C. Borman: Dental sensation in syphilis of the central nervous system, Arch. Neurol. & Psychiat., 16:629, 1926.

Quinlau, R. V.: The teeth in cases of congenital syphilis, Arch. Dermat. & Syph., 16:605, 1927.

Rein, C., & M. H. Feldman: A simple method for detecting syphilis in routine dental practice, J. A. D. A., 22:1203, 1935.

Rowntree, G. R., & J. R. Hendon: Extragenital transmission of syphilis among five persons in one family, J. A. M. A., 115:117, 1940.

Sarnat, B. G., I. Schour, & R. Hueppel: Roentgenologic diagnosis of congenital syphilis, J. A. M. A., 116:2745, 1941.

Sharon, J. P.: Role of the dentist in the program to stamp out syphilis, J. A. D. A. & Dental Cosmos, 25:2041, 1938.

Smith, C.: 1,000 cases of congenital syphilis, Arch. Dermat. & Syph., 15:527-49, 1927.

Smith, C. M.: Significant dental defects in congenital syphilis, Arch. Dermat. & Syph., 8:791, 1923.

Stathers, F. R.: Congenital syphilis and malocclusion of the teeth, Am. J. Orthodontics & Oral Surg., 28:138, 1942.

Stokes, J. H., & B. S. Gardner: Demonstration of unerupted Hutchinson's teeth by roentgen ray, J. A. M. A., 80:28, 1923.

Straith, F. E.: Chancre of the gingivae, J. A. D. A., 24:926, 1937.

Strakosch, E. A.: Postrhagadic scars, Arch. Dermat. & Syph., 43:664, 1941.

Strauss, I.: Masseter and temporal muscle tenderness in syphilitic trigeminal neuritis, J. Mt. Sinai Hosp., 8:1060-3, 1942.

Stumpf, F. W.: Symptoms of syphilis in the oral cavity, Dental Cosmos, 78:698, 1936.

Sutton, I. C.: The need for caution in the diagnosis of Hutchinson teeth, Am. J. Syph., Gonov. & Ven. Dis., 9:94, 1925.

Thurmon, F. M.: Clinical manifestations of primary syphilis, New England J. Med., 223:439-441, 1940.

Vonderlehr, R. A.: The role of the dentist in the control of syphilis, J. A. D. A., 24:1935-40, 1937.

Vonderlehr, R. A., & L. J. Usilton: Syphilis among men of draft age in the United States, J. A. M. A., 120:1369, 1942.

Wile, U. J., & H. H. Holman: A survey of 68 cases of extragenital chancres, Am. J. Syph., Gonor. & Ven. Dis., 25:58, 1941.

TUBERCULOSIS

Amiot, W. F.: Care and treatment of the teeth and oral cavity in tuberculous patients, Med. Bull. Vet. Admin., 7:1065, 1931.

Banyai, A. L.: Cod liver oil as local treatment for tuberculosis lesions, Brit. J. Tuberc., 34:107, 1940.

Berberich, J.: Oral tuberculosis treated with carbon dioxide snow, Am. Rev. Tuberc., 47:291-5, 1934.

Brodsky, R. H.: Grenz ray therapy in periodontoclasia and oral tuberculosis lesions, Dent. Items of Interest, 62:927-34, 1940.

Brodsky, R. H.: Tuberculous scrofuloderma, J. A. D. A., 32:459, 1945.

Brodsky, R. H., & J. S. Klatell: The tuberculous dental periapical granuloma, Am. J. Orthodontics & Oral Surg., 29:498, 1943.

Browning, C. C.: Dental infections and tuberculosis, Texas State J. Med., 21:650-52, 1926.

Cahn, L. R.: Observations on the effect of tuberculosis on the teeth, gums and jaws, Dental Cosmos, 67:479, 1925.

Cohen, Sumner S.: Tuberculosis of the cervical nodes, Journal-Lancet, 65:151, 1945.

Collins, L. H., & T. J. Cook: Oral tuberculosis as the initial manifestation of rapidly progressing fatal tuberculosis, J. A. D. A., 27:1608, 1940.

Cruickshank, D. B.: The natural occurrence of zinc in the teeth; variations in tuberculosis, Brit. Dent. J., 68:257-71, 1940.

Darlington, Chas. G., & I. Salman: Oral tuberculous lesions, Am. Rev. Tuberc., 35:147, 1937.

Duken, J.: Primary tuberculous lesion on the upper lip of a two-year-old child, J. A. M. A., 91:991, 1928.

Editorial: Dental lesions and systemic disease, J. A. M. A., 109:211, 1937.

Farber, J. E., et al.: Tuberculosis of the tongue, Am. Rev. Tuberc., 62:766, 1940.

Finney, J. M. T., & J. M. T. Finney, Jr.: Tuberculosis of the tongue, Surg. Gynec. & Obst., 40:743, 1925.

Fitzgerald, R. J., & A. L. Banyai: New treatment of oral tuberculosis, J. A. D. A., 27:1647, 1940.

Freeman, H. E.: Tuberculoma of the palate and right angle of the mouth, Arch. Dermat. & Syph., 41:1179, 1940.

Gelbenegger, F.: Air embolism in artificial pneumothorax—value of Liebermeister tongue phenomenon, Wien. med. Wchnschr., 81:159, 1931.

Gillette, H. W.: Dental care as an auxiliary in the treatment of tuberculosis, Monthly Health Quart., 1:24, 1931.

Gillette, H. W.: Dental service as an auxiliary in the treatment of tuberculosis, Am. Rev. Tuberc., 21:327, 1930.

Hatch, H. S.: The dentist and tuberculosis, Dental Digest, 40:417, 1934.

Ivy, R. H., & J. L. T. Appleton: Diagnostic importance of tuberculosis lesions of oral cavity, J. A. M. A., 81:1483, 1923.

Katz, H. L.: Tuberculosis of the tongue, Quart. Bull. of Sea View Hosp., 6:239, 1941.

Kramer, C. S.: Osseous trophic changes in the jaws and palate in the tuberculous, J. A. D. A., 12:1117-26, 1925.

Kreshover, S. J.: The histopathology of the incisor teeth of mice with experimentally produced tuberculosis, Jour. Dent. Research, 21:27, 1942.

MacPherson, G. T., & H. W. Gregg: Case of solitary tubercular ulcer of the lip, J. A. M. A., 82:966, 1924.

Martin, G. G., & S. W. Koepf: Tuberculosis of the gums and cheeks, Am. Rev. Tuberc., 37:381, 1938.

Michalowsky, E. H.: Anemic tongue phenomenon in arterial air emboli during artificial pneumothorax, Klin. Wchnschr., 9:2440, 1930.

Morrow, H., & H. E. Miller: Tuberculosis of the tongue, J. A. M. A., 83:1483-87, 1924.

Ormerod, F. C.: Tuberculous ulcerations of the mouth and pharynx, J. Laryng. & Otol., 52:675, 1939.

Rein, C. H., & M. H. Feldman: Non-ulcerative tuberculosis of the mouth following dental procedure, Arch. Dermat. & Syph., 31:858, 1935.

Rex, R.: Tuberculosis of the tongue, Boletin Odont. Mexicano, 21:238, 1940.

Rubin, E. H.: Tuberculosis of the buccal mucous membrane, Am. Rev. Tuberc., 16:39, 1927.

Schugt, H. P.: Tuberculosis of the tongue, Laryngoscope, 51:284-87, 1941.

Smith, A. W.: Case exhibiting Liebermeister's syndrome, following on air filling of left pleural cavity, Tubercle, 16:454-55, 1935.

Stafne, Edw. C.: Tuberculoma involving an upper molar tooth, J. A. D. A., 23:1694, 1936.

Stahler, C.: Tuberculosis of the lip, Ann. Surg., 42:419, 1938.

Tanchester, D., & S. Sorrin: Dental lesions in relation to pulmonary tuberculosis, J. Dent. Research, 16:69, 1937.

Tannenberg, Joseph: Tuberculosis of the oral cavity, New York J. Dent., 13:301, 1943.

Taylor, W. E.: Incidence of oral tuberculosis in pulmonary tuberculosis, J. Dent. Research, 18:287, 1939.

Weinberger, A. V.: Tuberculosis of the buccal mucous membrane, Am. J. Digest. Dis., 10:421, 1943.

MISCELLANEOUS INFECTIOUS GRANULOMATA

Actinomycosis

Ashley, R. E.: Primary actinomycosis of the nose with extension to the pharynx, hard and soft palate, and cervical vertebrae, with report of a case, Ann. Otol. Rhin. & Laryng., 43:248, 1934.

Bibby, B. G., & H. T. Knighton: Actinomyces of human mouth, J. Infect. Dis., 69:148-54, 1941.

(Cabot case 26391): Case report Mass. Gen. Hospital, New Eng. J. Med., 223:507-10, 1940.

Cameron, O. J.: Primary actinomycosis of the tongue with report of 2 cases, J. A. M. A., 99:1146-50, 1932.

Crowley, M. C.: Actinomyces in the normal mouth and in infectious processes, Am. J. Orth. & Oral Surg., 30:680, 1944.

Davis, M. I. J.: Analysis of 46 cases of actinomycosis with reference to its etiology, Am. J. Surg., 52:447-54, 1941.

Dieker, W.: Use of short wave radiation on localized forms of actinomycosis, Strahlentherapie, 61:338-45, 1938.

Dobson, L., E. Holman, & W. C. Cutting: Sulfanilamide in therapy of actinomycosis, J. A. M. A., 116:272-75, 1941.

Figi, F. A.: Actinomycosis of the tongue, Surg. Clin. N. Amer., 6:1343-57, 1926.

Ganner, H.: Actinomycotic infection of the submaxillary salivary gland, Arch. f. klin. Chir., 155:495-508, 1929.

Grythe, O.: The actinomycetes, and their occurrence in soil and in the organisms of warm-blooded animals, Acta. Odontol. Scandinavica, 1:155-69, 1939.

Henry, T. C.: A case of actinomycosis following dental extraction, Brit. Dent. J., 69:169-72, 1940.

Hollenbeck, W. F.: Actinomycosis treated with sulfadiazine, J. A. M. A., 123:1115, 1943.

Lord, F. T., & L. D. Trevett: Pathogenesis of actinomycosis; recovery of actinomyces-like organisms from normal mouth, J. Infect. Dis., 58:115-20, 1936.

Lyons, C., Cora R. Owen, & W. B. Ayers: Sulfonamide therapy in actinomycotic infections, Surg., 14:99, 1943.

MacCharles, M. R., & J. W. Kippen: Three cases of actinomycosis treated with sulfanilamide, Canad. M. A. J., 41:490-91, 1939.

McCloy, A.: Actinomycosis of the tongue successfully treated by sulphonamides, Brit. Med. J., July 24, 106, 1943.

McConnell, O. H.: Actinomycosis: report of case, J. Oral Surg., 2:173, 1944.

McHardy, G., & D. C. Browne: Primary bronchial actinomycosis, South. M. J., 36:674-76, 1943.

McLaughlin, W. J.: Actinomycosis, Am. J. Orthodontics & Oral Surg., 24:85-86, 1938.

Robinson, R. A.: Actinomycosis of the subcutaneous tissue of the forearm secondary to a human bite, J. A. M. A., 124:1049, 1944.
Sanford, A. H.: Distribution of actinomycosis in United States, J. A. M. A., 81:655-59, 1923.
Slack, J.: Source of infection in actinomycosis, J. Bact., 43:193-209, 1942.
Sudler, M. T., & C. B. Johnson: Treatment of actinomycosis with sulfanilamide, report of 2 cases, J. Kansas M. Soc., 40:330, 1939.
Wilkinson, E. E.: Actinomycosis treated with sulfanilamide, J. Pediat., 18:805-10, 1941.
Ziskin, D. E., J. Shohan, & J. M. Hanford: Actinomycosis—a report of 26 cases, Am. J. Orthodontics & Oral Surg., 29:193-201, 1943.

Monilial and Blastomycotic Infections

Albert, M.: A note on a case of blastomycosis cured by sulphapyridine and sulphathiazole, Brit. J. Dermat. & Syph., 55:294, 1943.
Bartels, H. A.: Significance of yeastlike organisms in denture sore mouths, Am. J. Orthodontics & Oral Surg., 23:90, 1937.
Downing, J. G., & J. B. Hazard: Cutaneous moniliasis associated with oral thrush, Arch. Dermat. & Syph., 31:636, 1935.
Engman, M. F., & R. S. Weiss: Monilia candida infection of mouth, Arch. Dermat. & Syph., 1:119, 1920.
Faber, H. K., & E. B. Clarke: Prevention and treatment of thrush (oidial stomatitis), Am. J. Dis. Child., 34:408, 1927.
Gardner, H. L.: Vaginal thrush, Texas State J. Med., 40:333, 1944.
Hardgrove, T. A.: Moniliasis developing following tooth extraction, J. A. D. A., 19:483, 1932.
Lorenz, E.: Thrush in a premature infant with cleft palate and hare lip, Ztschr. f. Kinderh., 47:164, 1929.
Ludlam, G. B., & J. L. Henderson: Neonatal thrush in maternity hospital, Lancet, 1:64, 1942.
MacGregor, A. R., & J. L. Henderson: Intestinal thrush, Arch. Dis. Childhood, 18:186, 1943.
Nussbaum, S., J. A. E. Sass, & H. Rascoff: Systemic thrush in neonatal period: report of case, Arch. Pediat., 58:689, 1941.
Waters, E. G., & E. W. Cartwright: Significance of vulvovaginitis in pregnancy, J. A. M. A., 113:30, 1939.
Wikler, A., E. G. William, & C. Wiesel: Monilemia associated with toxic purpura: report of case, Arch. Neurol. & Psychiat., 50:661, 1943.
Woodburne, A. R.: Moniliasis, J. Periodontol., 15:7, 1944.
Woodruff, P. W., & H. C. Hesseltine: Relationship of oral thrush to vaginal mycosis and incidence of each, Am. J. Obst. & Gynec., 36:467, 1938.
Zeisler, E. P.: Monilia infection of the tongue, Arch. Dermat. & Syph., 15:171, 1927.

Granuloma Inguinale and Lymphopathia Venereum

Anderson, K.: The cultivation from granuloma inguinale of organisms having the characteristics of Donovan bodies in the yolk sac of chick embryos, Science, 97:560, 1943.
Beeson, B. B.: Granuloma inguinale with lesion on the lower lip, Arch. Dermat. & Syph., 6:342, 1922.

Bezecny, R., & F. Sagher: Oral infection with lymphogranuloma inguinale, Med. Klin., 31:270, 1935.

Bloom, D.: Extragenital infection in lymphogranuloma inguinale, Arch. Dermat. & Syph., 27:687, 1933.

Bloom, D.: Lymphogranuloma of the tongue and cervical glands, Arch. Dermat. & Syph., 28:810, 1933.

Costello, M. J., & J. A. Cohen: Lymphogranuloma venereum affecting simultaneously the cervical and inguinal lymphatic glands, Arch. Dermat. & Syph., 41:557, 1940.

Coutts, W. E.: Glossitis marginata in Ihrer Beziehung zur Lymphogranulomatosis Inguinalis, Dermat. Wchnschr., 97:1664, 1933.

Coutts, W. E., & B. T. Banderas: Lymphogranulomatosis venerea and its clinical syndromes, Urol. & Cut. Rev., 38:263, 1934.

Coutts, W. E., & L. Opazo: Sindromas Linfogranulomatosis de la Cavidad Bucal del Intestino delgrado y Gruesa del Recto y del Ano, Rev. Chil. de Hig. y Med. Prev., 2:85, 1939.

Coutts, W. E., L. Opazo, & M. Montenegro: Digestive tract infections by virus of lymphogranuloma venereum, Am. J. Digest. Dis., 7:287, 1940.

Curth, W.: Extragenital infection with the virus of lymphogranuloma inguinalis, Arch. Dermat. & Syph., 28:376, 1933.

David, V. C., & M. Loring: Extragenital lesions of lymphogranuloma inguinale, Jour. Amer. Dent. Asso., 106:1875, 1936.

Dienst, R. B., et al.: Cultural studies on "Donovan bodies" of granuloma inguinale, J. Infect. Dis., 62:112-14, 1938.

Donovan, C.: Medical cases from Madras General Hospital, Indian Med. Gaz., 40:411, 1905.

Fox, H.: Granuloma inguinale: its occurrence in the United States, J. A. M. A., 87:1785, 1926.

Greenblatt, R. B., et al.: Extragenital granuloma inguinale, Arch. Dermat. & Syph., 38:358, 1938.

Hall, Thomas B.: Granuloma inguinale, Arch. Dermat. & Syph., 38:245, 1938.

Hunter, R. J.: Granuloma inguinale, with associated lesions of the lip, pharynx and larynx, Trans. Coll. Phys. (Phila.), 45:455, 1923.

Midana, A.: Bilateral submaxillary adenitis of poradenitic nature, Arch. ital. di. Chir., 53:88, 1938.

Pund, E. R., A. D. Smith, D. Y. Hicks, & R. E. Dienst: Extragenital granuloma venereum, South. M. J., 32:917, 1939.

Sharlit, H.: Surface lymphogranulomatosis confined to oral and penile mucosa, Arch. Dermat. & Syph., 24:288, 1931.

Shearer, W. L., & A. F. Tyler: Diseases originating at gum margin, J. Radiol., 6:352, 1925.

Sidlick, D. M.: Granuloma inguinale of the face and mouth, Arch. Dermat. & Syph., 15:703, 1927.

da Silva, Ramos and J.: Extragenital lymphogranuloma venereum on the tongue and cervical nodes, Arch. de dermat. e. syph. de São Paulo, 2:87, 1938.

Silva, F.: A case of buccal localization of venereal granuloma, Urol. & Cutan. Rev., 37:611, 1933.

Slaughter, W. B.: Lymphogranuloma venereum with special reference to head and neck lesions, Internat. Abstr. Surg., 70:43, 1940.

Miscellaneous Granulomatous Diseases

Boltjes, B.: Histoplasmosis: report of case with brief review of the literature, J. Kansas M. Soc., 44:226-29, 1943.

Brown, A. E., F. Z. Havens, & T. B. Magath: Histoplasmosis: report of case, Proc. Staff Meet. Mayo Clinic, 15:812, 1940.

Costa, O. G.: American (mucocutaneous) leishmaniasis (unusual location of initial lesion), Arch. Dermat. & Syph., 49:194-96, 1944.

Del Rio, A. L.: Clinical contribution to the study of leprosy of the ear, nose and throat, Ann. di. laring., Otol., 36:80, 1936.

Forkner, C. E., & L. S. Zia: Further studies on Kala-Azar. Leishmania in nasal and oral secretions of patients and the bearing of this finding on the transmission of the disease, J. Exper. Med., 61:183, 1935.

Humphreys, R. M.: Two cases of oral pharyngeal leishmaniasis treated with pentamidine, Ann. Trop. Med., 36:9, 1942.

Kemper, J. W., & Herbert J. Bloom: Histoplasmosis, J. Oral Surg., 2:167, 1944.

Levy, Barnet M.: Oral manifestations of histoplasmosis, J. A. D. A., 32:215, 1945.

Major, Ralph H., & L. H. Leger: Marked eosinophilia in Hodgkin's disease, J. A. M. A., 112:2601, 1939.

McCausland, D. J. M.: Hodgkin's disease in children, Arch. Dis. Childhood, 16:59, 1941.

Moore, M., & L. H. Jorstad: Histoplasmosis and its importance to otorhinolaryngologists. A review with report of a new case, Ann. Otol., Rhin., and Laryng., 52:779, 1943.

Palmer, A. E., et al.: Histoplasmosis with mucocutaneous manifestations, Arch. Dermat. & Syph., 45:912, 1943.

Pinkerton, F. J.: Leprosy of the upper respiratory tract, J. A. M. A., 111:1437, 1938.

Pinkerton, F. J.: Leprosy of the ear, nose and throat: observations on more than 200 cases in Hawaii, Arch. Otol., 16:469, 1932.

Prejean, B. M.: Manifestations of leprosy, Dent. Survey, 19:1153, 1943.

Simson, F. W., & J. Barnetson: Case of histoplasmosis, J. Path. & Bact., 54:299, 1942.

Parasitic Infections

Alvarez, R. S.: Red torula as cause of tongue abnormality, J. A. M. A., 87:1358-9, 1926.

Beatman, L. H.: Studies on trichomonas buccalis, J. Dent. Research, 13:339, 1933.

Bland, P. B., & A. E. Rakoff: Incidence of trichomonads in vagina, mouth and rectum, evidence that vaginal trichomonads does not originate in mouth or intestine, J. A. M. A., 108:2013-16, 1937.

Bonestell, A. E.: Inoculation experiments with trichomonas hominis, T. buccalis and T. vaginalis, J. Parasitol., 22:511, 1936.

Glaubach, N., & E. J. Guller: Pneumonia apparently due to trichomonas buccalis, J. A. M. A., 120:280-1, 1942.

Hogue, M. J.: Studies on trichomonas buccalis, Am. J. Trop. Med., 6:75, 1926.

Kofoid, et al.: Animal parasites of the mouth and their relation to dental disease, J. A. D. A., 16:1436, 1929.

Schilling, V.: Glossitis, allergy and marked eosinophilia from dead tapeworm, Arb. ü. Tropenkrankh. (Festschr. B. Nocht), pp. 481-84, 1927.

Shira, R. B.: Report of a case of oral myiasis, Mil. Surgeon, 92:57-8, 1943.

Simpson, R. E. H.: Mites infesting carcinoma of the jaw, Lancet, 1:740, 1944.

Stiles, C. W., & C. E. Baker: A 5th case of gongylonema hominis in man in the U. S., J. A. M. A., 91:1891, 1928.

Wenrich, D. H.: Comparative morphology of the trichomonad flagellates, Am. J. Trop. Med., 24:39, 1944.

FOCAL INFECTION, DENTAL PEDIATRICS AND GERODONTICS, HAZARDS OF DENTAL PRACTICE, DENTAL DISEASES OF OCCUPATIONAL ORIGIN

25

Focal Infection

GENERAL CONSIDERATIONS

Diseases of the teeth or gums have been considered as possible foci of infection from the early writings of Benjamin Rush. The modern concept of focal infection, which was introduced by Hunter in 1900, received strong support from Billings' clinical observations and Rosenow's extensive experimental studies, with the result that there was an unusual emphasis on this aspect of medicine during the 1920's. During this period many questionable teeth were removed with frequent disregard for less obvious, less readily diagnosed and eliminated foci of infection such as the nasal accessory sinuses, the gallbladder, the genito-urinary and the intestinal tracts.

While the concept of focal infection is generally accepted as a biologic possibility there still remain considerable doubt and controversy as to its clinical significance. Let us review briefly the evidence supporting this concept and how a focus of infection might theoretically affect the physiology of the organism in which it resides. The evidence supporting the concept of focal infection consists of: (1) clinical observations of exacerbations or the disappearance of the remote symptoms following the elimination of the suspected focus, (2) the common finding at necropsy of small primary foci of infection in cases of similar disease processes in more distant parts of the body, and (3) laboratory studies concerned with this problem.

A focus of infection may act: (1) as a depot from which bacteria or their products may be disseminated to remote areas of the body, (2) as an area where organisms from other parts of the body may localize, or (3) as an additional load on the general resistance of the individual. A focus of infection is important in one or more of the above-mentioned ways. In our discussion of oral foci of infection we must consider: (1) periodontal foci, (2) periapical foci including residual areas of infection in edentulous spaces (or jaws) and possibly (3) the infected vital pulp.

CLINICAL EVIDENCE SUPPORTING THE CONCEPT OF FOCAL INFECTION

A large mass of clinical evidence of the case report type has accumulated supporting the concept of focal infection. When this evidence is examined critically, it is found that controls are generally lacking or other factors which might give rise to the favorable clinical response have not been ruled out. The improvement which occasionally follows the elimination of a suspected focus furnishes at best only a casual relationship between the primary focus and the more distant disease process. Holman's critical analysis of the experimental and clinical evidence in support of this theory deserves careful study. Bierring's quarter of a century survey, Rieman and Havens' clinical evaluation of this subject and Darlington's review of the present status of dental foci of infection form a valuable background for the clinical appraisal of focal infection.

Attempts have been made to assess the importance of dental foci of infection (periapical lesions) on the general health status of the individual. While these studies represent only a static evaluation of a progressive biologic process, they are significant because the number of observations permit statistical analysis. Frankel analyzed the dental and systemic findings on 19,000 persons insured by the Metropolitan Life Insurance Company and found no correlation between any systemic disturbance and the extent of the dental restorations—which were considered to be an index of possible dental infection. Appleton's statistical study demonstrated no increase in the amount of systemic disease in those individuals with the greatest amount of periapical infection as judged by clinical and roentgenologic examination.

Arnett and Ennis studied the dental roentgenologic changes in connection with the past history and the physical examination of 800 college students. No relationship between periapical infection and any particular disease entity could be established. These authors assumed that all periapical radiolucent areas were infected.

Ziskin's analysis of the quantitative roentgenologic changes associated with systemic findings revealed no definite conclusion as to the type or size of the periapical radiolucent area and systemic disease. These observations failed to substantiate Price's theories concerning the size and type of periapical radiolucent area as indicating individual susceptibility or resistance. Internists who once emphasized the importance of focal infection and particularly dental foci, have in recent years developed a more conservative view.

The dental practitioner has also become more conservative in his recommendation for the removal of suspicious teeth in the hope of benefiting a wide variety of symptoms. Too frequently he has had to make artificial dentures for patients who no longer had their teeth but still experienced their symptoms. This conservatism has been misunderstood at times by the physician as representing a lack of appreciation for the well-being of the patient.

Summary: While isolated case reports appear to substantiate the concept of focal infection and the importance of dental foci, the more extensive studies do not uphold this concept. It should be mentioned that these studies considered only periapical foci of infection and it is now generally appreciated that periodontal foci of infection may represent a more widespread and potentially serious oral focus.

LABORATORY EVIDENCE SUPPORTING THE CONCEPT OF FOCAL INFECTION

Laboratory evidence supporting the concept of focal infection and particularly the importance of dental foci has not materially clarified the problem. Many of the studies have been inadequately controlled or performed under conditions which were not comparable to those occurring in man. The emphasis was placed on the pulpless tooth and those with apical granulomata. The interest in these specific lesions was due probably to the ease with which pathologic changes could be determined by roentgenologic examination and bacteriologic cultures secured. These studies were concerned with the bacterial flora of (1) the apices of extracted teeth which were associated with periapical radiolucent areas, (2) less frequently from the apices of extracted teeth which were not associated with periapical radiolucent changes and (3) a few attempts were made to culture the teeth *in situ,* employing a surgical approach to the apical area similar to that used for root amputations.

The majority of the studies fell in groups (1) and (2). Data were frequently lacking as to the technical or bacteriologic methods employed, and since widely variant results were obtained from the apical cultures of non-carious teeth, there was the possibility that the actual cultural findings of the periapical region were considerably modified by contamination from the mouth flora during the removal of the tooth.

The author studied the bacteriologic, roentgenologic, and histologic findings of 426 teeth obtained at necropsy, including non-carious teeth and those with periapical radiolucent areas. Teeth with marked periodontal involvement

530   FOCAL INFECTION

and those readily movable in the alveolar process were not considered suitable for culturing regardless of the clinical condition of the crown. All cultures were made in the bacteriologic laboratory with the teeth *in situ*. Under these conditions asepsis seldom attainable in clinical studies could be maintained routinely. Bacteriologic studies of the blood stream and viscera, also made at necropsy, were available for comparison with the periapical cultures and the clinical bacteriologic findings.

Histologic studies of the areas cultured revealed whether the periapical tissues were reached during the culturing technic.

The frequency of the organisms isolated from 206 periapical areas with positive bacteriologic findings is given in Table XXVIII. Streptococci of the alpha type were most frequently recovered.

TABLE XXVIII

FREQUENCY OF ORGANISMS ISOLATED FROM THE TWO HUNDRED SIX PERIAPICAL AREAS

	Pure and Mixed Cultures		Pure Cultures	
	No.	Per cent	No.	Per cent
Streptococcus viridans	127	61.2	58	28.0
Streptococcus hemolyticus	21	10.2	4	2.0
Non-hemolytic streptococcus	35	17.0	3	1.4
Staphylococcus aureus	66	32.0	31	15.0
Staphylococcus albus	4	2.0	2	0.97
Escherichia coli	9	4.4	8	3.9
Pneumococcus	6	2.9	4	2.0
Gram-negative coccus	9	4.4		
Gram-positive rod (unidentified)	5	2.4	3	1.4
Pseudomonas aeruginosa	4	2.0	4	2.0
Gram-negative rod (unidentified)	4	2.0	1	0.49
Eberthella typhosa	2	0.97	2	0.97
Diphtheroids	1	0.49	1	0.49
Haemophilus influenzae	1	0.49	1	0.49
Gram-positive coccus (unidentified)	1	0.49		
Micrococcus tetragenous	1	0.49	1	0.49

The per cent of positive cultures obtained from teeth with no observable periapical areas, (XN), those with a small periapical radiolucent change, (XPS), and those with a large periapical lesion (XPL) is given in Table XXIX.

TABLE XXIX

POSITIVE CULTURES OBTAINED FROM DIFFERENT ROENTGENOLOGIC GROUPS

Group	No.	Per cent
XN	283	30.6
XPS	65	76.0
XPL	71	60.8

A tabulation of the cultural results in the different clinical groupings of the teeth revealed some interesting findings. These are shown in Table XXX. With the advent of the carious process and the involvement of the pulp, the frequency of positive cultures from the periapical tissues, even in the absence of roentgenologic changes, increases markedly. The highest percentage of pure cultures was obtained from the teeth without periapical radiolucent areas.

TABLE XXX

POSITIVE CULTURES OBTAINED FROM DIFFERENT CLINICAL GROUPS

Group	No. of Teeth	Positive Per cent
Non-carious	92	43
Carious	144	38
Restorations	115	50
Exposures	50	68
Pulpless	28	72

Since all cultures were taken with the teeth *in situ*, it is believed that these findings represent the actual presence of bacteria in this region and not contamination from the oral flora. Alveolar bone marrow cultures obtained in a similar manner were negative in every instance.

The bacteriologic and histologic findings were compared with the roentgenologic changes about the apices of the teeth. The relation between the roentgenologic and histologic findings was closer than that of the bacteriologic and histologic findings. The x-ray changes in the periapical region could not be definitely associated with any particular bacterial type or with any characteristic pathologic process. The x-ray changes at times were not even a reliable guide as to the extent or location of the pathologic lesion.

The experimental focal infection studies of Miller, Genvert & Burn on the *Macacus rhesus* monkey simulated closely not only the anatomic relations but the natural history of development of the periapical lesion in man. These investigators found that positive periapical cultures were obtained from toothapices without roentgenologic changes and that negative cultural results were occasionally obtained from teeth with well-developed periapical radiolucent areas. The presence of these periapical lesions and their existence in the experimental animal failed to call forth any systemic response that was manifest by daily temperature records, frequent blood counts, blood cultures and erythrocyte sedimentation rate determinations.

Factors Governing the Dissemination of Bacteria from Dental Foci

Our knowledge concerning those factors which are responsible for the dissemination of bacteria from a dental focus is far from satisfactory. The mechanical factors responsible for postextraction bacteremias or those which occur following chewing can be easily understood if not so readily controlled. Certain experiments suggest that the allergic state of the individual may be of significance in the dissemination of organisms from a dental focus. Weisberger demonstrated that the hypersensitive state (in rabbits) prolonged the duration of positive blood and visceral cultures following an experimental bacteremia. More recent studies by the same investigator on the effect of sensitization have shown that organisms present in the periapical region can be disseminated at will by "shocking" an animal (rabbit) which has been sensitized previously with equine serum. A strain of *alpha* streptococcus which was isolated from a periapical lesion, was used in these experiments to produce an endocarditis. It is possible that the allergic reactivity of an individual should be considered when the significance of any focus of infection is being evaluated.

THE LOCALIZATION OF ORGANISMS IN THE PERIAPICAL REGION

While periapical granulomata are generally considered in terms of the bacteria they may harbor or disseminate, it should be remembered that the periapical granuloma and even the periapical region of teeth are sites where bacteria or particulate matter are prone to localize. Beretta showed that organisms from an experimental bacteremia may persist in the periapical region and spleen when they can be no longer demonstrated in the blood stream or other viscera. The author and Burn presented clinical and necropsy evidence which indicates that organisms which are present in the blood stream have a tendency to localize and persist in the periapical region of teeth, particularly those with large granulomatous lesions. Some peculiarity in the hydrodynamics of the periapical region may account in part for these observations. Csyzienski, Robinson & Boling, and others have called attention to the anachoretic effect of inflamed tissues, which might explain the localization of bacteria in the periapical tissues and the dental pulp which are the seat of inflammatory changes.

ORAL FOCI OF INFECTION: THEIR CLINICAL SIGNIFICANCE

Periodontal Foci

Within the last decade numerous clinical and laboratory studies have stressed the significance of diseases of the periodontium. These lesions not only are more prevalent than the periapical granuloma, but they contain a heavier bacterial flora and one which is composed of more potentially pathogenic organisms. The unprotected gums and the dental periosteum are more vascular and have an extensive lymphatic system, which favors the dissemination of bacteria or their products to other areas of the body. Furthermore, the periodontal tissues are not protected to the same extent as are the periapical tissues from external trauma and irritation. The periodontal tissues can be considered as the most important oral focus of infection.

The bacterial exudate from diseased periodontal tissues is in intimate relation with the gastro-intestinal and respiratory tracts. The possible sequellae in the gastro-intestinal and respiratory tracts have been discussed in detail in the sections concerned with the diseases of these organ systems. The gingival trauma incident to chewing and the pumping action of loosened teeth in their alveoli are recognized mechanisms whereby bacteria may gain entrance into the blood stream and be disseminated to more distant foci. When ulceration of the gums is present, the toxic absorption from the ulcerated areas may also be of clinical significance. It has been estimated that even in mild periodontal disease the total ulcerative area may exceed 8 square inches.

Okell and Elliot noted that the frequency of postextraction bacteremias was

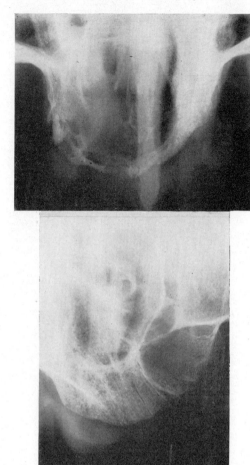

FIG. 255 (*Top*). Roentgenogram of edentulous maxilla showing a large cystic area in the left maxilla and a retained root fragment.

FIG. 256 (*Bottom*). Large cystic area in an edentulous right maxilla.

related to the health of the gums. It was later shown by the author and Burn that, if a test organism (*Serratia marcesens*) was applied to the gums prior to extraction, it could be demonstrated in the transient bacteremias. It has been shown by others that gingival massage or the chewing of hard candy or food by patients with diseased periodontal tissues will result in transient bacteremias. These studies emphasize the importance of securing and maintaining the best possible oral hygiene in all patients.

Periapical Foci Including Retained Roots or Residual Infection
in Edentulous Areas

The periapical dental granuloma or "blind dental abscess" has long been considered the most important oral focus of infection. This was due in part to the extensive bacteriologic studies made on this type of lesion and the ease (?) with which it could be diagnosed and removed. Retained root fragments and residual areas of "infection" in edentulous areas should also be included in this type of oral focus.

These lesions are fairly well protected by the alveolar process from the trauma associated with chewing. The degree of vascularity of the granuloma

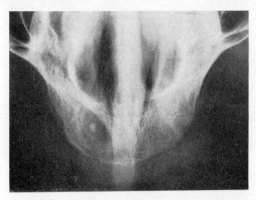

Fig. 257. Edentulous maxilla with retained root fragment and surrounding area of bone rarefaction suggestive of infection or cyst formation.

is variable and, when extensive, it presents a mechanism whereby bacteria or their products may be disseminated to more distant foci. Clinical proof is lacking of the dissemination of bacteria from this region, and no statistical correlation between the presence of periapical lesions and any particular disease process has been established. The bacterial flora of the periapical granuloma consists in most cases of *alpha* streptococci with occasional hemolytic strains.

The presence of a periapical radiolucent area is not diagnostic of "infection," any more than the absence of such an area indicates the absence of bacteria in the area. There are no characteristic periapical roentgenologic changes associated with the presence of infection or with any specific bacterial forms.

Retained root fragments or residual areas of infection constitute an important focus of infection because edentulous areas are too frequently not examined for hidden foci. The prevalence of retained roots, cysts or residual areas of infection will depend upon the age of the patient and the quality of his past dental care. Gardner found that about 33% of 10,000 patients examined in 1 year at the Mayo clinic had residual roots in areas of previously extracted teeth. A more recent study made at the same institution revealed a lower prevalence of retained roots, residual areas of "infection," etc. Logan, Molt and Cook have reported similar findings.

Schlack and Booth found roentgenologic areas suggestive of pathosis in 6% of the 1,075 roentgenograms of edentulous areas which were taken from the files of the Naval Dental School. Completely edentulous patients were not included in this study. Roentgenologic evidence of retained roots or "infection" is noted in approximately 25% of the edentulous patients who seek full denture service at the Dental School, University of Pennsylvania. It is evident that edentulous areas must always be examined roentgenologically in our search for oral foci of infection.

The Infected Vital Pulp

Considerable doubt exists as to the clinical significance of the infected vital pulp. At one stage in the pathogenesis of the periapical lesion, the pulp may become infected while it still manifests the attributes of vitality, but this fact does not establish the clinical significance of this dental focus. Because of the protection which the dentin and enamel afford this tissue, the absence of a well-defined lymphatic system and its lack of extensive vascular anastomoses, it should be regarded as a focus of minor importance. Certainly it is one that would be extremely difficult if not impossible to diagnose by conservative methods.

Most of the studies which have demonstrated the presence of bacteria in the vital pulp employed extracted teeth. The organisms recovered from the pulp in such cases may represent those which gained entrance into the circulation (and pulp) during the extraction of the tooth. The studies of Gunter et al. in which the vital dental pulp was cultured with the teeth in situ do not substantiate the high frequency of positive cultures obtained by investigators employing extracted teeth for their source of material. The author's pulpal cultures obtained at necropsy also failed to demonstrate a high prevalence of positive cultures.

Aids to the Diagnosis of Dental Foci of Infection of Systemic Importance

The actual bacteriologic examination of the periapical lesion is the only method of accurately determining whether bacteria are present in this area. The presence of a periapical radiolucent area is not always indicative of "infection" and bacteria may be isolated from the apical region of teeth without x-ray changes. There is no generally accepted procedure which will determine whether the infected area is serving as a focus of systemic importance.

Solis-Cohen and others have advocated the use of a pathogen-selective culturing technic for determining the clinical importance of a given focus. Theoretically the coagulable blood of a species, naturally resistant to infection by a given organism, kills that organism, while the blood of a species naturally susceptible to infection by it lacks this bactericidal power. Since this test requires the culturing of the suspected lesion, its value, conceding the theoretical implications, will depend upon the reliability of the culturing technic.

With the culturing technic which is generally employed, the bacteriologic examination of the root apex of an extracted tooth, may be seriously questioned as portraying the bacterial status of the periapical tissues *in situ*. Cultures of extracted teeth are of little if any significance even when a careful aseptic technic is employed. By the use of a bacterial indicator the author has shown that in spite of elaborate technical precautions, a high percentage of the periapical cultures made on extracted teeth are modified by the gingival flora. This lessens the diagnostic significance of such cultures as well as their immunologic importance if vaccine therapy is contemplated.

Appleton discussed the available methods of obtaining satisfactory periapical cultures. The Coriell dental trocar or a surgical approach to the periapical region with the tooth *in situ* are most satisfactory from a bacteriologic standpoint.

Skin-Testing Reaction. Kauffer described a test for determining whether teeth with periapical lesions are affecting the general health of the individual. This necessitates obtaining material from the periapical region, by way of the root canal, for culturing and then skin testing the individual with the cultured material. The clinical significance of this test has not been substantiated.

Short-Wave Provocative Radiation. Gutzheit and Küchlin described a diagnostic short-wave provocative test which, they claim, will differentiate dental infections which may cause systemic disorders from those which are purely local. They stated that, when an infected focus is responsible for systemic manifestations, the erythrocyte sedimentation rate is noticeably accelerated from 2 to 4 hours after short wave radiation. The diagnostic value of this test has not been established.

The sedimentation rate is known to be elevated in patients who harbor infectious processes such as focal infection. While this procedure may be of use in determining the presence or the absence of such a lesion, it is of little specific value in determining the existence of a specific focus, *i.e.*, infected teeth. Repeated sedimentation rate determinations furnish more valuable information than a single test. This procedure is of greater value to the physician than to the dentist. The variation of the sedimentation rate, associated with chronic dental infections such as the periapical granulomata, has not been established.

At one time an impression was held that the presence of focal infection anywhere in the body resulted in a reduction of the visual fields. There is no evidence substantiating this view.

DENTAL ASPECTS OF THE FOCAL INFECTION PROBLEM

Dental and medical co-operation is essential in searching for possible foci of infection. The dentist should be regarded as an oral consultant rather than a technician. His interpretation of the dental clinical and roentgenologic findings should be accepted as would those of any other medical specialist. An appreciation by the physician of the limitation of our knowledge in this field is also important. Of equal importance is the realization that oral foci may be treated and eliminated by other means than the extraction of teeth.

The patient who is seen by the dentist for an evaluation of possible oral foci, requires a detailed medical-dental history and a thorough clinical and roentgenologic examination of the oral structures. The clinical examination should include not only a careful mirror and explorer examination but a vitality test of all the teeth. If the latter is omitted many non-vital untreated teeth will be missed. The color, position and state of health of the gums should be noted and the gingival crevice should be carefully explored with a periodontal probe in the search for hidden pockets. The transient bacteremias which are frequently associated with infected periodontal tissues, make them a potentially serious oral focus.

Roentgenologic examination of the teeth and edentulous areas should be a routine procedure. These films will show the condition of the osseous tissues about the tooth apices and the amount of absorption of the interseptal alveolar bone. It is difficult to interpret the clinical significance of a periapical radiolucent area from a single x-ray film. Serial x-ray studies made over a period of years enable a more intelligent appraisal of a given lesion. Even when demonstrable x-ray lesions are present, it is not possible to tell whether they are of clinical significance. On the other hand not all pulpless or "infected" teeth will show periapical radiolucent changes and clinically significant periodontal pockets may exist in the absence of x-ray evidence of loss of interseptal bone. The roentgenologic demonstration of a periapical or periodontal area, suggestive of infection, represents only a step in evaluating the clinical significance of the lesion.

The increased radio-opacity which is associated with osteosclerotic areas, is not considered to be of pathologic significance. Such radio-opaque areas may represent the result of past infection and they can best be considered as bone scars which are indications of a satisfactory host reaction. Calcifications within the dental pulp are of no importance from a focal infection standpoint.

The dentist should report his findings and opinions, including the probability of eliminating any existent foci by conservative means, to the patient's physician. If a suspicious tooth is of strategic importance from a dental (clasp or abutment tooth) or masticatory standpoint, this fact should be stated. The physician is best equipped to integrate intelligently his clinical findings, the laboratory results and the reports from the various consultants and to determine the clinical importance of respective foci. The past history of the individual, the acuteness and duration of the present symptoms and the existence of other foci of infection are all important when evaluating a particular focus. More attention should be given to the patient, his reactions to disease processes in the past and also possibly to his familial background in this respect. The advice of the dentist should be followed as to the best method of eliminating the oral foci which may be present.

Lintz believed that in the face of a lesion commonly thought to be due to focal infection, which has not been ameliorated by good treatment, good results will be obtained in a large proportion of cases by the eradication of "dead" teeth irrespective of their roentgenologic findings. Both Grossman and Blayney have reviewed the pulpless tooth question and have come to the conclusion that the condemnation of teeth just because they are pulpless has no

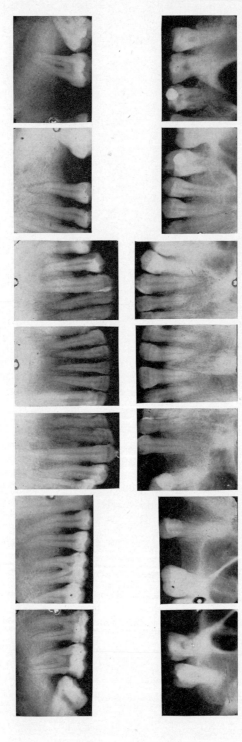

FIG. 258. Dental roentgenograms of patient shown in Fig. 253. Note the loss of the interseptal bone and the widening of the dental periosteal space.

clinical or laboratory justification. All oral foci, however, should be treated or eliminated even though they are not considered to be related etiologically to the primary disease process, but this does not mean necessarily the extraction of all pulpless teeth. Each patient will require individual consideration.

Even suspected foci of infection justify more radical consideration and treatment in certain systemic conditions. Acute infections involving the eyes, the heart, kidneys and joints are included in this category. The relation of oral foci to eye and joint involvement will be reviewed briefly in this section because of their frequency and clinical importance.

DENTAL FOCI OF INFECTION IN EYE LESIONS

The importance of oral foci of infection as etiologic or aggravating factors in acute eye lesions such as iritis, iridocyclitis and some forms of optic neuritis is well recognized by ophthalmologists. Roper-Hall believed that there is an intimate association between oral sepsis and diseases of the uveal tract and that severe eye conditions may be related to apparently trivial dental lesions. Patients requiring eye operations should first have the oral cavity placed in a good state of health before operation. Since these organs are so closely related anatomically and by means of numerous communicating vascular channels, the relative risks associated with the loss of sight or a tooth justify the immediate removal of all "infected" or suspicious teeth.

The eye lesions that may be associated with oral foci of infection include:

(1) Reflex neuroses of sensory, vasomotor or muscular nature such as may be manifested by dimness of vision, paralysis of the extra-ocular muscles and neuralgias. These are often associated with (a) periapical lesions and retained roots, (b) periodontal pockets, (c) (?) the infected vital pulp and (d) (?) impacted teeth.

(2) Inflammation of the eye tissues due to infection which may occur by means of: (a) direct extension of infection, or transmission to the eye from the mouth by means of the fingers; (b) infections from periapical or periodontal lesions which are carried by means of the vasomotor system or follow neural pathways, and (c) toxemias or allergic reactions resulting from oral foci.

There are many reports of the salutory effect on eye lesions associated with the elimination of oral foci of infection. The clinical response following the removal of oral foci has been dramatic in some of the cases observed by the author. Tichy reported a case of iridocyclitis which was apparently secondary to a dental focus. Following the removal of a retained dental root cyst in an edentulous area, there was an immediate exacerbation of the eye symptoms following which persistent clinical improvement occurred. This case also emphasizes the importance of examining all edentulous areas when searching for an oral focus.

DENTAL FOCI OF INFECTION IN THE ARTHRITIC PATIENT

Perhaps more suspicious teeth have been removed in the hope of eliminating "arthritic" symptoms than for any other condition. The elimination of pulpless or suspicious teeth results only occasionally in spectacular improvement. In the past, too much emphasis was given to pulpless teeth and those with periapical lesions and insufficient attention was paid to diseases of the periodontal tissues. The frequent occurrence of bacteremias which may arise from diseased periodontal tissues, might be of more importance in the causation of joint lesions.

A much more conservative attitude has crystallized in the last decade relative to the clinical significance of focal infection in the arthritic patient. The recent studies of Cecil and Angevine have minimized the significance of foci of infection and dental foci in rheumatoid arthritis. There are numerous factors which may be responsible for this lack of definite clinical evidence of the importance of foci of infection in this type of patient. The elimination of oral foci would only be expected to alter significantly the clinical course of those forms of arthritis which are associated with bacterial causative factors. As yet the causative agent of rheumatoid arthritis has not been clearly established although there is considerable evidence that a small proportion of the cases are closely associated with foci of infection.

In acute infectious arthritis of short duration the removal of all suspicious teeth may be justified when no other focus of infection can be found. The importance of a given tooth as a unit of the masticatory apparatus should always be weighed against its possible rôle in the causation of the joint symptoms. When immediate improvement of the joint symptoms follows the elimination of oral foci, the possibility of an allergic-dental-arthritic relationship should be considered. If an exacerbation of symptoms should be experienced following the extraction of teeth or gingival curettage, it should be regarded as clinical evidence of an etiologic relationship between the dental focus and the affected joints. The general prophylactic measures which should be taken before teeth are removed in patients with acute joint symptoms have been discussed in the section devoted to diseases of the joints.

Failure to note clinical improvement following the elimination of oral foci of infection may be due to numerous factors. Too frequently the patient seeks medical advice late in the course of the disease when secondary foci have already been established. The removal of an oral focus at this time serves only to increase the patient's general resistance. Too many teeth are still removed in the hope of curing some obscure joint lesion or myalgic pain which has not been adequately diagnosed. Under no circumstances should teeth be removed until a complete study of the patient has been made and other common foci of infection been searched for.

MULTIPLE FOCI OF INFECTION

The possible presence or known existence of multiple foci of infection, whether they are confined to the oral cavity or occur in other organs, is important in determining the treatment or prognosis in any patient. When multiple foci are present, any particular focus assumes less significance as a causative or aggravating factor of disease elsewhere. Which focus or foci should be eliminated presents a serious problem to the internist or dentist.

When multiple foci of the oral cavity or more remote organs are present they should be considered (ideally) as a single problem. The treatment should be directed against the elimination of all the foci. The removal of one or more secondary foci will have little effect on the general disease picture. Too frequently all suspicious teeth are eliminated first, or pulpless teeth are removed and little or no consideration is given the periodontal disease which may be present. It is desirable to treat simultaneously multiple oral foci such as several pulpless teeth or periodontal disease and pulpless teeth.

Infrequently a focus of infection may be of specific clinical importance but in general the elimination of foci of infection represents only an improvement in the general resistance and health of the patient which, however, may favorably affect the course of the remote disease process. The initial enthusiasm given to the concept of focal infection has not been substantiated by laboratory, clinical or mass statistical studies. The whole subject of focal infection must be viewed with both caution and conservatism.

SUMMARY OF DENTAL ASPECTS OF FOCAL INFECTION

The clinical significance of the concept of focal infection has not been clearly established nor has the relative importance of oral foci of infection been determined. The significance of oral foci of infection in respect to specific disease entities, such as rheumatoid arthritis, has not been clearly established. No fixed rules can be laid down concerning the importance of oral foci of infection, as each case represents an individual problem. Certain systemic conditions, such as acute eye and cardiac infections and joint lesions, may justify the early elimination of all foci of infection including suspicious teeth.

The oral foci of infection in the order of their probable importance include: (1) periodontal diseases; (2) periapical lesions including retained roots or residual areas of "infection" in edentulous spaces (or jaws) and (3) (?) the infected vital pulp. The presence of a periapical radiolucent area should not be considered as indicative of present "infection." The examination of serial roentgenograms made over a period of time is more informative. It should be remembered that bacteria have been isolated from teeth without periapical radiolucent areas.

There is no proven diagnostic test which will determine whether a given tooth is a focus of systemic significance. Bacteriologic cultures obtained from the apical region of extracted teeth are of little diagnostic or immunologic value even when a careful extraction technic is employed.

The dentist is most competent to evaluate whether an oral focus of infection is present and how it may best be eliminated. Many periapical dental foci can be treated successfully, using accepted surgical technics including bacteriologic controls without sacrificing the teeth, and many forms of periodontal disease may be satisfactorily eliminated by conservative methods of treatment.

26

Oral Pediatrics and Gerodontics

INTRODUCTION

The subdivision of the medical care of the patient into pediatrics and geriatrics permits an intelligent understanding of the functional and pathologic disturbances at these extremes of life, which enables more accurate diagnosis and effective treatment.

Oral disease in the early and later years of life manifests sufficient peculiarities and problems to justify a separate discussion. These peculiar problems are due to differences in the state of maturation of the oral tissues, their susceptibility to certain diseases and the functional demands made upon them at these periods of life.

The pediatrician rather than the dentist is better acquainted with oral diseases of early life and the oral manifestations associated with the usual childhood diseases, unless the dentist is on a hospital staff. Oral and dental disease in the aged, gerodontics, is mainly the responsibility of the dentist, although its problems are intimately related to those of geriatrics.

ORAL PEDIATRICS

It is common knowledge that the systemic response of the child is frequently exaggerated and at times abnormal as compared to the adult. The average practitioner is not aware that this holds true for oral diseases, since they are usually treated by the pediatrician. With the more widespread realization that the dental care of the child should commence with the eruption of the teeth, the dentist should see more oral lesions in the younger patients and his responsibilities of diagnosis and treatment will be increased.

Certain local environmental and developmental factors are present in the oral cavity of the infant which may predispose to disease or modify its course at this age. The pH of the oral cavity is more acid and the oral mucosa lacks a well-keratinized protective surface. There are also numerous problems associated with the mixed dentition which are not found in the adult.

542

Oral disease in infancy is usually more important because of its interference with the nutrition of the child than the actual tissue destruction which results. Oral disease in the infant prior to tooth eruption is usually exogenous in origin as exemplified by gonococcal stomatitis, moniliasis and the rhagades of prenatal syphilis. Herpetic stomatitis, noma (cancrum oris), and fusospirochetal infections affect the edentulous infant infrequently.

With the eruption of teeth, the local environmental conditions of the oral cavity approach those of the adult in respect to bacterial flora and salivary pH. The oral mucosa and the gums still lack a well-keratinized protective covering and they are susceptible to bacterial and mechanical irritation. Oral diseases in this period are more often the result of endogenous factors. The oral manifestations associated with scurvy and the other nutritional deficiencies and catarrhal stomatitis due to mechanical factors such as the eruption of teeth or the lack of normal oral hygiene are the most common causes of oral lesions. Herpetic stomatitis and fusospirochetal infections are uncommon.

From birth until 6 to 9 years of life there are numerous systemic diseases which may affect the odontogenesis of the permanent dentition. Rickets and rheumatic fever are frequently associated with enamel hypoplasia of the permanent teeth. Many of the exanthematous fevers such as measles, chicken pox and scarlet fever are also characterized by oral symptoms which in some instances are of diagnostic importance.

Oral disease of the child, apart from dental caries, may be grouped as follows:

(1) Congenital, hereditary or developmental anomalies.
(2) Pathologic teething.
(3) Oral and systemic manifestations of disease.
(4) Oral foci of infection in children.
(5) Habits.
(6) New growths.

Congenital, Hereditary or Developmental Anomalies

Harelip, cleft palate, ankyloglossia and other gross orofacial deformities are usually recognized at birth. Since an oral examination of the newborn is seldom a routine procedure, extensive developmental anomalies often escape recognition until other symptoms call attention to their presence. Failure of the infant to nurse may lead to the discovery of a cleft palate which is unassociated with a cleft lip. Infants so afflicted may require a special nursing nipple which mechanically closes the cleft of the palate, since surgical closure is not feasible at such an early age. The author observed a case of congenital ankylosis of the mandible which was first recognized by the infant's inability to nurse. Recurrent cyanotic attacks in infancy have been the symptom which led to the discovery of a marked lack of development of the mandible which permitted the tongue to fall back and block the air passage.

Many of the congenital, hereditary and developmental anomalies which affect the permanent teeth are not manifested clinically until these structures erupt. Partial or complete dental agenesia which at times may be associated with hereditary ectodermal dysplasia of the anhydrotic type can be verified by x-rays before the eruption of the permanent teeth. Syphilitic dental hypo-

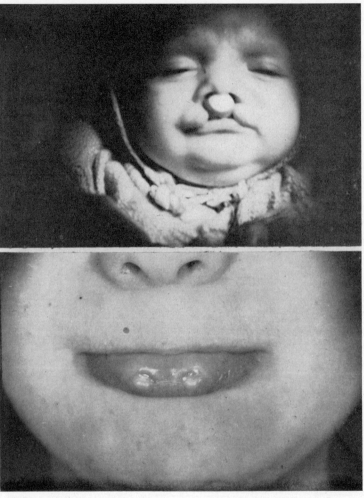

FIG. 259 (*Top*). Bilateral harelip. (Courtesy of Dr. Robert H. Ivy, Philadelphia, Pa.)
FIG. 260 (*Bottom*). Congenital lip pits in a 10-year-old girl.

plasias and the hypoplasias associated with rickets may also be similarly demonstrated but the usual anomalies or developmental changes involving the permanent teeth are not manifested until tooth eruption. The yellowish-green discoloration of the teeth in icterus gravis, hereditary opalescent dentin and brown hypoplasia of the enamel are anomalies which are manifested with the eruption of the permanent dentition.

Pathologic Teething

The physiologic process of tooth eruption or "teething," whether it occurs in infancy, childhood or adolescence (third molars), is frequently associated with painful local symptoms.

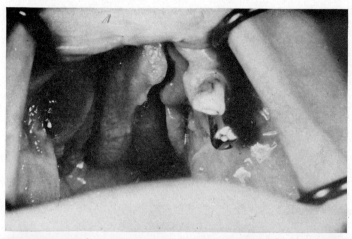

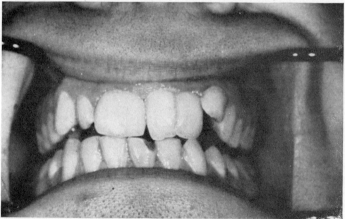

FIG. 261 (*Top*). Patient with extensive cleft of the hard and soft palates. The nasal septum and turbinate bones are plainly visible. The tooth with the gold crown serves as an abutment for an obturator.

FIG. 262 (*Bottom*). Unusual anomaly, true fusion of the maxillary right first incisor with a supernumerary tooth and false fusion of the maxillary left first incisor with a supernumerary tooth.

During the eruption of the teeth the infant is likely to be irritable, restless and to refuse to feed or to sleep properly. Salivary flow is markedly increased. The constant drooling of the saliva results at times in irritation of the skin about the mouth. The local oral symptoms are due to the pressure exerted by the erupting teeth against the overlying dense fibrous gum. This tissue normally atrophies spontaneously with the continued eruption of the tooth but in the unusual case it may be necessary to cut surgically (lance) the gum.

Schwartzmann's 5-year study of the dentitional disturbances included both private cases and those from the Metropolitan Hospital of N.Y.C. Dentitional disturbances were noted in 25% of the 378 pediatric cases encountered in private practice. Of the 2,193 examinations made on these patients 13.5% were concerned with the pathologic teething. The symptoms associated with dentitional disturbances were greatest in the winter and diminished progressively until the fall. The greatest number of derangements occurred with the lower incisors and other early erupting teeth.

The frequency of the symptoms observed in the private and hospital cases is given in the accompanying table.

TABLE XXXI

FREQUENCY OF SYMPTOMS

(153 cases—98 private and 55 hospital patients with dentitional disturbances)

Symptom	No. of Patients Presenting Symptom
Rhinitis	118
Fever	100
Anorexia	60
Vomiting	60
Cough	59
Irritability	57
Tonsillitis	56
Diarrhea	44
Otitis media	40
Constipation	22
Eruption	21
Drooling	14
Laryngitis and convulsions, each	8
Grinding of teeth	4
Pain in abdomen, polyuria, each	3
Drowsiness	3
Cervical adenitis, gingivitis with ulceration, halitosis, each	2
Thirst for water and perspiration, each	1

The rhinitis was unusual in that it was resistant to all local therapy and then cleared spontaneously when the teeth erupted. The convulsions occurred at the onset of the condition and they did not recur. In many cases the symptoms developed before there was definite redness or swelling of the gums. They persisted until the tooth was erupted.

The dietary or nutritional status of the patient did not appear to play any rôle in the "teething" difficulties. An interesting observation was that similar systemic symptoms were associated with repeated dental disturbances in the same patient. Sedation with phenobarbital and the use of aminopyrine for its analgesic effect were effective therapeutic measures.

Infection of the tissues immediately surrounding the erupting tooth occurs occasionally. This results in a painful condition which requires surgery. Such a mild infection and the increased irritability of the patient will result in a definite elevation of temperature. A gingivitis or a stomatitis, which is probably on a functional basis, may accompany the eruption of teeth.

The systemic aspects of pathologic teething are mainly those which are related to the lack of normal rest and nutrition. Patterson studied the systemic effect of "teething" on 100 children. Irritability, restlessness and the refusal to eat were commonly observed. He reported a flushing of the face on the side where the tooth was erupting. If the child had a tendency to eczema, this was aggravated during the "teething" period. A "teething" dermatitis without any eczematous background has been reported by dermatologists and seen by the author. In these cases the skin eruption could not be explained by the unusual irritability of the patient or by scratching.

A chronologic grouping of the common oral diseases of early life may assist the practitioner in their diagnosis. This age grouping is arbitrary and individual cases are expected to present departures from the average age range and symptomatology given.

Oral Lesions in Children Under 2 Years of Age

Attention is usually called to the oral lesions by (1) the failure to take food, (2) excessive dribbling of saliva and (3) undue restlessness or irritability.

(1) **Oral Moniliasis.** It was once believed that maternal vaginal moniliasis was an important source of this disease and that local trauma, debilitating diseases or prematurity were important predisposing factors. These views have largely been disproven and it has been shown that unpasteurized milk, infections from the throats and fingers of the nursing staff are more common sources of infection. The infrequent clinical recognition of moniliasis in the infant is actually due to the rarity of symptoms of sufficient severity to call attention to mild cases of the disease.

The cheeks, palate and tongue are commonly involved in moniliasis. The involved tissues appear similar to damp table salt. This whitish material is removed with difficulty and leaves a raw bleeding surface. The lesions present little or no ulceration or granulations. The topical application of an aniline dye usually results in a favorable clinical response.

(2) **Herpetic Stomatitis (Aphthous Stomatitis).** The development of herpetic stomatitis in infants represents an initial infection of the individual with the herpetic virus. Herpetic stomatitis is characterized by the sudden development of painful vesicular lesions (often unobserved) which rapidly undergo secondary change and appear as shallow erosive lesions which are frequently covered with a yellowish material. A marked increase in salivary flow, gastro-enteritis and a mild febrile reaction with an elevation of the leukocyte count is commonly experienced.

(3) **Fusospirochetal infections** at this age are uncommon. The conditions Black and McNair-Scott discussed under the name of Vincent's infection of virus etiology are examples of herpetic stomatitis.

(4) **Scurvy** is more common in the edentulous child, but the oral symptoms are less marked because of the absence of teeth. The symptoms consist of petechiae and submucosal ecchymoses. With the eruption of the teeth the prevalence of scurvy becomes less because of the more varied diet but, when the disease does occur, the oral lesions are more marked. They are characterized by hypertrophic, ulcerative, bluish-purple gingival lesions which bleed on the slightest provocation. *Fetor ex ore* is marked.

(5) **Developmental anomalies** of the oral structures are usually manifested in this period. They include ankyloglossia, cleft palate, harelip, the fissural clefts and possible dental agnesia of the deciduous dentition.

(6) **Noma** is uncommon in the edentulous child, but it may occur during this period.

(7) **A granulomatous lesion** affecting the lingual frenum may develop following the eruption of the mandibular incisors. The irritation to the lingual frenum from the sharp incisal edges of the newly erupted teeth is believed responsible. Secondary infection of the irritated frenum is associated with the production of granulation tissue and a pseudo-membrane. This symptom complex, known as Riga-Fede's disease, is common in southern Italy. It is treated by excision.

Oral Lesions in Children 2 to 6 Years Old

Gingival lesions are more common than the diffuse stomatitides and in this age range cervical adenopathy is more frequently experienced. The dentist will be required to differentiate between cervical swellings and adenopathy of dental origin and those associated with systemic disease. The swellings in this region associated with acute tonsillitis, mumps, tuberculosis, infectious mononucleosis, Hodgkin's disease, leukemia and scarlet fever must be differentiated from those of dental origin.

(1) **Herpetic Stomatitis.** Herpetic stomatitis is the most common acute oral infection in this age group. It represents the characteristic symptoms discussed previously. Occasionally a more severe form of the disease occurs in which the oral lesions precede by several days conjunctival involvement and a generalized body eruption of the erythema multiforme type (Stevens-Johnson disease).

(2) **Oral lesions** associated with the common childhood diseases of measles, chicken pox, and scarlet fever are common. They are discussed under their respective diseases at the end of this section.

(3) **Hemophilia** may be first manifested during this period by the protracted hemorrhage which is associated with the exfoliation or extraction of the deciduous teeth. Other blood dyscrasias, thrombocytopenic purpura, the childhood anemias—particularly Cooley's anemia—may manifest their presence during this age period.

(4) **Fusospirochetal infections** are more common than in the preceding age group. When present, they usually call forth a definite and at times a marked systemic response.

Oral Lesions in Children 6 to 12 Years Old

During this period the oral tissues begin to assume their adult characteristics. Gingival lesions are more common and they are related in most in-

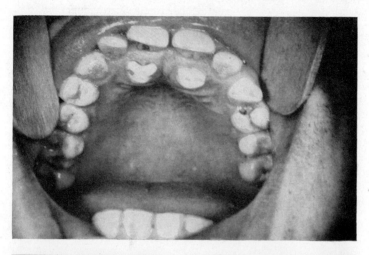

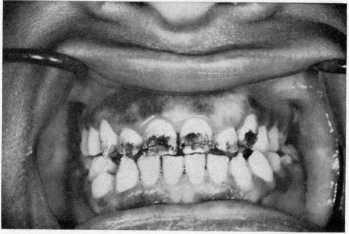

Fig. 263 (*Top*). Two supernumerary teeth which are erupting palatally to the maxillary anteriors. The patient's mother
had the same anomaly.

Fig. 264 (*Bottom*). Enamel hypoplasia associated with
childhood rickets.

stances to the exfoliation of the deciduous teeth and the eruption of the permanent teeth. The dental hypoplasias associated with prenatal syphilis and
the common childhood diseases become manifest during this period with the
eruption of the permanent dentition. Calculus is usually first observed and

becomes an important local predisposing cause for catarrhal and fusospiro-chetal gingivitis.

Hypertrophic gingival changes are also frequent during this period. They may be due in part to faulty oral hygiene, but frequently a hormonal or endocrine background can be established. Endocrine dysfunction may also be manifested by delayed or premature eruption of the permanent teeth. Marked periodontal disturbances at this age are highly suggestive of juvenile diabetes, which is characterized by rapid alveolar resorption, delayed wound healing

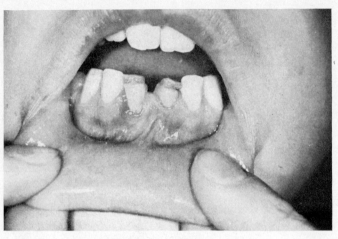

FIG. 265. Dilaceration in the lower first incisors result-ing from traumatic injury to the deciduous incisors at ap-proximately two years of age.

and the rapid deposition of calculus. The basis for periodontal disturbances of later life can be frequently traced to gingival disturbances or poor dental health habits formed during this age period.

Oral Lesions in Children After the Age of 12 Years

By 12 years of age the oral tissues have assumed their adult characteristics. Fusospirochetal infections are numerous and hypertrophic gingival changes are not uncommon. The former is less frequently accompanied by systemic reactions than in the younger age group. Solitary herpetic lesions are com-monly observed.

Oral Foci of Infection in Children

The common presence and the important significance of oral foci of infec-tion in the child has not been sufficiently appreciated. If oral foci of infection are considered to be of clinical importance in the adult, their significance in the child is obvious. Focal infection at this period of life often results in acute systemic reactions which may promptly regress, following the removal of the focus. The age of the patient lessens the possibility of multiple primary foci of infection. The acute systemic response to foci of infection results usually in an early diagnosis before secondary foci have been established, which cannot be readily eliminated. The failure to eliminate foci of infection in childhood may result in serious damage to the affected organ which may exist throughout life.

Periapical and periodontal foci must be considered in the child. Abscessed deciduous teeth should not be disregarded or their significance minimized as an oral focus of infection. The bacterial flora of abscessed deciduous teeth is composed of pathogenic staphylococci and streptococci. They have a copious vascularity about their roots which affords a ready avenue by which bacteria or their products can be disseminated to more distant parts of the body. Furthermore, the deciduous teeth are usually slightly loose, particularly when they become abscessed, and during chewing a mechanical element furnishes an additional mechanism by which bacteria may be forced into the circulation.

Many practitioners are hesitant about removing abscessed deciduous teeth in the belief that their premature loss favors malocclusion of the permanent dentition. The health of the child is certainly more important than possible malposed teeth which can be prevented by space retainers or corrected in later years by orthodontic treatment. McBride felt that too much emphasis has been placed on the maintenance of teeth for space retention and that many times infected deciduous teeth have been retained at the expense of the child's health.

Such important conditions as rheumatic fever, acute hemorrhagic nephritis, acute iritis, acute articular rheumatism, osteomyelitis, infections of the accessory nasal sinuses, meningitis, recurrent tonsillitis, streptococcal sore throat and otitis media are systemic conditions which may be associated with oral foci of infection. The author has observed instances of all of the above which, on clinical grounds, were closely related to oral foci. In cases of cavernous sinus thrombosis, pansinusitis and meningitis necropsy findings established the etiologic rôle of dental foci of infection. The favorable and rapid clinical response following the elimination of oral foci in cases of acute hemorrhagic nephritis, acute articular rheumatism and acute iritis constitute clinical proof of a causative rôle.

In these acute conditions in children, when permanent damage to the heart, kidneys or joints may be the consequence of the continuance of the process, the dentist is justified in the removal of dental foci at a time when their elimination may be most beneficial. Appropriate prophylactic measures should be taken to prevent transient bacteremias. Children with rheumatic heart involvement or congenital vascular or cardiac anomalies should receive special care. The recommended prophylactic procedures are discussed in the sections concerned with rheumatic fever and subacute bacterial endocarditis.

Measles (Rubeola)

Measles is an acute, highly contagious eruptive fever caused by a filtrable virus. The virus has been demonstrated in the saliva 48 hours after the appearance of the rash. Transmission may occur by means of salivary droplets.

It is rarely a dangerous disease in itself but it may lead to serious complications in infants and children. Most children in urban areas have measles before the 12th year. A mild infection is desirable to establish a permanent immunity.

The average incubation period is 8 to 15 days. Prodromal symptoms include drowsiness, irritability or malaise and more rarely nausea and vomiting. The classical symptoms are fever of 101° to 103° F., a catarrhal inflammation of the eyes and upper respiratory passages, photophobia, hoarseness and the Koplik's spots on the oral mucosa. The Koplik's spots precede the rash by 2 or 3 days.

The characteristic rash or exanthem begins as flattened, irregularly shaped reddish macules which increase gradually in size and become slightly elevated above the unchanged normal skin. The lesions either remain discrete or become confluent. They blanch on pressure. The exanthem appears first on the forehead and spreads gradually to the entire body in the course of several days. In 4 to 5 days a branny desquamation of the skin overlying the lesions takes place. The eruption clears in 14 to 21 days. During the acute phase of the disease there is a leukopenia.

Secondary respiratory infections, such as bronchitis, bronchopneumonia, are the most important complications of this disease. Otitis media, persistent adenitis, a reactivated tuberculous infection and more rarely meningitis and encephalitis are other sequellae.

Measles is diagnosed on the basis of a possible history of exposure, the characteristic prodromal symptoms and the rash. Koplik's spots permit an early diagnosis, while the typical branny desquamation is useful in making a diagnosis in the later stages of the disease. Measles must be differentiated from German measles, scarlet fever and chicken pox. Convalescent immune serum, immune globulin and placental extract are used to modify, or to prevent when indicated, the disease in exposed individuals and reduce the risk of complications.

Oral Aspects. The oral aspects of measles include: (1) the Koplik's spots or the enanthem and (2) the various oral complications that follow occasionally. Koplik's spots are important diagnostic signs as they appear several days before the appearance of the rash. They are present during the most infectious stage of the disease. Koplik's spots are found on the cheek mucosa along the line of closure of the teeth in the molar region. The patient may be aware of their presence and complain of a hot burning sensation in this area. The lesions appear as pin-head white or bluish-white spots which are surrounded by an area of erythema. Adequate illumination is essential for their detection. The spots fade gradually as the oral mucosa becomes congested and the exanthem appears. Koplik's spots are found less frequently on other mucosal areas.

An unusual aversion to the dental operating light in a restless young patient with coryza should cause the operator to suspect early measles. A thorough examination of the cheek mucosa may show the typical Koplik's spots.

Cervical adenopathy is commonly present. It may be associated erroneously with diseased teeth. Osteomyelitis of the jaw and noma have been reported following epidemic measles. Infection of tooth sockets and the alveolar process are often encountered. These complications represent secondary bacterial invasion of tissues whose resistance has been lowered by measles.

Scarlet Fever

Scarlet fever is an acute, contagious disease caused by any one of a variety of serologic types of beta streptococci. It is important because of its many serious complications. Scarlet fever is commonest between the ages of 1 and 6. It occurs sporadically or in small epidemics in the fall and winter. Infection results usually in permanent immunity. The causative organism, the *Streptococcus scarletinae* produces a soluble toxin which is responsible for the characteristic rash.

The incubation period in scarlet fever is between 2 to 7 days in 90% of the cases. The initial symptoms consist of a fever of 101° to 103° F., sore throat and vomiting. The pulse rate is out of all proportion to the temperature. The redness of the cheeks is accentuated by the pallor of the surrounding tissues, producing the characteristic circumoral pallor. Tonsillitis and pharyngitis are common symptoms. The membrane covering these areas, when present, is usually easily removed. The tongue lesions will be discussed under the oral aspects of this disease. The polymorphonuclear leukocyte count varies from 10,000 to 40,000 cells c. mm. depending on the severity of the infection.

The exanthem or rash appears 18 to 36 hours following the onset of symptoms. The initial pin-point reddened areas fuse to form a marked flush which is first noted on the head and neck but soon involves the entire body. The eruption fades gradually in 7 to 10 days and desquamation or peeling of the skin, including the palms of the hands and the soles of the feet, takes place in about 2 weeks. Tonsillitis and streptococcal sore throat may be a mild expression of scarlet fever without the rash.

The complications of scarlet fever develop between the 2nd and 3rd weeks. In about 10% of the cases, there is a marked cervical adenitis. In former years 10% to 15% of all cases developed otitis media or mastoiditis with deafness persisting in a small proportion of the cases. When the suppurative process involves the facial canal facial paralysis results commonly. Acute nephritis and cardiorespiratory complications occur less frequently.

The diagnosis can usually be made on the basis of the history, the appearance of the eruption and one or more of the following diagnostic aids.

Diagnostic aids include throat cultures, the Dick test, the Schultz-Charlton extinction reaction and the tourniquet test. Measles, German measles, diphtheria, drug and serum rashes must be considered in the differential diagnosis.

The disease can be prevented by the proper immunizing procedures in childhood. Convalescent serum or antitoxic equine serum is used for the acute infection. Sulfanilamide or penicillin is of special value in the treatment of the septic complications such as otitis media or mastoiditis.

Oral Aspects. Poor oral hygiene and carious teeth may predispose to scarlet fever. Carious teeth are said to serve as a focus of this disease in carriers or immune individuals. Fones reported a reduction of scarlet fever from 14.1% to 0.5% in the school children of Bridgeport, Connecticut, following the introduction of mouth hygiene. These figures do not take into consideration other preventive health measures which were also taken. The causative organisms are known to be dispersed in ill individuals by salivary droplets. During the height of the eruption, the oral mucosa is uniformily congested. Fine points of submucosal hemorrhage may appear on the palate.

The tongue presents characteristic changes in scarlet fever. At first the dorsum is uniformly and heavily coated but in about 24 hours the coating clears along the margins of the tongue and at the tip. The swollen, hyperemic, fungiform papillae appear as bright red spots through the coating. The entire coating clears gradually, leaving a smooth, glazed surface studded with the swollen fungiform papillae, producing the so-called "strawberry tongue" which is a characteristic finding in scarlet fever.

A severe stomatitis, noma, perforation of the palate, ulcerative glossitis and osteomyelitis of the jaws have been reported as complications of scarlet fever. The cervical adenitis and facial paralysis associated with this disease have already been discussed. The usual oral lesions require no attention. Ice compresses are helpful in relieving the tenderness and swelling of cervical adenitis. The less common oral complications are treated as similar conditions due to other causes.

Diphtheria

Diphtheria is an acute infectious disease which is characterized by a marked toxemia and the formation of a fibrinous exudate (membrane) on the involved mucosal surfaces. Diphtheria occurs commonly between the 1st and 5th years. Children with measles and scarlet fever are particularly susceptible. Artificial active immunization has reduced markedly the incidence. A positive Shick test denotes susceptibility. Transmission is usually by direct contact, coughing, sneezing or kissing. The organisms are present in the saliva and mucous secretions. They may be found at times in the pharynx of immune carriers. Diphtheria is caused by the *Corynebacterium diphtheriae,* the Klebs-Loeffler bacillus. This organism produces a potent exotoxin at the site of the local lesion. Diphtheria is a classical example of a toxemia.

The incubation period of diphtheria is from 2 to 5 days. Prostration, headache, a fever of 101° to 103° F., body aches and occasionally vomiting are the initial symptoms. The pulse, which is rapid, irregular and feeble, is increased out of proportion to the temperature. There is a polymorphonuclear leukocytosis.

There are marked pain and redness of the throat, accompanied by dysphagia. A grayish-white membrane is characteristically found over the tonsillar and pharyngeal region. This "membrane" consists of fibrin, leukocytes, bacteria and epithelial cells which have undergone coagulation necrosis. The membrane is removed with difficulty, leaving a raw bleeding surface which reforms rapidly. Its extent is no indication of the severity of the infection. The soluble toxins which are produced at the site of the membrane may give rise to a myocarditis, otitis media, lesions in the liver, the kidneys and other serious complications. Seventh nerve involvement secondary to otitis media may result in facial paralysis. Asphyxia is a fatal complication in laryngeal diphtheria.

Diphtheria is diagnosed on the basis of the clinical symptoms, the physical examination and the culture of the Klebs-Loeffler bacillus from the "membrane." The sodium tellurite throat swab is not an established diagnostic procedure. Tonsillitis, streptococcal sore throat, thrush, pharyngeal ulcerations in the blood dyscrasias, agranulocytic angina and Vincent's angina must be considered in the differential diagnosis. In Vincent's angina the lesions are usually unilateral and they are an ulcer rather than a membrane. Toxic symptoms are less striking in Vincent's angina.

Once the diagnosis is established, antitoxic serum should be administered at once. This is a prophylactic rather than a curative measure, as it neutralizes only the formed toxin. Hence, its early administration is important.

Oral Aspects. Diphtheritic involvement of the oral mucosa is rare. It has been reported at the site of erupting deciduous teeth and in the fissures of the oral commissures. Lavender and Squires reported a case of diphtheria confined to the oral cavity which began with a swelling of the lower lip. Eight hours later two-thirds of the lower lip and the labial mucosa had a granular appearance and were covered with a tough whitish membrane. Stained smears from the "membrane" showed cocci but no fusiform bacilli. Cultures of the lesion were also negative for the Klebs-Loeffler bacillus at this time. Thirty-six hours later, organisms which were morphologically similar to the Klebs-Loeffler bacillus were obtained from the lip lesion although the nose and throat cultures were negative for this organism.

The lower lip, the lower gums and the cheek mucosa were involved. Two lower incisors became loose and were extracted. Cultures from the sockets were positive for the Klebs-Loeffler bacillus. The lesions healed and the cultures became negative for this organism 45 days after the onset of the disease.

Varicella—Chicken Pox

Varicella is an acute contagious virus disease which is characterized by a cutaneous eruption. Constitutional symptoms are mild or absent. The disease may be related to herpes zoster.

The incubation period varies from 10 to 21 days. The rash consists of successive crops of scattered, itching papules which develop later into vesicles. The vesicles dry up commencing in the middle and form crusted lesions. Papules, vesicles and encrusted lesions are in close proximity on the same body area (diagnostic). The eruption is prominent on the face and scalp. Permanent scarring does not result unless there is secondary infection. Serious sequellae and complications are rare. There is no specific treatment. The itching may be relieved by lotions. Inoculation of contacts with the serum of convalescent patients is a fairly successful preventive measure.

Oral Aspects. Transitory painless vesicles are frequently present on the oral and pharyngeal mucosae 12 to 24 hours before the cutaneous eruption. The oral mucosal vesicles are of varying size and they are surrounded by an erythematous base. A shallow eroded area surrounded by mucosal tags is most frequently seen.

Erythroblastosis Fetalis (Icterus Gravis—Kernicterus)

This rare form of jaundice was once thought to be hereditary. Recent studies have shown that this disease may result from iso-immunization by the Rh factor. In 90% of the cases studied by Levine *et al.* the mother was Rh— and the fetus and father were Rh+. It is the continuous intra-uterine passage and action of the anti-Rh agglutinins on the susceptible Rh— blood which is the cause of the abnormal red blood cell hemolysis.

In erythroblastosis fetalis, the physiologic jaundice of the new born fails to disappear and the jaundice increases in severity. The condition usually terminates fatally within a few days and certain neurologic manifestations including convulsions are common in such patients. Advantage is taken of the recent knowledge of the Rh antigen relationship in this disease in its treatment and the response of the affected infant to Rh— transfusions has been almost dramatic.

Oral Aspects. A permanent yellowish-green discoloration of the permanent teeth has been noted in recovered cases of icterus gravis. Kreshover demonstrated histopathologic changes in the developing teeth of infants with icterus gravis which are characteristic. Because of its rarity, this disease is of little practical dental significance.

GERODONTICS

The jaws, the teeth and their supporting structures, the oral mucosa, the tongue and salivary glands are all affected by senescence. Changes in tooth morphology, in the supporting tissues and oral mucosa at this age modify considerably the treatment planning of the elderly patient. Many of these changes, such as the loss of teeth, the loss of normal intermaxillary space with the resulting undue prominence of the chin are preventible, or can be compensated for, by adequate and timely treatment. These changes are esthetically undesirable but, what is more important, they result in decreased efficiency of the masticatory apparatus. The average dental practitioner gives inadequate consideration to the effects of senescence on the dental structures during treatment planning.

An adequate functioning masticatory apparatus is more essential in the aged than at any other period of life because of the inability of the gastrointestinal tract to compensate for the improper comminution of food. Failure to replace lost members of the dental apparatus not only reduces the efficiency of the remaining teeth, but it places an additional strain on them for which the supporting tissues are not adapted at this period of life. The physician and the dental practitioner fail to realize that the loss of a single tooth also results in the functional loss of its antagonist. An individual with a complement of 24 teeth, who had 4 scattered missing teeth, has a masticatory efficiency of only 66%.

In many of the organ systems, a compensatory and protective mechanism is observed in senescence by decreased functional demands. For example, a diminished cardiac reserve is in part compensated for by the decreased work output demanded of this organ and diseased joints are called upon for less strenuous function. The teeth and their supporting structures do not share in such a compensatory mechanism. Moreover, the teeth remaining at this period of life are frequently called upon to function as bridge abutments or rests for prosthetic appliances replacing teeth which have succumbed to the exodontist's skill—or the physician's zeal. The functional demands made on the teeth remaining at this period of life are often greater than in early adult life before senile gingival recession and alveolar atrophy have weakened the support of these teeth. When periodontal disease is present, still less favorable conditions exist and the rapid breakdown of the supporting tissues of the abutment teeth results in overfunction of the remaining teeth and their premature loss. Now, in addition to the many other problems of later life, the individual must adapt himself to "plates."

A consideration of gerodontics includes:

(1) The changes in the teeth and supporting tissues.
(2) The changes in the intermaxillary space and the temporomandibular joint.
(3) The changes in the efficiency of the masticatory system.
(4) The changes in the oral mucosa, tongue and associated structures.
(5) Oral foci of infection in the aged.

Changes in the Teeth and Supporting Tissues

Many of the changes in the hard dental tissues associated with senescence have their analogy in the deciduous teeth, which erupt, lose their morphologic characteristics through normal wear or abrasion and are eventually exfoliated. In later life the permanent teeth become drier and more brittle and darker. This clinically observed increase in dryness, hardness and calcification has been verified by careful laboratory studies. The apparent decrease in the prevalence of dental caries in the elderly patient is largely the result of a reduction in the number of susceptible carious areas due to previous dental restorations and the loss of teeth.

Under theoretically "ideal" conditions, the occlusal and morsal surfaces of the posterior teeth gradually lose their characteristic form and, the cuspal angles becoming less and less, approach a flat surface. With these changes in the posterior teeth there is a tendency for an "edge to edge" bite to develop in the incisor region. These changes are the rule in primitive peoples and they are thought to compensate for the increased extra-alveolar lever arm of the tooth resulting from the senile atrophy of the supporting structures.

Dental restorations that fail to take into consideration changes in tooth anatomy occurring with increasing age, may result in abnormal destructive stresses being placed on the teeth. Fillings, crowns or bridges should not have steep cuspal angles and deep fossae. The occlusal surfaces of crowns and bridges should be narrowed buccolingually in order to prevent vertical overloading of the teeth. The contact points of the teeth become flattened due to the slight physiologic tooth movement which occurs during chewing. This results in a general mesial movement of the teeth. Degenerative changes in the dental periosteum due to pressure and the decreased blood supply may take place.

Years of improper tooth brushing technic may be manifested in the aged by the presence of "V"-shaped horizontal grooves in the teeth just apical to the enamel-cemental junction. In severe cases this abrasive grooving extends into the dentin to areas formerly occupied by the dental pulp chamber. Pulpal exposure occurs occasionally but in most instances sufficient secondary dentin has been formed to prevent exposure of the pulp or even to obliterate the pulp chamber. These grooved teeth are unsightly and at times they fracture at the site of the notching. Fortunately, pain is rarely a distressing symptom.

The senile gingival and alveolar atrophy in conjunction with the continuous eruption of the teeth results in exposure of the root to the oral environment. These exposed root surfaces frequently permit the transmission of painful stimuli when thermal changes take place within the oral cavity.

Changes in the Intermaxillary Space and the Temporomandibular Joint

Certain changes in the dentofacial characteristics of the aged are generally regarded as a normal accompaniment of senescence. These include the prominent and protruding chin, the wrinkling which extends downward from the oral commissures and the obtuse angle of the mandible. These esthetic considerations are of secondary importance to the disturbed physiologic function and pathologic changes which may result in the temporomandibular joints. These changes, which are secondary to a loss of the normal intermaxillary space, can be largely prevented through proper dental care, which includes not only good restorative dentistry and the replacement of lost dental structures, but frequent denture servicing. Few dentists and patients are sufficiently impressed with the need for periodic denture servicing, which includes either rebasing or complete denture reconstruction to maintain a near normal intermaxillary space and to compensate for the resorption of the osseous tissue.

Failure to maintain the intermaxillary space, due either to abnormal wear of the teeth or failure to restore adequately lost dental structures, results frequently in undue stresses being placed on the temporomandibular joints. This results at times in a syndrome, described by Costen, which consists of pain in the temporomandibular joint region, catarrhal deafness and neuralgias of the tongue, pharyngeal and cephalic regions.

Changes in the Efficiency of the Masticatory Apparatus

While technics for estimating the masticatory efficiency are limited as to their practicability and accuracy, both Paulsen and Claunsen demonstrated that a deficient number of teeth or disturbed occlusal relations result in a decreased comminution of food as compared with the comminution obtained when the occlusal relations are normal or when there are adequate prosthetic appliances. In the elderly individual, the gastro-intestinal tract is less able to compensate for defective oral comminution of food because of the frequent occurrence of relative achlorhydria and impaired gastric function.

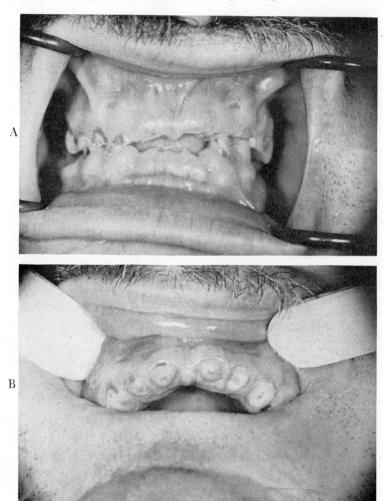

FIG. 266. (A) Extreme degree of tooth abrasion (attrition) which resulted from the habit of chewing tobacco. The patient, a 68-year-old male, was a railroad worker. (B) Same patient showing wear of the maxillary anterior teeth even with the gums. (Fourth degree of attrition.)

Quantitative deficiencies in the masticatory apparatus can be compensated for in part by prolonged chewing and the manner in which the food is prepared. The efficiency of artificial dentures in food partitioning is low as compared with natural dentures, being probably not more than one-fifth as efficient. For this reason, the artificial denture-wearing patient must chew his food much longer. In the aged patient, the failure to receive periodic denture servicing will reduce still further the masticatory efficiency of the artificial dentures until their usefulness is chiefly one of esthetics.

Changes in the Oral Mucosa and Tongue

The lips, the oral mucosa and the tongue in senescence present changes which are comparable with those observed in other tissues. They become atrophic; there is a loss of elasticity and a decrease in the *tunica propria*. The characteristic stippling of the healthy gingival and oral tissues seen in adult life is absent in the aged. The mucosa now has a satiny, wax-like or edematous appearance. The tissues lack frequently a protective layer of keratinized cells, which renders them more susceptible to mechanical, chemical or bacterial irritation, although these tissues are still subjected to the same or increased insults. Similar atrophic mucosal changes are observed frequently after the menopause. Atrophy of the underlying connective tissue results in a loss of resilience and elasticity which may contribute to further difficulties in denture retention.

A decreased salivary flow is a common complaint of the aged. With the decreased salivary flow the ptyalin content of the saliva is also reduced. Approximately 60% of the ingested cooked starch is digested in the mouth of a young adult but in the aged, relatively little starch digestion takes place in the mouth. The pancreatic amylase is usually able to compensate for this ptyalin deficiency of the saliva. Hamperl observed histologic changes in the salivary glands of the aged, although their clinical significance was not determined. The reaction of the saliva becomes more neutral and slightly alkaline with age, this being particularly true in the edentulous patient.

The diminished salivary flow frequently results in an annoying stickiness which may lead to mechanical irritation. The loss of the normal cleansing and protective action of the saliva renders the tissues more susceptible to infection.

Insufficient salivary flow also makes denture retention more difficult. Both the quality and the quantity of saliva are important in denture retention. In the aged, the small solitary mucous glands of the palate, cheeks and lips secrete a thick ropy saliva with a high mucin content which makes denture retention difficult.

The tongue loses its normal muscle tone and offers less resistance when palpated bidigitally. The normal papillary coating becomes decreased in amount and the dorsum of the tongue has an atrophic appearance as judged by its appearance in middle life. The decreased salivary flow often results in considerable irritation to the sides of this organ where it comes in contact with the teeth or prosthetic appliances. Glossodynia or glossopyrosis is a common complaint in senescence and many times no satisfactory explanation can be found.

Foci of Infection in the Aged

The importance of focal infection in the aged is not minimized but the clinical response following the removal of any one focus is seldom impressive.

The decreased reparative potentialities of the tissues at this age and the long duration of the foci, which has resulted frequently in permanent damage to the affected structures, lessen the likelihood of clinical improvement following the removal of any focus of infection.

For these reasons, when questionable oral foci are being considered for elimination, the value of the dental members as units of the masticatory apparatus, as bridge abutments or clasp anchorages must be weighed against the questionable benefits which might follow their removal. This does not sanction the retention of definitely diseased teeth but there is no reason why the teeth should be indiscriminately condemned just because of their ease of removal and other less accessible foci be allowed to remain.

27

Occupational Diseases of Dental Practice

PYOGENIC INFECTIONS OR TRAU-MATIC INFECTIONS	FEET
	X-RAY
RESPIRATORY INFECTIONS	AMALGAM
EYES	DERMATITIS
SEDENTARY ASPECTS	ACCIDENTALLY ACQUIRED SYPHI-LITIC INFECTIONS
POSTURE	

While permanent disability or death of a dentist is rarely ascribable to incidents of dental practice, this profession entails occupational risks of a wide diversity and considerable importance. Every dental practitioner will do well to consider these possible hazards and take the appropriate preventive measures.

PYOGENIC INFECTIONS OR TRAUMATIC INFECTIONS

At all times, except when the rubber dam is used, the dentist is working in a field containing large numbers of pathogenic organisms. The urologist and even the proctologist, who work in a "dirty field," hesitate to examine the mouth without wearing rubber gloves. The dentist's job moreover consists of working on carious or broken-down teeth with sharp instruments which offer numerous opportunities for traumatic injury and secondary infection. The possibility of receiving tooth-inflicted wounds should not be overlooked or minimized when working on incorrigible children, epileptics or mental patients or those under general anesthesia. It is remarkable that pyogenic infections are not encountered more frequently in dentists. The importance of the antibacterial property of the saliva as a protection against such infections may not be sufficiently appreciated.

RESPIRATORY INFECTIONS

The nature of dental practice and the type of the services rendered necessitate a close proximity with the patient's exchange of air, even when the rubber dam is used. This affords frequent exposure to the usual upper respiratory infections, as well as to the more serious pulmonary diseases. Practitioners who are susceptible to colds should not work on patients with upper respiratory infections unless a mask or an intranasal filter is worn. The risk of acquiring more serious pulmonary disease is greater in the dental practitioner than in the physician, as the latter is usually aware of any systemic background which the patient may have, while the dentist all too frequently treats his patients "blindly" without first taking a medical summary of the case. This is to be deplored. The dentist should know, and he has the right to know, the general physical background of the patient, for his personal protection as well as for planning the most effective treatment for the patient.

EYES

The dentist's eyes are as important as his fingers in the performance of his professional duties. Too many dentists neglect their eyes (and their teeth). As a profession, Dentistry makes rather severe demands on the vision and furthermore the risk of infection or inflammations of these organs due to foreign bodies, drugs or chemicals is great.

The visual concentration which is required for the satisfactory performance of dental operations, many times under suboptimal lighting conditions, produces a severe strain on the eyes. In the past, the dentist has been too self-satisfied with "light" and he has not been sufficiently concerned about "illumination." The modern scientific illumination of dental offices, with the reduction in light contrasts and with the better control of reflected light, is doing much to prevent eyestrain due to this cause.

The dentist requiring bifocal lenses can wear to advantage a form of "reversed" bifocals in which there is a larger field for close vision and a small field for distant vision.

The dentist runs a considerable risk of eye infections from salivary droplets, blood, or broken fragments of teeth or pieces of calculus. While no exact figures are available concerning the accidental loss of sight, they are sufficiently large to warrant serious consideration. Eye glasses offer a reasonably effective means of prevention. If corrective lenses are not required, plane ones should be worn at least when extractions or dental prophylaxes are being done. They will prevent fragments of tooth or calculus from entering the eye and one need only look through the lenses at the end of a morning's or afternoon's work to see the finer particles and salivary droplets that have been prevented from entering the eye.

It is not uncommon for the eye to be contaminated with some anesthetic solution when giving a local anesthetic. While the solution itself is relatively harmless it is usually contaminated with the mouth flora. The eye so contaminated should be washed out with boric acid and 1 or 2 drops of a fresh 20% argyrol solution instilled in the eye. This procedure can be repeated in one-half hour.

If medicaments or drugs should come in contact with the eyes, they should be washed out with sterile physiologic saline. The dilution of the agent and the mechanical flushing action will usually prevent serious complications. If a foreign body (fragment of enamel, calculus or root) should be encountered, the eyes should be washed with boric acid and argyrol instilled and a competent ophthalmologist seen at once!

SEDENTARY ASPECTS

Dental practice is confining. The general practitioner is restricted to his office during working hours and frequently afterwards when laboratory work must be completed. He does not obtain the fresh air, the exercise or change of scenery that his medical colleague does when he makes his house calls or ward rounds. The dentist spends the major portion of his working day standing in an unphysiologic position at the dental chair with most of his weight on one foot. Dentists can often be "spotted" because of a moderate scoliosis and the characteristic "droop" of their right shoulder.

POSTURE

Of necessity, the dentist's field of activity is restricted to his operating chair, but with proper positioning of the patient and by working with the mouth mirror a more erect, less tiring and more physiologic working posture can be obtained. A large proportion of the chair work can be performed while seated on an operating stool. This affords a change of position, rests the lower extremities and enables one to accomplish satisfactorily with less fatigue many dental operations.

FEET

In addition to being tiresome, the dentist's relatively fixed position at the chair predisposes to defective arches, varicose veins and possibly hemorrhoids. The constant weight bearing, frequently on one foot, causes a flattening of the pedal arches. The prevalence of defective arches among dentists is attested to by the lasts some shoe manufacturers are marketing to give adequate support for the dentist's feet. While the immediate symptoms due to "flat feet" are not as a rule striking, these changes may be manifest by a variety of obscure neuralgias and pains.

Lelyveld has made the following recommendations for proper foot care for the dentist:

(1) Select shoes which are generous in length and width. They should be of flexible leather, including the soles.
(2) Select socks at least ½ size longer than the foot. If you wear woolen socks, wear cotton ones inside.
(3) Keep the feet parallel in standing. Toeing in or out weakens the ankles and the arches.
(4) Bathe in water of comfortable temperature. Some sea salt added to the water may be refreshing. Massage the feet at night with lanolin, and dust with boric acid powder in the morning.
(5) Cut toe nails straight across—do not round the corners. Do not cut corns or calluses yourself.

(6) Elevate the feet to rest them. Change to a fresh pair of shoes and socks at midday.

The fixed position, with constant weight bearing on the feet, predisposes to varicosities of the veins of the lower extremities and also to hemorrhoids. The muscular contractions of the leg muscles are not sufficient to press the blood from the lower extremities where it stagnates in the veins and favors the formation of varicosities. The modern electric dental chairs do not even afford the exercise of "pumping" the chair. Occasionally placing one's feet on the desk or laboratory bench is physiologically, if not professionally, sound. The venous stasis in the lower extremities also affects the venous drainage of the hemorrhoidal veins, predisposing to hemorrhoids. Working in both the standing and in the sitting positions, with frequent "resting" of the feet and legs by placing them as high as possible for a few minutes, aids in preventing varicose veins and hemorrhoids.

X-RAY

The average dentist does not adequately appreciate the serious dangers arising from the careless use of the dental x-ray. Modern x-ray equipment may be shockproof but it is not foolproof and it must be used with full knowledge of the hazards incident to undue exposure to the roentgen rays. Ennis repeatedly called attention to the pernicious habit of the operator holding the films during exposure. The accumulative effect of this practice is likely to result in serious x-ray burns of the fingers if not actual malignant degeneration. Many individuals have been professionally incapacitated because of a

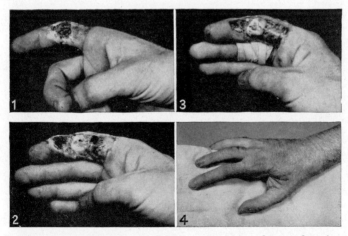

FIG. 267. Hyperkeratosis of right index finger that increased progressively to extend from the distal interphalangeal joint to the base of the index finger on the palmar surface, ultimately requiring removal of the entire diseased area by amputation. (Courtesy of Dr. George E. Pfahler.) (Ennis, Dental Roentgenology, Lea & Febiger.)

few minutes' carelessness every day. X-ray burns are serious and the repeated operations on the affected fingers result in scarring and contractions and at times loss of one or more fingers, a hand, or a life.

In recent years a small dental fluoroscopic screen somewhat similar to a large mouth mirror has been marketed. An absolutely dark room and almost complete dark adaptation are required for the efficient use of the dental fluoroscope—conditions rarely obtainable or practical in the dental office. The use of this screen is particularly dangerous as the operator must be exposed to the direct radiation. The size and the quality of the fluoroscopic image are not of sufficient detail to permit the diagnosis of any but the most gross types of pathosis which could be detected by easier, quicker and less dangerous methods of examination. The dental fluoroscopic screen should not be used under any circumstances.

The effects of exposure to the x-rays are cumulative, and in time, if this practice is continued, the tissues will have received a damaging amount of radiation. A period of 4 to 14 years may elapse before malignant changes appear. At first there is dryness of the skin, increased hardness of the tissues with eventual formation of fissures and ulcers. Squamous cell carcinoma is a common sequel to x-ray dermatosis. The index finger is most commonly affected.

AMALGAM (MERCURY)

There has been considerable controversy concerning the technical advisability and the toxicologic dangers of "working" or "kneading" the silver amalgam prior to its use as a filling material. A few cases of mercurialism have been reported in dentists, which were believed due to this practice. The exposure to mercury vapors is much more serious. While the dangers due to vapors result mainly from the heating of copper amalgam, amalgam dies or mercury-containing substances, it is desirable to keep the waste amalgam in a closed container. The possible dangers of silicosis from the polishing compounds which are used in the dental laboratory are discussed under diseases of the respiratory system.

DERMATITIS

Dermatitis, especially of the hands, is a serious disease for the dental practitioner. The appearance of his hands may be objectionable to his patients, and the dermatitis may be so aggravated by working in the moist oral cavity with its bacterial population that dental practice is impossible.

There are numerous solutions, drugs and compounds which are used by the dentist that may cause a dermatitis. A partial list of these agents has been included in the tabulation of some of the causes of stomatitis venenata (in the patient), due to medicaments or restorative materials used in dental practice. Because of his more frequent and prolonged contact with these substances, it is surprising that occupationally acquired dermatitis does not occur more frequently in dentists.

Procaine dermatitis is an additional cause of dermatitis in the dentist. In some cases, this is limited to the right hand, especially the index and first fingers and the finger webs. The procaine solution comes in contact with these structures when the dentist expels the air bubbles from the syringe. Procaine dermatitis begins as a slight redness, itching and desquamation of the tissues which come in contact with this substance. Vesiculation occurs in a more acute type of reaction. Drying, cracking and fissuring of the involved tissues take place later when the lesions may be so severe as to prevent practice. Procaine dermatitis develops only in individuals who are unusually sensitive to this substance.

Dermatitis due to formalin-containing cold sterilizing fluids gives rise to skin lesions similar to procaine dermatitis. One dentist was treated for procaine dermatitis for several months before the lesions were correctly diagnosed as lichen planus. The dentist with suspected procaine dermatitis should consult a competent dermatologist for diagnosis and treatment.

The dentist with a high sensitivity to procaine can wear rubber gloves when procaine is used, or they can absorb the procaine that is expelled when the air bubbles are eliminated by sterile gauze or cotton. Better yet, the assistant can prepare the syringe for the injection. The author knows of one dentist with severe procaine dermatitis who used monocaine hydrochloride without difficulty. Substitution of monocaine for procaine may be a simple and effective solution to procaine dermatitis.

Formalin-containing cold sterilizing solutions are more frequently the cause of dermatitis in dentists than procaine. Many of the commercial cold sterilizing solutions contain this substance, which may be so effectively masked that the odor is not recognizable. The dermatitis is likely to develop if the instruments are removed with the fingers (a poor practice), or if the sterilization solution is not washed off thoroughly before the instruments are used.

Formalin dermatitis has the same general distribution as that due to procaine. Formalin has a marked hardening and drying effect on the tissues, which result in the development of deep, painful cracks or fissures, especially on the tips of the fingers. Once the cause of the condition is recognized, the treatment is obvious.

Any of the medicaments used in dental practice may give rise to dermatitis in sensitive individuals. The aromatic oils such as eugenol and eucalyptol, phenol, creosote or their derivatives, proprietary drugs (if used), iodine-containing preparations, mercury and acrylic materials may be possible causes of dermatitis in dentists. Moody experienced a severe reaction due to the acrylic monomer which was used in processing a denture. It requires real detective work at times to determine the agent responsible for the dermatitis.

One other cause for dermatitis in dentists should be mentioned. Sensitivity to soaps as a cause of dermatitis is not generally appreciated by the dentist. The frequent washing of the hands, which is so necessary in dental practice, affords a ready opportunity for the development and continuation of the dermatitis. One young dentist was treated, more or less symptomatically, for more than a year for dermatitis of the hands, which finally prevented practice. The dermatitis cleared up within 3 weeks, when a non-saponifying cleansing agent was used. This dentist had been patch-tested with the medicaments used in his office, but the hand soap had been omitted. Numerous similar cases have been observed.

The author urges again that the dentist with dermatitis consult early a competent dermatologist for advice and treatment, rather than follow personal experimentation in treatment or that of his well-wishing friends.

Certain specific diseases may be acquired by the dentist during the performance of his professional services. Upper respiratory infections and tuberculosis have already been alluded to. When working on a case of "open" tuberculosis, the dentist should wear an efficient mask. The individual with undiagnosed tuberculosis is the more dangerous patient. A medical summary of each case prior to treatment will afford some protection against unknowingly treating such patients.

ACCIDENTALLY ACQUIRED SYPHILITIC INFECTIONS

Accidental syphilitic infections are fortunately uncommon, but when they arise they represent a serious personal and professional problem.

There are numerous instances where the dentist, or the physician, has acquired syphilis "innocently" during the performance of his professional services. It has been said that the incidence of *syphilis insontium* is higher in dentists than in any other professional group.

In some series of cases 35% of all chancre of the fingers occurred in dentists. Appleton and Salzmann reported 31 cases of syphilis which were acquired accidentally by dentists and an additional case acquired by a hygienist. In 18, data were given as to the site and location of the primary lesion. It was found that 15 developed the chancre on the left hand, particularly on the tips of the fingers. When one considers the frequent use of the left hand for retracting the cheek tissues and for holding the mouth mirror during operative procedures the more common occurrence on the left hand is easily understood. Dentists have also been infected by holding instruments between their teeth, by scratches from a jagged tooth or dental instruments. The lesions which develop are usually less painful than those due to a pyogenic infection and they are accompanied by adenopathy at the elbow or the axilla.

Leifer treated 2 cases of professionally acquired syphilis in dentists. The initial lesion in both patients developed on the nail fold of the left index finger. The lesions, which were initially diagnosed as paronychiae, were fortunately soon interpreted correctly and effective treatment was instituted with a satisfactory result. This author believed that paronychia in dentists should be considered as possible luetic infection until proven otherwise.

In the past, dentists have neglected to examine routinely the oral cavity for lesions which might arouse a suspicion of syphilis. If these lesions are not identified etiologically, other patients, one's professional associates and even members of the dentist's family may be innocently infected. It is recognized that it is impractical and impossible to have a serologic test for syphilis made on every patient seeking dental treatment because of the social and moral implications involved. However, the possibility of a professionally acquired syphilitic infection can be greatly minimized by a careful oral examination, a knowledge of the usual site of development and the clinical manifestations of the oral luetic lesions. Contrary to common opinion, the dentist runs a risk of infection even in the absence of demonstrable lesions if the patient has early syphilis in which a spirochetemia is present.

Dental care should not be withheld in luetics, as the elimination of oral foci of infection as well as the maintenance of optimum oral hygiene is particularly important in the treatment of the syphilis.

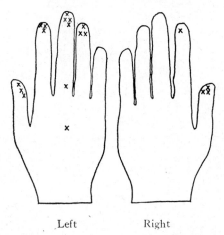

Left   Right

FIG. 268. Relative frequency of location of points of entry, palmar view. (Salzmann and Appleton, N. Y. Jour. Dent., 2:269-76, 1925.)

Appleton and Salzmann recommended the following preventive measures against the accidental contraction of syphilis.

(1) The dentist must be more suspicious of all mouth lesions and should become familiar with the clinical appearance of the oral manifestations of syphilis. If the presence of syphilitic lesions is suspected, it is well to consult with the patient's physician.

(2) The mouth should be examined under a good light with care. With the mouth closed, the lips should be examined. With the teeth occluded but the lips apart, examine the inner surfaces of the lips, commissures, and buccal mucosa. Have patient extend the tongue as far as possible, move it from side to side, and try to moisten the upper lip; this affords an opportunity for thorough examination. With the tongue drawn back, inspect the fauces, tonsils, nasopharynx, palate and uvula.

(3) It is important for the dentist to keep the skin of his hands intact. Those subject to novocaine dermatitis with its attendant fissuring of the finger-tips should wear gloves when administering this anesthetic.

(4) Wear rubber gloves when working on a known syphilitic. Oral surgeons should insist on serologic tests for syphilis in patients on whom they are about to perform extensive surgical operations.

(5) Needle pricks received while working on a known syphilitic may be laid open and 33.33% mercurous chloride rubbed in. This should be done immediately after the needle wound is received, otherwise this and similar prophylactic measures are of no avail and merely lead to a false sense of security. A serologic test of the operator should be taken weekly for at least 6 weeks following the wound, and monthly thereafter for at least a year.

(6) Indolent sores on the fingers, especially if indurated and if there is enlargement of the lymph nodes draining the area, should be investigated to rule out syphilis.

(7) If a cut is received while working on a patient, an antiseptic should be applied immediately. If suspicious of syphilis in the patient, calomel ointment should be rubbed on the hands before operating and if a wound is received, the operator should immediately place himself under the care of a syphilologist.

Some of these recommendations seem somewhat strict for the patient who is receiving luetic treatment, since it is extremely difficult to perform efficiently many of the dental operative procedures while wearing rubber gloves.

On rare occasions, it may be necessary to give emergency dental treatment to a syphilitic patient who has not received intensive treatment. Rubber gloves should be worn and all possible precautions taken to preclude the possibility of acquiring the infection. The use of calomel ointment before putting on the rubber gloves is an additional protective measure in case the gloves should become perforated. A thick soapy lather which is allowed to dry on the hands is also a good protective measure. The hands should *not* be scrubbed with a brush prior to or following working on such patients. Scrubbing may produce minute abrasions which serve as portals of entry for *Treponema pallidum*.

Following 3 or more injections of arsphenamine or at least 1 course of treatment, the luetic patient can be generally considered non-infectious, at least for oral operations. Patients who have bismuth pigmentation of the gums are usually non-infectious.

If any suspicious lesions should develop upon the hands of the dentist, particularly the left, he should immediately consult an experienced dermatologist. This is a protection to the dentist, his patients and his family. If the lesion is nonspecific, it will avoid needless worry and, if a syphilitic infection has been acquired, it will enable early treatment when the results are most successful.

28

Industrial Dentistry and Oral Manifestations of Occupational Origin

The detrimental effects of mouth infection, as they relate to the industrial health problem, were recognized more than 25 years ago, but the important contributions of industrial dentistry to the general industrial health program have been appreciated only in recent years. This has been evidenced by an increased emphasis on mouth health and by the establishment of industrial low-cost complete dental service clinics for the worker. In addition to the industrial dental clinic's responsibility for the diagnosis and treatment of dental diseases, it has efficiently cared for traumatic surgical conditions of the mouth and jaws. The health education functions of the industrial dental service deserve special mention.

A comprehensive industrial dental service benefits not only the worker but also industry. Fisher, Goldhorn and Hooper believe that oral sepsis is a major, if not the major, underlying cause of a large proportion of employee absenteeism. The relation of oral foci of infection to the various degenerative diseases has been discussed elsewhere. Good oral health has been shown to minimize the complications arising from nondental injuries.

In former years, the loss of teeth was not considered a compensatable item because it was possible to supply adequate substitutes. Compensation was granted only when the jaw was injured to such an extent that teeth could not be supplied. Schour and Sarnat quoted a recent decision of the Wisconsin State Industrial Commission in which an employer was ordered to pay an upholsterer for restorations which were required to correct a dental disability resulting from holding tacks in the mouth.

ORAL MANIFESTATIONS OF OCCUPATIONAL ORIGIN

Schour and Sarnat and Salzmann made extensive studies of the oral manifestations of occupational origin. The reader is referred to these authors for a more complete discussion of the subject.

Occupational diseases of the teeth and oral structures can be conveniently grouped into (1) those which are due to direct action of the occupational causative agent on the oral structures and (2) those in which the oral structures are affected as a part of a systemic disturbance. In a few instances, the typical and characteristic symptoms of an occupational disease are manifested in the mouth, but for the most part the oral changes are of secondary importance. Poor oral hygiene renders the oral tissues particularly vulnerable to many of the diseases of occupational origin. The rôle of good oral hygiene in preventing the development of the more common oral manifestations of occupational origin deserves special emphasis.

The oral manifestations of occupational diseases can be grouped according to their local or systemic mode of production.

OCCUPATIONS RESULTING IN DIRECT DAMAGE TO THE ORAL TISSUES

Abrasive Action on Hard Tissues.
(1) Glass blowers.
(2) Cigar makers.
(3) Upholsterers, cobblers, carpenters, seamstresses.
(4) Stone cutters, sand blasters.
Corrosive or Caustic Action on Hard and/or Soft Oral Tissues.
(1) Acid fumes.
    Welders.
    Manufacturers of acids.
    Storage battery workers.
    Chrome platers.
(2) Cement workers—alkalies.
(3) Chemical workers—chemists.
Increased Incidence of Dental Decay.
(1) Bakers, millers.
(2) Candy makers.

OCCUPATIONS RESULTING IN DAMAGE TO THE ORAL TISSUES THROUGH SYSTEMIC ABSORPTION

Absorption of Metals.
    Radium.
    Mercury.
    Lead.
    Bismuth.
Absorption of Non-metallic Substances.
    Phosphorus.
    Fluorine.
Absorption of Organic Substances.
    Benzene compounds—blood dyscrasias.
    Aniline compounds.

OCCUPATIONS CAUSING ABRASION OF THE HARD DENTAL TISSUES

Numerous trades result commonly in abnormal tooth wear. While much of the present-day glass industry is mechanized, skilled glass-blowers are still widely employed. The contact and rotation of the blow pipe against the teeth, usually the second incisors and canines, result in abrasion of the edges of these teeth. The dental deformity is similar to that occurring in clay-pipe smokers, except that it is circular rather than oval in form. Glass-blowers experience at times a pneumatocele of the parotid gland due to the high intra-oral pressure which is required for blowing large objects. The pain and discomfort disappear gradually if no more air is forced into the gland. It is the common, although unhygienic, habit of cigar wrappers to trim

ORAL MANIFESTATIONS OF OCCUPATIONAL DISEASE
ACCORDING TO OCCUPATION.

Occupation	Active Agent	Possible Oral Manifestation
Abrasive Powder Workers	Dust	Generalized Abrasion of Teeth Calculus
Acid Dippers	Fumes	Decalcification of Teeth Stomatitis
Arsenic Roasters and Handlers	Arsenic	Osteomyelitis and Necrosis of Mandible
Aviators	Variation in Atmospheric Pressure	Hemorrhage from Gums
Bakery Workers	Flour, Sugar	Calculus-Periodontitis Caries
Candy Workers	Sugar	Caries
Carpenters	Nails	Localized Abrasion
Coal Tar Contacts	Tar	Malignancy
Cryolite Workers	Fluorine	Osteosclerosis
Electrotypers	Lead	Lead Line - Gums
Explosive Workers	Benzol	Hemorrhage from Gums
Garment Workers	Chemicals - Dyes, Foreign Bodies in Mouth	Stomatitis Abrasion of Teeth
Glass Workers	Hydrofluoric Acid, Increased Intraoral Pressure	Decalcification Pneumatocoele -Abrasion
Lead Workers	Lead	Lead Line-Gums
Metal Workers	Dust (Iron, Copper, Chromium, etc.)	Staining of Enamel. Pigmentation of Oral Mucosa
Mercury Workers	Mercurial Compounds	Gingivitis, Periodontitis, Ulcerations, Ptyalism, Osteomyelitis
Photographic Workers	Mercurial Compounds, Chromium	Gingivitis
Polishers and Blasters	Dusts	Abrasion Pigmentation
Stoneworkers	Dusts	Abrasion Gingivitis
X-Ray Technicians	X-Ray (Radium)	Xerostomia

LOCAL ORIGIN

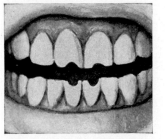

Abrasion—Nails

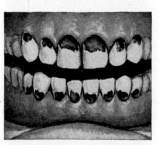

Caries—Sugar

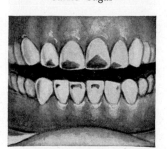

Decalcification—Acids

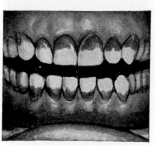

Staining—Metals

Oral Manifestations of Occupational Diseases
MODE OF ACTION• STRUCTURES AFFECTED •ETIOLOGIC AGENTS

			POSSIBLE ORAL MANIFESTATIONS
LOCAL	TOOTH	ENAMEL AND DENTIN	DUSTS / DUSTS / PREHENSION OF INSTRUMENTS / ACIDS / SUGAR
	SUPPORTING STRUCTURES	GUMS AND GINGIVAE	DUSTS / DUSTS
		PERIODONTAL MEMBRANE	VARIATIONS IN ATMOSPHERIC PRESSURE / ACIDS / DUSTS
		ALVEOLAR BONE AND JAWS	As-Cr-Hg-P-Ra / FLUORINE
SYSTEMIC	ORAL CAVITY	LIPS	LOW HUMIDITY / ANILINE
		ORAL MUCOSA	TAR / DUSTS / CHEMICALS
		TONGUE	FOOD TASTERS
		SALIVARY GLANDS	MERCURY COMPOUNDS / X-RAY / RADIUM / INCREASED INTRA ORAL PRESSURE

MERCURY COMPOUNDS / HEAVY METAL / MERCURY COMPOUNDS / FLOU / CARBON MO

	POSSIBLE ORAL MANIFESTATIONS
...TERS· METAL REFINERS · INSECTICIDE MAKERS	NECROSIS OF BONE.
...POWDER MAKERS	BLUE PIGMENTATION OF GUMS & ORAL MUCOSA · GINGIVOSTOMATITIS
...TERS SMITHS	GREEN STAINING OF TEETH· PIGMENTATION OF GINGIVAE · GINGIVOSTOMATITIS
...UE PRINTERS· CHROME WORK...ER MIXERS· STEEL WORKERS	ORANGE STAINING OF TEETH · NECROSIS OF BONE · ULCERATION OF ORAL TISSUES. OSTEOSCLEROSIS
...ERS· LEAD REFINERS· PRINT-...RAGE BATTERY MAKERS· ...Y MAKERS· DETONATOR -...RY SALTS WORKERS· PAINT MIXERS.	BLUE BLACK PIGMENTATION OF GINGIVAE · GINGIVOSTOMATITIS GINGIVOSTOMATITIS · OSTEOMYELITIS SALIVATION.
...ERS· FIREWORKS MAKERS· ...SPHOR-BRONZE WORKERS.	GINGIVOSTOMATITIS·ULCERATION OF ORAL TISSUES OSTEOMYELITIS
...ANS. ETC.	GINGIVITIS· PERIODON TITIS OSTEOMYELITIS
...ROLEUM REFINERS ...RS· GALVANIZERS	BLEEDING STOMATITIS DECALCIFICATION OF ENAMEL & DENTIN
...PHOSGENE MAKERS· SUGAR-...INFECTANT, LAUNDRY WORKERS.	STOMATITIS
...S ELECTROTYPERS·...STONE CUTTERS.	STAINING· ABRASIVE · GINGIVITIS BLEEDING · CALCULUS.
...AWMILL, TEXTILE AND...ERS.	STAINING· ABRASIVE · GINGIVITIS BLEEDING · CALCULUS.
...E WORKERS· PAINTERS·...LCANIZERS.	BLUE COLORATION OF LIPS · AND GINGIVAE.
...KERS· SOAP MAKERS·...SH BOILERS.	STOMATITIS.
...SHELLAC WORKERS·...OWDER WORKERS.	STOMATITIS.
...ANERS· LACQUER WORKERS·...POWDER MAKERS	HEMORRHAGE FROM GUMS· STOMATITIS BLUE COLORATION OF LIPS.
...T MAKERS· RUBBER WORKERS·...ICAL DRESSING WORKERS.	STOMATITIS.
...RKERS· FISHERMEN·...D PRESERVERS.	STOMATITIS · MALIGNANCIES OF LIPS AND MUCOSA
...MAKERS.	CARIES
	CALCULUS · PERIODONTITIS
	ANESTHESIA & PARESTHESIA OF TONGUE
...LASS BLOWERS·...SEAMSTRESSES	ABRASION.
CAISSON WORKERS	BLEEDING FROM GUMS.
...RS	BLEEDING FROM GUMS.
...INTERS· RESEARCH MEN	GINGIVITIS· PERIODON TITIS · OSTEOMYELITIS & NECROSIS· XEROSTOMIA

PRINTED IN U. S. A.   "DENTISTRY, A DIGEST OF PRACTICE," SCHOUR AND SARNAT, DECEMBER, 1942,

FIG. 269.

roughly the ends of the cigars with their teeth. This repetitious act, performed on a material which contains fine abrasives, results in abnormal wear of the incisors.

Carpenters, roofers, upholsterers and cobblers customarily hold nails or tacks in their mouths and pass them between their teeth and lips with their tongue as they are required. Over a period of years abnormal tooth wear occurs. Occupational habits of this nature not only produce objectionable abrasion of the teeth but also periodontal disturbances which may result in loss of the involved teeth.

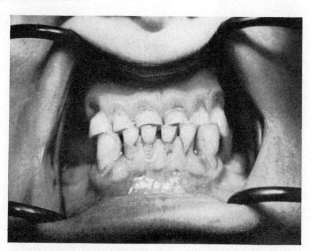

Fig. 270. Marked abrasion of the anterior teeth in a cigar maker who performed the rough trimming of the ends of the cigar by biting. Also note the cervical notching of the teeth due to an incorrect method of tooth brushing.

Tailors and seamstresses who are in the habit of cutting their thread with their teeth may show a characteristic tooth defect which consists of sharp "V"-shaped notches in the middle of the incisal edge of the incisors. The notching is most prominent in the upper incisors. This tooth defect develops at times first on one pair of incisors. When it is no longer possible to cut the thread because of the loss of tooth structure, then the teeth on the opposite side of the jaw are utilized.

Stone-cutters, sand-blasters, quarrymen and workmen in an atmosphere of abrasive dusts may show abnormal wear of the morsal surfaces of the teeth. These workmen are commonly heavy tobacco chewers, which may also account for the abnormal tooth wear.

The author has seen several cases of abnormal tooth wear and severe periodontal disturbances occurring in metal pattern makers and galvanized iron workers due to the habit these workmen have of holding the heavy blue marking chalk between their anterior teeth. Several "beauticians" have also been treated who, no doubt without their customers' knowledge, have held hair pins and bobby pins in their teeth. Over a long period of time this habit has resulted in abnormal wear of the incisal edges of the teeth.

A

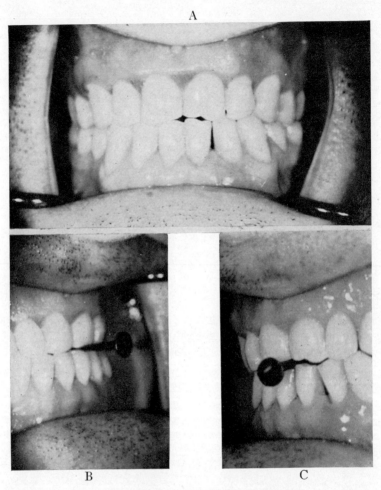

B   C

Fig. 271. (A) Occupational notching of the incisors in an up-holsterer caused by holding tacks in the mouth. There was considerable osseous destruction about these teeth. (B) Original manner of holding tacks. When the left first incisors became so worn that the tacks could not be held satisfactorily the upholsterer started holding them between all four first incisors as in (C).

Metal galvanizers may develop constitutional symptoms due to the absorption of zinc. In mild cases, these consist of a low-grade fever and chills—the "zinc shakes." The more severe constitutional reactions resemble those of an acute anaphylactic reaction. Individuals exposed to metal galvanizing fumes develop at times a chronic marginal gingivitis which is characterized by a purplish-red edematous appearance. Ulceration is not a prominent feature. This type of gingivitis is resistant to the usual forms of treatment. The author has not had the opportunity to make gingival biopsy studies, but it is probable that the pathologic process is similar to that present in bismuth stomatitis, except that no discoloration of the gum margin is produced by the white zinc sulfide.

Occupations Causing Oral Lesions Due to Corrosive or Caustic Agents

Many corrosive and caustic agents can produce undesirable changes in both the hard and soft dental tissues. In most instances, the occupational dental

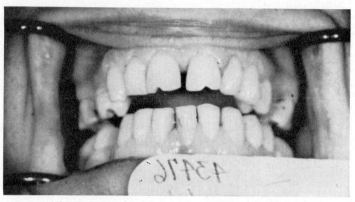

Fig. 272. Occupational notching of the maxillary first incisors in a seamstress caused by biting threads with her teeth. When the left first incisors could no longer be used for this purpose the patient began using the maxillary right first incisors.

hazard is recognized and preventive measures are known, but due to negligence or indifference, the workmen do not avail themselves of these measures. In acid-manufacturing plants, commercial metal plating establishments and storage battery repair shops, the continued exposure to the acid-containing droplets of moisture may result in discoloration, etching and at times decalcification of the teeth. In the case of chrome platers, the chrome salts are especially irritating to the mucosae. If respirators are not worn, indolent perforating ulcers of the nasal septum, lips and oral mucosa are likely to develop. Reed & Harcourt found that blond and red-haired individuals were more susceptible than brunettes to the action of chrome compounds.

A characteristic gingivostomatitis has been observed in welders, particularly electric arc welders. This type of stomatitis has many of the clinical features of fusospirochetal infection. Pain and ulceration of the marginal and interdental gum areas are prominent symptoms. In addition, the alveolar gum and to some extent the cheek mucosa have a white cauterized appearance with a tendency to slough. This type of gingivostomatitis does not respond satisfactorily to the usual treatment for fusospirochetal stomatitis or any other local treatment unless the fumes associated with the welding operation are prevented from coming in contact with the oral tissues. This can be accomplished by wearing a welding hood and by keeping the lips closed.

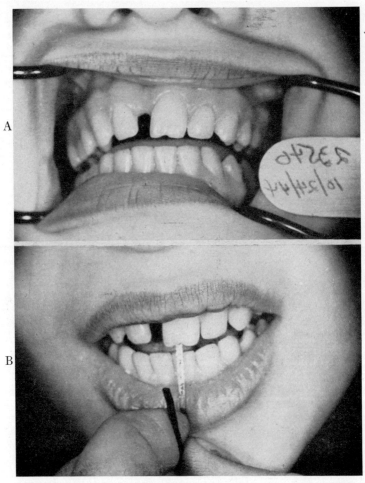

FIG. 273. (A) A hairdresser with a congenitally missing upper right first incisor and an incisal edge defect of the upper left first incisor. The notching of the upper left first incisor resulted from the habit of opening bobby pins with her teeth. (B) Method which was employed in opening the bobby pins. The loss of tooth substance on the palatal surface was greater than that on the incisal edge.

The metallic oxides arising from the surface coating of the metals being welded and the acid substances (fluxes) contained in the welding rods which are volatized during the welding process, appear to be the irritating agents. According to Johnstone the nitrogen peroxides which are produced during the welding operation are also irritating to the mucosae. Lead or zinc plated or painted metals or alloys containing these elements, may be oxidized during the welding or cutting operation. If sufficient lead or zinc absorption occurs, plumbism or symptoms of zinc toxicity will develop.

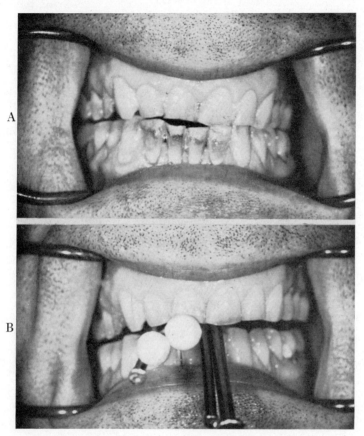

Fig. 274. (A) Occupational wear of anterior teeth in a carpenter caused by holding nails in his mouth. (B) Manner in which teeth were used to hold nails.

Strong alkalies have an irritating action on the oral mucosa. Cement workers commonly experience a dermatitis and inflammation of the oral mucosa because of the alkaline nature of cement dust. A workman in a caustic potash manufacturing plant was recently treated. He had a dark brown adherent coating on the lips, which resulted from the contact of the moist mucosal surfaces with caustic potash containing dust. These lip lesions and a mild conjunctivitis are regularly experienced by the workers in this particular stage of caustic potash manufacturing.

Chemists occasionally experience a gingivostomatitis from the exposure to fumes or chemicals which accidentally or intentionally come into contact with the oral tissues. A persistent, low-grade gingivostomatitis which is more marked in the anterior part of the mouth may be the only change that is present.

Occupations Associated with an Increased Incidence of Dental Decay

An increased incidence of dental decay is a common occurrence in individuals engaged in certain occupations. Flour millers, bakers and candy makers have a high caries experience. Flour millers and bakers have an unusually high incidence of cervical decay which is believed due to the accumulation of flour dust at this region. The flour dust-mucin plaques furnish a favorable site for bacterial growth and acid production. The increased dental decay noted in candy makers is believed due to the habit they have of sampling their products. There is a close relationship between the consumption of highly refined carbohydrates, such as candy, and the incidence of dental decay.

Occupations Causing Oral Lesions Due to Systemic Absorption of Metallic and Non-metallic Substances and of Toxic Organic Compounds

The oral manifestations resulting from occupational absorption of metals or their compounds constitute an important group of dental diseases of occupational derivation. The bone, joint and oral lesions associated with exposure to radium-containing compounds were at one time a serious occupational problem. Workers who painted watch dials with radium-containing luminous paints frequently developed radium osteonecrosis of the jaws. The jaw necrosis and severe anemia occurred 4 to 6 years after the initial symptoms. It was originally believed that the jaw lesions were due to the local effect of the radio-active substance (from pointing the paint brushes in the mouth), but it was later shown that the destructive process occurs in other bones. Osteosarcomas developed sometimes in individuals with radium osteonecrosis.

Occupational exposure to lead and mercury may result in the oral symptoms discussed in the chapter devoted to the metallic stomatitides. Metallic stomatitis of occupational origin is uncommon because of better appreciation of the occupational hazards and more knowledge about effective preventive measures. The individual worker and those in small manufacturing establishments are more likely to develop these occupational diseases. Reed and Harcourt reported a general reddish-brown discoloration of the oral mucosa in cases of mercurialism.

There are 2 important dental diseases of occupational origin due to the non-metallic elements phosphorus and fluorine. Phosphorus (yellow) necrosis of the jaws is uncommon now, but at one time it was an important occupational disease. Phosphorus is used in the alloying of certain metals and in the manufacture of fire works. Phosphorus poisoning was originally believed to affect only the jaws, rendering them more susceptible to pyogenic infection and to the development of periostitis of the mandible and massive necrosis of the jaw bones. Phosphorus necrosis was especially serious since the tissues would suppurate again even after resection of the involved area. Red phosphorus is not important as an occupational hazard.

Fluorine intoxication is recognized as an occupational hazard. Art glass workers, dyers, etchers, workers in insecticide and fertilizer plants are exposed to fluorine as an occupational hazard. The waste gases and dusts from aluminum factories contain a high concentration of fluorine.

Johnstone described mottling of the teeth in chronic fluorosis of occupational derivation but, considering our knowledge of mottled enamel, this is difficult to understand unless the individual was exposed at an unusually early age or to an unusually high concentration of fluorides.

Exposure to high concentrations of fluorine in the adult cannot cause mottled enamel. A child nursed by a woman working in a cryolite decomposing factory is reported to have had dental fluorosis, although the water supply did not contain significant amounts of this element. Individuals with fluorine intoxication complain of gastric disturbances, stiffness and indefinite rheumatic pains. X-ray examinations reveal sclerotic changes in the bones in four-fifths of the cases with particular involvement of the spinal column and pelvis.

Many organic substances, particularly those derived from, or closely related to, benzol or the benzene ring may result in severe oral lesions as a part of a generalized reaction. Dryness of the oral mucosa, with bleeding from the gums, is typical of benzene poisoning. Severe ulcerative lesions of the gums and oral tissues develop at times in an aplastic anemia, secondary to occupational exposure to this substance and many other organic compounds.

The author has seen several patients with a persistent chronic gingivitis who were employed in a particular operation in a patented dry-cleaning process. It was impossible to learn the exact organic compound used in this stage of the dry-cleaning process but it was generally known that the employees in this operation had "inflamed gums."

REFERENCES

FOCAL INFECTION

Appleton, J. L. T.: Statistical contribution to the problem of focal infection, Dent. Cosmos, 66:739, 1924.

Arnett, J. H., & L. M. Ennis: Dental infection and systemic disease, Am. J. Med. Sc., 185:777, 1933.

Austin, L. T., & T. J. Cook: Bacteriologic study of normal vital teeth, J. A. D. A., 16:894, 1929.

Balding, Grant: Relation of teeth to inflammation of the eyes, Northwest Med., 41:100, 1942.

Beretta, A.: Mikrobenlokalisation in der Zahnpulpa auf dem Wege der Blutbahn, Centralbl. f. Bakteriol., 76:124, 1915.

Berwick, C. C.: The bacteriology of periodontal tissues radiographically suggesting infection, J. Infect. Dis., 29:537, 1921.

Billings, Frank: Chronic focal infections and their etiological relations to arthritis and nephritis, Arch. Int. Med., 9:484, 1912.

Blayney, J. R.: Present-day evaluation of the pulpless tooth, J. A. D. A., 23:533, 1936.

Brown, J. B.: Types of chronic infection about mouth, Internat. J. Orthodontia, 19:59, 1933.

Bulleid, A.: Bacteriology of apical infection, Brit. Dent. J., 49:855, 1928.

Burket, Lester W.: Studies of apices of teeth. Correlation of bacteriological, roentgenological, and gross anatomical findings in human necropsies, Yale J. Biol. & Med., 9:271, 1937. Part II. Ibid., 9:287, 1937.

Burket, Lester W.: Recent studies in relation to periapical infection, including data obtained from human necropsy studies, J. A. D. A. & Dent. Cosmos, 25:260, 1938.

Cecil, R. L., & D. M. Angevine: Clinical and experimental observations on focal infection, with an analysis of 200 cases of rheumatoid arthritis, Ann. Int. Med., 12:577, 1938.

Clagett, H. Henry: The relation of oral infections to the circulatory system, Mil. Surgeon, 88:662, 1941.

Clagett, A. H., & E. H. Smith, Jr.: Subacute bacterial endocarditis and dental extraction, J. A. D. A., 28:1841, 1941.

Cole, G. H.: Tic douloureux: report of case, J. A. D. A., 18:2402, 1931.

Cook, T. J.: Dental granuloma, J. A. D. A., 14:2231, 1927.

Cook, T. J.: Statistics obtained by clinical and roentgenologic examinations of 500 edentulous and partially edentulous mouths, Dental Cosmos, 69:349, 1927.

Corriell, L. D.: Dental trocar, Dental Cosmos, 60:1154, 1919.

Cotton, H. A.: Relation of oral infection to mental diseases, J. Dent. Research, 1:269, 1919.

Darlington, C. G.: Dental foci of infection, New York Acad. Med., 17:618, 1941.

Editorial: Dental lesions and systemic disease, J. A. M. A., 109:211, 1937.

Ellingham, G. H.: Bacteriological investigation into some filled teeth, Brit. Dent. J., 58:108, 1935.

Elliot, S. D.: Bacteremia and oral sepsis, Proc. Roy. Soc. Med., 32:747, 1939.

Fralkis, N. F.: Cardiac disease—focal infection, Ohio Med. J., 37:1045, 1941.

Frankel, L. K.: Consideration of evidences on oral sepsis in relation to systemic disease, Dental Cosmos, 66:35, 1924.

Fuendeling, M. J., & T. L. Cartney: The roentgenographic diagnosis of vital pulp infection as confirmed by bacteriologic examination, Am. J. Roentgenol., 40:386, 1938.

Genvert, H., H. Miller, & C. G. Burns: Experimental production of apical lesions of teeth in monkeys and their relation to systemic disease, Yale J. Biol. & Med., 13:649, 1941.

Goldberg, H. A.: Prostatitis and multiple arthritis of dental origin, J. A. D. A., 30:1378, 1943.

Grace, J. D.: Extensive alopecia areata of dental origin; evidence that isolated areas of alopecia may be due to ipsilateral foci of infection, Arch. Dermat. & Syph., 45:349-52, 1942.

Gross, E. R.: Flare up of sycosis vulgaris, possibly referable to the extraction of teeth, Arch. Dermat. & Syph., 39:938, 1939.

Grossman, L. I.: Apicostomy: method to obtain cultures from the periapical tissues, J. Dent. Research, 12:595, 1932.

Grossman, L. I.: Changing concept regarding pulpless teeth, J. A. D. A., 24:1928, 1934.

Grossman, L. I.: The present status of the pulpless tooth, Ann. Int. Med., 13:1805, 1940.

Gutzeit, K., & W. Kuchlin: Short wave provocative method in diagnosis of dental infection, Munchen. med. Wchnschr., 84:961, 1937.

Haden, R. L.: Radiographic diagnosis of periapical dental infection in light of bacteriologic findings, Dental Cosmos, 67:380, 1925.

Hatton, E. H.: Evaluation of the theory of focal infection, J. A. D. A., 21-A:463, 1934.

Hatton, E. H., et al.: Comparison of xray, transillumination and bacteriologic examinations of pulpless and infected teeth, J. A. D. A., 23:190, 1936.

Hunter, W.: Oral sepsis as a cause of disease, Brit. M. J., 2:215, 1900.

Jones, N. W., & S. J. Newsom: Experimentally produced focal (dental) infection in relation to cardiac structure, Arch. Path., 13:392, 1932.

Kauffer, H. J.: A consideration of the pulpless tooth in focal infection, Dental Cosmos, 68:544-49, 1926.

Kirby, D. B.: Dental infection and the eye, Ann. Dent., 6:65, 1939.

Kolmer, John A.: The cooperative management of focal infection of dental origin, Dental Cosmos, 78:403, 1936.

Levinthal, D. H.: Oral sepsis and its relation to orthopedic conditions, J. A. D. A., 24:1618, 1937.

Lintz, Wm.: Focal infection in dentistry and its relation to general medicine, Dent. Items of Interest, 64:1079, 1942.

Main, L. R.: Nerve reflex disturbances of dental origin, J. A. D. A., 20:877, 1933.

Marquez, H. G.: Studies of the blood picture in paradental infections, J. A. D. A. & Dent. Cosmos, 24:691, 1937.

Matis, E. I.: Two unusual cases of postanginal sepsis, Ann. Otol. Rhin. Laryng., 49:559-63, 1940.

Mentzer, W. E., & E. L. Tuohy: An attempt to unify and harmonize points of view of medical and dental professions toward the constitutional influence of dental pathology, Minn. Med., 4:305, 1921.

Meyer, Otto: Focal infection and idiopathic epilepsy, Dent. Digest, 49:396, 1943.

Molt, F. F.: Value of roentgenogram in edentulous mouths, J. A. D. A., 12:788, 1925.

Morgenroth, E.: Methods and evaluation of blood sedimentation test in stomatogenic infection, Deut. Zahn. Wchnschr., 41:1137, 1938.

Murphy, F. D.: Heart disease and circulatory disturbances in dental practice, Jour. Wisconsin State Dent. Soc., 17:163, 1941.

Nisenson, A.: An appraisal of the advantage of teeth extraction in arthritis, Med. Bull. Vet. Admin., 18:57, 1941.

Northrop, P. M., & M. C. Crowley: Further studies on the effect of the prophylactic use of sulfathiazole and sulfamerazine on bacteremia following extraction of teeth, J. Oral Surg., 2:134, 1944.

Okell, C. C., & S. D. Elliott: Bacteremia and oral sepsis with special reference to the aetiology of subacute bacterial endocarditis, Lancet, 2:869, 1935.

Oveido, G. F.: Paradental infections as related to prostatic infection: a preliminary report, J. A. D. A. & Dental Cosmos, 24:696, 1937.

Paquin, O.: Bacteremia following the removal of diseased teeth, J. A. D. A., 28:879, 1941.
Piperno, A.: Anisocoria of dental origin, J. A. D. A., 21:1459, 1934.
Post, W. E.: Oral infection in relation to systemic disease, J. A. D. A., 21:623, 1934.
Price, W. A.: Dental infections, oral and systemic. Vol. 1. Cleveland: Penton Publishing Co., 1923.
Queries and Minor Notes: Reduction in visual field for green not sign of focal infection, J. A. M. A., 111:1870, 1938.
Rabkin, A.: Current reactions to the concept of focal infection, Cinn. J. Med., 22:510, 1942.
Rault, C. V.: Value of routine blood sedimentation tests in dental patients, Northwest. Univ. Bull. Dent. Research, 39:9, 1938.
Reimann, Hobart A., & W. P. Havens: Focal infection and systemic disease: critical appraisal, J. A. M. A., 114:1, 1940.
Richards, John H.: Bacteremia following irritation of foci of infection, J. A. M. A., 99:1496, 1932.
Robinson, H. B. G., & L. R. Boling: Anachoric effect in pulpitis, J. A. D. A., 28:268, 1941.
Roper-Hall, H. T.: Oral sepsis in relation to ophthalmology, Dent. Gaz., 8:389, 1942.
Rosenow, E. C., & J. G. Meisser: The production of urinary calculi by the devitalization and infection of teeth in dogs with streptococci from cases of nephrolithiasis, Arch. Int. Med., 31:807, 1923.
Schurr, E. G.: Association between ocular disease and oral sepsis, Brit. Dent. Jour., 52:333, 1931.
Seybold, J. W.: Pulp stones and devitalized and impacted teeth as factor in systemic disease, J. A. D. A., 26:1627, 1939.
Solis-Cohen, Myer: The relation of dental to other foci of infection, Dent. Cosmos, 78:573, 1936.
Sprague, C. H.: Hemorrhage in pulmonary tuberculosis—focal infection as primary cause, Northwest Med., 38:475, 1939.
Stiles, M. H., et al.: Attempts to better results with bacterial antigen ("vaccine") therapy of low grade chronic ("focal") infection, J. Lab. & Clin. Med., 28:1447, 1943.
Sweet, A. Porter: The edentulous mouth and focal infections, J. A. D. A. & Dental Cosmos, 24:546, 1937.
Thoma, K. H.: Infected vital dental pulp; an important focus of systemic disease, J. Dent. Research, 8:529, 1928.
Tichy, F. S.: Iridocyclitis apparently of dental origin, report of case, J. Oral Surg., 1:265, 1943.
Waggener, D. T., & L. T. Austin: Dental structures remaining in 1,948 edentulous jaws: a statistical study, J. A. D. A., 28:1855, 1941.
Warner, George R.: The pathologic vital tooth; with report of cases, J. A. D. A., 29:1791, 1942.
Weisberger, David: Influence of hypersensitive state in experimental streptococcus viridans bacteremia, Proc. Roy. Soc. Exper. Biol. & Med., 29:445, 1932.
Weisberger, David: Relation of hypersensitivity to localization in and dissemination of streptococcus viridans from incisor teeth of rabbits, Yale J. Biol. & Med., 9:417, 1937.

Wendell, Lehman: Three pulpless teeth: a case history and a conclusion, J. A. D. A., **29**:558, 1942.

Ziskin, D. E.: Dental infections: comparative systemic effects of quantitative apical changes, J. Dent. Research, **11**:285, 1931.

ORAL PEDIATRICS AND GERODONTICS

Abramson, M., & James O. Dowrie: Sublingual granuloma in infancy (Riga-Fede's disease), J. Pediat., **24**:19, 1944.

Anderson, Manuel: Faucial and labial diphtheria, Brit. M. J., **22**:104, 1943.

Black, W. C.: Acute infectious gingivostomatitis, Am. J. Dis. Child., **56**:126, 1938.

Buddingh, C. J., & K. Dodd: Stomatitis and diarrhea of infants caused by a hitherto unrecognized virus, J. Pediat., **25**:105, 1944.

Ellis, R. C., & M. Luten: Deciduous teeth and diseases of childhood, J. A. D. A., **22**:1117, 1935.

Ellis, R. W. B.: Green teeth following icterus gravis, Brit. J. Child. Dis., **34**:85, 1942.

Fawdry, A. L.: Erythroblastic anemia of childhood in cyprus, Lancet, **1**:171, 1944.

Greenbaum, S. S.: Dermatitis diphtheritica, Am. J. Dis. Child., **28**:51, 1924.

Koplik, H.: Diagnosis of the invasion of measles, from a study of the exanthema as it appears on the buccal mucous membrane, Arch. Pediat., **13**:918, 1896.

Lavender, H. J., & J. B. Squires: Diphtheric involvement of the lips with absence of signs in the nose and throat, J. A. M. A., **111**:915, 1938.

Lowenburg, H., & E. L. Grimes: Ectodermal dysplasia of the anhydrotic type, Am. J. Dis. Child., **63**:357, 1942.

Lynch, H., & E. G. Dovey: Nasal diphtheria invading the paranasal sinuses, with curious history, Med. Bull. Vet. Admin., **20**:212, 1943.

MacFarlane, L. H.: Cancrum oris following measles, Brit. J. Child. Dis., **33**:275, 1936.

McBride, W. C.: Juvenile dentistry, Phila., Penn., Lea & Febiger, Ed. 3.

McKhann, C. F., & F. T. Chu: Antibodies in placental extracts, J. Infect. Dis., **52**:268-77, 1935.

Mumford, P. B., & A. G. Heppleston: An epidemic in children, characterized by diversity of lesions in skin and mucous membranes, probably caused by streptococcus pyogenes, Brit. J. Dermat. & Syph., **55**:143-53, 1943.

Murphy, J. P., G. S. Bozalis, & E. J. Bieri: Blood diastase in mumps, Am. J. Dis. Child., **66**:264-66, 1943.

Oxenius, K.: Diphtheria at site of erupting teeth, Deutsche med. Wchnschr., **61**:1803, 1935.

Rake, G., & M. F. Shaffer: Studies on measles; use of chorio-allantois of developing chicken embryo, J. Immunol., **38**:117-200, 1940.

Robinson, E. S., & C. F. McKhann: Immunological application of placental extracts, Am. J. Pub. Health, **25**:1353-8, 1935.

Ronaldson, G. W., & W. H. Kelleher: Palatal paralysis in extrafaucial diphtheria, Brit. M. J., **1**:1019, 1935.

Sanford, H. N., & I. Shmigelsky: Purulent parotitis in newborn, J. Pediat., **26**:149, 1945.

Stitzel, E. W.: Pediatrist's study of focal infection in children, Penn. Med. J., **35**:395-97, 1932.

Wilkins, L., & W. Fleischman: Diagnosis of hypothyroidism in childhood, J. A. M. A., **116**:2459, 1941.
Zerbino, V.: Dermatosis from eruption of dentition; three infants, Rev. med. del Uraguay, **26**:524-31, 1923.

OCCUPATIONAL DISEASES OF DENTAL PRACTICE

Astrachan, G. D.: Unsuspected syphilis, Dental Outlook, **29**:348, 1942.
Bower, R. L.: Care of the dentist's eyes, J. A. D. A., **25**:1236, 1938.
Ennis, L. M.: X-rays are still fraught with danger, Proc. D. Centenary, pp. 91-101, 1940.
Houston, Trim: Syphilis as the dentist sees it, J. A. D. A., **26**:1362, 1939.
Johnstone, R. T.: Occupational diseases, Phila., W. B. Saunders Co., 1941.
Jones, T. R., & J. A. Lockhart: Occupational disease of electric welders, Texas State J. Med., **39**:532, 1944.
Kramer, L. R.: Silicosis: a potential hazard in dental laboratories, J. A. D. A., **27**:1503, 1940.
Kulstad, H. M.: Place of dentistry in industry, California & Western Med., **62**:11, 1945.
Leifer, W.: Accidental syphilitic infection of dentists: report of two cases, J. A. D. A., **29**:435, 1942.
Lelyveld, J.: Foot care for the dentist, J. A. D. A., **24**:1900, 1937.
Note: Etched teeth in a battery repairman, New England J. Med., **223**:303, 1940.
Pfahler, G. E.: Danger of injury to dentist in roentgenography, J. A. D. A., **26**:949, 1939.
Reed, J. V., & A. K. Harcourt: The essentials of occupational diseases, C. C. Thomas, 1941.
Salzman, J. A., & J. L. T. Appleton, Jr.: Syphilis insontium: acquired by the operator during dental treatment, New York J. Dent., **2**:269-76, 1932.
Shaw, C.: Accidental inoculation with spirochaeta pallida, Arch. Dermat. & Syph., **44**:878, 1941.
Siltzbach, L. E.: The silicosis hazard in mechanical dentistry, J. A. M. A., **113**:1116, 1939.
Thompson, W. S.: Detrimental biological effects of roentgen rays, Proc. D. Centenary, pp. 86-91, 1940.

SECTION NINE

ORAL ASPECTS OF AVIATION MEDICINE

by ALVIN A. GOLDHUSH, D.D.S., M.S., Major, Dental Corps, A.U.S.

29

Introduction

HISTORICAL REVIEW
PHYSIOPATHOLOGIC FLYING DISORDERS

Flying brought a challenge to dentistry. Exposure to high altitudes sometimes causes subjective dental symptoms which are not experienced on the ground. Attention has been called to problems in periodontia, oral surgery, prosthetics, occlusion, caries and pulp pathology. These dental problems have been grouped under the subject "Aviation Dentistry," a parallel term to the well-established specialty of Aviation Medicine. Most observations on the oral aspects of aviation medicine have arisen as a result of military operations. Some problems will remain applicable only to military personnel; others, however, will affect the future flying public. When a few airmen were flying at high altitudes, their problems were of concern to a few physiologists interested in the basic principles of aviation medicine. Now, with thousands of men in military aviation and with the prospect of tremendous expansion of civilian aviation, the physical and mental reactions to flight conditions are of concern to all clinicians. An understanding of the oral phases is essential to all dentists. Flight conditions are subjecting diagnostic procedures, operating methods and dental materials to new critical tests. The dental profession must accept the challenge to deal with the problems of modern flying by assisting in conditioning the body to withstand the demands of the new environment, by offering effective corrective treatment of dental difficulties occurring in flight, and by keeping research in oral aspects of aviation medicine abreast of advances in aeronautics. This section is a summary and analysis of the observations in this new and relatively unexplored field; the general principles of the theoretical and practical aspects are expected to be modified and extended by future observations and research.

HISTORICAL REVIEW

A review of the early literature reveals few significant studies. Twenty years ago, the demands of flying on the body were limited. Aircraft were not capable of high speeds, high ceilings or rapid rates of ascent or descent. The dental studies of those days were appropriate for the flying conditions

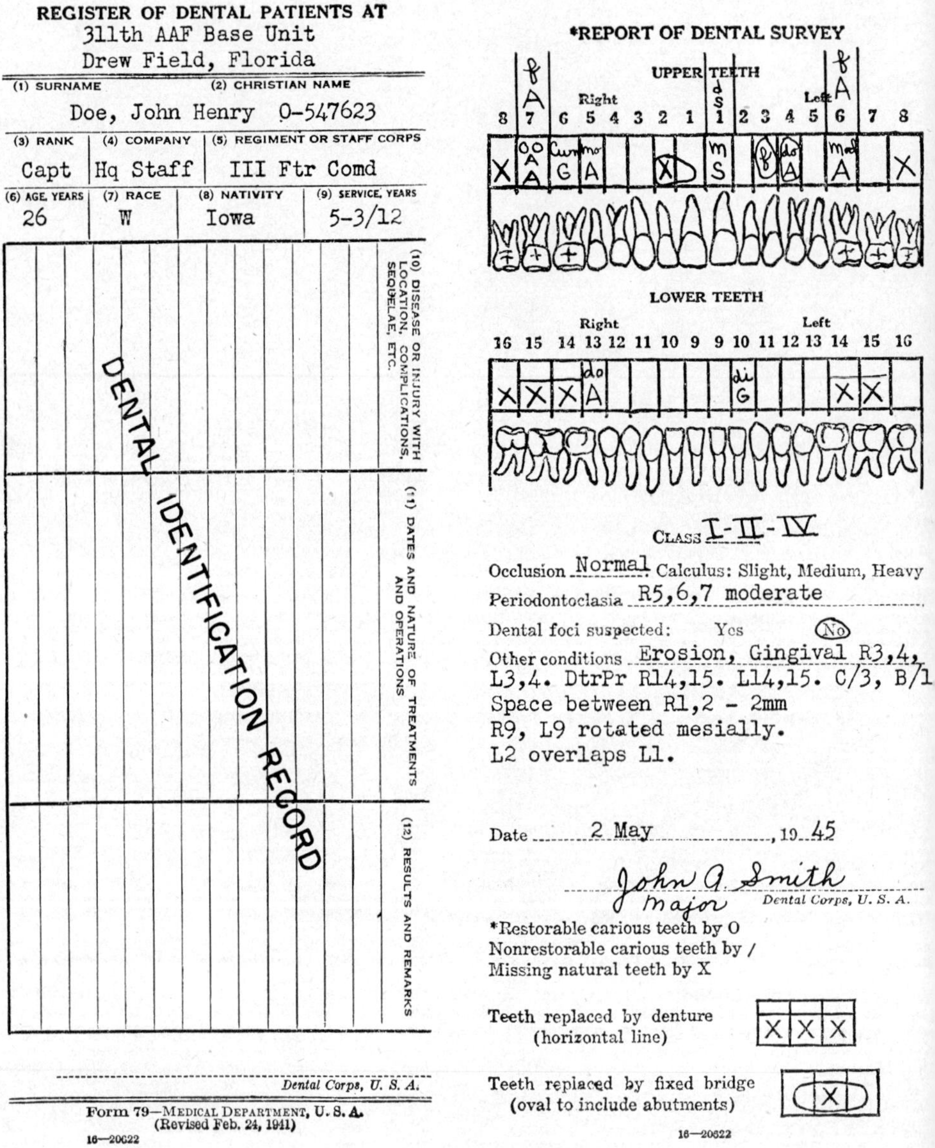

REGISTER OF DENTAL PATIENTS AT
311th AAF Base Unit
Drew Field, Florida

(1) SURNAME	(2) CHRISTIAN NAME	
Doe, John Henry 0-547623		

(3) RANK	(4) COMPANY	(5) REGIMENT OR STAFF CORPS
Capt	Hq Staff	III Ftr Comd

(6) AGE, YEARS	(7) RACE	(8) NATIVITY	(9) SERVICE, YEARS
26	W	Iowa	5-3/12

(10) DISEASE OR INJURY WITH LOCATION, COMPLICATIONS, SEQUELAE, ETC.

(11) DATES AND NATURE OF TREATMENTS AND OPERATIONS

(12) RESULTS AND REMARKS

DENTAL IDENTIFICATION RECORD

Dental Corps, U. S. A.

Form 79—MEDICAL DEPARTMENT, U. S. A.
(Revised Feb. 24, 1941)

16—20622

***REPORT OF DENTAL SURVEY**

UPPER TEETH
Right 8 7 6 5 4 3 2 1 | 1 2 3 4 5 6 7 8 Left

LOWER TEETH
Right 16 15 14 13 12 11 10 9 | 9 10 11 12 13 14 15 16 Left

CLASS I-II-IV

Occlusion Normal Calculus: Slight, Medium, Heavy
Periodontoclasia R5,6,7 moderate
Dental foci suspected: Yes (No)
Other conditions Erosion, Gingival R3,4, L3,4. DtrPr R14,15. L14,15. C/3, B/1
Space between R1,2 - 2mm
R9, L9 rotated mesially.
L2 overlaps L1.

Date 2 May, 19 45

John A. Smith
Major
Dental Corps, U. S. A.

*Restorable carious teeth by O
Nonrestorable carious teeth by /
Missing natural teeth by X

Teeth replaced by denture (horizontal line)

Teeth replaced by fixed bridge (oval to include abutments)

16—20622

FIG. 275. Dental identification record used by the U. S. Army Air Forces.

of the times. The early investigators emphasized the importance of dental examinations and records, and called attention to the oral hygiene of aviators as an important factor in flying safety. With the relatively low speed of planes of that period, most non-fatal crashes resulted in a fracture of either jaw because of the pilot's position in the plane. Fischer suggested that models of the teeth and jaws of aviators be available to simplify the construction of dental splints in cases of accidental fracture of the jaw. Charlet pointed out the need of dental records as a means of identification in cases of accidents. Today, dental identification records are compiled and maintained on all flying personnel in the Army Air Forces. In 1923, Neblett pointed out the possible connection between oral infection and "staleness" in pilots. Apical abscesses and periodontoclasia were found in pilots whose general symptomatology indicated neurocirculatory disturbances. Diminished visual acuity was frequently observed, sometimes only demonstrable on the side of the involved teeth.

In the past decade, the advances in aeronautics have resulted in the development of highly maneuverable planes which can fly more than five miles a minute, climb a mile a minute, and operate above 30,000 feet. These advances ushered in new physiologic problems, including new dental problems. In 1937, the first case history of aerodontalgia, toothache at altitude, appeared in the literature. Dryfus described a case of a flyer who had violent pains in one of his teeth at about 5,000 feet. The pain subsided on landing. Examination revealed a subacute pulpitis in a lower first molar and, following pulpectomy, the pilot could resume flying at high altitudes without pain. Willhelmy pointed out that malocclusion of the teeth in selected cases may impair the function of the eustachian tube, resulting in ear symptoms. Many investigators speculated on the causes of the loosening of dental fillings as a result of flying. These problems will be discussed in detail later in the section.

PHYSIOPATHOLOGIC FLYING DISORDERS

The human body constantly makes adjustments for changes in its terrestrial environment. Compensatory mechanisms, such as changes in respiration, in the activity of the sweat glands, and in the desire for rest or physical activity, maintain the body within narrow limits of fluctuation. The demands of flying upon the compensatory mechanisms of the body are of considerable magnitude. Effective operation of highly developed planes demands the utmost in physical and mental performance and, even then, artificial and mechanical aids must be employed to assist the compensatory mechanisms of the body in making the necessary adjustments to the new environment. In flight, apart from the emotional stress, airmen are subject to the following environmental changes of great physiologic significance: (1) changes in barometric pressure; (2) changes in temperature, and (3) movement at high speed in three dimensions. A brief introduction to the general flying disorders resulting from these environmental changes will serve as a background for any possible correlation with problems of aviation dentistry.

Effects of Oxygen Deficiency ("Anoxia")

As the barometric pressure and the density of the atmosphere decrease with altitude, likewise the oxygen partial pressure and density in the lungs decrease, and therefore the blood absorbs less and less oxygen. The first and principal effect of oxygen-want is an anesthesia-like reaction in which the senses are dulled. Thought and memory processes, vision, muscular control and respiration are affected. If oxygen-want continues, unconsciousness intervenes; and, if not soon relieved, prolonged oxygen-want results in permanent injury.

Effects of Evolved Gases (Aero-embolism or Bends)

At high altitudes the pressure of nitrogen in solution in the body fluids becomes greater than that of atmospheric nitrogen. When ascents, especially at a rapid rate, are made to 20,000 feet or more, the nitrogen tends to come out of solution and form bubbles in the tissues and the blood. The nitrogen bubbles appear usually in joints and fatty tissues and the result is pain of a deep, boring character, at times so severe as to become intolerable.

Effects Due to Entrapped Gases

During ascent, the volume of any free gas tends to increase in accordance with Boyle's Law, which states that the volume of a gas is inversely proportional to the pressure. The gradual lowering of barometric pressure during ascent results in the expansion of free gases in certain body cavities, from which escape is not readily available. On descent, the equalization of the pressure in body cavities with the external pressure is impeded. The resultant disorders include gastro-intestinal pain, aerosinusitis, aero-otitis media, and possibly toothache.

Effects of Low Temperatures

Exposure to the extremely low temperature encountered at high altitudes results in injuries, physical suffering and resultant lowering of efficiency.

Effects of Motion in Space

Air sickness, characterized by such symptoms as nausea, vomiting, pallor, sweating and dizziness, is caused by motion and acceleration experienced in flight.

Effects of Centrifugal Forces

When planes are in curved flight, the occupants are subject to centrifugal forces. The centrifugal force of an inside loop causes the blood to move away from the head. This is called "blacking-out," which is a loss of vision without loss of consciousness. Recovery is rapid when the force abates. Pilots are recommended to increase muscular and nervous tension when pulling out of a dive or a tight turn to prevent, to some extent, the flow of blood from the head. In performing an outside loop, the centrifugal force pulls the blood to the head, causing ocular and cerebral congestion. The eyeballs feel as if they would pop out of their sockets and there is a throbbing pain in the head. This unpleasant syndrome is called "redding-out."

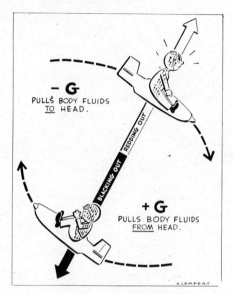

FIG. 276. Effects of centrifugal force
in plane maneuvers.

Data on flying disorders from actual flight are limited. Most research is carried out during simulated flights in large steel chambers, in which barometric pressure is controlled. A few decompression chambers are equipped to simulate temperature conditions at high altitude. The effects of centrifugal forces are studied in the laboratory in a human centrifuge.

30

Aerodontalgia

Toothache is one of the significant indispositions occurring in actual flight and in simulated flight in the decompression chamber. In military aviation, aerodontalgic pain has resulted in many disconcerting experiences; in future commercial and civilian flying, it will bring many patients from the airfield directly to the dental office. Clinical studies of this problem have been made by the dental services of the air forces of many nations. Although we have a knowledge of the etiologic factors, differences of opinion exist on the methods of treatment and the theories of the actual mechanism which causes the pain.

INCIDENCE

Toothache ranks fifth in frequency of all complications from exposure to low barometric pressures. Of 62,160 men receiving altitude indoctrination in the decompression chamber at a large Army Air Force installation, the incidence of complications was as follows:

	Per Cent
Bends	13.00
Aero-otitis	7.86
Abdominal distress	4.00
Sinus pain	1.10
Toothache	1.02
Skin reactions	1.00
Vasomotor instability	.33
Chokes	.28
Anoxia	.25
Visual disturbance	.15
Hyperventilation	.05

Reports from Army and Navy air stations indicated that 1 to 3% of all personnel given altitude training in the decompression chamber suffer toothaches. The incidence of dental pain among civilian subjects exposed to simulated flights in the chamber was 5.8%. The lower incidence among military personnel was presumed to be due to their better-than-average dental health.

Significant as these figures are, dental difficulties occurring during actual flight cannot be adequately evaluated on the results of one or a few simulated flights in the pressure chamber. Such experiences are at best only a substitute for actual flying experiences. Data, based on the entire flying experience of many pilots, present a more complete picture of the frequency and tactical significance of aerodontalgia.

In response to a questionnaire, 79 of 603 experienced fighter pilots, or 13.1%, voluntarily submitted past or current accounts of dental pain while flying. For clarification, each case of different etiology, whether experienced once or many times, was considered one case history. Considering the reluctance of pilots to divulge freely medical or dental complications involved in flying, 13.1% must be adjudged a minimum. This percentage is high as compared to the 1 to 3% occurrences reported on many series of pressure chamber runs. However, it must again be emphasized that this survey encompassed the entire flying experience of each pilot, not one pressure chamber run. The aggregate flying time of these pilots was approximately 600,000 hours. During this time, 79 pilots experienced aerodontalgic pain. During the two months these pilots were under observation, the 603 pilots flew approximately 35,000 missions, or 53,000 hours. In this period, 16 pilots complained of aerodontalgic pain. Although these figures indicate that aerodontalgic pain does not occur frequently, a large percentage of flyers have experienced aerodontalgic pain during their flying careers. Any distraction, which impairs a flyer's efficiency, is of utmost significance.

ETIOLOGY

Aerodontalgia is due to the presence of some pre-existing pathologic disturbance of the pulp or periapical tissues. The physical changes associated with high altitudes result in an exacerbation of symptoms previously experienced, an accentuation of subclinical symptoms or an early revelation of symptoms which would eventually appear in the course of the pre-existing lesion. High altitude environment, in itself, does not affect a normal pulp using pain as the criterion.

Case History Classification

Case histories of aerodontalgia can be conveniently classified on the basis of the clinical etiologic findings into three categories:

Class I. Pain in teeth with acute or chronic pulpitis, apical pathosis, pulp exposure or pulp necrosis.

Class II. Pain in teeth with a recently inserted filling, a deep-seated filling without an underlying base material, a defective filling, recurrent caries under a restoration, a high spot on a filling, hypersensitive dentin, or a developing cavity. The pulps of these teeth have been irritated and hyperemia of the pulp is the probable pre-existing pathologic disturbance. These cases are differentiated from the cases of pulpitis (Class I) by observing the effects of treatment.

Class III. Pain referred to the teeth from aerosinusitis, aero-otitis media, ear infections, unerupted or partially erupted third molars or pericoronitis. Differences of opinion may arise as to whether referred pain should be classified under aerodontalgia. It is included here for completeness and convenience.

The incidence of various pathologic conditions as causative factors in aerodontalgia is dependent upon the entire dental history of the individuals under consideration. Teeth with pulp exposure, a subclinical pulpitis, a filling without a base, a recently inserted filling and apical pathosis are the most common offenders. Reports indicate no significant difference in the etiologic factors between actual flight and decompression chamber findings.

DIAGNOSIS

While data on the altitude of incidence and relief of pain based on numerous cases of aerodontalgia is available, many variations occur. Pain in vital teeth usually occurs on ascent; pain in non-vital teeth and referred pain from aerosinusitis usually occur on descent. Aerodontalgia rarely occurs below 5,000 feet. Pain in a given tooth in a specific individual may show remarkable constancy in the altitude at which it first becomes manifest. Pain usually decreases as ground level is approached, and it is not uncommon for the toothache to subside on descent at the same altitude at which pain began.

The subjective symptoms of aerodontalgia are as varied as human symptoms can be, but again a few generalized findings will serve as diagnostic aids. Sharp pain during ascent indicates a hyperemic or acutely inflamed pulp; dull pain during ascent indicates a chronically inflamed pulp; dull pain during descent directs suspicion to a pulpless tooth or aerosinusitis. Pain which persists on the ground may disclose a pulpless tooth with periapical involvement. These cases may develop a cellulitis shortly after the flight.

The localization of the tooth involved is usually difficult. The patient cannot always be relied upon to locate the exact source of the pain, although the quadrant involved can usually be defined. Roentgenograms of the suspected area should be taken, but not relied upon entirely in selecting the offending tooth. The electric pulp tester and sensitivity to hot and cold are valuable aids. Orban and Ritchey described the response to stimulation with ice as the most reliable single clinical aid. Prolonged pain to irritation with ice, as compared to the reactions of the neighboring teeth, will help localize the offending tooth. Percussion tests and examination for high spots on fillings often reveal the offending tooth. A complete dental history should be taken, including the age of fillings, the pain involved during the filling operation, post-filling reactions and any recent dental disturbances. The history may direct suspicion to recently filled teeth, deep-seated fillings, defective fillings and unfilled cavities.

If diagnosis cannot be established after exploiting all routine diagnostic procedures, removal of suspected fillings, and removal of decay is indicated, except in some cases of aerodontalgia in recently filled teeth. Examine carefully for minute exposures, especially of the pulp horns. Staining the cavity with an aqueous iodine solution, or with silver nitrate, will often mark the exposed area as a small unstained spot. Recently filled teeth, even those with cement bases, are offenders at high altitude. If one is certain that there is no pulp exposure, it is advisable to defer treatment until after a few additional flights. In many cases, the pain does not recur, or may recur once or twice and then disappear. On subsequent examination, these teeth respond normally to clinical tests.

Repeated flights may be used to confirm the diagnosis and to determine the efficacy of the treatment. However, a single, uneventful re-run in the pressure chamber or an actual flight is not indicative of successful diagnosis and treatment in all cases. A specific case of aerodontalgia can occur on one flight and not occur on the next 10 or 20 flights. This is also true of other flying disorders. Then perhaps on the 11th or 21st flight, the pain involving the same tooth reappears. A recall of the patient and an interview after many flights is a more accurate checkup. The use of zinc oxide and eugenol as a base distorts further the true picture in some cases because its action on the pulp may conceal temporarily the effects of the flight. Although the action and the duration of action of zinc oxide and eugenol on the pulp is not clear, a mixture of zinc oxide and eugenol has been recommended by many clinical investigators as an effective base material in teeth which have been painful in flight or the decompression chamber.

DIFFERENTIAL DIAGNOSIS

Approximately 4% of the aerodontalgia cases are attributable to aerosinusitis. If the openings into the maxillary sinuses are normal, air passes into and out of these cavities without difficulty during ascent and descent, thus assuring equalization of pressure at all times. Obstruction of the maxillary ostia by swelling of the mucosal lining, caused by inflammation, an allergic condition or redundant tissue, makes it difficult for the air pressure in the maxillary sinus to become equalized with changing atmospheric pressure. Maxillary aerosinusitis may produce pain referable to the teeth of the upper jaw, especially molars and premolars, thus giving rise to a problem in differential diagnosis. Pain usually occurs on descent and often continues at ground level. It appears that on ascent, air can usually escape through the partially obstructed openings, but on descent, air may be prevented from entering the sinuses. The patient usually reveals a history of a chronic sinusitis or an acute nasopharyngitis, and should be referred to the otolaryngologist for treatment. Subsequent flights, after a cold or sinusitis has cleared up, will determine the accuracy of the diagnosis.

Aero-otitis media or a severe ear infection, complicated by difficulty in equalizing pressure in the middle ear, will cause referred pain to the teeth and jaws. An associated temporary "locking of the jaw" probably is the result of muscle spasm due to the severity of the pain. Dental pain is generally secondary to severe ear pain and diagnosis can usually be made from the history.

Unerupted or partially erupted third molars, with or without pericoronal inflammation, may cause referred pain during simulated or actual flight. Pain may arise from the expansion of gases in the surrounding sac of an unerupted tooth. Frequently, pericoronal inflammations are accentuated by the impingement of the oxygen mask. In some cases, diagnosis is obvious; in others, the diagnosis is arrived at by eliminating all possible sources of pain by routine diagnostic procedures.

ACTIVATING FACTORS

During ascent, temperature decreases approximately $2°$ C. every 1,000 feet and the low oxygen partial pressure above 10,000 feet requires the use of an artificial supply of oxygen. Before the advent of the oxygen mask, aviators used a pipe-stem mouthpiece from which issued a jet of extremely cold oxygen, which impinged upon the teeth and mucous membranes. Frostbite of the cheek as a result of this has been described, so that one readily realized why dental pain while flying was first attributed to the low temperatures at high altitudes. Oxygen masks, some equipped with heaters, have replaced the pipe-stem, thus providing dispersion of oxygen before inhalation.

Harvey inserted thermocouples in oxygen masks, dental fillings and various places in the mouth and, at external temperatures up to $-40°$ C., measured the temperature at these loci under varying conditions of oral and nasal breathing, intermittent and constant oxygen flow, and still air and draft. The temperature never dropped below $20°$ C. during the experiments and pain occurred only after iced water was used to reduce the tooth temperature to $12°$ C. The teeth are normally well insulated by the cheeks, lips, tongue and saliva against cold and the standard equipment used in high altitude flights provides an additional measure of protection. Harvey stated that the range of tooth temperatures while flying is between $20°$ and $45°$ C., which is well within the limits which occur in everyday life. He finds his experimental results supported by the fact that men in the coldest aircraft or in the most exposed positions are not those who complain of dental pain while flying.

It has been suggested that the dental pulp, due to the valveless condition of its veins, is susceptible to "blacking-out" as a result of the centrifugal forces experienced during radial accelerations. Permanent damage to the tooth is implied because of the lack of any recoil mechanism whereby recovery could be complete and rapid. Reports from 603 experienced fighter pilots, who on every flight are exposed to centrifugal forces, did not reveal any case histories which indicate that centrifugal forces produce acute dental symptoms. Sognnaes exposed a group of flyers, each with a high incidence of periapical abscesses, necrotic pulps, root canal fillings, cavities, impactions or periodontal disease, to accelerations in a human centrifuge equal to and more than those tolerated in actual flight. These experiments failed to reveal subjective symptoms referable to the teeth. In view of the completely negative reports, it appears that centrifugal forces are not a factor in the production of the acute symptoms of aerodontalgia.

Two environmental changes of physiologic significance encountered in flight, low temperature and motion in space, appear to play no significant rôle as activating factors in aerodontalgia. The majority of the reports of aerodontalgia are from decompression chambers in which temperature and motion play no part. The aerodontalgic findings from actual flights appear to coincide in symptomatology and etiology with those from decompression chambers. Exposure to low barometric pressure, the remaining environmental change of physiologic significance, appears to be the activating factor in toothaches at high altitude. However, the exact mechanism is complicated by the many effects of low barometric pressure: oxygen-want, expansion of free gases, liberation of gases from solution and vascular changes.

Toothache occurs in the decompression chamber with and without the use of oxygen. There is no evidence that oxygen-want results in any pain during the deficiency period. Since oxygen is supplied in all flights over 10,000 feet, it does not appear likely that oxygen-want is an activating factor in aerodontalgia.

It has been suggested that aerodontalgia may be caused by the expansion of air entrapped under fillings. Numerous investigators have experimentally produced air bubbles under dental restorations and exposed these patients to low barometric pressure. No symptoms were experienced in these cases. Theoretical consideration of this problem reveals that one of two conditions exist: either the entrapped air is in communication with the atmosphere or it is completely trapped by the non-expandable walls of the tooth and the filling material. In the former case, the pressure would be quickly equalized and any pain incurred would rapidly subside while altitude is maintained. We know this does not occur. In the latter case, the air being in no communication with the environment, there could not possibly be any volume or pressure change in view of the fact that barometric pressure changes are incommunicable through inelastic walls. All investigators have concluded that air under fillings is not a likely cause of dental pain while flying.

In a study on a large group of pilots, x-rays revealed 39 periapical abscesses, but only 8 elicited pain during actual flight. In addition, the x-rays revealed hundreds of pulpless teeth with varying qualities of root canal fillings. None of these teeth gave symptoms at any time in the flying careers of these pilots. Apparently, the pathosis of the pulpless tooth, with or without apical involvement, which causes symptoms in flight, is at a stage where exposure to low barometric pressure is the "straw which breaks the camel's back." Expansion of gas occurring during ascent in putrescent pulps or periapical abscess cavities may be related to aerodontalgia. The exacerbation of these teeth during flight is frequently followed by a marked cellulitis. Kennon and Osborn stated that a few hours or days after completing a flight in the decompression chamber without incident, patients report frequently to the clinic suffering from toothache. The patient attributes the subsequent ailment to the experience at simulated high altitude in the chamber, although no pain was present during the "flight." This complaint is consistent with the observation that similar reactions may occur after travelers cross mountains by land conveyance. Necrosis of the contents of the root canal has been found in many of these cases. Kennon and Osborn suggested that gases from a necrotic pulp, expanding under reduced atmospheric pressure, expel septic material through the root canal into the surrounding tissues, resulting in an acute abscess or an exacerbation of a chronic condition.

Recently filled teeth which react at high altitudes may be explained on the basis that a mild hyperemia exists because of reaction to overheating during drilling, drugs of unproven value and filling materials. Manley has shown that when the dentinal tubules are not occluded by secondary dentin, there is a vascular and cellular reaction in the pulp, due to the irritant action of oxyphosphate and silicate cements. Harvey has pointed out that heat production

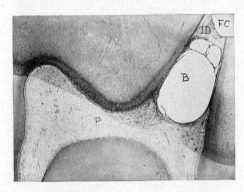

FIG. 277. Histologic section of a lower molar which was painful at 2,000 feet, intolerable at 10,000 feet: Large bubbles (B) in pulp horn; P, pulp; ID, irregular dentin; FC, floor of cavity cut into irregular dentin. (Orban and Ritchey, Jour. Amer. Dent. Asso., 32: 145-180, 1945.)

while burring is likely to cause damage to the pulp. These conditions result in the indisposition of the pulp, which is a prerequisite for tooth reaction at high altitudes. The provocative condition necessary to activate this subclinical entity may be vascular changes due to high altitudes.

There is evidence that ascent to altitudes of 30,000 feet is accompanied by vascular changes in the arterioles. Knisely pointed out that prolonged arteriolar spasm, which may be a factor in aero-embolic symptoms, causes a local anoxia, resulting in pain. Although toothache may occur at much lower altitudes than the altitudes at which vascular changes have been observed, the possibility that the existing pathologic disturbance in the pulp may predispose to vascular changes at lower altitudes cannot be overlooked. Moreover, the blood vessels of the pulp, without a collateral circulation, and enclosed in rigid walls are an ideal setting for vascular disturbances. Research on vascular changes at high altitudes is in its earliest stages; perhaps further work will reveal findings which can be correlated with those of aerodontalgia.

Orban and Ritchey, by correlating clinical and histologic findings, maintained that the predisposing pathologic process in all cases of toothache at high altitude is a circulatory disturbance in the pulp that prevents the equalization of the pressures of fluids or gases in the vessels and tissues. In edema of the pulp and acute or chronic pulpitis, there is a predisposition to high altitude toothaches due to an impaired circulation. Capillary permeability and dilation of blood vessels may be further aggravated during decompression by an increased intrapulpal pressure. It is implied that nitrogen released during decompression is an added impact on the circulation, throwing it into disorder and resulting in pain. In 6 of the 75 teeth sectioned, empty bubble-like spaces were observed. These are attributed either to gas formation as a result of tissue decomposition or nitrogen liberation due to decompression. These teeth were not exposed to altitudes at which nitrogen is usually liberated, but the authors consider it possible that nitrogen is liberated at a much lower level in diseased teeth. Orban and Ritchey concluded that extraction or root canal therapy is the only treatment indicated for teeth which are painful during decompression.

Wald minimized the importance of the evolution of nitrogen bubbles in the pulp as a factor in aerodontalgia. He pointed out that pain is often elicited at altitudes far below those at which nitrogen bubbles are normally released and that denitrogenation of an individual suffering from symptoms of aerodontalgia causes no change in the threshold of stimulation. Wald maintained that the decreased barometric pressure is transmitted to the circulatory system of the body through the volumetric expansion of the body during ascent. This force, transmitted undiminished throughout the system, communicates with all its ramifications. In most places, there is sufficient collateral circulation to maintain tissue exchange. However, at points of terminal circulation, as in the pulp of the tooth, the transmitted pressure tends to evacuate these terminal vessels. Osmotic changes take place as a result of the tendency of the fluid elements to be drawn to the apex of the tooth. A space, described by Orban and Ritchey, may appear most distal to the apex, the point of communication, as the vessels are evacuated. This space is not a "bubble of nitrogen"—it is a space containing all the volatile elements normally present in the blood (nitrogen, oxygen, carbon dioxide and water vapor) in equilibrium with these same elements in the tissues which surround the space. The space is exerting no more pressure on the surrounding pulp tissue than the tissue itself is exerting on the space, for if there were any difference, a new equilibrium would be established. To summarize Wald's theory, pain due to decreased barometric pressure is brought about by an evacuation of the fluid elements at a point of terminal circulation through the point of communication, thus cutting off or decreasing the circulation to a state where tissue metabolism and osmotic equilibrium are upset.

In summary, the activating factors in aerodontalgia still await adequate and complete explanation. Early research indicates that the majority of cases of aerodontalgia are probably due to circulatory disturbances brought about by reduced barometric pressure in an already diseased or irritated pulp. The variety of case histories indicates other factors play a rôle, but only in a small percentage of cases.

31

Periodontal Aspects

INCIDENCE	PRESSURE HABITS
ETIOLOGY	VINCENT'S STOMATITIS

Various sources have reported a relatively high incidence of gingival diseases, especially acute gingivostomatitis (Vincent's) among flying personnel. Many clinicians have noted the persistent nature of periodontal disease among flyers and find it less responsive to treatment. In addition to the usual etiologic factors of dental origin, these periodontal disturbances have been attributed to factors peculiar to flying conditions and flying personnel. Flying fatigue, use of oxygen, nervous tension, reduced atmospheric pressure, lack of oral hygiene and other conditions ascribed to the transient existence of flyers have been suggested as factors predisposing flying personnel to a high incidence of gingival disease. There is a widespread superstition among flyers that high altitude and continued use of oxygen have a deleterious effect on teeth, fillings, gums, and the mouth in general. As concerns periodontal aspects, the literature does not reveal any detailed studies to verify or repudiate these beliefs.

Many aspects of the section on periodontal disease are derived from the author's (A.A.G.) original survey. A brief description of the methods employed and the personnel studied is essential. Through pilot interviews and exhaustive dental examinations, a comprehensive series of subjective and clinical findings on aviation dentistry were compiled from 500 experienced fighter pilots. "Your Teeth in Flight," a pamphlet which discusses problems in aviation dentistry and in which space is provided for answers to pertinent questions, was used to stimulate the flyer's interest and to provide a background for the pilot's interview with the dental officer. Pilots were interviewed on flying experience, combat service, aerodontalgic experiences, gingival disorders, habits during flight, fit of the oxygen mask, ear pains and flying time lost due to dental difficulties. Their opinions were sought on the effect of flying on the teeth, fillings and gums. In conjunction with the compiling of subjective information during the interviews, a complete oral examination, including x-rays, was accomplished.

The personnel studied was an unselected group of experienced fighter pilots engaged in the final phase training of fighter pilot trainees. The average flying time per pilot was 973 hours. The youngest was 20, the oldest was 36 and the average age was 25. Seventy-eight % of these pilots had served 1 or 2 tours of overseas duty. They were all officers and the average rank was Captain. All planes flown by these pilots were combat, fighter-type aircraft, capable of the highest altitudes and speeds.

A complete periodontal examination of the 500 pilots was accomplished. The oral hygiene of each pilot was evaluated during the interview and the clinical examination. The color and surface of the gums were noted; the condition of the gingival margins and papillae was described; periodontal pockets, food impaction and mobility were charted; x-ray findings were noted and the probable etiologic factors were listed. Full mouth x-ray and bitewing films were taken in 352 of the 500; bitewing and individual films were taken of the remaining 148 pilots.

INCIDENCE

The incidence of periodontal disturbances varies among different groups of airmen. The type of assignment, whether fighter, bomber or transport, and the station, whether overseas or in the United States, are influencing factors. Statistical data of this nature are completely lacking. However, opinions of dental officers stationed at different types of air force installations have been collected and upon the consensus of opinions, a few generalized statements can be made. The prevalence of gingival disturbances is greater in air crews than in ground crews, and is greater in transient than in permanent personnel. Combat pilots and ferry pilots, especially those who have served overseas, have a high incidence of periodontal disturbances. A comparative study of the periodontal problem in air corps personnel and infantry or ground force personnel is not available.

A study of the incidence of bleeding gums among R.A.F. personnel revealed that 18% of the airmen and 21% of the airwomen exhibited some degree of bleeding gums. This survey was made incident to a study on the value of ascorbic acid treatment. These figures are presented as an indication of the incidence of one symptom usually associated with gingival disturbances.

The dental survey of 500 fighter pilots revealed that 146 or 29.2% had some form of periodontal disease. No attempt was made to classify each case, but the etiologic factors involved in each case were noted and will be discussed later. Without statistics on a comparable group of Army Air Force ground personnel, it is difficult to evaluate the 29.2% incidence of periodontal disease among these pilots. However, by considering other factors, this figure assumes new proportions. These fighter pilots are a select group, physically and mentally. Their average length of service was more than 3 years and during this time they have undoubtedly received better than average dental attention. The oral hygiene of the 500 pilots was considered average or above average in 92.8%. Considered in this light, the incidence of periodontal disease among these men is relatively high. Although the etiologic factors of dental origin play the major rôle as causative factors, the relatively high prevalence of periodontal disease in this select group indicates that other etiologic factors must be involved.

ETIOLOGY

Periodontal disturbances are caused by a combination of factors which lower tissue resistance. The basic etiologic factors which cause periodontal disease in pilots are the same as those we see in everyday practice, namely calculus, occlusal trauma, faulty dentistry, habits, etc. However, in combination with these basic factors are etiologic factors peculiar to flying and to the living conditions which result from military aviation operations. It is apparent that these factors, to date intangibly judged, play at least a secondary rôle as causative agents and are largely responsible for the persistent or chronic nature of many periodontal disturbances among airmen. Failure to take these factors into account results in unsuccessful treatment.

All stages of periodontal disease from the incipient to the advanced state were evident among the 146 fighter pilots with periodontal disturbances. In 18 or 12% of the pilots with periodontal disease, a pathologic degree of tooth mobility could be demonstrated. Fusospirochetal (Vincent's) organisms were considered a probable etiologic factor in 10 cases. Of these cases, the description of the gums of only 5 indicated the presence of an acute ulcerative gingivitis. Soft tissue trauma and abrasion of the teeth due to improper toothbrushing methods were evident in many cases. Poor diet and avitaminoses played a rôle in the cases of a few pilots returned from overseas. The number of times each basic etiologic factor was deemed of probable significance in the 146 cases was as follows:

Oral hygiene—improper tooth brushing, poor oral hygiene............... 72
Calculus—supragingival, subgingival..................................... 69
Exciting factors—tissue trauma, fusospirochetal (Vincent's) organisms, other bacterial forms.. 41
Abnormal anatomy—tooth form, tooth position......................... 41
Overfunction—occlusal trauma, insufficient periodontal support, too powerful musculature.. 29
Mechanical irritants—faulty cavity margins, clasps, bridges, dentures..... 25
Food impaction... 23
Systemic factors—dietary and nutritional deficiencies, allergies, etc........ 16
Underfunction—non-occlusion, premature wear......................... 6
Mouth breathing.. 3

There is no evidence at the present time of the effect of lowered atmospheric pressure or the continued use of oxygen on the oral tissues. Mitchell, reporting experiments from the AAF School of Aviation Medicine, found no demonstrable changes in the rate of flow, pH, and *Lactobacillus acidophilus* count of the saliva of subjects breathing 100% oxygen at a simulated altitude of 25,000 feet for $5\frac{1}{2}$ hours on two consecutive days. Problems worthy of consideration are the effects of vascular changes and aeroembolic phenomena associated with low pressure on normal and diseased periodontal tissue.

Circumstances incident to the everyday life of flying personnel cannot be overemphasized as probable etiologic factors in periodontal disease. Air crews, especially bomber and ferry crews, lead unbalanced existences due to the transitory nature of their jobs. Irregular meals, unbalanced and inadequate diet, neglect of hygiene when traveling from one station to another, lack of proper rest and excessive smoking and drinking stemming from the stress of aerial warfare contribute to a generalized lowering of tissue resistance. Long bomber or ferry missions and brief, but strenuous fighter missions, day after day, are extremely fatiguing. Nervous tension involved in combat maneuvers, formation flying and gunnery are an added impact after physical strain has exhausted a large part of the available energy. Even the most experienced flyers are under tension, for flying requires continuous alertness. The fact that nervous tension interferes with digestion and assimilation of essential foods cannot be overlooked. Flying fatigue is recognized as an entity by the flight surgeon and is reason for temporary grounding.

PRESSURE HABITS

A psychosomatic factor, related to nervous tension and plane maneuvers, which consistently remains unrecognized and uncontrolled, is the habit of clamping or grinding of the teeth, often referred to as bruxism or bruxomania. The significance of dental pressure habits in periodontal disease and, as will be discussed later, in the ventilation of the middle ear, cannot be over-emphasized. During the fighter pilot dental survey, 45% of the pilots volunteered information concerning their diurnal, nocturnal, and flight habits. Of the 146 men with periodontal disease, 77 admitted practicing pressure habits. It was not recognized until the survey was completed that the use of the word "habit" confused many pilots. Not all pilots interpreted clamping during linear and radial accelerations as a habit. Moreover, pilots are prone to deny or belittle this factor. A more likely figure on the incidence of habits in fighter pilots is 60 to 70%.

Many pilots admitted that these habits were the result of the tension they are under while flying, not only in combat, formation flying or maneuvers, but at all times in the air. A few mentioned that these habits started during combat duty. Pilots are advised to increase muscular and nervous tension when subjected to centrifugal force to prevent to some extent the flow of blood from the head. In this procedure, pilots usually clamp their jaws together and exert tremendous pressure. Stewart of the R.C.A.F. pointed out that clenching the jaws is a common complication of the Valsalva procedure (pinching the nostrils and blowing) in the decompression chamber when attempting to equalize pressure in the middle ear. Pressure habits are more common in fighter pilots than in bomber pilots and more prevalent among pilots than their crews.

Leof pointed out that the majority of periodontal cases in everyday practice have some pressure habits as a cause or as a contributing factor. Although pressure habits are as multiple and varied as there are individuals, he classified them into categories, which are applicable to the habits found in flight during the fighter pilot dental survey.

Class I. Habits involving a foreign object, such as oxygen pipe-stem biting. No Class I flight habits were uncovered in the survey.

Class II. Habits involving the teeth and other tissues such as cheek biting and sucking on interproximal spaces. Pilots inflict severe trauma on their oral tissues during flight and are completely unaware of the damage or pain until landing. Chapped lips, cuspal and incisal indentations, scars on the buccal mucosa and papillomas resulting from the constant chewing of the cheeks were uncovered during the survey. A few pilots complained that the oxygen mask forced the cheeks between the teeth, thus inviting tissue trauma. Class II habits may result in periodontal disease, *e.g.*, constant sucking on interproximal spaces will lead to tissue breakdown; or Class II habits may be the result of periodontal disease, *e.g.*, sucking on periodontal pockets and food-impacted areas. These habits, though harmful, result in little periodontal damage because the pressure involved is not great.

Class III. Clamping or grinding habits, such as clamping at the expense of all or a few of the teeth, grinding excursions, rhythmic tapping or clicking of the teeth. These habits are the most common in flight and result in the greatest damage. They may be practiced continuously throughout all flights, in maneuvers only, and both in flight and on the ground. Pilots who practice these habits are aware of a throbbing soreness or develop a consciousness of the teeth on landing, which disappears quickly. Tired jaw muscles are a common subjective sign. The prolonged tension and compression resulting from clamping and grinding habits cause congestion and irritation of the periodontal tissues, as differentiated from the stimulating effect of the intermittent forces of normal function. These habits can in time damage the periodontal membrane, causing periodontal disease, or they may become a secondary factor in an already existing periodontal disturbance.

Habits are one of the important factors responsible for the persistent nature of periodontal disease among flyers. Leof's explanation of pressure habits as a complication in periodontal disease is directly applicable to this problem in flying personnel. The larger group of periodontal cases among flyers present an etiologic picture wherein local irritational factors, calculus, mechanical irritants, etc., are not the whole story. These cases present missing teeth, tilted teeth, deep overbites, mutilated occlusion and other forms of traumatogenic occlusion. Functional occlusion has been lost. Simultaneously there develops hyperfunction of certain or all remaining teeth. With the accompanying pressure of clamping or grinding habits, this increases many fold. Having decided that hyperocclusal stress is the important etiologic factor, the dentist must reduce this not only by equilibration of the occlusion, but also by habit control.

VINCENT'S STOMATITIS

The prevalence of Vincent's stomatitis among air crews is greater than among ground crews. Coons observed that Vincent's infection develops quickly in persons subject to gingival lesions on long-sustained flights at comparatively low altitudes, as well as at high altitudes during flights of short duration. He maintains that there is a change in the resistance of the gums

accompanied by bleeding and the return of active infection. Pockets condu-
cive to the incubation of the organisms were undoubtedly present in the
mouth, but such rapid development of the infection did not occur at ground
level. Clinicians attribute the high incidence of acute gingival disturbances
to poor oral hygiene during long trips, fatigue and nervous strain, inadequate
diet and a cumulative predisposition of oral soft tissue to infection after continuous flying status. Erupting or impacted third molars, complicated by
pericoronal inflammation, are common in the age group of the personnel in
military aviation. Third molar flaps are an ideal incubation pocket for organisms and, with lowered tissue resistance due to predisposing factors, poor
oral hygiene and, in many cases, trauma incurred as a result of habits and
the oxygen mask, an acute infection develops. Discomfort due to the slight
pain and excessive bleeding is aggravated by the wearing of an oxygen mask
and such indispositions in flight interfere with the efficiency of the individual.
Observations indicate that the breathing of pure oxygen at high altitudes is
neither beneficial nor detrimental in cases of Vincent's infection.

Penicillin mouth washes have been successful in bringing relief from the
acute symptoms in a short period, but acute gingivostomatitis appears to
lapse into the chronic state in many cases. This is due to failure to follow
up treatment, lack of co-operation on the part of the patient in home care,
failure to eliminate or control systemic predisposing factors as fatigue, emotional factors, over-indulgence in smoking and drinking, and inadequate diet,
and in part may be due to certain intangible factors associated with high
altitudes.

32

Relation of Malocclusion to Ear Symptoms

The effect of flight on the ear is the most frequent cause of discomfort among flying personnel. Changes in atmospheric pressure are a source of constant trauma to the ear. Aero-otitis media, already recognized as an occupational disease, is an acute or chronic traumatic inflammation caused by a pressure difference between the air in the middle ear and that of the surrounding atmosphere. This physiopathologic entity is characterized by pain, deafness, tinnitus and occasionally vertigo. The fundamental cause of aero-otitis media is a failure of ventilation of the middle ear. As the atmospheric pressure is reduced during ascent, the expanding air in the middle ear passes out intermittently through the eustachian tube to the nasopharynx, thereby equalizing pressure within the ear with the outside pressure. During descent, the changes in pressure in the ear do not occur automatically, due to the fact that the pharyngeal opening of the eustachian tube acts as a flutter valve, allowing air to pass out easily but resisting its passage into the ear cavity. With an increase in atmospheric pressure during descent, the pressure of the outside air rises above that in the middle ear and the ear drum is forced into the middle ear. Unless the eustachian tube is opened, this condition results in increasing pain and further increased pressure differential may rupture the ear drum. Normally, however, there is no difficulty in relieving ear block during descents. This can be accomplished by swallowing or yawning, procedures which result in opening the pharyngeal orifice of the eustachian tube by muscle action. If relief is not obtained this way, then air can be forced into the ear by pinching the nose, closing the mouth and blowing (Valsalva movement). Aero-otitis media occurs most frequently when inflammation or infection of the nose, throat, ear, or sinuses affects the eustachian tube and its pharyngeal orifice.

The cause of chronic aero-otitis media in some cases has been ascribed to stenosis of the eustachian tube as a result of malposition of the mandible. Willhelmy in 1936 was the first to apply to flying the relationship between ear symptoms and the loss of vertical dimension of the jaws. By opening the bite in 6 selected cases, presumably relieving the pressure on the eustachian tube, symptoms of ear pains, dizziness and temporary deafness were relieved. A few investigators have made similar reports, but none of these papers contain otolaryngologic histories of any of the cases treated. The restoration of vertical dimension as related to ear symptoms, especially deafness, has been advocated and condemned alternately for years. Willhelmy and other investigators associated ear pains, dizziness, and deafness in flyers with Costen's syndrome, which included a multitude of ear and sinus symptoms associated with disturbed function of the temporomandibular joint. They attributed these ear symptoms to obstruction of the eustachian tube, which, according to Costen, is due to pressure on its anterior membranous wall, transmitted

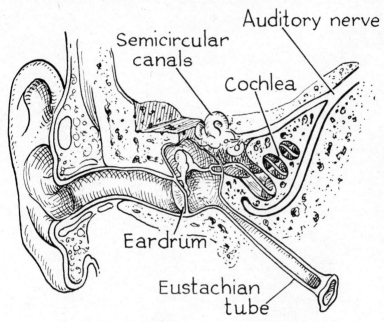

FIG. 278. Schematic representation of the ear.

through soft tissue from the relaxation of the pterygoid muscles and associated sphenomandibular ligaments during overbite. Many anatomists and otolaryngologists are not impressed with this explanation of passive obstruction of the eustachian tube. At the present time, Costen, formerly the foremost proponent of a causal relationship between malocclusion and deafness, after critical analysis of 400 cases, admits that audiometric tests fail to confirm improvement of hearing after bite-opening.

Overclosure of the mandible may interfere with ventilation of the middle ear, resulting in chronic ear pain and a stuffy sensation in the ear, but recent reports indicate that these cases are rare. Temporary ear blocks must be accepted as an everyday effect of flying; however, this difficulty is easily overcome. Failure to open the eustachian tube occurs most often among trainees and passengers, due to ignorance, inexperience or carelessness. Ear symptoms are a common complaint of cadets and trainees experiencing their initial altitude indoctrination run in the decompression chamber. After instruction in the methods of ventilating the ear and experience in these procedures have been acquired, the incidence of ear symptoms is markedly reduced. Harvey, reporting on the decompression tests of 1,000 R.A.F. personnel, found 89 men who developed symptoms in their ears. When decompressed 3 times, there were only 7 men of these 89 who had pain on each occasion. Of the 7, there were only 3 whose otolaryngologic history offered no contributory factor; and in only 1 of these men, malocclusion may have been a factor—he had an Angle Class II, division I type of occlusion.

Persistent ear blocks, not associated with nasopharyngitis, are uncommon. Interviews with 500 experienced pilots revealed that 22 suffered ear pains, not associated with nasopharyngitis, chronically or occasionally during their flying careers. Of these, 9 cases were in the realm of the otolaryngologist and in no way associated with overclosure of the mandible. Of the remaining 13 pilots, 7 had deep or very deep overbites. No other significant occlusion findings were revealed. Judged on the frequency and extent of this handicap, corrective procedure to open the bite was indicated in only 1 case. A report on more than 50,000 decompression tests of RCAF personnel pointed out that in only 1 case, bite opening was necessary to facilitate ventilation of the middle ear. It is possible that malocclusion of various types may interfere with the function of the eustachian tube. However, bite-opening appliances are unnecessary when flyers can obtain the same result by learning the routine methods of equalizing pressure in the ears.

One of the major difficulties in equalizing pressure in the ears is tension on the muscles of the jaw and throat. Muscles do not function as separate entities, but rather as "kinetic chains." Tension on the muscles of mastication during clamping habits in flight interferes with the function of the muscles of the throat. Clenching of the jaws, associated with nervous tension and plane maneuvers, markedly handicaps the methods of ventilating the ear, namely, swallowing, yawning, and the Valsalva movement. This is a common difficulty not only in actual flight, but also in the pressure chamber as was pointed out by Stewart on more than 50,000 runs. Habit control and training to relax these muscles during the Valsalva movement will invariably result in easy and rapid relief from uncomplicated ear blocks.

33

Considerations Involving Dental Materials, Prosthetics, and Personnel Care

EFFECTS ON TOOTH STRUCTURE AND FILLING MATERIALS	PROSTHETIC ASPECTS DENTAL CARE OF FLYING PERSONNEL

EFFECTS ON TOOTH STRUCTURE AND FILLING MATERIALS

There is a widespread conviction among aviators that flight at high altitudes and the use of oxygen have a detrimental effect on teeth and dental restorations. Some believe that fillings fall out at high altitude and, on a few occasions, this has been confirmed. Koelsch attributed the loss of fillings to the breathing of cold air or oxygen due to the difference in the coefficient of expansion between the filling material and tooth structure, or to air trapped under fillings. He added that the difference in expansion and contraction may cause fissures between tooth structure and fillings which may result in recurrent caries. McDowell exposed extracted teeth with dental restorations to extreme changes of temperature and concluded that a sudden change of temperature of the magnitude tolerated by the oral cavity will not dislodge restorations. Harvey, whose experiments are described in the section on aerodontalgia, found that the range of tooth temperature while flying is between 20° and 45° C., which is well within the limits which occur in everyday life. Therefore, the contraction and expansion of fillings is just as likely to occur on the ground as in the air. Many investigators have experimentally produced air bubbles under fillings and concluded that they do not affect the pulp or restorations. Armstrong and Huber studied the effect of decreased barometric pressure, decreased temperature and increased oxygen percentages, separately and combined, on teeth and filling materials clinically and in the laboratory. They concluded that the environmental conditions encountered at altitudes between 10,000 and 40,000 feet, in addition to the inhalation of oxygen cooled to a maximum of −60° F., have no deleterious effect on human teeth or dental restorations. Restarski studied *in vitro* the effects of low barometric pressure on dental restorations constructed of properly and improperly manipulated filling materials. His results indicate that during ascents and descents, oral fluids could be forced under leaking fillings or fillings with air spaces. Restarski concluded that displacement of properly inserted dental fillings and restorations, constructed with improperly manipulated filling materials or with air spaces, seems improbable.

The probable explanation for the loss of fillings in flight is that they were defective and unable to withstand the force of the bite. It is reasonable to assume that the biting force, which is limited, not by muscle power, but by the threshold of pain of the tooth-supporting tissues, can be greater in flight than the biting force normally applied on the ground. Pilots frequently inflict severe trauma on the oral tissues and are completely unaware of the damage or pain until landing. Pilots are frequently aware of a soreness or consciousness of the teeth or a tiredness of the masticatory muscles after landing. They are usually not conscious of these symptoms in flight. These symptoms are the result of the excessive biting force in flight associated with clamping or grinding habits, nervous tension, or muscle tension when counteracting the effects of maneuvers. Whereas the normal or even the maximum biting force on the ground will have no effect on a defective filling or a filling with inadequate retention, the excessive biting force in flight is likely to dislodge it.

PROSTHETIC ASPECTS

New thoughts on the problem of denture retention have been aroused by studies stemming from the prosthetic aspects of aviation dentistry. A recent study on the effect of reduced atmospheric pressure upon the retention of dentures reported findings which are at variance with the mucostatic theory of denture retention. The purely physical forces related to denture retention are adhesion, atmospheric pressure and gravity. The proponents of the mucostatic theory contend that atmospheric pressure plays little or no part in denture retention. Using a small spring hand scale attached to specially prepared baseplates and full upper dentures and taking measurements at sea level and at altitude simulating 30,000 feet in the decompression chamber, Snyder et al. found that a reduction of 70% in atmospheric pressure was followed by a loss of retention of full dentures of approximately 50%. They maintained that in order to take the greatest possible advantage of that part of retention produced by atmospheric pressure, the periphery and postdam areas of impressions be fully muscle-trimmed and adapted as closely as possible, and maximum available tissue area be covered by the impression.

Sognnaes discussed the handicaps associated with the use of loose dental appliances by aviators exposed to radial accelerations. In testing the retention of dentures, he found many dentures satisfactory with regard to their efficiency in chewing and speech, but their retention was insufficient to tolerate the load applied by the centrifugal forces of radial accelerations. As a result of these studies, Sognnaes recommended that fixed bridgework be used wherever possible in place of removable appliances, partial dentures be securely retained and full dentures be as light in weight and as thin as possible.

DENTAL CARE OF FLYING PERSONNEL

Dentistry must assist in conditioning the body to withstand the demands of flying and must offer effective corrective treatment to alleviate dental difficulties occurring in flight. The knowledge already gained from clinical and research studies in aviation dentistry can be applied to the dental service of flying personnel, with the reservation that future work may modify or extend these practical points. Dental difficulties associated with flight can be prevented, corrected or, if necessary, eliminated by surgical intervention. Major efforts, however, in the care of flying personnel must be concentrated on prevention. The following procedures are recommended:

(1) A program of dental education through lectures, posters, pamphlets, motion pictures and personal contact with the dentist, should serve to debunk the superstitions concerning the effect of flying on the teeth and to emphasize the need for good oral hygiene and periodic dental checkups.

(2) All flying personnel should have complete and periodic oral examinations, including roentgenograms.

(3) The elimination of foci of infection and incipient dental disease will remove the pre-existing conditions which cause dental difficulties in flight.

(4) Flying personnel should receive periodic dental prophylaxes.

(5) Periodontal disturbances should be treated in the incipient stages with due regard to the etiologic factors peculiar to flight conditions and flying personnel.

(6) In cavity preparations and filling operations, good retention form is essential; filling materials must be properly manipulated and inserted; and protective bases should be placed under all fillings.

(7) Root canal therapy should be limited to teeth with the most favorable prognosis.

(8) Impacted third molars, frequently complicated by inflammation and subsequent generalized gingival disturbances, should be removed.

(9) Fixed bridges should be used as replacements wherever possible; removable appliances should be securely retained.

(10) The dentist can assist the otolaryngologist in relieving ear symptoms incident to flight by pointing out that clamping or grinding habits handicap the methods of ventilating the ear and, rarely, by constructing appliances to open the bite.

Since aerodontalgia, in many cases, is caused by an exacerbation of a previously undetected pathologic condition, exposure to high altitude can be considered a new diagnostic procedure. The effects of exposure to high altitude has afforded research a new method of critically testing our methods and materials. These studies will not only be of value in the oral aspects of aviation medicine, but will reveal information which will affect everyday dental practice.

REFERENCES

ORAL ASPECTS OF AVIATION MEDICINE

Armstrong, H. G., & R. E. Huber: Effect of high altitude flying on human teeth and restorations, Dent. Dig., 43:132-134, 1937.
Batson, O. V.: The closed bite and related clinical problems, J. A. D. A., 25:1191-1196, 1938.
Charlet, R.: Les fiches d'identification buccodentaires et le personnel de l'aeronautique civil et militaire, Presse Medicale, 41:17-19, 1933.
Coons, D. S.: Aeronautical dentistry, J. Canad. D. A., 9:320-323, 1943.
Costen, J. B.: Reflex effects produced by abnormal movement of the lower jaw, Arch. Otolarygn., 36:548-554, 1942.
Costen, J. B.: A syndrome of ear and sinus symptoms dependent upon disturbed function of the temporomandibular joint, Ann. Otol., Rhinol. and Laryngol., 43:1-15, 1934.
Devoe, K., & H. L. Motley: Aerodontalgia, Dent. Dig., 51:16-18, 1945.
Drefus, H.: Les dents des aviateurs, l'Odontologie, 75:612-613, 1937.
Fischer, W. C.: The advisability of recording the models of the jaws of aviators, J. A. Milit. Dent. Surgeons U. S., 2:169-179, 1918.
Goldhush, A. A.: A dental survey of fighter pilots. To be published in The Air Surgeon's Bulletin.
Harvey, W.: Some aspects of dentistry in relation to aviation, Proc. Roy. Soc. Med., 37:465-474, 1944.
Harvey, W.: Tooth temperature with reference to dental pain while flying, Brit. Dent. J., 75:221-228, 1943.
Kennon, R. H., & C. M. Osborn: A dental problem concerning flying personnel, J. A. D. A., 31:662-667, 1944.
Knisely, M. H.: Quoted by Harvey.
Koelsch, F.: Handb. d. Berufskrankh., 1st Ed. Verlag Gustav Fischer, Jena, 1935.
Leof, M.: Clamping and grinding habits: their relation to periodontal disease, J. A. D. A., 31:184-194, 1944.
Lipson, H. J., & S. G. Weiss: Biologic approach to problems in aviation dentistry, J. A. D. A., 29:1660-1663, 1942.
Manley, E. B.: Some clinical, histological and biological observations on the acidity of dental cements, Brit. Dent. J., 77:126-129, 1944.
McDowell, R. M.: The loss of dental fillings by aviators engaged in high altitude flights, Dent. Bull., 6:195-196, 1935.
Medical Safety Division, Office of Flying Safety, Headquarters, A.A.F.: Flying and dentistry, The Air Surgeon's Bull., pp. 1-4, 1944.
Mitchell, D. F.: Aerodontalgia, Bull. U. S. Army Med. Dept., 73:62-67, 1944.
Mitchell, D. F.: 1945 effects of oxygen and decompression on saliva, project No. 392, report No. 1, A.A.F. school of aviation medicine, Randolph Field, Texas.
Neblett, H. C.: Chronic infections of teeth and gums as cause of staleness in air service pilots, Mil. Surgeon, 53:224-229, 1923.
Orban, B., & B. T. Ritchey: Toothaches under conditions simulating high altitude flight, J. A. D. A., 32:145-180, 1945.
Pigott, J. B.: Dental pain at high altitude, Report No. 38, Yale Aeromedical

Research Unit, Yale University School of Medicine, New Haven, Conn., October, 1944.

Restarski, J. S.: Effect of changes in barometric pressure upon dental fillings, U. S. Nav. M. Bull., 42:155-157, 1944.

Sognnaes, R. F.: Studies on aviation dentistry, Associate Committee on Aviation Medical Research, National Research Council, Ottawa, Canada, 1944.

Stamm, W. P., T. F. Macrae, & S. Yudkin: Incidence of bleeding gums among R.A.F. personnel and the value of ascorbic acid in treatment, Brit. M. J., 2:239, 1944.

Stewart, C. B.: Personal communication, February, 1945.

Synder, F. C., H. D. Kimball, W. B. Bunch, & J. H. Beaton: Effect of reduced atmospheric pressure upon retention of dentures, J. A. D. A., 32:445-450, 1945.

Wald, A.: Personal communication, April, 1945.

Willhelmy, G. E.: Ear symptoms incidental to sudden altitude changes and the factor of overclosure of the mandible—preliminary report, U. S. Nav. M. Bull., 34:533-541, 1936.

SECTION TEN
COLOR ATLAS

Fig. 1. Chancre of the lower lip. This primary luetic lesion is moderately painful. It has the translucent coating commonly associated with lesions of acute syphilis. The local induration of the lip is clearly shown. Regional adenopathy was also present. Dark field examination of material from this lesion was positive for *Tr. pallidum*. The blood Wassermann was negative.

Fig. 2. Acute herpetic stomatitis. The acute herpetic stomatitis in this patient was of allergic causation. Eroded areas (ruptured or macerated herpetic vesicles) were present on the cheek mucosa, the palate and the tongue. This condition must be differentiated from erythema multiforme and early pemphigus.

Fig. 3. Severe erythema multiforme of the oral mucosa which occurred in a 13-year-old girl. The lesions were of sudden onset and acutely painful. She has experienced two other attacks in the last six months. Same patient as shown in Fig. 58.

Fig. 4. Oral mucosal lesions in acute pemphigus vulgaris. The gingivae were not involved. The oral mucosal involvement preceded the dermal manifestations of this disease for many weeks. The history of recurring crops of bullae, which developed painlessly and then became painful, in conjunction with the marked systemic symptoms aided in making the clinical diagnosis. Same patient as shown in Fig. 52.

Fig. 5. Bismuth pigmentation of the gingiva. The discrete bluish-black bismuth line in the marginal gingival tissue is clearly depicted in this patient. There are four areas of pigmentation on the inner surface of the upper lip. The small yellow spots on the vermilion border of the upper lip are Fordyce's granules.

Fig. 6. Allergy to acrylic denture material. There is superficial necrosis of the denture supporting and contacting areas. The lesions developed during a period of five days and they were intensely painful. Dermal patch tests made with the denture base and the monomer were strongly positive. The patient has worn a denture processed of highly refined acrylic materials for over two years without any trouble.

PLATE I

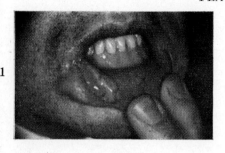

1

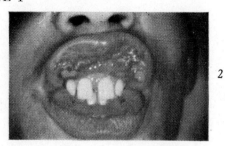

2

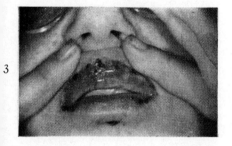

3

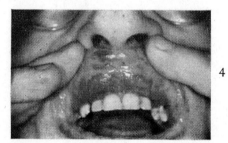

4

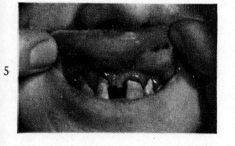

5

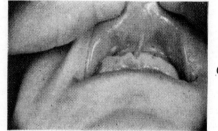

6

FIG. 7. Acute fusospirochetal gingivitis of two days' duration. This 12-year-old colored girl has an acute fusospirochetal gingivitis which is characterized by loss of the interdental papillae, ulceration of the marginal gingivae, pain, salivation and gingival hemorrhage. The hematologic findings were essentially normal.

FIG. 8. Acute fusospirochetal gingivitis. This 27-year-old woman has used a sodium perborate mouth wash for three months on the advice of her physician, without controlling the disease. Note the destruction of the interdental papillae. This case of fusospirochetal stomatitis responded rapidly to local therapy and instrumentation.

FIG. 9. Streptococcal stomatitis. The diffuse, red, inflamed appearance of the gingiva and oral mucosa is characteristic of this disease. It can be differentiated from fusospirochetal stomatitis by the absence of ulceration and necrosis of the marginal gingiva and interdental areas, and the bacterial smear and cultural findings. Streptococcal stomatitis must be differentiated from the stomatitis associated with nicotinic acid deficiency.

FIG. 10. Localized gingivitis and marginal periodontitis. The acute inflammation of the marginal gingiva and periodontal tissues about the lower left first premolar resulted from the accidental retention of a small band of rubber dam material. Toothbrush bristles, corn husks, small fishbones and toothpick fragments may produce similar lesions.

FIG. 11. Dilantin gingival hyperplasia. The gingival enlargement which is associated with the administration of dilantin sodium is stippled in appearance and light pink in color. It has a dense fibrous consistency. It does not bleed readily nor is it susceptible to infection. Recurrence is common even after surgical removal.

FIG. 12. Acute monocytic leukemia. This 27-year-old female exhibits the typical gingival changes of acute leukemia. There is generalized swelling of the gingival tissues, most marked at the interdental papillae, and extensive areas (greenish-black) of necrosis. Spontaneous gingival hemorrhage is common. The mouth odor is putrid in character. The white blood cell count was 86,000 c.mm. with 90% monocytes.

PLATE II

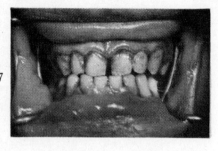
7

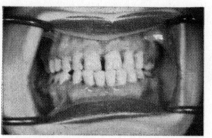
8

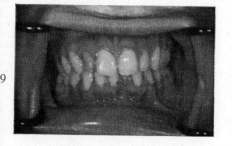
9

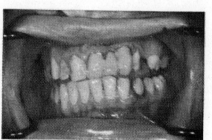
10

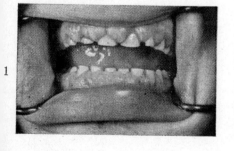
1

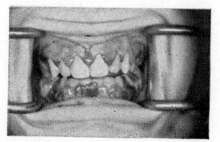
12

Fig. 13. Glossitis rhombica mediana. This developmental anomaly of the tongue gives rise commonly to much diagnostic speculation. The location of the lesion in the midline, just anterior to the circumvallate papillae, is an important aid in the diagnosis. Glossitis rhombica mediana may have a smooth or a tufted, nodular surface similar to that illustrated.

Fig. 14. Geographic tongue. The typical irregular depapillated areas with their red and raised yellow margins are illustrated. Few subjective symptoms are experienced.

Fig. 15. Hairy tongue associated with the use of sodium perborate mouth wash. Same case as Fig. 8. The continued use of sodium perborate produces frequently an unusual growth of the filiform papillae of the tongue. This abnormal coating will disappear when the irritating mouth wash is stopped and normal physiology of the oral cavity prevails.

Fig. 16. Lichen planus of the tongue. The lesions of lichen planus of the tongue have commonly a central, plaque-like distribution. The purplish color of the lesion, the presence of purplish-white radiating lines and associated lesions on the cheek mucosa are an aid to diagnosis.

Fig. 17. Carcinoma of the tongue. Advanced squamous cell carcinoma of the tongue with associated hard yellowish-white patches of leukoplakia.

Fig. 18. Syphilitic gumma, leukoplakia and carcinoma of the tongue. Syphilitic gumma of the tongue is frequently associated with leukoplakia and malignant degeneration. The characteristic bluish-purple color of a syphilitic gumma, the yellowish white areas of leukoplakia, surrounded by the light-colored neoplastic tissue can be plainly seen in this figure.

PLATE III

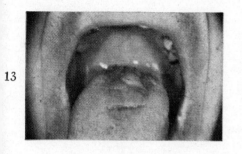

13

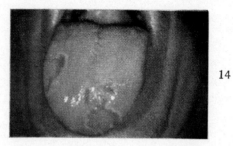

14

15

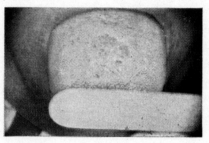

16

17

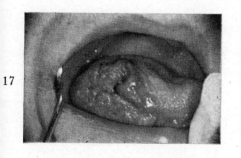

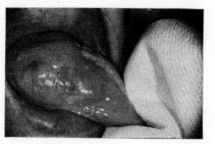

18

FIG. 19. Mottled enamel—chronic endemic dental fluorosis. The consumption of drinking water containing over 2 p.p.m. fluorine may give rise to a characteristic brown discoloration of the enamel which is formed during this period. The patient illustrated is a 48-year-old native of Sicily. Observe the relative freedom from dental decay and the excellent condition of the periodontal tissues.

FIG. 20. Dental hypoplasia. Extensive hypoplasia of the enamel and staining of the dentin observed in a 13-year-old negress whose early history and physical findings suggested severe rickets in the early years of life. There is well-developed racial pigmentation of the gums.

FIG. 21. Dental changes in prenatal syphilis and bismuth line. The notching of the incisor teeth and the underdevelopment of the premaxilla are characteristic of prenatal syphilis. A definite bismuth line is present in the marginal gingival tissues labial to the lower incisors.

FIG. 22. Paget's disease with oral involvement. A progressive enlargement of the superior maxilla, especially in the molar region, may represent the first symptom of Paget's disease. The depression in the left maxillary molar area is the site of a localized osteomyelitis which followed a dental extraction.

FIG. 23. Case of acute bismuth stomatitis. This patient shows the intense, discrete, blue-black pigmentation in the marginal gingivae and also contact areas of pigmentation on the inner surfaces of the lower lip. The white sloughing area on the right alveolar gingiva is a chemical burn produced by a crushed aspirin tablet.

FIG. 24. Same case as is shown in Fig. 23 following local treatment without interruption of the bismuth injections. The pigmentation has almost entirely disappeared.

PLATE IV

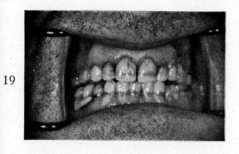
19

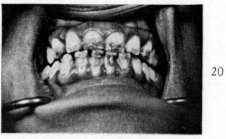
20

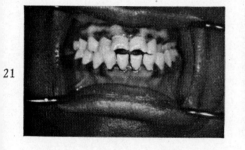
21

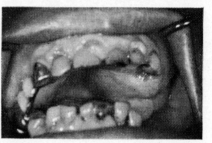
22

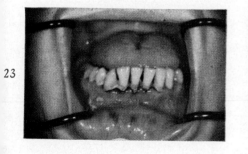
23

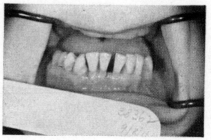
24

FIG. 25. Tuberculous lesions of the palate. The entire left side of the palate was enlarged. The tissues had a doughy consistency and they were intensely painful. A large area of necrosis was present adjacent to the maxillary left second molar. This 27-year-old female has bilateral pulmonary tuberculosis. Same patient as Fig. 40. (Courtesy of Dr. Victor Frank, Philadelphia, Pa.)

FIG. 26. Acute herpetic stomatitis. This example of acute herpetic stomatitis developed in a patient who had experienced previously a severe upper respiratory infection which was accompanied by extensive dermal lesions of herpes simplex. The lesions were present on the lips, the palate, cheek mucosa and tongue. This condition must be differentiated from erythema multiforme and early pemphigus.

FIG. 27. Stomatitis venenata. The acute contact stomatitis illustrated resulted from the chewing of several poison ivy leaves in the hope of producing an immunity to this plant. There is superficial necrosis of the tissues. Small ruptured vesicular lesions are present on the lips.

FIG. 28. Syphilitic gumma of the palate. The palate is a common site for syphilitic gumma. The bluish-purple color of the tissues surrounding this gumma of the palate is typical. There was a complete perforation of the palate in spite of intensive luetic therapy.

FIG. 29. Lichen planus—erosive type. This patient has recurring lichen planus of the erosive type. The lesions are painful and prevent the wearing of the denture. The fine white lines radiating from the periphery of the lesion aid in the clinical diagnosis. Biopsy study is frequently required.

FIG. 30. Fissured epulis and pseudo-cheilosis. The cauliflower-like mass of tissue resulted from the failure to receive adequate denture servicing. As the bony supporting tissues resorbed, a fold of soft tissue became interposed between the denture flange and the supporting tissues. Traumatic irritation of the tissue resulted in hypertrophy and fissuring. Note the bilateral angular cheilosis which is associated with a loss of the intermaxillary space. This lesion must be differentiated from true cheilosis which is associated with a nutritional deficiency.

PLATE V

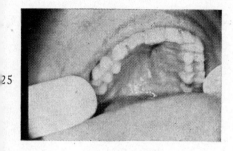

25

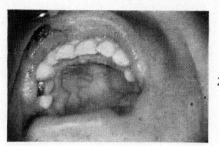

26

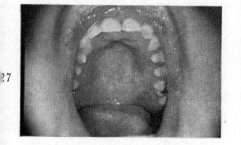

27

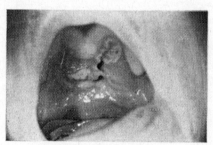

28

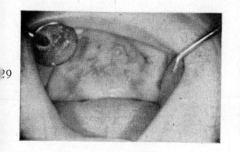

29

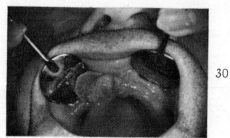

30

FIG. 31. Lichen planus of the cheek mucosa. The typical irregular, slightly raised, radiating bluish-purple lesions of lichen planus are shown in this figure. There were no painful subjective symptoms. Same patient as shown in Fig. 16.

FIG. 32. Lichen planus of the cheek mucosa. This female patient presents the typical early manifestations of lichen planus. The delicate white intersecting lines can be seen on the cheek mucosa in the molar region. This lesion must be differentiated from leukoplakia, cheek biting and Fordyce's disease.

FIG. 33. Aspirin burn. This patient has a painful, sloughing chemical burn of the cheek mucosa and gingival tissues in the lower right molar area resulting from contact with a crushed aspirin tablet which was placed in this area in the hope of relieving odontalgia of the lower right second molar.

FIG. 34. Lugol's solution as an aid in the diagnosis of leukoplakia. The hyperkeratinized epithelial cells comprising an area of leukoplakia have a reduced glycogen content. Normal epithelial tissue takes a deep-brown stain due to the action of the iodine and glycogen. Fig. 34 shows the appearance of an area of leukoplakia of the buccal mucosa before (*left*) and after (*right*) the application of Lugol's solution.

FIG. 35. Sodium perborate burn. Sodium perborate gives rise frequently to irritative lesions of the oral mucosa even when it is used in the proper concentration. These sodium perborate burns are painful and they heal slowly. Observe the diffuse redness and edema of the oral mucosa and the small eroded areas in the mucobuccal fold.

FIG. 36. Fordyce's "disease." This figure illustrates the raised, yellowish granules which are commonly found beneath the cheek mucosa in the molar region and on the vermilion border of the lips. These granules produce at times a definite nodular surface to the cheek. They result from plugged ectopic sebaceous glands.

PLATE VI

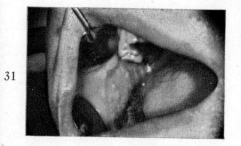

31

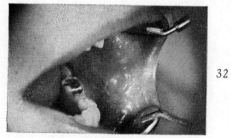

32

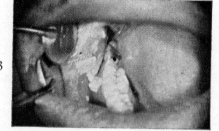

33

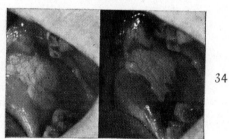

34

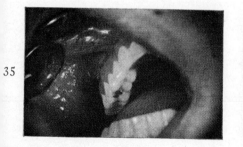

35

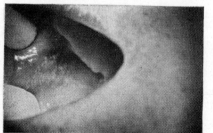

36

FIG. 37. Herpetic vesicle. A typical herpetic (simplex) vesicle of the vermilion border of the lip is pictured. Herpetic vesicles are rarely seen on the oral mucosa, where they are readily broken. The broken vesicles appear as eroded areas which are covered with a cheesy yellow opaque material.

FIG. 38. Chancre of the lower lip. The chancre of the lip in this patient was originally diagnosed as herpes simplex. The persistence of the lesion, the regional adenopathy and the dark field microscopic examination established the diagnosis. Oral chancres are less painful than oral herpetic lesions, and they are not preceded by symptoms of burning or itching.

FIG. 39. Oral and dermal manifestations of acute syphilis. Several of the characteristic manifestations of acute (secondary) syphilis are shown in this figure. The ham-colored macular lesion on the chin is typical of the dermal eruption. A "split papule" is present on the left commissure of the mouth. Mucous patches can be seen on the inner surface of the lower lip between the dental mirrors and on the ventral surface of the tongue.

FIG. 40. Diffuse superficial tuberculous lesions of the oral mucosa and gingiva. The oral mucosa of the lower lip and the gingiva are covered with a superficial membranous lesion which is intensely painful. In spite of the diffuse involvement of these tissues and the gingival enlargement, this condition was first treated as a fusospirochetal infection. Same patient as shown in Fig. 25. (Courtesy of Dr. Victor Frank, Philadelphia, Pa.)

FIG. 41. Mucous patch (syphilitic). A typical mucous patch of acute syphilis can be seen on the mucosal surface of the lower lip. This mucous patch has the usual oval outline, raised and translucent appearance. Where the mucous patch involves the vermilion border of the lower lip, the lesion has a brown crusted appearance. The lesions on the upper lip and the left oral commissure are also luetic.

FIG. 42. Angular cheilosis associated with a nutritional deficiency. Angular cheilosis is commonly associated with a nutritional deficiency of the B complex (riboflavin and pyridoxine). One feature of this form of cheilosis aids in differentiating it from the angular cheilosis associated with a decrease of the intermaxillary space. The macerated, painful lesions associated with a B complex deficiency extend characteristically onto the cheek mucosa as illustrated in this figure.

PLATE VII

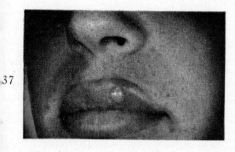

37

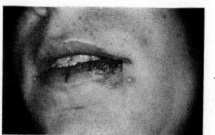

38

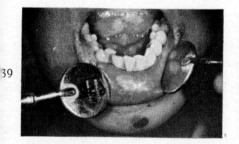

39

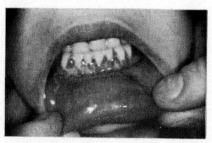

40

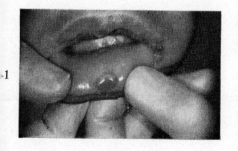

1

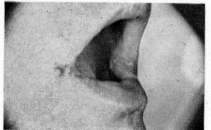

42

Fig. 43. Leukoplakia of the sublingual space. Leukoplakia of the sublingual space and ventral surface of the tongue is common in pipe smokers. This white, verrucous area of leukoplakia is typical in appearance. A slight opacity of the mucosa covering the left sublingual space is indicative of developing leukoplakia.

Fig. 44. Leukoplakia of the inner surface of the lip. The location and distribution of oral leukoplakia is modified by local predisposing factors, as in this case pipe smoking. The puckered area of leukoplakia corresponds to the place where the pipe stem was customarily held.

Fig. 45. Erythema multiforme with oral lesions. Severe oral lesions are commonly found in patients with generalized erythema multiforme. The oral mucosal lesions can be differentiated from oral mucous patches by their irregular outline and the hemorrhagic and yellowish opaque covering.

Fig. 46. Tuberculous ulcer of the tongue. A deep central tuberculous ulcer of the tongue is one of the typical secondary oral manifestations of a tuberculous infection. The base of this indolent, painful ulcer is covered with a glairy yellow mucous material.

Fig. 47. Thrombocytopenic purpura. Persistent gingival hemorrhage is a frequent and serious complication of thrombocytopenic purpura. (Courtesy of Dr. Abram Cohen, Philadelphia, Pa.)

Fig. 48. Oral lesions of the B complex deficiency—ariboflavinosis. In ariboflavinosis and B complex deficiencies the soft tissues have a magenta or purple color. There is a painful marginal periodontitis and at times a superimposed fusospirochetal infection. The oral mucosa has a glazed opalescent appearance.

PLATE VIII

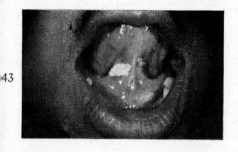

43

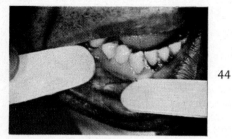

44

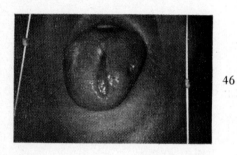

45

46

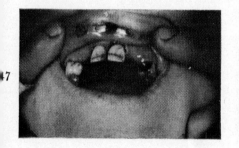

47

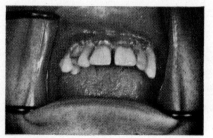

48

Fɪɢ. 49. Stomatitis in an electric arc welder. This patient presented many of the clinical symptoms of a fusospirochetal infection with ulceration, necrosis and hemorrhage of the marginal gingiva and interdental papilla. In addition, the buccal and labial alveolar gingiva had a cauterized appearance. The case did not respond satisfactorily to treatment until the patient's occupation was changed.

Fɪɢ. 50. Oral changes associated with ovarian dysfunction. In postmenopausal patients or those with gynecologic disorders oral soft tissue changes are commonly observed. The tissues have a bright red color, they bleed easily and the patient complains frequently of a burning type of pain. Whitish patches are commonly found on the tissues. These tissue changes respond to female sex hormone therapy.

Fɪɢ. 51. Marginal glossitis in pernicious anemia. An intensely red, painful inflammation of the tip and lateral margins of the tongue represented the first clinical symptom of pernicious anemia in this 52-year-old negress.

Fɪɢ. 52. Pemphigus vulgaris of the tongue. The tongue is a frequent site of oral manifestations of pemphigus vulgaris. Bullous lesions are transitory and hence are rarely seen. These extremely painful lesions must be differentiated from those of erythema multiforme and acute herpetic stomatitis. Same patient as shown in Fig. 4.

Fɪɢ. 53. Pigmentation of the cheek mucosa. This pigmentation of the cheek mucosa simulates that observed in Addison's disease. The cause for the pigmentation in this patient could not be determined.

Fɪɢ. 54. Aspirin burn of the oral mucosa. The white cauterized oral mucosa opposite the molar teeth was the result of a crushed aspirin tablet in the mucobuccal fold.

PLATE IX

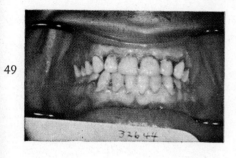
49

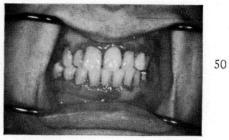
50

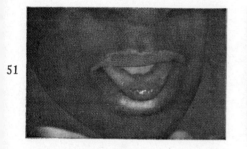
51

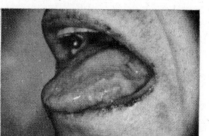
52

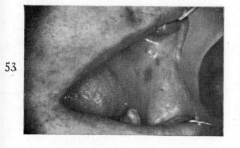
53

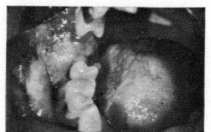
54

FIG. 55. Abnormally coated tongue. This patient has an abnormally coated tongue. The elongated filiform papillae can be easily parted in the midline.

FIG. 56. Tongue changes in B complex deficiency. The oral tissue changes associated with a deficiency of a particular fraction of the B complex are seen occasionally. The rose-pink color of the tongue and the unusually prominent fungiform papillae were associated with a thiamine deficiency. (Courtesy of Dr. John H. Gunter, Philadelphia, Pa.)

FIG. 57. Mucous patch of the tongue. Mucous patches on the tongue are common. This figure illustrates an early and typical mucous patch of the tongue. Observe the oval outline, the reddened margin and the raised appearance of the lesion. The notching of the upper right first incisor resulted from the habit of opening bobby pins with the teeth.

FIG. 58. Erythema multiforme localized to the mouth. This 13-year-old girl has had two previous episodes of acute stomatitis. The history of repeated attacks, the clinical appearance and the distribution of the lesions established the diagnosis of erythema multiforme. A satisfactory clinical response was obtained following high vitamin therapy, topical penicillin therapy and frequent mouth irrigations of hot bicarbonate of soda solution. Same patient as shown in Fig. 3.

FIG. 59. Advanced leukoplakia of the tongue. This 54-year-old male has had leukoplakia of the tongue for over twenty years. He is a heavy pipe smoker. Areas of fissuring, cracking and irritation are present. The extensive, advanced leukoplakia of the tongue led to the making of serologic tests for syphilis which were found to be strongly positive. The lesion responded to antiluetic treatment and conservative therapy.

FIG. 60. Advanced leukoplakia of the ventral surface of the tongue and sublingual space. This is an example of advanced leukoplakia with widespread distribution in an 82-year-old woman. No predisposing cause could be found. The area of leukoplakia had been previously fulgurated without permanent improvement. High vitamin A therapy and female sex hormone therapy were also ineffective.

PLATE X

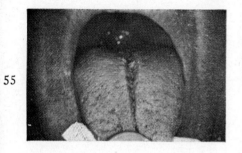

55

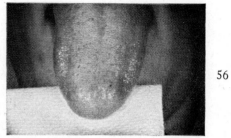

56

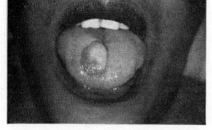

57

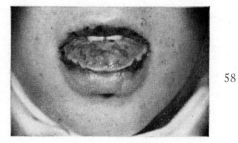

58

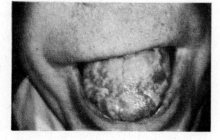

59

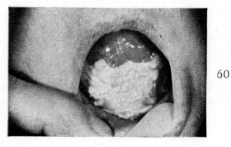

60

SECTION ELEVEN
REGIONAL DIAGNOSTIC INDEX

The oral manifestations of many of the diseases of local and systemic causation appear typically on certain areas of the lips, oral mucosa or tongue. A knowledge of the more common sites of involvement of a disease assists in its diagnosis and differential diagnosis.

The most authoritative and complete reference book is of little value to the practitioner if he does not know the general nature of the disease process under consideration. A listing of the characteristic sites of appearance of the oral and systemic diseases will at least furnish a basis for a study of the likely diagnostic possibilities.

This regional diagnostic index is not intended to supplant the taking of a careful history and the performing of a complete and thorough oral examination. It represents only an aid to the application of the diagnostic procedures which have been discussed in Chapter 3. No diagnostic index or outline can take into consideration the capriciousness of a disease or the different reactions of an individual host to a disease. The clinical appearance and characteristics of the lesion, the history of the development of the disease and the laboratory findings should always determine the final diagnosis.

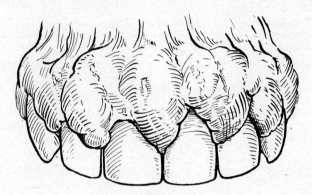

FIG. 279. INCREASE IN SIZE

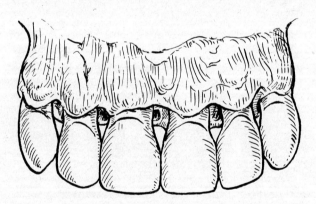

FIG. 280. DESTRUCTION, ULCERATION OR ATROPHY

THE GINGIVAE

LOCAL ORIGIN	SYSTEMIC BACKGROUND
(See Figure 279)	
Poor oral hygiene	**Pregnancy** gingivitis or hypertrophy, pregnancy tumors
Calcareous deposits	Endocrine dysfunction, especially at time of puberty, hyperthyroidism
Local irritation due to: cavity margins overhanging fillings orthodontic appliances drugs	Nutritional disturbances of the B complex and vitamin C
Food impaction (early)	Hypertrophied tissue in uncontrolled diabetes
Overfunction (early)	Hyperplasia associated with barbiturate or dilantin therapy (early)
Mouth breathing	Leukemia (early)
	Epuli

(See Figure 280)	
Fusospirochetal disease, acute and chronic	Malignant neutropenia (early)
Overfunction (late)	Aplastic anemia
Food impaction (late)	Leukemia (late)
Habits	Nutritional deficiencies—pellagra, secondary fusospirochetal disease
Long-continued use of caustic drugs in treatment of fusospirochetal infection	Malignant growths
	Secondary to alveolar resorption from any cause

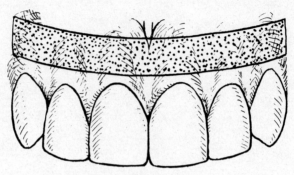

FIG: 281. ALVEOLAR

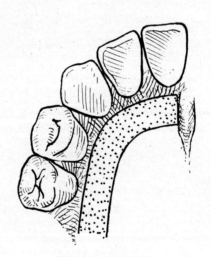

FIG. 282. PALATAL

THE GINGIVAE

LOCAL ORIGIN   SYSTEMIC BACKGROUND

(See Figures 281 and 282)

INCREASE IN SIZE

Poor oral hygiene	Endocrine disturbances, especially during puberty
Extensive calcareous deposits	Hyperplasia associated with barbiturate and dilantin administration
Periodontal abscess	
Hematoma	Scurvy
Diffuse fibromatosis of the gingivae	Leukemia (early)

DESTRUCTION, ULCERATION OR ATROPHY

Trophoneurotic ulcer	Leukemia (late)
Severe burns	Malignant neutropenia
Radio-osteonecrosis	Diabetic gangrene
Noma	Mercury, arsenic or phosphorous necrosis
	Syphilitic ulceration

ACUTE INFLAMMATION

Acute reactions to mouth washes, tooth pastes, denture creams, stomatitis venata	Nutritional deficiencies of the B complex
Staphylococcal stomatitis	Gonadal and menopausal changes in the tissues
Streptococcal stomatitis	Enanthem in measles, scarlet fever
Gonococcal stomatitis	Acute reactions to administration of mercury, bismuth or other drugs, stomatitis medicamentosa
	Acute reactions to foods
	Erythema multiforme
	Lichen planus—erosive type

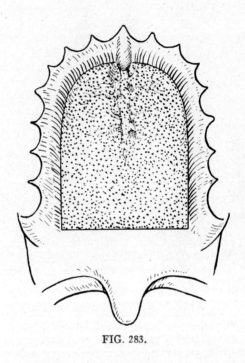

FIG. 283.

THE PALATE

LOCAL ORIGIN	SYSTEMIC BACKGROUND
Torus palatinus	**Syphilitic gumma**
Leukoplakia	**Necrotic lesions** associated with the blood dyscrasias, malignant neutropenia, leukemia
Palatal gland irritation and hypertrophy due to smoking, suction and relief chambers	Tuberculous ulcers
Irritation of palatine (incisive) papilla due to mechanical causes, cysts in the same structure	Lichen planus, particularly of the erosive type
Herpes—especially following novocaine injections	Purpuric, ecchymotic phenomena associated with jaundice, subacute bacterial endocarditis, etc. On both the hard and soft palate.
Malignant growths	Color changes associated with anemia, jaundice and subacute bacterial endocarditis—especially on the soft palate
Congenital and developmental anomalies. Partial or complete cleft palate, high palatal arch.	Necrosis of the palate following extraction, especially in the uncontrolled diabetic
	Syphilitic mucous patches—especially on the soft palate
	Allergic manifestations
	Pemphigus

Disease	Age Group			Extent of Involvement
	Under 20	20-40	Over 40	
Periapical, pericoronal or pericemental infection.	**	*		Unilateral regional nodes. Edema may cause enlargement to appear more extensive.
Syphilis.		**	*	Regional and unilateral with chancre. May be generalized in generalized stage of disease.
Carcinoma.		*	**	Variable, depending on the site and extension of the primary growth.
Acute follicular tonsillitis. Streptococcal sore throat. Scarlet fever.	**			Extensive unilateral or bilateral adenopathy.
Actinomycosis	*	**	**	Usually unilateral. Extensive change in surrounding tissues, dull red subcutaneous nodules.
Hodgkin's disease	*	**		Unilateral at first and then bilateral. May be very extensive in advanced cases.
Infectious mononucleosis.	*	**		Variable, may be slight cervical enlargement.
Tuberculosis.	***	*		Bilateral submaxillary and deep cervical adenopathy.
Lymphosarcoma.	*	**	*	Extensive bilateral.
All acute leukemias. Monocytic leukemia.	**	*		Variable, may be none, when present usually secondary to necrosis of the oral tissues.
Lymphatic leukemia.	*	*	**	Usually bilateral and may be extensive.
Myelogenous leukemia.		**	*	Variable, may be secondary to oral ulcerative processes.

* to *** indicates frequency of occurrence in different age groups.

Painful Response	Consistency or Discreteness	Tendency to Break Down	Temperature Reaction	Diagnostic Aid
Very painful.	Varies as to stage, fluctuant or non-fluctuant.	Untreated, tend to break down.	Elevated 102°-103° F.	History, pulp testing, x-ray.
Slight if secondary infection.	Hard, firm and discrete.	No.	Usually none.	Dark field examination of lesion and/or S.T.S., depending on stage of disease.
Moderate to marked, depending on the secondary infection which is present.	Stony hard, firm.	Yes, in later stages.	None at early stages, variable later.	Biopsy, history.
Usually painful, may be marked.	Firm, usually discrete.	None, as a rule.	Variable to 103° F. or higher.	Blood counts, bacterial cultures, fibrinolysin tests.
Slight to moderate.	Soft, putty-like, may be matted together.	Yes, gradually with multiple discharging fistulae.	Variable.	X-rays, smears and cultures.
Generally not.	Firm consistency, discrete.	Little tendency to break down.	Slightly elevated.	Biopsy study, chest and abdominal x-rays.
May be slightly.	Discrete, firm.	No.	101° F.	Heterophile antibody test.
Only slightly.	Caseous or putty-like. Discrete at first, then becomes matted.	Yes, numerous fistulae, may calcify.	None, variable.	Smears, biopsy study, animal injections, x-rays.
Not in early stages.	Firm and matted together.	No.	Slight.	Biopsy and x-ray studies.
Variable, due to oral infection.	Firm, discrete.	No.	Variable to 102-103° F.	Complete blood count.
Not usually.	Firm and diffuse enlargement.	No.	Variable.	Complete blood count.
Not usually.	Usually discrete.	No.	Variable.	Complete blood count.

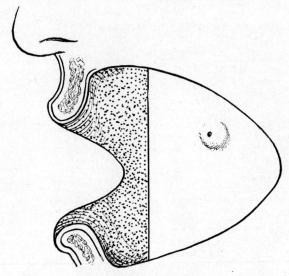

FIG. 284. ANTERIOR

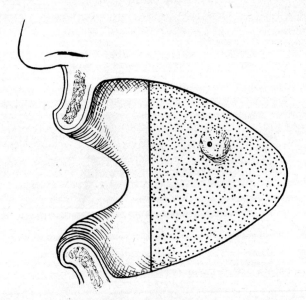

FIG. 285. POSTERIOR

CHEEK MUCOSA

LOCAL ORIGIN	SYSTEMIC BACKGROUND
(See Figure 284)	
Leukoplakia	Intra-oral continuation of chei-
Herpes—solitary lesions and diffuse involvement	losis of nutritional origin
Traumatic injury—cheek biting	Syphilitic chancre, mucous patch or split papule
Burns including those associated with dental practice	Erythema multiforme
Carcinoma	Pemphigus
Mucous cysts, varices	Racial pigmentation

(See Figure 285)	
Fordyce's disease	Lichen planus
Traumatic irritation due to poor occlusal relations, restorations or appliances	Koplik's spots
Habits—cheek biting	Lesions associated with B complex deficiency
Contact fusospirochetal ulcerations and metallic contacting pigmentations and irritations	Necrotic lesions associated with leukemia and malignant neutropenia
Herpes simplex	Erythema multiforme
Streptococcal stomatitis	Pemphigus
	Thrush
	Allergic reactions
	Pigmentation associated with Addison's disease
	Racial pigmentation

THE LIPS

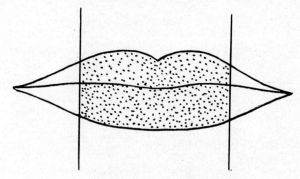

FIG. 286. VERMILLION BORDER
CENTRAL PORTION

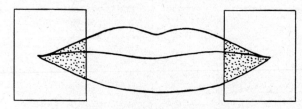

FIG. 287. VERMILLION BORDER
LATERAL PORTION

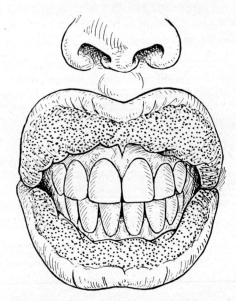

FIG. 288. INNER SURFACE OF THE LIPS

THE LIPS

LOCAL ORIGIN	SYSTEMIC BACKGROUND
(See Figure 286)	
Fordyce's disease	**Cheilosis** and minute cracking due to nutritional deficiencies
Leukoplakia (smoker's patch)	**Generalized lesions of acute syphilis**
Herpes simplex	**Carcinoma**
Cheilosis due to chapping	Syphilitic chancre
Contact cheilosis—sensitivity to lip sticks, dentifrice, etc.	Manifestations of drug eruptions
Traumatic injuries	Erythema multiforme
Burns, thermal and chemical	Lichen planus
Congenital anomalies, lip pits, hare lip, macrocheilia	Pemphigus
	Angioneurotic edema

(See Figure 287)	
Herpes simplex	**Angular cheilosis** due to a nutritional deficiency
Angular cheilosis due to decreased intermaxillary space—excess salivation	**Syphilitic split papule**
	Tuberculous ulcerations
Burns and trauma associated with dental operations	Syphilitic rhagades
	Erythema multiforme

(See Figure 288)	
Traumatic injuries	Syphilitic mucous patch
Herpes simplex	Pemphigus
Fusospirochetal contact ulcerations	Erythema multiforme
Metallic contact pigmentations	Generalized form of herpetic stomatitis
Mucous cysts	
Irritation of the solitary glands of the lips	

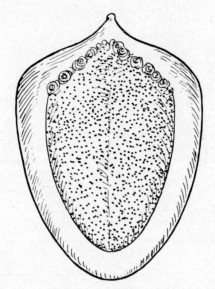

FIG. 289. CENTRAL AREA

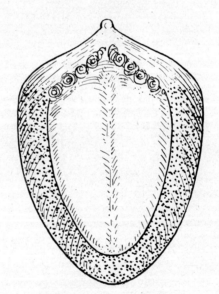

FIG. 290. MARGINAL AREA

THE TONGUE

LOCAL ORIGIN	SYSTEMIC BACKGROUND

(*See Figure 289*)

LOCAL ORIGIN	SYSTEMIC BACKGROUND

Geographic tongue
Leukoplakia of the tongue—also with carcinoma and syphilitic sclerous glossitis
Herpes, especially the recurrent form
Carcinoma—also see leukoplakia
Abnormally coated tongue with or without abnormal staining due to tobacco, candies, or drugs
Congenital and developmental anomalies
  Ankyloglossia, micro- and macroglossia
  Fissured tongue
  Congential absence of papillae
  Glossitis rhombica mediana
	Papillary atrophy and irritation
	  B complex deficiency
	  Pellagra
	  Plummer-Vinson syndrome
	  Secondary anemia
	  Cardiac decompensation
	  Hypochlorhydria
	  Dry, red tongue of uncontrolled diabetes
	Lichen planus
	Syphilis
	  mucous patch
	Gumma—**sclerous glossitis**
	Tuberculous ulcer
	  Central fissure type
	Drug eruptions
	Erythema multiforme
	Angioneurotic edema
	Pemphigus

(*See Figure 290*)

LOCAL ORIGIN	SYSTEMIC BACKGROUND
Trauma—due to rough teeth or restorations, calculus, prosthetic appliances Bites in epileptic patients **Herpetic lesions,** especially recurrent form Leukoplakia Contact fusospirochetal ulcerations and metallic contact pigmentations and irritations Carcinoma Fibromas and papillomas	**Tongue changes in pernicious anemia** **Crenated margins** associated with B complex deficiency Hypothyroidism Diabetes—uncontrolled Tuberculous ulcerations Glossopyrosis Drug eruptions Erythema multiforme Pemphigus

Index

NOTE: Text pages are in Roman type, illustrations in italic, and colored illustrations have "c" after page number.

Anesthesia, eye, danger to, 563
for cardiac patients, 229-230, 232, 235
for diabetics, 421
general, precautions of, 123, 130, 227, 230, 232
resulting in death, 311
use of, 220
for hypertension, 239
for hyperthyroids, 308
for jaw dislocation, 330-331
local, carrier of infection, 246
in pregnancy, 297
Anesthesia-like reaction in flyers, 588
Anesthetic troches, 448
Angina, agranulocytic, 438-442
pectoris, 227-230
and coronary occlusion, comparison of, 232
syphilitic, 471
"Vincent's," 41, 59
Angle, gonial, 263
Angular cheilosis, 392, 392-393, 623 c, 627 c
Aniacinosis, 395
Aniline dyes for fusospirochetal infectioris, 53, 56
Animal inoculation for tuberculosis, 496
Anisocytosis, 15, 423
Ankyloglossia, 119, 120, 543
Ankylosis of temporomandibular joint, 331
Anodontia, uncompensated, 332
Anomalies, congenital, 543-544, 544, 545
developmental, 544, 548
renal, 279-280
Anoxia of flying, 588, 596
Anti-gray hair vitamin, 400
Antirachitic vitamin, 404-408
Anuria, 281
Aorta, coarctation of, 240
Apical pathosis in flyers, 591
Apnea, voluntary test, 306
Appendicitis, 270-271
A P plates for sinus x-rays, 215
Appliances, dental, see dentures
Aphthae, Mikulicz's, 146
Arches, faucial, chart for, 8
Argyl-Robertson pupils, 472, 488
Argyria, 80-83, 81
Ariboflavinosis, 392, 394, 629 c
Arrhythmias, cardiac, 242
Arsenic intoxication, 82-83, 139
Arteriosus, persistent ductus, 239
Arteritis, diabetic, 420
nodosa, peri-, 240
Arthritis, classification of, 317-318
degenerative, 325-327, 325, 326

Arthritis—(Continued)
dental focal infection, 540
gonococcal, 516
gouty, 425-426
hypertrophic, 325-327, 325, 326
osteo-, 325-327, 325, 326
rheumatoid, 318-324, 320, 321
senile, 325-327, 325, 326
traumatic, 329-330
Articular meniscus, 328, 330
Aschheim-Zondek test for pregnancy, 35, 292
Ascorbic acid, 400-404
Asialorrhea, 249, 251-252
Aspirin burn of oral tissue, 94, 94, 185-186, 185, 621 c, 625 c, 631 c
Asthma, 90-91, 219
cardiac, 244
Attrition, 4th degree, 559
Auditory canal, furuncles of, 216
Auto-inoculation, 508-509
Autopsy, bacteriologic studies at, 530, 532, 535
leukemia, acute, 449-450
Aviation, oral aspects of, 585
dentistry, 585-609
A virus of influenza, 223
Avitaminosis, 385

Bacillary dysentery, 273
Bacteremia, demonstration of, 29
experimental, 531-532
postextractive, 234-236, 237, 532-533
Bacteria in mouth, 174, 221
from periapical areas, 530-531, 534-535
in urine, 25
Bacterial cultures for tooth apices, 28-29
endocarditis, subacute, 232, 237
flora of teeth, 529-532
smears, stained, 25-28
Bacterium Fusiformis, 38
Balanitis, 298
fusospirochetal, 38
Band, orthodontic, 454
Banti's syndrome, 269
Barbiturate derivatives, effects of, 95
Basal metabolic rate, 34
Basedow's disease, 305-310, 306
Beard growth in pemphigus, 154
Bell's palsy, 358-359, 359
Bence-Jones protein, 350
Bends in flyers, 588
Benedict's Qualitative test, 24
Benzene, reaction to, 579
Benzol, reaction to, 579
Beri-beri, 389

Jaundice—(*Continued*)
obstructive, surgery precaution, 410
Jaw, bone cysts of, 314-315
indexes, 263
fracture in planes, 587
lumpy, 498
malformation in scleroderma, 162-163, *163, 164*
necrosis, radium, 578
porosity of, 428
Joint, Charcot, destruction of, 488
diseases of, 317-351
exostoses of, *326,* 327
"marginal lipping" of, 326-327
proximal interphalangeal, deformity of, *320, 326*
temporomandibular, changes in, 558
diseases of, 328-333
dislocation of, 329, 330-331
involvement in arthritis, 322-323
gonococcal arthritis of, 516
terminal phalangeal, involvement in osteo-arthritis, *325, 325, 326, 327*

Kala-azar, 506-507
Kahn test for syphilis, 32
Keratosis, 387
Kernicterus, 556
Kidney, amyloidosis of, 283
horseshoe, 280
"Kinetic chains," 606
Klebs-Loeffler bacillus, 554
Kline test for syphilis, 32
Keloid reaction, 197
Koplik's spots, 552

Labio-glosso-pharyngeal paralysis, 353-354
Laboratory, evidence, focal infection, 529-532
examinations, 4-36
Laceration of tongue, 123
Lactation, 297
Lactobacillus acidophilus, 600
Laryngitis, 217-218
Lead intoxication, 71-73, 577
line, 72
Leishmania donovani, 506
Leishmaniasis, 506-507
Leprosy, 504-506, *505, 506*
nodular, 505, *506*
Lesions, *see also* specific conditions
Boeck's sarcoid, 169
congenital heart, 239-240
galvanic, 167-169
genital, 38
granulomatous, *508*
in children, 548

Lesions—(*Continued*)
herpes zoster, 152
herpetic, 50, *146, 148, 149, 615* c, *622* c, *627* c
compared with syphilitic, 480
oral, in children, 547-550
histologic study of, *31, 32*
perlèche, 393
traumatic, staining of, 138
compared with leukoplakia and lichen planus, 145
vegetative, *233*
vulval, 38
Leukemias, 443-452
acute, 444-448, *444*
lymph node enlargement, 642-643
asymptomatic, 448
lymphatic, acute, hemogram for, 463
chronic, 450-451
monocytic acute, 444-448, *444, 445, 617* c
case report, 449-450
hemogram for, 463
lymph node enlargement, 642-643
monocytic, chronic, 451-452
myelogenous, lymph node enlargement, 642-643
myeloplastic, acute, hemogram for, 463
various forms, 443
Leukocyte count, 13
normal values of, 15
differential, 13-17
Leukocytosis, conditions associated with, 16
Leukopenia, conditions associated with, 16
Leukoplakia buccalis, 131-139, *133, 135-137, 337,* 484, *485, 625* c, *629* c, *633* c
crusted form, *135*
due to galvanism, 169
lichen planus and traumatic lesions of cheek compared, 145
of tongue, 126, *135, 619* c
torus palatinus, *337*
in World War I, 132
Lichen planus, 139-145, *140-144, 619* c, *623* c, *625* c
Line, bismuth, 63-64, 66, *67, 621* c
copper, 84
lead, 72
mercury, 74
zinc, 85
Lingua nigra, 124, *125*
Linguomaxillary reflex, 360-361
Lips, angioneurotic edema of, *92*